MULTIMETHOD CLINICAL ASSESSMENT

MULTIMETHOD CLINICAL ASSESSMENT

edited by
Christopher J. Hopwood
Robert F. Bornstein

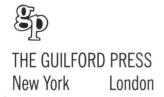

THE GUILFORD PRESS
New York   London

© 2014 The Guilford Press
A Division of Guilford Publications, Inc.
72 Spring Street, New York, NY 10012
www.guilford.com

Printed in the United States of America

This book is printed on acid-free paper.

Last digit is print number: 9   8   7   6   5   4   3   2   1

The authors have checked with sources believed to be reliable in their efforts to
provide information that is complete and generally in accord with the standards
of practice that are accepted at the time of publication. However, in view of the
possibility of human error or changes in behavioral, mental health, or medical
sciences, neither the authors, nor the editors and publisher, nor any other party
who has been involved in the preparation or publication of this work warrants
that the information contained herein is in every respect accurate or complete,
and they are not responsible for any errors or omissions or the results obtained
from the use of such information. Readers are encouraged to confirm the
information contained in this book with other sources.

Library of Congress Cataloging-in-Publication Data

Multimethod clinical assessment / edited by Christopher J. Hopwood,
Robert F. Bornstein.
        pages cm
    Includes bibliographical references and index.
    ISBN 978-1-4625-1601-8 (hardback : acid-free paper)
    1. Psychoanalysis.   2. Personality assessment.   I. Hopwood, Christopher J.,
1976– editor of compilation.   II. Bornstein, Robert F., editor of compilation.
    BF698.5.M85 2014
    616.89′075—dc23
                                                                2014011934

To Sullivan
—C. J. H.

To Mary, with love
—R. F. B.

About the Editors

Christopher J. Hopwood, PhD, is Assistant Professor of Psychology at Michigan State University, Director of the Michigan State University Psychological Clinic, and a licensed psychologist in Michigan. Dr. Hopwood has published numerous articles, book chapters, and books on personality processes and psychological assessment. He is Associate Editor for *Assessment* and the *Journal of Personality Disorders* and Consulting Editor for several other journals in the areas of personality, personality disorders, and assessment. Dr. Hopwood's research has been funded by the National Institute of Mental Health and the National Institute on Drug Abuse. He is a board member of the Society for Interpersonal Theory and Research and the North American Society for the Study of Personality Disorders. He received the 2011 Samuel J. and Anne G. Beck University of Chicago Early Career Award for Outstanding Research in Personality Assessment from the Society for Personality Assessment.

Robert F. Bornstein, PhD, is Professor of Psychology at Adelphi University. Dr. Bornstein has published numerous articles and book chapters on personality dynamics, assessment, diagnosis, and treatment. He wrote *The Dependent Personality* and *The Dependent Patient: A Practitioner's Guide*; coauthored (with Mary Languirand) *When Someone You Love Needs Nursing Home Care, How to Age in Place*, and *Healthy Dependency*; and coedited (with Joseph Masling) seven volumes of the *Empirical Studies of Psychoanalytic Theories* series, as well as *Scoring the Rorschach: Seven Validated Systems*. Dr. Bornstein is a Fellow of the American Psychological Association, the Association for Psychological Science, and the Society for Personality Assessment. His research has been funded by grants from the National Institute of Mental Health and the National Science Foundation. He received the 2005 Theodore Millon Award for Excellence in Personality Psychology from Division 12 (Society of Clinical Psychology) of the American Psychological Association and the American Psychological Foundation and is a five-time recipient of the Walter G. Klopfer Award for Outstanding Statistically Based Research Article from the Society for Personality Assessment.

Contributors

R. Michael Bagby, PhD, ABAP, CPsych, Departments of Psychology and Psychiatry, University of Toronto, Toronto, Canada

Iruma Bello, PhD, First Episode Psychosis Program, Department of Psychiatry, New York University Langone Medical Center/Bellevue Hospital, New York, New York

Mark A. Blais, PsyD, Department of Psychiatry, Massachusetts General Hospital/ Harvard Medical School, Boston, Massachusetts

Daniel M. Blonigen, PhD, Center for Innovation to Implementation, VA Palo Alto Health Care System, Menlo Park, California

Robert F. Bornstein, PhD, Derner Institute of Advanced Psychological Studies, Adelphi University, Garden City, New York

Danielle Burchett, PhD, Division of Social, Behavioral, and Global Studies, California State University, Monterey Bay, and United States Air Force Psychology Research Service Analytic Group, Department of Defense Center–Monterey Bay, Seaside, California

Alex Cogswell, PhD, Children's Psychiatry Clinic, University at Buffalo, State University of New York, Buffalo, New York

Christy A. Denckla, MA, Derner Institute of Advanced Psychological Studies, Adelphi University, Garden City, New York

Kimberly Marie Dunbeck, BS, Department of Psychology, Case Western University, Cleveland, Ohio

Natalie Emmert, BA, Children's Psychiatry Clinic, University at Buffalo, State University of New York, Buffalo, New York

Stephen E. Finn, PhD, Center for Therapeutic Assessment, University of Texas at Austin, Austin, Texas

Janine Galione, MA, Department of Psychology,
Washington University in St. Louis, St. Louis, Missouri

Robert A. Graceffo, MA, Department of Psychology, University of Toledo,
Toledo, Ohio

Shawn Harrington, MA, Department of Psychology, University of Windsor,
Windsor, Ontario, Canada

Christopher J. Hopwood, PhD, Department of Psychology,
Michigan State University, East Lansing, Michigan

Spee Kosloff, PhD, Department of Psychology, California State University, Fresno,
Fresno, California

Anthony D. Mancini, PhD, Department of Psychology, Pace University,
Pleasantville, New York

Molly Maxfield, PhD, Department of Psychology, University of Colorado
Colorado Springs, Colorado Springs, Colorado

Joni L. Mihura, PhD, Department of Psychology, University of Toledo,
Toledo, Ohio

Jason S. Moser, PhD, Department of Psychology, Michigan State University,
East Lansing, Michigan

Suzanne O'Brien, PhD, California Forensic Assessment Project,
San Diego, California

Thomas F. Oltmanns, PhD, Department of Psychology,
Washington University in St. Louis, St. Louis, Missouri

Antonio Pascual-Leone, PhD, Department of Psychology, University of Windsor,
Windsor, Ontario, Canada

Aaron L. Pincus, PhD, Department of Psychology, Pennsylvania State University,
University Park, Pennsylvania

Amy Przeworski, PhD, Department of Psychology,
Case Western Reserve University, Cleveland, Ohio

Michael J. Roche, MS, Department of Psychology, Pennsylvania State University,
University Park, Pennsylvania

Pamela Sadler, PhD, Department of Psychology, Wilfrid Laurier University,
Waterloo, Ontario, Canada

Hans S. Schroder, BS, Department of Psychology, Michigan State University,
East Lansing, Michigan

Terence Singh, PhD, Early Psychosis Treatment Service, Foothills Medical Centre,
Calgary, Alberta, Canada

Justin D. Smith, PhD, Department of Psychology and Neuroscience, Baylor
University, Waco, Texas

Sheldon Solomon, PhD, Department of Psychology, Skidmore College,
Saratoga Springs, New York

Michael L. Stanfill, PhD, Jail Health Services, Public Health–Seattle and King County, and Department of Health Services, University of Washington, Seattle, Washington

Katherine M. Thomas, MS, Department of Psychology, Michigan State University, East Lansing, Michigan

Rachel L. Tomko, MA, Department of Psychological Sciences, University of Missouri, Columbia, Missouri

Timothy J. Trull, PhD, Department of Psychological Sciences, University of Missouri, Columbia, Missouri

Donald J. Viglione, Jr., PhD, California School of Professional Psychology at Alliant International University, San Diego, California

Erik Woody, PhD, Department of Psychology, University of Waterloo, Waterloo, Ontario, Canada

Aidan G. C. Wright, PhD, Department of Psychology, University of Pittsburgh, Pittsburgh, Pennsylvania

Amy Wytiaz, PhD, VA Palo Alto Health Care System, Menlo Park, California

Nikita Yeryomenko, MA, Department of Psychology, University of Windsor, Windsor, Ontario, Canada

Contents

Introduction to Multimethod Clinical Assessment

Robert F. Bornstein and Christopher J. Hopwood

Suppose you developed numbness in your left leg, along with back pain and balance problems—a worrisome situation to say the least. You go to your physician and describe your symptoms; after listening carefully and asking some questions, your physician renders a diagnosis, writes a prescription, and sends you on your way. You're surprised that the doctor didn't order additional tests, but you assume she must know what she is doing, so you let it go.

A week has gone by and the symptoms have not remitted, so you decide to consult a different physician. As you start to explain your problem, the physician stops you. He doesn't want to hear your take on things, he says—tests will provide all the information he needs. He writes out several orders and sends you off to the lab.

These scenarios illustrate a fundamental difference between psychology and medicine. In medicine, multimethod assessment is so firmly entrenched that we hardly notice it: Virtually every clinical decision reflects an integration of the patient's self-report with data obtained in other modalities. A very different situation characterizes contemporary psychology. Here the clinician often relies primarily—sometimes completely—on tests from a single modality (e.g., a series of questionnaires), and neither patient nor referent is likely to question this approach. To be sure, many clinicians draw upon evidence from multiple modalities in formulating an assessment, but in psychology, unlike medicine, this is neither expected nor required. It depends on the background, attitudes, and preferences of the clinician.

We believe it is time for multimethod clinical assessment to become the norm—an expectation rather than an option. Just as physicians cannot gain complete understanding of a patient's problem unless they integrate evidence from multiple modalities (e.g., self-report, behavioral, physiological), psychologists cannot gain complete understanding of a patient's difficulties without evidence from multiple modalities (e.g., self-report, behavioral, performance-based). Moreover, just as the particular combination of tests that is most useful to an assessing physician will depend on the nature of the patient and that patient's symptoms, the particular combination of tests that will be useful to the assessing psychologist will vary from problem to problem and from patient to patient.

What Is Clinical Assessment?

Psychologists, psychiatrists, and others often use the terms *diagnosis* and *assessment* interchangeably, but in fact these terms mean different things. Diagnosis involves identifying and documenting a patient's symptoms to classify that patient into one or more categories whose labels represent shorthand descriptors of complex psychological syndromes (e.g., bulimia nervosa, schizoid personality disorder). Assessment, in contrast, involves administering a series of psychological tests to disentangle the complex array of dispositional and situational factors that combine to determine a patient's subjective experiences, core beliefs, emotional patterns, motives, traits, defenses, and coping strategies.

As a number of writers have noted, diagnosis is key to understanding a patient's *pathology*; assessment is key to understanding the *person* with this pathology (Finn, 2005; Hopwood, 2010; Weiner, 2000). Although assessment data by themselves are not adequate to render a diagnosis, these data can be useful in refining diagnoses, in supporting a tentative diagnosis, and in making a differential diagnosis (such as when marked discontinuities in a patient's performance on more structured versus less structured tests suggest borderline pathology; see Carr & Goldstein, 1981). Beyond refining diagnostic decisions, assessment data play an important role in risk management (VandeCreek & Knapp, 2000) and treatment planning (Clarkin, 2012; Livesley, 2005), as well as in forensic settings (e.g., custody and competency hearings; Hilsenroth & Stricker, 2004), fitness for duty evaluations (Anfang & Wall, 2006), psychiatric disability evaluations (Gold et al., 2008), and myriad other domains.

As is true for diagnosis and assessment, clinicians and researchers often use the terms *psychological testing* and *psychological assessment* interchangeably, but in fact these terms also mean different things. Handler and Meyer (1998) provided an excellent summary of the conceptual and practical differences between psychological testing and psychological assessment. They wrote:

> Testing is a relatively straightforward process wherein a particular test is administered to obtain a particular score or two. Subsequently, a descriptive meaning can be applied to the score based on normative, nomothetic findings. . . . Psychological assessment, however, is a quite different enterprise. The focus here is not on obtaining a single score, or even a series of test scores. Rather, the focus is on taking a variety of test-derived pieces of information, obtained from multiple methods of assessment, and placing these data in the context of historical information, referral information, and behavioral observations in order to generate a cohesive and comprehensive understanding of the person being evaluated. (pp. 4–5)

Handler and Meyer's (1998) insightful analysis has been echoed and elaborated by numerous clinicians and clinical researchers (e.g., Groth-Marnat, 1999; Widiger & Samuel, 2005). Cates (1999, p. 637) put it well when he noted that in the realm of psychological assessment, "art rests on science." Psychological testing requires precision, objectivity, and the kind of scientific detachment that facilitates accurate data gathering. Psychological assessment involves integration, synthesis, and clarification of ambiguous—even conflicting—evidence obtained during the testing process. As Bornstein (2010) noted in describing the complexity of clinical assessment:

> The competent tester must be (at least for that moment) a staunch behaviorist, understanding the contingencies that define the testing situation and using this knowledge to maximize the validity and generalizability of test data. Once these data are gathered the behavioral tester must transform into a psychodynamically informed assessor, able to combine dynamic concepts with research findings from other areas of psychology to interpret test results in the context of referral information, life history information, and behavioral observations made during testing. (p. 147)

On Test Score Convergences and Discontinuities

Several decades ago psychological assessment almost invariably included a comprehensive test battery consisting of measures designed to tap different domains of adaptation (e.g., trait scales and intellectual tests), and different levels of functioning and experience (e.g., questionnaires and performance-based measures; see Allison, Blatt, & Zimet, 1968; Rapaport, Gill, & Schafer, 1945, 1968). Owing in part to the demands of managed care (Sperling, Sack, & Field, 2000), assessment now consists primarily of the administration, scoring, and interpretation of questionnaires. This trend extends beyond clinical assessment to research settings as well:

When Bornstein (2003) conducted a systematic survey of personality disorder studies published in five major journals between 1991 and 2000, he found that over 80% of published investigations relied exclusively on self-report data, both in quantifying personality pathology and in measuring its correlates and consequences (only 4% of published studies assessed actual behavior).

Even when test batteries include measures from multiple modalities, they are not always integrated in a way that is maximally heuristic and clinically useful. Following the tradition established by Campbell and Fiske (1959), during the past 50 years psychological assessment research has focused primarily on documenting the convergence of scores on different measures of the same construct, even when the measures use very different methods to quantify these constructs (see Messick, 1989, 1995; Slaney & Maraun, 2008). Most clinicians intuitively value converging results from different tests, in part because converging results are reassuring and increase one's confidence in test-derived clinical predictions. In the early 1990s, psychologists began to write more extensively on the systematic interpretation of test score divergences as well as convergences (e.g., Archer & Krishnamurthy, 1993a, 1993b; Meyer, 1996b, 1997). As Meyer et al. (2001) noted, when different personality assessment tools use different formats and engage different psychological processes in the testee, divergences in scores on these tests can be particularly informative.

Consider, for example, a series of studies wherein Bornstein and his colleagues found that discontinuities between self-report and performance-based dependency test scores provided information regarding personality dynamics that neither test alone could provide (Bornstein, 1998; Bornstein, Bowers, & Bonner, 1996a, 1996b; Bornstein, Rossner, Hill, & Stepanian, 1994). These studies were all based on an often observed pattern: Although many patients obtain consistently high (or consistently low) scores on self-report and performance-based dependency tests (and are therefore classified as *high dependent* or *low dependent*), some patients score high on one type of test but low on the other (see Bornstein, 2002, 2012). Those who obtain high performance-based but low self-report dependency scores have a personality style characterized by *unacknowledged dependency*; those who obtain the reverse pattern—low performance-based but high self-report dependency scores—have a *dependent-self presentation*, exaggerating dependent feelings and urges as a means of obtaining rewards in social and work relationships. Moreover, college students who score high on both self-report and performance-based dependency tests have high levels of dependent personality disorder symptoms, whereas students who obtain high performance-based but low self-report dependency scores tend to have histrionic rather than dependent features (Bornstein, 1998). Similar conclusions have emerged in studies contrasting self-report and performance-based measures of other personality traits, including need for achievement (McClelland, Koestner, & Weinberger, 1989), power (Koestner, Weinberger, & McClelland, 1991), and intimacy (Craig, Koestner, & Zuroff, 1994).

Process and Outcome in Clinical Assessment

Findings like these point to the importance of considering process as well as outcome in clinical assessment: Only by understanding the psychological processes engaged by different types of tests can test score convergences and divergences be interpreted meaningfully. Although a comprehensive analysis of psychological processes that underlie the broad spectrum of tests in use today has yet to be written, Meyer and Kurtz (2006) and others (e.g., Schultheiss, 2007) contrasted the processes engaged by two of the more widely used types of measures: self-report and performance based. As Bornstein (2009) noted, when people genuinely engage a typical self-report test item (e.g., "I would rather be a follower than a leader," "I often feel depleted"), three processes occur in sequence. First, testees engage in *introspection*, turning their attention inward to determine if the statement captures some aspect of their feelings, thoughts, motives, or behaviors. Second, a *retrospective memory search* occurs, as testees attempt to retrieve instances wherein they experienced or exhibited the response(s) described in the test item. Finally, testees may engage in *deliberate self-presentation*, deciding whether, given the context and setting in which they are being evaluated, it is better to answer honestly or to modify their response to depict themselves in a particular way. Typically, these efforts are aimed at "faking good" (i.e., attempting to portray oneself as healthier than is actually the case) or "faking bad" (attempting to portray oneself as unhealthy and exaggerate pathology), depending on the person's self-presentation goals.

Contrast this set of psychological processes with those that occur as people respond to stimuli from a performance-based measure such as the Rorschach Inkblot Method (RIM). Unlike a self-report test, here the fundamental challenge is to create meaning in a stimulus that can be interpreted in multiple ways. To do this, patients must direct their attention outward (rather than inward) and focus on the stimulus (not the self); they then attribute meaning to the stimulus based on properties of the inkblot and the associations primed by these stimulus properties. Once a series of potential percepts (or *stimulus attributions*) is formed, patients typically sort through these possible responses, selecting some and rejecting others before providing their description (see Exner & Erdberg, 2005; Meyer, Viglione, Mihura, Erard, & Erdberg, 2011).

With this as context, Bornstein (2009, 2011) provided a preliminary process-based classification of widely used psychological tests. In an updated version of this classification, these tests may be divided into five broad categories, as follows.

Self-Attribution Tests

Self-attribution (or *self-report*) test scores reflect the degree to which the person attributes various traits, feelings, thoughts, motives, behaviors, attitudes, or experiences to him- or herself. Because they are efficient and cost effective, self-attribution tests are far and away the most widely used type of test in both research and clinical settings. The Beck Depression Inventory, the Personality Assessment Inventory, and the NEO Personality Inventory (NEO-PI) would all be included in this category, as would questionnaire measures of attitudes, interests, and values.

Stimulus Attribution Tests

Traditionally called *projective tests*, and more recently *performance-based tests*, in stimulus attribution tests the respondent attributes meaning to an ambiguous stimulus, with attributions determined in part by stimulus characteristics and in part by the person's cognitive style, emotions, motives, and need states. The RIM is the most widely used and well-known stimulus attribution test; others include the Thematic Apperception Test and the Holtzman Inkblot Test.

Constructive Tests

In constructive tests, generation of test responses requires the person to create or construct a novel image or written description within parameters defined by the tester. The Draw a Person Test (and other projective drawings) would be classified in this category, as would various open-ended self-descriptions (e.g., Blatt's Qualitative and Structural Dimensions of Object Representations).

Behavioral Tests

In some behavioral tests, scores are derived from indices of a person's behavior exhibited and measured *in vivo*, as in spot sampling (a technique wherein researchers sample behavior at randomly selected times, in multiple contexts). Behavior may also be examined in a controlled setting (e.g., using joystick feedback tasks wherein moment-by-moment behaviors are rated as they occur). Other behavioral tests assess the person's unrehearsed performance on one or more structured tasks designed to tap attentional resources, working memory, and other cognitive skills (e.g., the Bender Visual–Motor Gestalt Test, the Attentional Capacity Test).

Informant-Report Tests

Scores on tests in this category are based on informants' ratings or judgments of a person's characteristic patterns of responding (e.g., the therapist version of the Shedler–Westen Assessment Procedure, the Informant Report version of the NEO-PI). In contrast to observational measures, which are based on direct observation of behavior, informant-report tests are based on informants' retrospective, memory-derived conclusions regarding characteristics of the target person.[1]

Dispositional and Contextual Influences on Psychological Test Responses

Scrutiny of these five categories and the processes engaged by tests within each category suggests two things. First, scores on each type of test not only reflect aspects of the construct that the test is designed to assess (e.g., narcissism, self-esteem, introjects, cognitive skills), but are also influenced by an array of dispositional and contextual variables, not all of which are conceptually linked with the construct in question. Second, in many instances these extraneous variables—typically considered confounds in clinical assessment—will differentially influence scores derived from tests in different categories, even when these tests purport to quantify the same construct.

Among the key dispositional influences on psychological test responses are self-perception biases (i.e., distortions in the respondent's view of him- or herself; Oltmanns & Turkheimer, 2009), and memory distortions (e.g., selective recall of trait-relevant behaviors). The individual's cognitive (information-processing) style also plays a role: Some people tend to focus primarily on details when thinking about themselves, other people, or test stimuli (e.g., inkblots); others emphasize overall patterns and global impressions at the expense of detail. Self-attributions and informant reports are both influenced by various heuristics inherent in self-perception and perceptions of others (e.g., confirmatory bias, actor–observer effects, the fundamental attribution error). Finally, studies confirm that self-presentation needs (e.g., the desire to present oneself in a positive or negative light) often influence psychological test responses (Horvath & Morf, 2010), as do the

---

[1]Certain psychological tests have characteristics of more than one category and may be best conceptualized as "hybrid tests" that engage multiple processes. For example, structured clinical interviews involve patient self-report (and therefore engage the processes characteristic of self-attribution tests), as well as clinician observation of patient behavior (and therefore engage the processes of behavioral tests). Broad-range neuropsychological tests like the Halstead–Reitan may engage processes from multiple categories (see Reitan & Wolfson, 2000).

person's previous testing experiences and the expectations that these earlier experiences produce (Garb, 1998).

Beyond dispositional influences, several state and contextual variables have been shown to play a role in moderating test scores. For example, variations in the respondent's mood or anxiety level influence test responses in at least two ways. First, variations in mood influence retrieval of episodic memories, as people tend to retrieve mood-congruent memories more readily than mood-incongruent ones (Rholes, Riskind, & Lane, 1987). Second, anxiety captures attentional capacity (as does negative mood), impairing respondents' performance on various behavioral and cognitive measures (Arnell, Killman, & Fijavz, 2007). In addition, sometimes particular concepts or motives are inadvertently primed during a testing situation, influencing test performance: Masling and others have shown how the gender of the examiner influences RIM responses (see Masling, 1966, 2002, for reviews); even seemingly minor stimuli such as an examiner's clothing, his or her age, and the layout of the testing room may affect test performance (Bargh & Morsella, 2008; Weiner, 2004).

Quantifying Dispositional and Contextual Influences

There are at least three ways of assessing the impact of various dispositional and contextual variables on psychological test scores. First, researchers can examine naturally occurring (*in vivo*) influences (e.g., variations in mood or in anxiety level). This was the approach used by Hirschfeld, Klerman, Clayton, and Keller (1983) to examine the impact of changes in severity of depressive symptoms on traits theoretically linked with depression (e.g., dependency, self-esteem). Second, researchers can examine changes in test scores over time due to the effects of maturation (in children) or aging (in older adults). This was the approach used by Jansen and Van der Maas (2002) to detect Piagetian developmental shifts in children's reasoning, and that used by Baltes (1996) to assess age-related changes in the expression of underlying dependency needs in older adults (see also Roberts & DelVecchio, 2000, for additional findings in this area).

A third approach—the least widely used but potentially the most informative—is to introduce experimental manipulations that deliberately alter the processes engaged by different psychological tests. This approach allows the researcher to (1) confirm that altering these processes does in fact change test scores as expected; and (2) illuminate the processes involved in two tests that measure parallel constructs using contrasting methods. This was the approach used by Bornstein et al. (1994, 1996a) to examine the differential impact of instructional set and mood state on self-report and performance-based dependency scores. As hypothesized, deliberately inducing a negative mood state increased performance-based (but not self-report) dependency scores, whereas an instructional set that framed interpersonal dependency in negative terms increased self-report (but not performance-based) dependency. Along somewhat similar lines, Morf and her colleagues have examined the impact of threats to self-esteem on self- and other-evaluations in narcissistic and control participants (see Morf & Rhodewalt, 2001). Arntz and his colleagues assessed the impact of manipulating stress level and mood on schema-related responding in patients with and without borderline pathology (e.g., Arntz et al., 2009).

Maximizing the Value of Multimethod Assessment: A Framework for Test Score Integration

In many—perhaps most—testing situations, multimethod assessment will yield richer, more clinically useful data than assessment that relies exclusively on tests from a single modality. From a psychometric standpoint, multimethod assessment helps minimize the negative impact of reliability and validity limitations inherent in different types of measures, because these limitations tend to vary across test modality. Although they can never be entirely eliminated, to some degree these limitations can be balanced out by deliberately selecting tests with contrasting strengths and weaknesses. From a clinical standpoint, when test data from different modalities are integrated, and test score convergences and divergences are explored, multimethod assessment allows aspects of a patient's dynamics that might otherwise go unrecognized to be scrutinized directly (e.g., conflicts, defenses, unconscious motives, and emotional responses, areas wherein the patient has limited insight or is overtly self-deceptive).

Thus, in our view, the central issue regarding multimethod clinical assessment is not *why* but *how*. In the following sections we outline a six-step framework for multimethod assessment and test score integration.

1. *Understand the strengths and limitations of different methods.* In part, these methods reflect the psychometric properties of each measure (see Messick, 1989, 1995) and the degree to which scores derived from that measure fulfill established criteria for validity (convergent, discriminant, concurrent, predictive), and reliability (retest, internal, interrater). The strengths and limitations of different methods are also a product of the psychological processes engaged by measures within that particular test category (Bornstein, 2011), since different processes (e.g., self-attributions, online responding, judgments of others' behavior) are differentially influenced by various extraneous variables (e.g., self-presentation goals, testing milieu).

2. *Know when to collect data using multiple methods.* Although critics of the RIM have often cited its modest correlations with self-report test scores as evidence of poor RIM validity (e.g., Wood, Nezworski,

Lilienfield, & Garb, 2003), given the different processes engaged by self-report and performance-based tests, such modest correlations—far from being problematic—actually represent evidence supporting the discriminant validity of both measures (Bornstein, 2002; McGrath, 2008). Similarly, while modest correlations between scores on the NEO-PI and indices of observable behavior have occasionally been cited as evidence of limitations in the measure (Block, 2010), given respondents' self-presentation needs and inherent limitations in our ability to describe ourselves accurately, correlations (effect sizes) between self-report test scores and behavior in the medium range are precisely what one would expect for trait-focused scales.

Any time two tests that measure parallel constructs using different methodologies fulfill established criteria for reliability and validity, each test has the potential to add incremental validity—unique predictive value—to a test battery. Thus, use of two tests that measure a particular construct via contrasting methods is potentially useful any time a complete and nuanced understanding of this construct is needed (see Meyer et al., 2001). Given cost and efficiency concerns, multimethod assessment of a construct is most easily justified when a complex clinical or empirical question merits particularly close scrutiny (e.g., when assessing impulse control, suicidality, parental fitness, or competence to stand trial).

3. *Decide which methods to use.* The choice of assessment method will be based in part on the referral question, the patient's history, and results from previous evaluations if these are available. The domains of behavior and mental functioning most salient to the assessment (e.g., stress tolerance, potential to benefit from psychotherapy) are also relevant here: Because different measures are best suited for predicting different forms of behavior, it is important to tailor the battery to match tests with outcome. (See, e.g., findings demonstrating that performance-based measures of interpersonal dependency and need for achievement predict spontaneous behavior in those domains, whereas self-report measures of these constructs tend to predict goal-directed rather than spontaneous behavior; Bornstein, 2002; McClelland et al., 1989.) Meyer (1996a) suggested that—even within a category—psychological tests can be distinguished with respect to the degree of *conscious penetration* associated with the processes engaged by that test (i.e., the degree to which test responses reflect deliberate, mindful responding versus reflexive, automatic processing). Erdelyi (2004) has shown that conscious awareness of internal states may also vary over time, waxing and waning in response to external events and environmental contingencies.

4. *Select appropriate measures.* Beyond the referral question itself, initial test selection decisions should be based on validity evidence, an understanding of underlying processes engaged by different tests, cost effectiveness, and clinical utility. Given that clinical assessment is a dynamic process

(Finn, 2005; Hopwood, 2010; Hopwood & Huprich, 2011), and that new questions arise as data accumulate, in many instances the assessor must adjust "on the fly," modifying the test battery as preliminary results reveal new issues that merit scrutiny. For example, a patient may produce an unremarkable Minnesota Multiphasic Personality Inventory (MMPI) clinical scale profile, but if scrutiny of that patient's validity scales suggests defensive responding, it may be useful to follow up with a performance-based test that includes well-validated indices of psychopathology and subjective distress. In general, scales with high face validity are more susceptible to dissimulation and self-presentation effects than are scales with low face validity (Shedler, Mayman, & Manis, 1993); as Bornstein et al. (1994) and McGrath (2008) noted, performance based tests in general tend to have low face validity. Self-report tests also vary with respect to face validity, however, and even within a particular scale items may vary considerably with respect to susceptibility to dissimulation and self-presentation effects (Sartori, 2010).

5. *Implement a framework for integrating data from different sources.* How can we integrate data we acquire from multiple sources? First, we must develop an overarching framework for understanding convergences and divergences among scores from tests that measure parallel constructs using different methods (see Finn, 2007). Bornstein's (1998, 2012) four-cell model of interpersonal dependency based on the integration of self-report and performance-based test patterns may be useful in this context; in this model respondents are classified into *low dependent, high dependent, unacknowledged dependency*, and *dependent self-presentation groups* (see Bornstein, 2012, Fig. 1). A parallel framework was developed by Shedler et al. (1993) when they used responses to the Eysenck Neuroticism Scale and raters' evaluations of open-ended descriptions of early memories to classify respondents into *genuinely healthy, genuinely distressed, "illusion of mental illness"* (exaggerations in self-reported distress), and *"illusion of mental health"* (defensively healthy) groups (see Shedler et al., 1993, Fig. 1).

Second, we must develop a framework for integrating test data across domains as well as across methods. Carr and Goldstein's (1981) finding that marked discontinuities in patient performance between more structured versus less structured tests is useful in identifying underlying borderline pathology is an example of this strategy (see also Hopwood et al., 2008, for evidence regarding the contrasting dynamics of questionnaires and structured interviews). This is also the general approach used by neuropsychologists to identify areas of cognitive deficit by contrasting patients' performance across tests that capture different skills and capacities. Along slightly different lines, Hopwood et al. (2011) contrasted circumplex-derived indices of interpersonal sensitivities across three types of relationships (romantic, platonic, and non-close) to elucidate the degree to which consistent interpersonal patterns emerged across relationship domains.

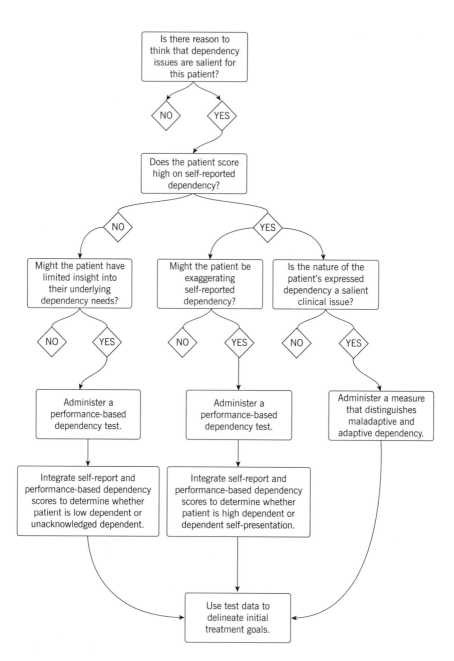

FIGURE 1. Decision tree for using multimethod dependency test data in treatment planning. Initial assessment of the patient's self-reported (self-attributed) dependency may be followed by administration of a performance-based dependency test, if there is reason to believe the patient may be either underreporting or exaggerating his or her dependency. If the nature of the patient's expressed dependency is a salient clinical issue, then initial assessment of self-reported dependency may be followed by administration of a measure that distinguishes maladaptive from adaptive expressions of underlying dependency needs.

Similar logic holds when integrating personality and psychopathology test data with data derived from a patient's life records, and with that provided by knowledgeable informants; in both areas convergences and discontinuities may be informative.

6. *Use assessment data to enhance treatment planning.* Moving from assessment to treatment planning is a stepwise process: The initial clinical (or referral) question will guide the clinician's preliminary choice of tests, after which the initial test results—interpreted in the context of the patient's life history, presenting problem, and other salient information—will determine the next test(s) to be administered, and how test results may be integrated most usefully. Figure 1 summarizes this process, illustrating how initial test results guide subsequent clinical decisions when assessing patient dependency.

Multimethod Clinical Assessment: Looking Forward

A plethora of empirical research indicates that use of multiple assessment methods in clinical and research settings provides important incremental information that cannot be obtained when a single assessment modality is used. Nevertheless, many psychologists continue to utilize unimodal rather than multimethod assessment in their practice and research, in part because empirically validated, clinically useful models for integrating multimethod data have not been presented in a comprehensive, systematic, transtheoretical way. The goal of this volume is to strengthen links between evidence-based multimethod assessment and clinical practice by providing systematic reviews of how to incorporate diverse assessment techniques in the laboratory, clinic, and consulting room.

The volume includes 14 chapters by leading clinical researchers. Within each chapter we asked authors to (1) discuss the assessment approaches that are particularly useful for assessing key constructs relevant to a particular clinical issue, along with a rationale for integrating data within this domain; (2) review empirical evidence supporting the integration of these methods, including evidence regarding their interrelations and the incremental validity provided by each method; and (3) describe a case in which assessment using these assessment methods was clinically useful. Chapters are organized into three broad domains, as follows.

The first five chapters focus on *Personality and Individual Differences*, opening with a discussion of multimethod assessment of personality traits by Galione and Oltmanns. Pincus, Sadler, Woody, Roche, Thomas, and Wright review research on multimethod assessment of interpersonal dynamics, followed by Tomko and Trull's review studies of affective processes. Kosloff, Maxfield, and Solomon discuss existential concerns. This section closes with Cogswell and Emmert's discussion of implicit processes, one of the most challenging areas in contemporary psychological assessment and one that helped impel many of the current integrative approaches used in this area.

The next four chapters discuss multimethod assessment of *Psychopathology and Resilience.* Here authors address the opportunities and challenges faced in assessing several variables of particular relevance in the clinical setting: anxiety (Moser, Przeworski, Schroder, & Dunbeck), externalizing disorders (Blonigen & Wytiaz), thought quality (Blais & Bello), and resilience (Denckla & Mancini). Chapters in this section illustrate nicely the range of assessment modalities used to assess psychopathology and protective factors, and the contrasting strategies that are useful in integrating assessment data when different constructs are examined.

The final section includes chapters on *Clinical Management.* Mihura and Graceffo review research on multimethod assessment and treatment planning, followed by Pascual-Leone, Singh, Harrington, and Yeryomenko's discussion of how assessment can illuminate the treatment process. Burchett and Bagby review research on detecting and evaluating distortion and dissimulation in patient responding, followed by Stanfill, O'Brien, and Viglione's discussion of the complexities of multimethod risk assessment. The volume closes with Smith and Finn's review of the therapeutic presentation of multimethod assessment results, which brings us full circle, as Smith and Finn demonstrate how assessment data not only inform the clinician, but may also facilitate patient motivation and engagement.

As these brief descriptions illustrate, this volume addresses a diverse array of clinical issues. A broad range of methods are used to address these various issues, including self-reports, performance-based tests, behavioral measures (both laboratory-based and *in vivo*), archival data, and observer reports. Despite this diversity in topic, method, and integration strategy, contributors share a fundamental belief in the value of multimethod assessment in contemporary clinical psychology. As a result, these chapters not only bring together the best work on multimethod clinical assessment available today, but help set the stage for continued refinement of empirically validated integrative assessment methods that will enhance this important area of clinical practice and research during the coming years.

REFERENCES

Allison, J., Blatt, S. J., & Zimet, C. N. (1968). *The interpretation of psychological tests.* New York: Harper & Row.

Anfang, S. A., & Wall, B. W. (2006). Psychiatric fitness for duty evaluations. *Psychiatric Clinics of North America, 29,* 675–693.

Archer, R. P., & Krishnamurthy, R. (1993a). Combining the Rorschach and MMPI in the assessment of adolescents. *Journal of Personality Assessment, 60,* 132–140.

Archer, R. P., & Krishnamurthy, R. (1993b). A review of MMPI and Rorschach interrelationships in adult samples. *Journal of Personality Assessment, 61,* 277–293.

Arnell, K. M., Killman, K. V., & Fijavz, D. (2007). Blinded by emotion: Target misses follow attention capture by arousing distractors in RSVP. *Emotion*, 7, 465–477.

Arntz, A., Roos, D., & Dreesen, L. (2009). Assumptions in borderline personality disorder: Specificity, stability, and relationship with etiological factors. *Behaviour Research and Therapy*, 37, 545–557.

Baltes, M. M. (1996). *The many faces of dependency in old age.* Cambridge, UK: Cambridge University Press.

Bargh, J. A., & Morsella, E. (2008). The unconscious mind. *Perspectives on Psychological Science*, 3, 73–79.

Block, J. (2010). The five-factor framing of personality and beyond: Some ruminations. *Psychological Inquiry*, 21, 2–25.

Bornstein, R. F. (1998). Implicit and self-attributed dependency needs in dependent and histrionic personality disorders. *Journal of Personality Assessment*, 71, 1–14.

Bornstein, R. F. (2002). A process dissociation approach to objective–projective test score interrelationships. *Journal of Personality Assessment*, 78, 47–68.

Bornstein, R. F. (2003). Behaviorally referenced experimentation and symptom validation: A paradigm for 21st century personality disorder research. *Journal of Personality Disorders*, 17, 1–18.

Bornstein, R. F. (2009). Heisenberg, Kandinsky, and the heteromethod convergence problem: Lessons from within and beyond psychology. *Journal of Personality Assessment*, 91, 1–8.

Bornstein, R. F. (2010). Psychoanalytic theory as a unifying framework for 21st century personality assessment. *Psychoanalytic Psychology*, 27, 133–152.

Bornstein, R. F. (2011). Toward a process-focused model of test score validity: Improving psychological assessment in science and practice. *Psychological Assessment*, 23, 532–544.

Bornstein, R. F. (2012). From dysfunction to adaptation: An interactionist model of dependency. *Annual Review of Clinical Psychology*, 8, 291–316.

Bornstein, R. F., Bowers, K. S., & Bonner, S. (1996a). Effects of induced mood states on objective and projective dependency scores. *Journal of Personality Assessment*, 67, 324–340.

Bornstein, R. F., Bowers, K. S., & Bonner, S. (1996b). Relationships of objective and projective dependency scores to sex role orientation in college students. *Journal of Personality Assessment*, 66, 555–568.

Bornstein, R. F., Rossner, S. C., Hill, E. L., & Stepanian, M. L. (1994). Face validity and fakability of objective and projective measures of dependency. *Journal of Personality Assessment*, 63, 363–386.

Campbell, D. T., & Fiske, D. (1959). Convergent and discriminant validation by the multitrait–multimethod matrix. *Psychological Bulletin*, 56, 81–105.

Carr, A. C., & Goldstein, E. G. (1981). Approaches to the diagnosis of borderline conditions by the use of psychological tests. *Journal of Personality Assessment*, 45, 563–574.

Cates, J. A. (1999). The art of assessment in psychology: Ethics, expertise, and validity. *Journal of Clinical Psychology*, 55, 631–641.

Clarkin, J. F. (2012). An integrated approach to psychotherapy techniques for patients with personality disorder. *Journal of Personality Disorders*, 26, 43–62.

Craig, J. A., Koestner, R., & Zuroff, D. C. (1994). Implicit and self-attributed intimacy motivation. *Journal of Social and Personal Relationships*, 11, 491–507.

Erdelyi, M. H. (2004). Subliminal perception and its cognates: Theory, indeterminacy, and time. *Consciousness and Cognition*, 13, 73–91.

Exner, J. E., & Erdberg, P. (2005). *The Rorschach: Advanced interpretation* (3rd ed.). New York: Wiley.

Finn, S. E. (2005). How psychological assessment taught me compassion and firmness. *Journal of Personality Assessment, 84*, 29–32.

Finn, S. E. (2007). *In our client's shoes: Theory and techniques of therapeutic assessment.* New York: Routledge/Taylor & Francis.

Garb, H. N. (1998). *Studying the clinician: Judgment research and psychological assessment.* Washington, DC: American Psychological Association.

Gold, L. H., Anfang, S. A., Drukteinis, A. M., Metzner, J. L., Price, M., Wall, B. W., et al. (2008). AAPL practice guideline for the forensic evaluation of psychiatric disability. *Journal of the American Academy of Psychiatry and the Law, 36*, S3–S50.

Groth-Marnat, G. (1999). Current status and future directions of psychological assessment. *Journal of Clinical Psychology, 55*, 781–785.

Handler, L., & Meyer, G. J. (1998). The importance of teaching and learning personality assessment. In L. Handler & M. J. Hilsenroth (Eds.), *Teaching and learning personality assessment* (pp. 3–30). Mahwah, NJ: Erlbaum.

Hilsenroth, M. J., & Stricker, G. (2004). A consideration of challenges to psychological assessment instruments used in forensic settings: Rorschach as exemplar. *Journal of Personality Assessment, 83*, 141–152.

Hirschfeld, R. M. A., Klerman, G. L., Clayton, P. J., & Keller, M. B. (1983). Personality and depression: Empirical findings. *Archives of General Psychiatry, 40*, 993–998.

Hopwood, C. J. (2010). An interpersonal perspective on the personality assessment process. *Journal of Personality Assessment, 92*, 471–479.

Hopwood, C. J., Ansell, E. B., Pincus, A. L., Wright, A. G. C., Lukowitsky, M. R., & Roche, M. J. (2011). The circumplex structure of interpersonal sensitivities. *Journal of Personality, 79*, 707–739.

Hopwood, C. J., & Huprich, S. K. (2011). Introduction to the Special Issue on personality assessment in the DSM-5. *Journal of Personality Assessment, 93*, 323–324.

Hopwood, C. J., Morey, L. C., Edelen, M. O., Shea, M. T., Grilo, C. M., Sanislow, C. A., et al. (2008). A comparison of interview and self-report methods for the assessment of borderline personality disorder criteria. *Psychological Assessment, 20*, 81–85.

Horvath, S., & Morf, C. C. (2010). To be grandiose or not to be worthless: Different routes to self-enhancement for narcissism and self-esteem. *Journal of Research in Personality, 44*, 585–592.

Jansen, B. R. J., & Van der Maas, H. L. J. (2002). The development of children's rule use on the balance scale task. *Journal of Experimental Child Psychology, 81*, 383–416.

Koestner, R., Weinberger, J., & McClelland, D. C. (1991). Task-intrinsic and social-extrinsic sources of arousal for motives assessed in fantasy and self-report. *Journal of Personality, 59*, 57–82.

Livesley, W. J. (2005). Principles and strategies for treating personality disorder. *Canadian Journal of Psychiatry, 50*, 442–450.

Masling, J. M. (1966). Role-related behavior of the subject and psychologist and its effect upon psychological data. In D. Levine (Ed.), *Nebraska symposium on motivation* (pp. 67–104). Lincoln: University of Nebraska Press.

Masling, J. M. (2002). Speak, memory, or goodbye Columbus. *Journal of Personality Assessment, 78*, 4–30.

McClelland, D. C., Koestner, R., & Weinberger, J. (1989). How do self-attributed and implicit motives differ? *Psychological Review, 96*, 690–702.

McGrath, R. E. (2008). The Rorschach in the context of performance based personality assessment. *Journal of Personality Assessment, 90,* 465–475.

Messick, S. (1989). Validity. In R. L. Linn (Ed.), *Educational measurement* (3rd ed., pp. 13–103). New York: Macmillan.

Messick, S. (1995). Validity of psychological assessment: Validation of inferences from persons' responses and performances as scientific inquiry into score meaning. *American Psychologist, 50,* 741–749.

Meyer, G. J. (1996a). Construct validation of scales derived from the Rorschach method: A review of issues and introduction to the Rorschach Rating Scale. *Journal of Personality Assessment, 67,* 598–628.

Meyer, G. J. (1996b). The Rorschach and MMPI: Toward a more scientific understanding of cross-method assessment. *Journal of Personality Assessment, 67,* 558–578.

Meyer, G. J. (1997). On the integration of personality assessment methods: The Rorschach and MMPI. *Journal of Personality Assessment, 68,* 297–330.

Meyer, G. J. (2000). Incremental validity of the Rorschach Prognostic Rating Scale over MMPI Ego Strength Scale and IQ. *Journal of Personality Assessment, 74,* 356–370.

Meyer, G. J., Finn, S. E., Eyde, L. D., Kay, G. G., Moreland, K. L., Dies, R. R., et al. (2001). Psychological testing and psychological assessment: A review of evidence and issues. *American Psychologist, 56,* 128–165.

Meyer, G. J., & Kurtz, J. E. (2006). Advancing personality assessment terminology: Time to retire "objective" and "projective" as personality test descriptors. *Journal of Personality Assessment, 87,* 223–225.

Meyer, G. J., Viglione, D. J., Mihura, J. L., Erard, R. E., & Erdberg, P. (2011). *Rorschach Performance Assessment System: Administration, coding, interpretation, and technical manual.* Toledo, OH: Rorschach Performance Assessment System.

Morf, C. C., & Rhodewalt, F. (2001). Unraveling the paradoxes of narcissism: A dynamic self-regulatory processing model. *Psychological Inquiry, 12,* 177–196.

Oltmanns, T. F., & Turkheimer, E. (2009). Person perception and personality pathology. *Current Directions in Psychological Science, 18,* 32–36.

Rapaport, D., Gill, M. M., & Schafer, R. (1945). *Diagnostic psychological testing.* Chicago: Yearbook.

Rapaport, D., Gill, M. M., & Schafer, R. (1968). *Diagnostic psychological testing* (rev. ed.). New York: International Universities Press.

Reitan, R. M., & Wolfson, D. (2000). The neuropsychological similarities of mild and more severe head injury. *Archives of Clinical Neuropsychology, 15,* 433–442.

Rholes, W. S., Riskind, J. H., & Lane, J. W. (1987). Emotional states and memory biases: Effects of cognitive priming and mood. *Journal of Personality and Social Psychology, 52,* 91–99.

Roberts, B. W., & DelVecchio, W. F. (2000). The rank-order consistency of personality from childhood to old age: A quantitative review of longitudinal studies. *Psychological Bulletin, 126,* 3–25.

Sartori, R. (2010). Face validity in personality tests: Psychometric instruments and projective techniques in comparison. *Quality and Quantity, 44,* 749–759.

Schultheiss, O. C. (2007). A memory systems approach to the classification of personality tests: A response to Meyer and Kurtz (2006). *Journal of Personality Assessment, 89,* 197–201.

Shedler, J., Mayman, M., & Manis, M. (1993). The illusion of mental health. *American Psychologist, 48,* 1117–1131.

Slaney, K. L., & Maraun, M. D. (2008). A proposed framework for conducting data-based test analysis. *Psychological Methods, 13,* 376–390.

Sperling, M. B., Sack, A., & Field, C. L. (2000). *Psychodynamic practice in a managed care environment.* New York: Guilford Press.

VandeCreek, L., & Knapp, S. (2000). Risk management and life threatening patient behaviors. *Journal of Clinical Psychology, 56,* 1335–1351.

Weiner, I. B. (2000). Using the Rorschach properly in practice and research. *Journal of Clinical Psychology, 56,* 435–438.

Weiner, I. B. (2004). Rorschach Inkblot Method. In M. E. Maruish (Ed.), *The use of psychological testing for treatment planning and outcomes assessment* (3rd ed., pp. 553–588). Mahwah, NJ: Erlbaum.

Widiger, T. A., & Samuel, D. B. (2005). Evidence-based assessment of personality disorders. *Psychological Assessment, 17,* 278–287.

Wood, J. M., Nezworski, M. T., Lilienfeld, S. O., & Garb, H. N. (2003). *What's wrong with the Rorschach?* San Francisco: Jossey-Bass.

PART I

Personality and Individual Differences

CHAPTER 1

Multimethod Assessment of Traits

Janine Galione and Thomas F. Oltmanns

Personality is a complex concept that represents the integration of multiple components. To fully understand the meaning and utility of personality, it is necessary to consider an individual's pattern of cognitions, emotions, behaviors, perceptions, aspirations, values, interpersonal interactions, and self-knowledge. Advances in technology have allowed personality researchers to measure these patterns using not only self-report methods but also behavioral, physiological, and cellular approaches. As a result, the field has started to move beyond a unidimensional perspective of personality. It seems natural that a multifaceted definition of personality warrants a multifaceted approach to measurement and analysis. In this chapter, we will review the common mechanisms used to assess personality traits, including self and observer perspectives, and standardized interviews, behavioral ratings, and life narratives. We will then discuss the benefits of combining multimethod measurements of personality traits to maximize the validity of assessments.

Following the introduction of the multitrait–multimethod matrix (MTMM) by Campbell and Fiske (1959), psychologists sanctified the notion of confirmatory evidence. Multiple measurements of the same trait, or similar constructs, are expected to reflect similar findings across methods. Conversely, measures of different constructs are expected to diverge. For example, if we were to measure Trait A using three methods—a semistructured interview, an informant-report questionnaire, and ambulatory assessment measures—then we would expect all three measurements to correlate robustly with each other. Measures for Trait A would not be expected to correlate highly with parallel measures of Trait B.

The commitment to validating psychological constructs by utilizing multiple methods has become a fundamental cornerstone in psychological assessment. In some circumstances, however, psychologists may overvalue shared variance and the sense of security that comes along with corroborative evidence. Taken literally, high agreement between measures could not succeed as a suitable benchmark because of the complexity of personality itself and the empirical fact that measures of the same trait rarely correlate strongly. Rather, empirical data indicates that correlations among alternative methods of personality assessment are typically modest at best (Klonsky, Oltmanns, & Turkheimer, 2002). Instead of recognizing the importance of nonredundant information, researchers have tended to focus on comparisons regarding the validity of parallel instruments and alternative sources of information. For example, one occasionally contentious debate in the field of personality psychology is whether self or others have a better understanding of the target's traits. Those who have sided with the self have argued that others do not have access to or fully understand the target's experiences, while those who believe peers are more accurate claim that informants have less self-serving biases and observe behavior objectively.

There is a fundamental problem in sizing one method up against the other because both represent an incomplete portrait of personality. Meyer and colleagues (Meyer, Finn, Eyde, & Kay, 2001) offered the following thoughtful summary: "First, at best, any single assessment method provides a partial or incomplete representation of the characteristics it intends to measure. Second, in the world of applied clinical practice, it is not easy to obtain accurate or consensually agreed on information about patients" (p. 145). Researchers have advised that it would be unwise to wager our understanding of a scientific construct on just one, narrow measure due to the limitations of a single assessment (Eid & Diener, 2006; Fiske, 1978). Fortunately, we can expand our knowledge by combining measures, so that the deficits from one approach are accounted for by the other. Therefore, using multiple methods is justified when alternative measurements account for new insight into personality that the first measure was unable to exploit. In other words, the second (and third) measures would incrementally add to the success of determining and understanding personality traits (Klein, 2003; Miller, Pilkonis, & Clifton, 2005).

Recent evidence indicates that alternative measures may not be identical, but likely complement each other and are a useful feature in the detection and understanding of abnormal personality (Clifton, Turkheimer, & Oltmanns, 2004). This approach is ostensibly different from the idea that inconsistencies are shortcomings and should be labeled as error. Instead, the current direction in the field of personality embraces the variance that multiple measures provide, to the extent that it increases validity. From this approach, we will review the evidence that indicates alternate assessment measures provide independently valid information about personality that is strengthened when combined with other measures.

The purpose of this chapter is to present several of the most commonly used assessments in the study of personality. We begin by discussing the strengths and weaknesses of each method, while highlighting evidence that each approach contributes unique and valid information about a target's personality and that not one in particular is superior. We will then discuss factors that influence discrepancies and agreement between measures of personality and the implications of convergent and divergent measures. We hope to make the case that relying too much on either redundant or nonredundant data may lead to biased or inaccurate conclusions about personality, which may have practical implications about diagnosis, prognosis, and treatment planning for mental disorders (Fournier et al., 2008; Shea & Yen, 2005; Widiger & Samuel, 2009). For example, more exhaustive and accurate assessments of personality disorders , which may be achieved using multiple sources, contribute to increased treatment satisfaction and outcome of other mental disorders (Jensen-Doss & Weisz, 2008; Zimmerman, 2003). In the final section of the chapter, we provide case examples to illustrate the importance of combining self and informant data and utilizing both shared and nonshared variance between reports.

Assessment Methods

In this section we will discuss various methods for assessing personality traits. We will focus primarily on self and informant reports, but will also introduce other trait measurements including behavioral observations, structured interviews, and life narratives. Of course, each of these personality measures may be better suited for addressing particular hypotheses, depending on the researcher's or clinician's goal, and we will review these circumstances.

The structure of personality is composed of *traits*, which are clusters of characteristics (e.g., cognitions, affect, behaviors) that reliably differ between individuals across time and situations (Funder, 1991). Descriptions of traits are relatable and relevant to all people in day-to-day life. While there has been considerable debate about how many global dimensions are optimal for describing personality, it is beyond the scope of this chapter to consider the relative merits of alternative models. Instead of discussing assorted organizations of personality, we will refer to several trait scales throughout this chapter, but frequently refer to the most commonly used approach (i.e., the five-factor model).

While proceeding through the chapter, it is important to keep in mind that many of the points we raise about assessing normal-range personality are relevant for abnormal personality as well. Although there is considerable controversy in the field about how to assess and define personality disorders (Pilkonis, Hallquist, Morse, & Stepp, 2011), there seems to be consensus in favor of a dimensional model. Put simply, personality traits are thought to fall on a continuum that ranges from normal to abnormally high or low (O'Connor, 2002; Trull & Durrett, 2005; Widiger & Simonsen, 2005). While we plan to focus on approaches for assessing adaptive personality traits, it is important to acknowledge that extreme variations of general traits are considered maladaptive and many personality assessments attempt to capture the whole range of personality. We intend to mention maladaptive traits, but a more focused assessment of personality disorders is beyond the scope of this chapter.

Self-Reports

When collecting self-report data on personality, the target person makes judgments about his or her own traits and/or behavior. These judgments are traditionally recorded using a rating scale and in response to standardized questions. The target has a clear advantage while making these ratings, having experienced every cognition, emotion, behavior, and interpersonal relationship to which the questions refer. Since the self has a more extensive knowledge of his or her personal history, it is reasonable to think that the self's perspective on his or her own personality would be different from that of others. However, the self is still subject to the same perceptive biases as someone who did not have these first-hand experiences, because judgment about personality is not intuitive. We make inferences about the nature of our own traits based on internal (e.g., thoughts) and external (e.g., behaviors) information we have access to, but conclusions about our own personality are just that, an interpretation (McCrae & Costa, 1999).

Self-reports of personality are capable of predicting various outcome measures, including morbidity, subjective well-being, physical health, spirituality, identity, interpersonal relationships, occupation, volunteerism, and criminality, indicating that part of what is being measured reflects actual trait differences (Bogg & Roberts, 2004; Ozer & Benet-Martínez, 2006; Roberts, Kuncel, Shiner, Caspi, & Goldberg, 2007; Terracciano, Lockenhoff, Zonderman, Ferrucci, & Costa, 2008). Of course, extraneous factors and subjective biases may distort the target's end response. These factors make dependence on a single source of information a major limitation and explain why self-reports have less than ideal validity (Meyer, 2002). The reasons for response biases can be broken down into two varieties: those that are specific to the test setting, and those that transpire in day-to-day life, typically without most of us realizing it. Within the test setting, targets may have a difficult time interpreting or understanding the meaning of the question or the rating scale. Widespread confusion about abstract concepts or technical language (e.g., psychological terms) would understandably produce unreliable or inaccurate answers. A clear solution to this problem is to apply everyday language during questionnaire development; at this point the most common personality assessments fulfill this criterion. However, there is no standard for assigning a quantitative rating to a qualitative judgment. Raters may gauge the magnitude for descriptions on response scales differently. In other words, ratings are subjective, so targets may assign the same value for essentially different presentations. What one person rates as "moderate" or "sometimes," another person may consider "severe" or "frequently" (Fiske, 1978; Hoyt, 2000).

If the target person is able to interpret and understand the questionnaire well enough, some individuals may not be willing to divulge honest information about their personality. The desire to portray oneself in a positive light, commonly referred to as the social desirability bias, is a concern among personality assessors because of the challenge to differentiate between real and tailored responses (Paulhus & John, 1998). The reasons for withholding information from researchers and clinicians vary but may involve shame, preservation of self-esteem, belief systems, boredom, or lack of motivation. Evidence indicates that concerns about social desirability bias are realistic because the desirability and observability of a behavior significantly predicts the reported frequency of that behavior (Gosling, John, Craik, & Robins, 1998). The relationship between social desirability and target-informant agreement may also provide insight into the influence of self-serving bias on assessments, but the evidence is mixed. Some findings suggest no relationship, whereas others indicate a significant curvilinear relationship (Ready & Clark, 2002). In other words, agreement between target and informant reports is weaker for highly desirable and undesirable traits when compared to more neutral traits (John & Robins, 1993).

While some individuals may not be willing to present accurate information, others are sincerely unable to do so. Similar to the social desirability bias, unconscious or self-deceiving biases may also be self-serving (Paulhus & John, 1998), but not necessarily so (Christensen, Stein, & Means-Christensen, 2003; Swann, 1997). Targets with abnormal personality may be especially vulnerable to reporting bias because many of the defining traits are characterized by lack of insight or forthrightness. Some maladaptive traits that may influence the accuracy of self-report include inhibition in new interpersonal situations due to feeling inadequate or suspiciousness, fear of disapproval, deceitfulness, unstable or grandiose self-image, suggestibility, distorted thinking patterns, and exaggerated response style.

Another factor that might influence trait ratings unconsciously is access to and interpretation of memories. Memory accuracy is important because targets are being asked to assess the persistence and pattern of characteristics over time, even though memories are vulnerable to biases. For example, attention management when the event occurred, interpretation of the event while it is occurring, and integration and interpretation of the memory are all factors that may result in memory failure. Evaluations of traits are based on blanket impressions (i.e., semantic memories) that are converted from specific behaviors that occurred (i.e., episodic memories). It appears that memory biases about personality can occur as early as encoding specific behaviors. Gosling and colleagues (1998) measured how reliably targets were able to report the frequency of specific behaviors retrospectively. Their results imply that self-report of behavior is biased before it can be incorporated into semantic memory. In addition to memory biases, Huprich and colleagues (Huprich, Bornstein, & Schmitt, 2011) noted that self-report measures ineffectively discriminate the impact of momentary mood states and priming effects from trait impressions. In fact, when targets rate their personality while depressed, self-informant correlations become weaker (Ball, Rounsaville, Tennen, & Kranzler, 2001), indicating that mood states impact the accuracy of self-reports (Griens, Jonker, Spinhoven, & Blom, 2002).

Due to response biases and distorted self-perceptions, self-report validity is undermined by higher error variance. For this reason, researchers have argued that self-reports on their own are insufficient for assessing personality traits (Ganellen, 2007; Huprich et al., 2011; Klonsky et al., 2002; Miller et al., 2005).

Informant Reports

It should be clear that humans are predisposed to biases and that these biases impact personality assessment. While people tend to downplay their own biases, they are also prone to recognize biased behavior in others (Pronin & Kugler, 2007). In fact, targets tend to ignore their own behavior and rely excessively on their thoughts and motivations, thereby justifying their self-favoring behavior (Pronin, Lin, & Ross, 2002). Although internal thoughts can undoubtedly provide useful information, it is also important to assess behavior without giving too much weight to the rationale. Informants are a useful resource for these circumstances.

Similar to self-reports, informant reports demonstrate good predictive validity (Kolar, Funder, & Colvin, 1996) and considerable incremental validity when added to self-report measures predicting academic achievement, first impressions of strangers, and job performance (Connelly & Ones, 2010). In some cases, when the predictive ability of self- and informant reports is compared, informants are more accurate. For example, spouse ratings of hostility are better able to predict the occurrence of coronary heart disease after accounting for heart disease risk factors and self-reports (Kneip et al., 1993; Smith et al., 2008). Wagerman and Funder (2007) persuasively found that informant ratings of conscientiousness predicted target grade point averages better than did the target's self-ratings. In addition, some evidence indicates that informants are more useful for rating observable or externalizing traits, whereas targets are more attuned to internal experiences (e.g., mood, cognitions) (Fiedler, Oltmanns, & Turkheimer, 2004; Spain, Eaton, & Funder, 2000).

Informants may also be in a better position to evaluate the target's interpersonal relationships. Rodebaugh and colleagues (Rodebaugh, Gianoli, Turkheimer, & Oltmanns, 2011) demonstrated that incorporating an interpersonal source (i.e., informant) with self-reports of personality traits better predicted interpersonal problems than either source independently. In addition, Klein (2003) measured the comparative validity of self- and informant reports of personality disorders in predicting external criteria over 7.5 years. Ratings from both sources predicted elevated depressive symptoms, but only informant reports predicted social adjustment at follow up. The investigator concluded that both sources of information make important contributions in predicting clinical outcomes.

Although predictive validity is essential for evaluating the overall accuracy of informant reports, it is also important to consider whether accurate judgments from one informant predicts judgments from another informant. Analyzing interrater reliability accounts for whether informant reports are less valuable under certain conditions. In general, interjudge agreement is higher than informant–self correlations (John & Robins, 1993), and scores range from 0.32 to 0.43 (Connelly & Ones, 2010). Family members and close friends tend to have the strongest interrater reliability with other informants. However, factors other than informant accuracy may influence high rater consensus, such as estimating a "stereotypical" or average personality while rating the target. Incidental accuracy is especially a concern for less acquainted informants.

Just like all humans, informants suffer from the same biases described in the self-report section (Srivastava, Guglielmo, & Beer, 2010), but there are also informant-specific biases that need to be brought to attention. For example, the length of the relationship between self and informant enhances the accuracy of informant personality rating (Kurtz & Sherker, 2003). This relationship appears to be a result of intimacy and not frequency of contact (Connelly & Ones, 2010; Watson, Hubbard, & Wiese, 2000). Informants have a higher susceptibility to bias when the traits that are being rated are abstract or require a degree of inference (e.g., friendliness). Some traits are easily objectified (e.g., conscientiousness, extraversion; Zillig, Hemenover, & Dienstbier, 2002) and are influenced less by biased perspectives (Fiske, 1978). A study by John and Robins (1993) confirmed this idea, reporting that interjudge agreement was highest for observable and less evaluative traits.

Some findings suggest that self-selected informants provide more positive reports than informants not selected by the target (Leising, Erbs, & Fritz, 2010). In other words, targets tend to pick informants who are familiar to them and like them. A bias that has been called the "letter of recommendation" effect occurs when self-selected informants rate their target positively. When this bias occurs, trait variability is low, and little incremental validity is added to self-report ratings. Incorporating informants that targets do not prefer into assessments may therefore be beneficial.

Another informant-specific bias is the self-based heuristic. This refers to the possibility that informants are projecting some perceptions of their own personality onto the target, especially when traits are perceived to be difficult to rate (Ready, Clark, Watson, & Westerhouse, 2000).

It is important to consider how many informants are to be used for assessing one target's personality. People develop unique relationships depending on their role and time spent with the other person; thus single-informant ratings may be substantially idiosyncratic. For example, it seems likely that a man usually behaves differently around his mother than with his golf buddies. Each of these informants is exposed to different behaviors, expressions, and thought processes. In addition, informants share differences in preference, tolerance, and evaluation of characteristics, especially for maladaptive traits (Ganellen, 2007). Therefore, relying on one informant may weaken the reliability of the measure and self–other correlations. Although some researchers believe that using multiple informants strengthens assessment measures (Achenbach, Krukowski, Dumenci, & Ivanova, 2005; Connelly & Ones, 2010), Kraemer and colleagues (2003) note that if informants show high collinearity, then quantity does not matter as much as using other reports to compensate for measurement deficiencies.

Despite promising findings on informant reports, Paunonen and Neill (2010) have argued that informants cannot replace targets. If the overlap between informant and target ratings was extensive enough that they became redundant, then it would be appropriate to rely only on one report or the other. Instead, both self- and informant reports provide unique and valid information, suggesting the application of both perspectives.

Standardized Interviews

Instead of using empirically supported techniques to assess personality traits, the majority of clinicians across orientations rely on informal interviews and clinical observations (Westen, 1997). When conducting informal clinical interviews, most clinicians (unconsciously) seek confirmatory evidence for their initial impressions and fail to systematically assess alternative explanations (Rogers, 2003). Researchers may even be inclined to assess for their "pet" personality type before anything else. As a result, clinicians are inclined to undervalue inconsistent evidence, even though findings demonstrate that alternative perspectives improve validity (Hunsley & Meyer, 2003). Standardized assessments have the added benefit of being comprehensive, which is a substantial advantage for psychologists considering the breadth of items needed to assess personality. Not surprisingly, agreement between informal interviews and standard evaluations is considered low to moderate (Rettew, Doyle-Lynch, Achenbach, Dumenci, & Ivanova, 2009).

Standardized interviews increase reliability when they are used by trained interviewers, have clear language, and have an established sequence and protocol to rate items (Rogers, 2003). These factors better control for interviewer bias. Semistructured interviews have the added benefit of allowing the interviewer opportunities to incorporate relevant follow-up questions and to use clinical judgment. It is important to note that responses derived from interviews are provided from the target's perspective. Thus, if the interviewer were simply to record the participant's initial response, interviews would be restricted from obtaining unique information that could not already be collected by questionnaires. In other words, a source overlap artifact may distort the relationship between interviews and self-reports. For this reason, raters are allowed some latitude when rating personality traits. Nevertheless, reasonable evidence is necessary to support deviating from the target's response. This may be especially beneficial in clinical subjects where personality disorders are more prevalent and doubt may be cast on the target's credibility. A useful tool for targets that may be unwilling or unable to acknowledge maladaptive traits is using an interview that employs a conversational interview style (e.g., the SIDP-IV).

Testing the incremental validity of interviews while controlling for self-reports is essential considering source overlap (Hunsley & Meyer, 2003). However, the majority of personality interviews exclusively measure maladaptive traits; thus the number of studies that demonstrate validity for normal personality interviews is limited. One measure, the Structured Interview for Five-Factor Model (SIFFM), was developed to measure normal and pathological traits. Stepp, Trull, Burr, Wolfenstein, and Vieth (2005) used the SIFFM to illustrate that normal personality was related to a relevant outcome measure after controlling for self-report trait scores. Interviews meant to assess personality disorders have also demonstrated incremental validity when controlling for self-reports (Galione & Oltmanns, 2013). Thus, interviews provide an alternative method for assessing personality and help us provide a more comprehensive description of traits by providing unique diagnostic information.

Behavioral Observations

In an effort to minimize the influence of bias associated with self-report and interview methods, investigators may also use "objective criteria" or behavioral observations as outcome measures. Even though objective ratings of behavior are sometimes called the gold standard of personality traits, it is rarely considered a personality measure on its own because it disregards emotions and cognitions. Because of the reduced subjective influence on ratings (i.e., in comparison to interviews, self, and informant reports), this method can reasonably be expected to account for trait variance that is not recovered by more common instruments. However, observations still require an observer, so human or technology error is not obsolete. In this chapter we describe several studies that illustrate the growing research on the relationship between personality traits and behavioral observations.

Vazire and Mehl (2008) used portable electronic devices to assess in the moment daily activities. After collecting self- and informant reports on how much the target engages in specific behaviors compared to the average person, results showed that both informants and targets predicted actual behavior. Each source provided unique and overlapping information. This suggests regularity in behaviors and traits that others observe and predict. In a related study, Funder and Sneed (1993) videotaped social interactions and had strangers use the Q sort to rank behaviors they had observed. Results revealed that strangers rated relevant behaviors highest and that these behaviors validly described three domains of the target's personality: extraversion, agreeableness, and conscientiousness.

Upon meeting someone new, individuals rely on quick, self-presentation cues and observations; thus strangers are beneficial to research as impartial assessors. For example, strangers show significant agreement with self-reports on extraversion, conscientiousness, and intelligence, signifying the importance of initial impressions (Borkenau & Liebler, 1993). In addition, perceived firm handshakes are positively correlated with high scores on extraversion (and openness in women) and low scores on neuroticism and shyness (Chaplin, Phillips, Brown, Clanton, & Stein, 2000). In one study strangers observed bedrooms and offices and then rated the target's personality. Even though the observers never met the targets, they achieved high accuracy when rating openness, but lowest correlations when rating agreeableness. Except for emotional stability, observing personal environments yielded more accurate ratings than long-term acquaintance relationships (Gosling, Ko, Mannarelli, & Morris, 2002).

Although there appears to be a relationship between behavioral observations and personality surveys, they do not overlap completely. Correlations tend to be moderate with both self- and informant reports (mean $r \approx .26$). We conclude that measuring specific behaviors can tell us things about personality that we would not necessarily know through generalized descriptions of traits.

Life Narratives

Life narratives (McAdams, 1993) are extended interviews in which targets are prompted to describe significant life events, analogous to a CliffsNotes version of their biography. Autobiographical recollections and life stories are collected to gain a better understanding of the target's evolving personality and identity. The narrator has freedom to carve out the trajectory of their development, and the examiner does little to interfere with recording the qualitative data. Researchers typically use videos or transcripts to analyze thematic content in the target's life stories, such as communion, resilience, and agency. Information elicited from the life narrative is considered related but distinct from the Big Five and other lower-level traits (McAdams, 1995; McAdams & Pals, 2006). Features from the life narrative, including information on the person's high points, low points, and transitional stages in life, are related to several trait-relevant outcome measures, including physical health, life satisfaction, and depression (McAdams, Reynolds, Lewis, Patten, & Bowman, 2001).

Empirical evidence collected by Wilt, Cox, and McAdams (2010), demonstrated that the life narrative predicted psychosocial adaptation above and beyond demographic characteristics (e.g., age, gender, income) and the Big Five self-reported traits. For example, healthy interpersonal relationships and themes of generativity during adulthood (i.e., care for one's family, contributions to society) predicted social connectedness. By adding unique variance to the personality profile, the life narrative should be considered a valuable assessment.

Implicit Measures

Huprich and colleagues (2011) argue that personality traits are more than what we are consciously aware of or remember. Implicit processes occur without our conscious knowledge and include various cognitive pathways that implement behaviors and emotions automatically. There is now a body of cognitive driven research that says people do make inferences about their environment without having conscious awareness. Research using amnesic patients reveals a distinction between conscious and unconscious influences on memory. For example, amnesiacs score poorly when explicitly asked to recall words from a list, but they achieve near-normal results using indirect methods (Schacter, 1987). Similar to memory tests, implicit measures of traits attempt to recognize portions of personality that the target or informant may not be aware of such as motives, self-perceptions, and emotional regulation. Performance-based tests offer access to information about personality that direct questioning is unable to access, and may explain commonly known discrepancies between self-reports and physiological measures (Shedler, Mayman, & Manis, 1993).

Implicit traits not only have practical implications for the validity of traditional assessments, but also impact how we define personality. For example, priming informants with a list of personality traits unconsciously increases the chances of informants rating targets with those characteristics (Moskowitz & Roman, 1992), challenging the validity of these scales. Accordingly, implicit measures should be less susceptible to unconscious or intentional biases. Evidence supports a distinction between implicit and explicit motives and suggests that the two types of measures account for different aspects of personality. In an influential article, McClelland, Koestner, and Weinberger (1989) suggested that implicit motives are mostly responsible for a person's automatic, unconscious behavior and are largely influenced by natural incentives, whereas explicit motives are deliberate and influenced by social incentives. Their analysis indicated that implicit measures do in fact predict spontaneous achievement and that explicit measures are a better predictor of attention-focused achievement. Another example of the implicit–explicit distinction comes from a review of the literature on 86 projective and explicit tests measuring dependency. Using implicit measures predicted dependent behavior equally well as explicit measures, but the scales diverged, showing only modest intercorrelations (Bornstein, 2002). Thus, even though implicit and explicit measures are intended to measure the same construct (i.e., personality traits), they tap into different facets and thereby should be aggregated.

Integration of Methods

Convergence

Convergence between methods measuring the same personality trait is considered vital. If measures do not converge, then we may begin to question whether they are measuring the same construct. Hofstee (1994) even defines personality in terms of multimethod agreement and makes a plea for increased use of informant reports in order to ultimately aggregate data across informants.

Review articles on multimethod assessments conclude that agreement between independent measures designed to tap the same trait is typically low to moderate across sources (Blackman & Funder, 1998; Klonsky et al., 2002; McCrae, 1982; Paulhus & Bruce, 1992; Watson & Clark, 1991; Watson et al., 2000; Zimmerman, Pfohl, Coryell, Stangl, & Corenthal, 1988). Correlations between target and informant reports on the Big Five traits typically range from .30 to .50 (McCrae, 1994; Ready & Clark, 2002). The five trait domains display moderate agreement when comparing self and romantic partners: Neuroticism (mean $r = .46$), Extraversion (mean $r = .52$), Conscientiousness (mean $r = .47$), Agreeableness (mean $r = .42$), and Openness to Experience (mean $r = .53$; Watson, Hubbard, & Wiese, 2000). Levels of agreement are maintained across settings, including college, community, and psychiatric samples (John & Robins, 1993; Ready & Clark, 2002; Watson et al., 2000). Meyer et al. (2001) noted that agreement between methods is weak, and so they strongly recommended combining measures in order to improve predictive validity and reliability. Response biases, method variance, and distorted perceptions about the self and others likely explain why agreement between measures is not more substantial.

Divergence

In this chapter, we refer to divergence when two measures that are meant to measure the same construct do not overlap. In this case, if we used a Venn diagram to represent two methods of trait assessment, the convergence of methods would be represented by the intersection of the overlapping circles, while the divergence would be represented by the portions of the circles along the outer edges that are unique to each shape. From this perspective, the amount of shared and nonshared information between measures is inversely related. Since reviews on the convergence of trait measures typically conclude that shared variance is moderately good, it would make sense to conclude that each measure also contributes a considerable amount of unique information. The question then is, what should we do with these data? Hunsley and Meyer (2003) believe that using multiple methods and the ensuing nonconvergent data improves assessment accuracy and future clinical recommendations. In fact, its application in clinical settings would only be justified if it added to the prediction of clinically relevant criteria (e.g., daily functioning) over and above data obtained by one measure. Accordingly, we have attempted to highlight the incremental validity of each measurement we reviewed above as a rationale for using multiple assessments. In addition, when predicting a structured interview diagnosis of personality disorders, normal personality measurements explained up to an additional 8% of the variance when predicting, after controlling for maladaptive trait scores (Quirk, Christiansen, Wagner, & McNulty, 2003). Furthermore, Lawton, Shields, and Oltmanns (2011) examined the incremental validity of NEO-PI-R prototype informant scores and cluster B prototypes, and they demonstrated significant predictive validity after controlling for variance accounted for by self-reports.

Measurement divergence has further clinical implications because self-reports from individuals with psychopathology are often unreliable and correlate poorly with clinicians, informants, and objective reports (Meyer et al., 2001). One study demonstrated this by having clinicians assess for and diagnose personality disorders based on information provided by patients. After obtaining informant data, the initial diagnosis was changed 20% of the time, usually because the informant provided pathological information not reported by the patient (Zimmerman, Pfohl, Stangle, & Corenthal, 1986). Not surprisingly, nonredundant information is typically related to the presence of maladaptive personality traits. For example, self-informant discrepancies are predominantly related to facets of neuroticism (e.g., shy, hostile, and depressed; Mosterman & Hendriks, 2011).

If both shared and nonshared information is valid, then it is up to the clinician to interpret what differences between measures might mean. McCrae (1994) suggested an underutilized formula for determining whether different sources agree or disagree. If sources are clearly in agreement, it may be best to average scores. If ratings are inconsistent, however, then average scores would not be representative. Instead, gathering additional information or referring to the life narrative may allow the investigator to draw conclusions about the discrepancies. Even though target and informant ratings are not completely redundant, alternative perspectives tend to be harmonious. It does not appear that self- and informant reports are incompatible, even though they describe the target's personality profile differently. In a study by Clifton et al. (2004), informants and targets filled out questionnaires about the target's maladaptive personality. When the informant's ratings indicated the presence of a personality disorder, targets were more likely to report traits that complemented the informant's profile description. The same was true when self-reports indicated a diagnosis and informant trait descriptions were analyzed. For example, when informant reports diagnosed the target with obsessive–compulsive personality disorder, the targets were more likely to claim, "Other people sometimes have trouble keeping up with the pace I set." The authors concluded that informants provide relevant incremental information and that differences between informant and target reports are systematic. Further examples of this phenomenon are provided in the case studies.

Case Examples

Distinct methods of measuring traits share a certain amount of variance with each other, but tests of incremental validity show that they also account for unique information. Shared and unique information among methods provide valuable information about personality for predicting relevant outcome data. A theoretical model incorporating both types of variance into assessments and systematic care has yet to be established, leaving practical concerns about the diagnosis and treatment of personality disorders unanswered. Case studies may be beneficial for researchers and clinicians, enabling them to better recognize how to conceptualize personality from a multimethod perspective and to illustrate many of the concepts from this chapter. Below we present two case studies from the St. Louis Personality and Aging Network (SPAN; Oltmanns & Gleason, 2011) study in an attempt to highlight the complexity and importance of using multiple instruments for assessment purposes. The cases differ regarding the extent to which self- and peer reports agree, forcing us to consider how to systematically handle various response patterns between sources (e.g., conflicting and/or converging evidence). By anticipating multimethod trait patterns in advance, using empirically derived data, we may be able to avoid reliability problems resulting from using similar information in decidedly different ways.

The people described in these cases were participants in a longitudinal community study. The SPAN study was designed to evaluate personality using both self- and informant reports from a representative sample of adults between the ages of 55 and 64 living in a Midwestern metropolitan area. We will report information collected during the baseline phase of the study. All subjects completed a 3-hour assessment battery that included a brief life narrative interview (adapted from McAdams, 1993), the Structured Interview for DSM-IV Personality (SIDP-IV; Pfohl, Blum, & Zimmerman, 1997), the Multisource Assessment of Personality Pathology (MAPP;

Oltmanns & Turkheimer, 2006), and the NEO Personality Inventory—Revised (NEO PI-R; Costa & McCrae, 1992), among other assessments of clinical disorders and health status. As part of the study, subjects were asked to identify an informant who knew them well. With permission from the subjects, we collected MAPP and NEO PI-R informant reports regarding the target person's personality. Our objective for the case studies is to compare personality and personality disorder scores between the interviewer, self, and informant reports to demonstrate how clinicians may use multiple methods to refine their conceptualization of the individual for diagnostic and treatment purposes. We have altered the participants' names and minor details of their narrative to protect their identity.

Case 1: Convergent Reports, Avoidant Prsonality Disorder

Adam is a Caucasian, 58-year-old, never-married male living alone. He is the youngest of three children, but despite having two older siblings, he reported growing up "alone" with his "extremely depressed and volatile" mother. Both of his parents died by the time he was 28 years old, and at one point in the interview he noted that a portion of his life was "dominated by people dying." Adam enrolled in college to evade the Vietnam draft and was admitted to graduate school "in another attempt to avoid serious employment" but did not complete his degree. He described "drifting" through his career in an attempt to "avoid actual jobs." For over 20 years he has been successfully self-employed as a remodeling contractor, and he acknowledged that expanding his business was a viable option, but he preferred less responsibility. In general, Adam works independently and will avoid jobs that involve coordination with peers, such as building inspectors. He admitted that he prefers to spend most of his time alone, both at work and recreationally.

Similar to his early career path, Adam retained his bachelor status throughout most of his life, in pursuit of avoiding any serious commitment. He reported two significant relationships in his life, but mostly his interactions were "sexually based . . . comfortable but not fulfilling." Most recently, Adam was involved with a woman he "truly loved," but he admitted it took "a few years" before he considered the relationship intimate and the commitment didn't last. Two years prior to his assessment, the woman died suddenly, soon followed by the death of his brother-in-law and sister. Regarding the loss of one of the few relationships he had invested in, he stated, "That won't happen again, not like that," suggesting that he does not plan on venturing into future relationships that make him feel vulnerable.

The results of Adam's SIDP-IV interview indicated that he satisfied DSM-IV criteria for avoidant and obsessive–compulsive personality disorders (American Psychiatric Association, 2013, pp. 672, 678). He reported the presence of several maladaptive traits that have interfered with his interpersonal relationships and qualified for at least subthreshold ratings on all seven avoidant personality criteria. The interviewer rated Adam positively on the following obsessive–compulsive personality disorder criteria: preoccupation with organization to the extent that the major point of the activity is lost; perfectionism that interferes with task completion; inability to discard worthless objects with no sentimental value; and a miserly spending style. He also qualified for subthreshold scores on borderline, dependent, and paranoid disorders that appeared to reflect his low self-confidence. For example, he described feelings of emptiness and difficulty disagreeing with others for fear of losing approval.

Quotations from his clinical interview revealed additional insight into his personality, relationships and rationality. Adam described himself as being "too introspected and analytical," and he expressed a longing for a "better sense of self-confidence." Related to intimate relationships, Adam stated, "I've always relied on the woman's desire for me to make itself very clear, so I was pretty much guaranteed to be accepted. I work off of cues. I hate rejection, so why risk rejection if you don't have to?" Unless he acquires "solid evidence that [his] affections are invited," he does not reveal his true feelings in order to prevent others from judging him harshly or from inadvertently insulting the other person. While Adam acknowledged that he can appear to be engaging and self-confident—traits that were evident throughout the interview process—he admitted to having "tremendous anxiety" about going to social functions and can be "painfully shy because there are so many times when [he's] not around people." He believes his true desire is to "just fit in," and he makes a conscious effort "not to draw attention" to himself.

For ease of interpretation, we converted NEO-PI-R domain and facet scores to z-scores based on the SPAN sample ($N = 1,630$) norms. Compared to the sample means, Adam's overall domain scores for extraversion ($z = 1.91$), agreeableness ($z = 2.22$), and conscientiousness ($z = 1.70$) were significantly low, and neuroticism ($z = 2.98$) was markedly elevated. Specific facets that were considered abnormal included anxiety (N1), depression (N3), self-consciousness (N4), vulnerability (N6), warmth (E1), positive emotion (E6), trust (A1), straightforwardness (A2), dutifulness (C3), and achievement seeking (C4) (valence was in the same direction for facets as domains). Consistent with his SIDP-IV profile, his composite scores on the self-rated MAPP for avoidant ($z = 3.22$), obsessive–compulsive ($z = 1.70$), and borderline ($z = 2.00$) personality disorders were significantly elevated.

Adam personally selected his informant, a friend whom he has known for over 40 years. Information from the informant generally converged with ratings from the self-report questionnaires and interview. Similar to the self-rated NEO-PI-R, his informant's ratings for the agreeableness ($z = 1.61$, $p < .06$) and extraversion ($z = 1.97$) domains were considered significantly low compared to the informant sample means. Scores on the informant's MAPP were elevated on items featuring avoidant, obsessive–compulsive, borderline, and schizotypal traits. His informant rated 35 (out of 106) maladaptive traits occurring at least 50% of the time, while Adam rated 29 items similarly, with a 33% overlap between the actual items. Figure 1.1 illustrates the comparison between Adam's self- and informant reports on the NEO-PI-R.

Case 2: Divergent Reports, Narcissistic Personality Disorder

Nancy is a 59-year-old, never-married, Caucasian female. She is the eldest of four children, and during her childhood she was the self-proclaimed favorite of her extended family. Both of her parents died four years prior to the interview, but she remains especially close to one of her sisters, who served as her informant for the study. Nancy received an "excellent" education from an all-girls Catholic high school; she considered these years the high point of her life, mostly due to what she described as a thriving social life. She did not flourish academically, but she managed to complete some education at a technical school. After feeling constrained by the margins of her salary, she furthered her education, earning herself an Associate's degree in nursing and started working an "elite" job in intensive care. Nancy held a series of nursing positions throughout her life and saw herself as "extremely adept" in each setting, and, according to her, thrives in management positions. She considers her financial independence as something of a triumph, referencing her "excellent" income several times, while her paperwork reflected a more modest account of her status. She has taken it upon herself to mentor the "aimless," younger generation by recommending the same path into nursing that she took.

As an adolescent, Nancy had a rich social network and established a role as a "mover and a shaker," a "pivotal figure" in her theater group, and editor of the yearbook. When reflecting on her time in high school, she stated, "I was a star." While the depth of her relationships was unclear, she was seemingly proficient in establishing connections, possessing "whole colonies" of friends throughout much of her young adulthood. During her 20s, Nancy dated a high school classmate, following a chance encounter while he was being treated on the same ward where Nancy worked. Two years into their "drama-filled" relationship, her boyfriend committed suicide. Emotionally scarred by the event, she has not pursued a romantic relationship since. Instead, she became involved with circles of gay men and found herself occupied by an intense, yet transitory, friendship involving a pattern of drug abuse. Nancy has failed to maintain her social network in later life and attributes this failure to the lack of interesting people living in the suburbs. She now defines her success through her career as opposed to her social life.

Nancy's responses during the administration of the SIDP-IV satisfied DSM-IV requirements for narcissistic personality disorder (American Psychiatric Association, 2013, p. 669). The interviewer rated her positively on

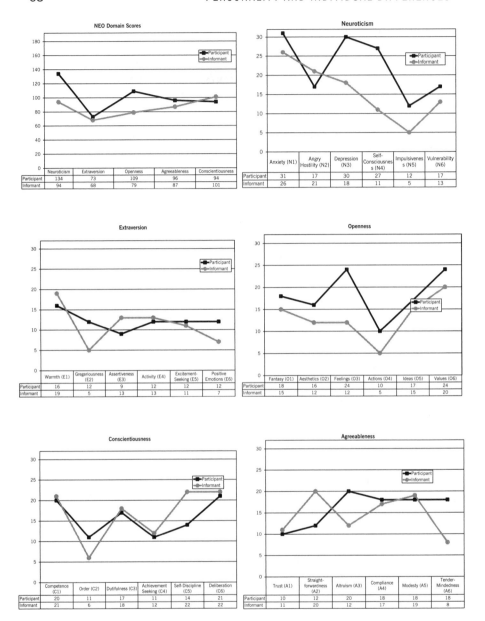

FIGURE 1.1. Case 1 self- and informant personality profile on the NEO-PI-R.

the following criteria: grandiose sense of self-importance, sense of entitlement, belief that others are envious of her, arrogant behaviors or attitude, and belief that she is special and can only be understood by other special or high-status people. And she was rated subthreshold on two items: requires excessive admiration and interpersonal exploitation. Nancy met the criteria for some other notable Cluster B traits, including unstable relationships involving "intense arguments and dramatic reunions," and a strong desire to be the center of attention and "gravitate to the stage."

To gain a deeper understanding of the interviewer's position, we decided to highlight some of her responses that were representative of her presentation. When asked, "Are you pretty good at getting people to do what you want?" she replied, "My relative tells me to 'stop barking orders,' to which I reply, 'If people would just follow my orders we wouldn't have any problems.' I can be pretty persuasive and I can bring people around to do things my way. I spearheaded my high school reunion even though there were 8 or 10 of us, and we were going to delegate certain things. I ended up having my finger in everything. . . . In my midcareer I did not hesitate to go over someone's head for what I thought was incompetence." Despite her apparent dominance over others, she stated, "I develop pretty good interpersonal relationships." When describing her success she described her "flawless" achievements and commented, "I tend to rise to the top, or at least the top 2 or 3." When asked if she is envious when others have more money than she does, she responded, "No, because most of them don't."

Nancy reported strikingly little personality pathology on the MAPP, compared to her SIDP-IV scores, and did not introduce any remarkable or new information. The self-rated personality disorder scores and total number of personality disorder criteria met did not differ from the sample means. Using the rest of the SPAN sample as a basis for comparison, her NEO-PI-R profile resembled normal functioning. Even though her self-rated conscientious score of 143 did not differ from the mean (M = 123.44, SD = 17.35), it was noticeably elevated. Noteworthy is her competence and order facet scores that are nearly 2-3 SD above their respective means. A selection of some of the items that embody her pattern of responses include: "I'm pretty set in my ways," "I feel capable of coping with most of my problems," "I keep myself informed and usually make intelligent decisions," "I am a very competent person," and "I tend to be somewhat fastidious or exacting."

In contrast to the target's self-ratings, many parallels can be drawn between Nancy's informant and the interviewer's ratings. The informant's total rating score on the MAPP displayed significant maladaptive functioning, primarily driven by the narcissistic, histrionic, paranoid, and schizoid composites. Four of the five narcissistic criteria that the informant rated positively were items that she also met on the SIDP-IV. In fact, the informant rated 33 maladaptive personality traits as being present at least 50%

of the time, while Nancy only endorsed twelve items on the self-report, with 25% overlap. The informant's narcissistic ($z = 2.72$), and schizoid ($z = 2.97$) scores were significantly elevated compared to the mean informant ratings. On the NEO-PI-R, her informant's ratings reflected substandard scores on the agreeableness and extraversion domains. More specifically, the facets her informant rated as significantly elevated included angry hostility (N2) and vulnerability (N6), while her lowest scoring facets included all of the agreeableness features (trust, straightforwardness, altruism, compliance, modesty, and tender-mindedness), warmth (E1), gregariousness (E2), positive emotions (E6), actions (O4), and dutifulness (C3). Her informant responded "strongly agree" to 15 of the 240 NEO items, including "She is dominant, forceful, and assertive," "Some people think she is selfish and egotistical," "At times she bullies or flatters people into doing what she wants them to," and "She has a very high opinion of herself." Figure 1.2 illustrates the comparison between Nancy's self- and informant reports on the NEO-PI-R.

Case Study Conclusions

The preceding case formulations provide a detailed description of two distinct personality profiles and illustrate the application of a multimethod approach to personality assessment. Findings were derived from assessment instruments completed by interviewers, the target, and informants. Although we understand that our interpretations of these cases are anecdotal and may not be entirely generalizable to other data, our hope is to highlight trends that may bridge the gap between clinical and empirical multimethod approaches to integrative personality assessments.

Consistent with other reports on avoidant personality disorder, Case 1 demonstrated strong convergence between measures (Lawton, Shields, & Oltmanns, 2011). Self- and informant ratings on the MAPP supported evidence gathered from the SIDP-IV. Adam qualified for a diagnosis of avoidant and obsessive–compulsive personality disorders and the presence of borderline traits on all three measures. In addition, informant and target ratings of normal personality traits were indicative of an abnormal presentation, considering the number of facets that significantly differed from the mean. However, this does not imply that personality assessments were identical and that researchers and clinicians should only rely on one source. Clinicians may use alternative sources to supplement evidence on the presence of personality pathology, but another advantage is that informants provide new insight into how to conceptualize the disorder. For example, both the self and informant may report that the target is avoidant, but one may interpret these qualities as cold and distant while the other may perceive their behavior as odd. Rodebaugh and colleagues (Rodebaugh, Gianoli, Turkheimer, & Oltmanns, 2011) reported findings on maladaptive traits

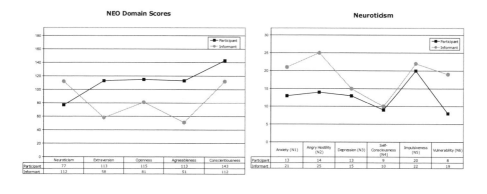

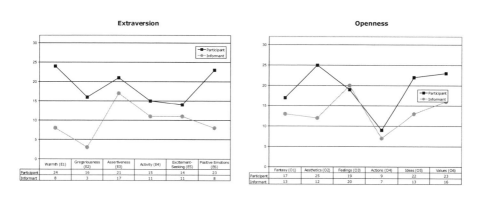

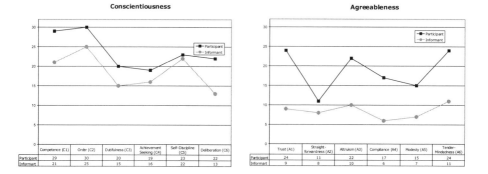

FIGURE 1.2. Case 2 self- and informant personality profile on the NEO-PI-R.

that would have been misleading if the analyses relied solely on informant or self-reports. To avoid spurious findings driven by rater error, the authors concluded that the shared-variance method produced optimal results by controlling for over- or underestimation of attributes. In the example of avoidant personality disorder, targets may be more likely to overestimate assertiveness, while informants tend to underestimate positive attributes such as warmth (Rodebaugh et al., 2011).

In Adam's case, information obtained from each source was complementary, but agreement was not uniform across items. Both Adam and his informant rated the target's extraversion and agreeableness as significantly low, but upon further inspection of the facets, their ratings differed as to how these personality traits manifested themselves. Specifically, the target endorsed low trust and straightforwardness, while his informant described his disagreeableness with low altruism, tender-mindedness, and trust. Because of the reasons described earlier in the chapter, it is impossible to determine whether either perception is accurate without further exploration from the clinician or researcher. One possible reason for the discrepancy is that self-informant ratings generally have stronger correlations when the traits involve observable behaviors (Naumann, Vazire, Rentfrow, & Gosling, 2009; Ready & Clark, 2002) and weaker agreement when internal states are assessed, such as emotions and thoughts. For example, Adam's neuroticism might be internally distressing, but it doesn't appear to be so on the surface. Ironically, the informant appears to be interpreting Adam's neuroticism as lack of emotion in light of the informant's abnormally low ratings on the openness to feelings ($z = 1.85$) and positive emotions ($z = 2.10$) facets. This demonstrates that informant reports may not accurately reflect reality but could be just as clinically valuable for setting treatment goals and planning. While this interpretation may explain the diverging neuroticism scores, it also raises other questions about personality assessment, such as whether we should weight informant or self-reports differently depending on internal processes versus external behaviors.

Due to the notoriously external nature of Cluster B personality traits, it came as no surprise that most of the dysfunction that emerged in Case 2, Nancy, was evidence gathered from informant reports and interview. Miller et al. (2005), for instance, reported that others perceive narcissistic individuals as socially aversive, but targets rate themselves as extraverted and interpersonally engaging. Nancy's informant report, including high neuroticism and low agreeableness/extraversion scores, is consistent with the narcissistic prototype informants reported in their study and others (Balsis, Eaton, Cooper, & Oltmanns, 2011; Lynam & Widiger, 2001; Miller et al., 2005). The supposed reason for the low agreement between self- and informant reports is that narcissistic individuals lack insight into their relationships. However, Carlson, Vazire, and Oltmanns (2011) did not find this to be the case. In fact, narcissists are aware of their negative impression on others and are capable of reporting this when asked directly, but their accurate metaperceptions do not interfere with their inflated self-evaluation, ultimately protecting the ego. Insight into others' perceptions was demonstrated several times by Nancy. For instance, when she reported negative characteristics, she started her sentences by stating, "My sister would say. . . ." Another possible explanation for Nancy's temperate ratings is that she is no longer cognizant or aware of her elitist impressions because it occurs so frequently (in comparison to rare events being vulnerable to overreporting).

As opposed to scoring herself low on modesty as her informant did (e.g., "She thinks she is a superior person"), Nancy perceives herself as highly competent and methodical ("I seem to be completely successful at everything"). Drawing on information from her interview and self-report, it appears that she has an incessant need to succeed. Measuring success is a common feature of narcissistic personality disorder, especially when competence is assessed relative to others (Morf, Weir, & Davidov, 2000). Nancy's desire to be extremely competent inevitably leads to exclusion and the inferiority of others. Farwell and Wohlwend-Lloyd (1998) reported that narcissists may overestimate their competence, but not with the direct intention of belittling others. Paulhus and John (1998) reports that the effects of egoistic bias and narcissism may be presented as exaggeration on ability dimensions and seek to stand out through achievements. Nancy's seemingly honest intentions are reflected in the following responses from her SIDP and NEO: "I'm not above blowing my own horn or pouring out my own successes but I don't think at the expense of anyone else," "I would rather praise others than be praised myself," and "I believe all human beings are worthy of respect." This case demonstrates that if researchers relied on self-reports alone, we would have an incomplete or inaccurate understanding of the individual. This is not surprising considering previous research from our lab (Lawton et al., 2011).

While analyzing individual cases is a powerful illustration of the importance of multiple sources, it also draws attention to the idiosyncratic complexities that interfere with the construction of a complete multimethod personality assessment framework. The process of personality assessment needs to be revised to include other forms of evaluation that do not depend on direct response from the target. In addition, discrepancies between self-reported and alternative instruments should not be automatically considered invalid, but considering their connection to PDs, they should be examined more closely. This is not only apparent in light of the above case examples, but is consistent with evidence presented by multiple reports stating that informants report significantly greater amounts of pathology for narcissistic personality disorder compared to targets and significantly underestimate for avoidant personality disorder (Miller et al., 2005; Clifton et al., 2004).

Closing Remarks

Despite a series of recent findings supporting multimethod assessments of personality pathology, assessment procedures in clinical settings still resemble those practiced thirty years ago (Watkins, Campbell, Nieberding, & Hallmark, 1995). In fact, a survey of clinician–researchers considered empirical research less influential and meaningful in their clinical practice compared to interactions with their clients (Safran, Abreu, Ogilvie, & DeMaria, 2011). Although it may be impossible to measure personality exhaustively, we may be able to optimize our ability to predict behavior by using reliable and valid measurements. We have introduced several personality assessment methods that demonstrate valid and unique sources of data. Further research should investigate the development of an empirical model that integrates multiple methods to maximize trait validity even further. Ideally, researchers and clinicians will be able to interpret redundant and nonredundant information from multiple personality assessments in a standardized and practical fashion. We are aware of the challenges this presents because of individual differences and the overwhelming number of covariates related to measuring behavior. Until that day, psychologists should strive to incorporate multiple sources into research and clinics to maximize the accuracy of personality assessments.

REFERENCES

Achenbach, T. M., Krukowski, R. A., Dumenci, L., & Ivanova, M. Y. (2005). Assessment of adult psychopathology: Meta-analysis and implications of cross-informant correlations. *Psychological Bulletin, 131,* 361–382.

American Psychiatric Association. (2013). *Diagnostic and statistical manual of mental disorders* (5th ed.). Arlington, VA: Author.

Ball, S. A., Rounsaville, B. J., Tennen, H., & Kranzler, H. R. (2001). Reliability of personality disorder symptoms and personality traits in substance-dependent inpatients. *Journal of Abnormal Psychology, 110,* 341–352.

Balsis, S., Eaton, N. R., Cooper, L. D., & Oltmanns, T. F. (2011). The presentation of narcissistic personality disorder in an octogenarian: Converging evidence from multiple sources. *Clinical Gerontologist, 34,* 71–87.

Blackman, M. C., & Funder, D. C. (1998). The effect of information on consensus and accuracy in personality judgment. *Journal of Experimental Social Psychology, 34,* 164–181.

Bogg, T., & Roberts, B. W. (2004). Conscientiousness and health-related behaviors: A meta-analysis of the leading behavioral contributors to mortality. *Psychological Bulletin, 130,* 887–919.

Borkenau, P., & Liebler, A. (1993). Convergence of stranger ratings of personality and intelligence with self-ratings, partner ratings, and measured intelligence. *Journal of Personality and Social Psychology, 65*(3), 546–553.

Bornstein, R. (2002). A process dissociation approach to objective-projective test score interrelationships. *Journal of Personality Assessment, 78*(1), 47–68.

Campbell, D. T., & Fiske, D. W. (1959). Convergent and discriminant validation by the multitrait-multimethod matrix. *Pschological Bulletin, 56,* 81–105.

Carlson, E. N., Vazire, S., & Oltmanns, T. F. (2011). You probably think this paper's about you: Narcissists' perceptions of their personality and reputation. *Journal of Personality and Social Psychology, 101*(1), 185–201.

Chaplin, W. F., Phillips, J. B., Brown, J. D., Clanton, N. R., & Stein, J. L. (2000). Handshaking, gender, personality, and first impressions. *Journal of Personality and Social Psychology, 79*(1), 110–117.

Christensen, P. N., Stein, M. B., & Means-Christensen, A. (2003). Social anxiety and interpersonal perception: A social relations model analysis. *Behaviour Research and Therapy, 41,* 1355–1371.

Clifton, A., Turkheimer, E., & Oltmanns, T. F. (2004). Contrasting perspectives on personality problems: Descriptions from the self and others. *Personality and Individual Differences, 36*(7), 1499–1514.

Connelly, B. S., & Ones, D. S. (2010). An other perspective on personality: Meta-analytic integration of observers' accuracy and predictive validity. *Psychological Bulletin, 136,* 1092–1122.

Costa, P. T., Jr., & McCrae, R. R. (Eds.) (1992). *Revised NEO Personality Inventory (NEO PI-R) and NEO Five Factor Inventory (NEO-FFI) professional manual.* Odessa, FL: Psychological Assessment Resources.

Eid, M., & Diener, E. (Eds.). (2006). *Handbook of multimethod measurement in psychology.* Washington, DC: American Psychological Association.

Farwell, L., & Wohlwend-Lloyd, R. (1998). Narcissistic processes: Optimistic expectations, favorable self-evaluations, and self-enhancing attributions. *Journal of Personality, 66,* 65–83.

Fiedler, E. R., Oltmanns, T. F., & Turkheimer, E. (2004). Traits associated with personality disorders and adjustment to military life: Predictive validity of self and peer reports. *Military Medicine, 169*(3), 207–211.

Fiske, D. W. (1978). *Strategies for personality research: The observation versus interpretation of behavior.* San Francisco, CA: Jossey-Bass.

Fournier, J. C., DeRubeis, R. J., Shelton, R. C., Gallop, R., Amsterdam, J. D., & Hollon, S. D. (2008). Antidepressant medications v. cognitive therapy in people with depression with or without personality disorder. *British Journal of Psychiatry: The Journal of Mental Science, 192*(2), 124–129.

Funder, D. C. (1991). Global traits: A Neo-Allportian approach to personality. *Psychological Science, 2,* 31–39.

Funder, D. C., & Sneed, C. D. (1993). Behavioral manifestations of personality: An ecological approach to judgmental accuracy. *Journal of Personality and Social Psychology, 64,* 479–490.

Galione, J. N., & Oltmanns, T. F. (2013). Identifying personality pathology associated with major depressive episodes: Incremental validity of informant reports. *Journal of Personality Assessment, 95,* 625–632.

Ganellen, R. (2007). Assessing normal and abnormal personality functioning: Strengths and weaknesses of self-report, observer, and performance-based methods. *Journal of Personality Assessment, 89*(1), 30–40.

Gosling, S. D., John, O. P., Craik, K. H., & Robins, R. W. (1998). Do people know how they behave? Self-reported act frequencies compared with on-line codings by observers. *Journal of Personality and Social Psychology, 74,* 1337–1349.

Gosling, S. D., Ko, S. J., Mannarelli, T., & Morris, M. E. (2002). A room with a cue: Personality judgments based on offices and bedrooms. *Journal of Personality and Social Psychology, 82*(3), 379–398.

Griens, A. M. G. F., Jonker, K., Spinhoven, P., & Blom, M. B. J. (2002). The influence of depressive state features on trait measurement. *Journal of Affective Disorders, 70*, 95–99.

Hofstee, W. (1994). Who should own the definition of personality? *European Journal of Personality, 8*, 149–162.

Hoyt, W. T. (2000). Rater bias in psychological research: When is it a problem and what can we do about it? *Psychological Methods, 5*(1), 64–86.

Hunsley, J., & Bailey, J. M. (2001). Whither the Rorschach?: An analysis of the evidence. *Psychological Assessment, 13*, 472–485.

Hunsley, J., & Meyer, G. J. (2003). The incremental validity of psychological testing and assessment: Conceptual, methodological, and statistical issues. *Psychological Assessment, 15*(4), 446–455.

Huprich, S. K., Bornstein, R. F., & Schmitt, T. A. (2011). Self-report methodology is insufficient for improving the assessment and classification of Axis II personality disorders. *Journal of Personality Disorders, 25*(5), 557–570.

Jensen-Doss, A., & Weisz, J. R. (2008). Diagnostic agreement predicts treatment process and outcomes in youth mental health clinics. *Journal of Consulting and Clinical Psychology, 76*(5), 711–722.

John, O. P., & Robins, R. W. (1993). Determinants of interjudge agreement on personality traits: The Big Five domains, observability, evaluativeness, and the unique perspective of the self. *Journal of Personality, 61*(4), 521–551.

Klein, D. N. (2003). Patients' versus informants' reports of personality disorders in predicting 7½-year outcome in outpatients with depressive disorders. *Psychological Assessment, 15*(2), 216–222.

Klonsky, E. D., Oltmanns, T. F., & Turkheimer, E. (2002). Informant-reports of personality disorder: Relation to self-reports and future research directions. *Clinical Psychology: Science and Practice, 9*, 300–311.

Kneip, R. C., Delamater, A. M., Ismond, T., Milford, C., Salvia, L., & Schwartz, D. (1993). Self- and spouse ratings of anger and hostility as predictors of coronary heart disease. *Health Psychology, 12*(4), 301–307.

Kolar, D. W., Funder, D. C., & Colvin, C. R. (1996). Comparing the accuracy of personality judgments by the self and knowledgeable others. *Journal of Personality, 64*, 311–337.

Kraemer, H. C., Measelle, J. R., Ablow, J. C., Essex, M. J., Boyce, W. T., & Kupfer, D. J. (2003). A new approach to integrating data from multiple informants in psychiatric assessment and research: Mixing and matching contexts and perspectives. *American Journal of Psychiatry, 160*(9), 1566–1577.

Kurtz, J. E., & Sherker, J. L. (2003). Relationship quality, trait similarity, and self–other agreement on personality ratings in college roommates. *Journal of Personality, 71*, 21–48.

Lawton, E. M., Shields, A. J., & Oltmanns, T. F. (2011). Five-factor model personality disorder prototypes in a community sample: Self- and informant-reports predicting interview-based DSM diagnoses. *Personality Disorders: Theory Research and Treatment, 2*(4), 279–292.

Leising, D., Erbs, J., & Fritz, U. (2010). The letter of recommendation effect in informant ratings of personality. *Journal of Personality and Social Psychology, 98*(4), 668–682.

Lynam, D. R., & Widiger, T. A. (2001). Using the Five-Factor Model to represent the DSM-IV personality disorders: An expert consensus approach. *Journal of Abnormal Psychology, 110*, 401–412.

McAdams, D. P. (1993). *The stories we live by*. New York: Guilford Press.

McAdams, D. P. (1995). What do we know when we know a person. *Journal of Personality, 63,* 365–396.

McAdams, D. P., & Pals, J. L. (2006). A new Big Five: Fundamental principles for integrative science and personality. *American Psychologist, 61,* 204–217.

McAdams, D. P., Reynolds, J., Lewis, M., Patten, A. H., & Bowman, P. J. (2001). When bad things turn good and good things turn bad: Sequences of redemption and contamination in life narrative and their relation to psychosocial adaptation in midlife adults and in students. *Personality and Social Psychology Bulletin, 27,* 474–485.

McClelland, D. C., Koestner, R., & Weinberger, J. (1989). How do self-attributed and implicit motives differ? *Psychological Review, 96,* 690–702.

McCrae, R. R. (1982). Consensual validation of personality traits: Evidence from self-reports and ratings. *Journal of Personality and Social Psychology, 43*(2), 293–303.

McCrae, R. R. (1994). The counterpoint of personality assessment: Self-reports and observer ratings. *Assessment, 1,* 159–172.

McCrae, R. R., & Costa, P. T., Jr. (1999). A Five Factor theory of personality. In L. A. Pervin & O. P. John (Eds.), *Handbook of personality: Theory and research* (2nd ed., pp. 139–153). New York: Guilford Press.

Meyer, G. J. (2002). Implications of information-gathering methods for a refined taxonomy of psychopathology. In L. E. Beutler & M. L. Malik (Eds.), *Rethinking DSM: A psychological perspective* (pp. 69–105). Washington, DC: American Psychological Association.

Meyer, G. J., & Archer, R. P. (2001). The hard science of Rorschach research: What do we know and where do we go? *Psychological Assessment, 13,* 486–502.

Meyer, G., Finn, S., Eyde, L., & Kay, G. (2001). Psychological testing and psychological assessment: A review of evidence and issues. *American Psychologist, 56*(2), 128–165.

Miller, J. D., Pilkonis, P. A., & Clifton, A. (2005). Self- and other-reports of traits from the Five-Factor model: Relations to personality disorder. *Journal of Personality Disorders, 19*(4), 400–419.

Morf, C. C., Weir, C., & Davidov, M. (2000). Narcissism and intrinsic motivation: The role of goal congruence. *Journal of Experimental Social Psychology, 36,* 424–438.

Moskowitz, G. B., & Roman, R. J. (1992). Spontaneous trait inference as self-generated primes: Implications for conscious social judgment. *Journal of Personality and Social Psychology, 62,* 728–738.

Mosterman, R. M., & Hendriks, A. A. J. (2011). Self–other disagreement in personality assessment: Significance and prognostic value. *Clinical Psychology and Psychotherapy, 18,* 159–171.

Naumann, L. P., Vazire, S., Rentfrow, P. J., & Gosling, S. D. (2010). Personality judgments based on physical appearance. *Personality and Social Psychology Bulletin, 35,* 1661–1671.

O'Connor, B. P. (2002). The search for dimensional structure differences between normal and abnormality: A statistical review of published data on personality and psychopathology. *Journal of Personality and Social Psychology, 83,* 962–982.

Oltmanns, T. F., & Gleason M. E. J. (2011). Personality, health, and social adjustment in later life. In L. B. Cottler (Ed.), *Mental health in public health: The next 100 years* (pp. 151–179). New York: Oxford University Press.

Oltmanns, T. F., & Turkheimer, E. (2006). Perceptions of self and others regarding pathological personality traits. In R. F. Krueger & J. L. Tackett (Eds.), *Personality and psychopathology* (pp. 71–111). New York: Guilford Press.

Ozer, D. J., & Benet-Martínez, V. (2006). Personality and the prediction of consequential outcomes. *Annual Review of Psychology*, *57*, 401–421.

Paulhus, D. L., & Bruce, M. N. (1992). The effect of acquaintanceship on the validity of personality impressions: A longitudinal study. *Journal of Personality and Social Psychology*, *63*, 816–824.

Paulhus, D. L., & John, O. P. (1998). Egoistic and moralistic biases in self-perception: The interplay of self-deceptive styles with basic traits. *Journal of Personality*, *66*(6), 1025–1060.

Paunonen, S. V., & Neill, T. A. O. (2010). Self-reports, peer ratings and construct validity. *European Journal of Personality*, *24*, 189–206.

Pfohl, B., Blum, N., & Zimmerman, M. (1997). *Structured Interview for DSM-IV Personality*. Washington, DC: American Psychiatric Press.

Pilkonis, P. A., Hallquist, M. N., Morse, J. Q., & Stepp, S. D. (2011). Striking the (im)proper balance between scientific advances and clinical utility: Commentary on the DSM-5 proposal for personality disorders. *Personality Disorders: Theory Research and Treatment*, *2*(1), 68–82.

Pronin, E., & Kugler, M. B. (2007). Valuing thoughts, ignoring behavior: The introspection illusion as a source of the bias blind spot. *Journal of Experimental Social Psychology*, *43*, 565–578.

Pronin, E., Lin, D. Y., & Ross, L. (2002). The bias blind spot: Perceptions of bias in self versus others. *Personality and Social Psychology Bulletin*, *28*, 369–381.

Quirk, S. W., Christiansen, N. D., Wagner, S. H., & McNulty, J. L. (2003). On the usefulness of measures of normal personality for clinical assessment: Evidence of the incremental validity of the Revised NEO Personality Inventory. *Psychological Assessment*, *15*(3), 311–325.

Ready, R. E., & Clark, L. A. (2002). Correspondence of psychiatric patient and informant ratings of personality traits, temperament, and interpersonal problems. *Psychological Assessment*, *14*(1), 39–49.

Ready, R. E., Clark, L. A., Watson, D., & Westerhouse, K. (2000). Self- and peer-reported personality: Agreement, trait ratability, and the "Self-Based Heuristic." *Journal of Research in Personality*, *34*(2), 208–224.

Rettew, D. C., Doyle-Lynch, A., Achenbach, T. M., Dumenci, L., & Ivanova, M. Y. (2009). Meta-analyses of agreement between diagnoses made from clinical evaluations and standardized diagnostic interviews. *International Journal of Methods in Psychiatric Research*, *18*(3), 169–184.

Roberts, B. W., Kuncel, N. R., Shiner, R., Caspi, A., & Goldberg, L. R. (2007). The power of personality: The comparative validity of personality traits, socioeconomic status, and cognitive ability for predicting important life outcomes. *Perspectives on Psychological Science*, *2*(4), 313–345.

Rodebaugh, T. L., Gianoli, M. O., Turkheimer, E., & Oltmanns, T. F. (2011). The interpersonal problems of the socially avoidant: Self and peer shared variance. *Journal of Abnormal Psychology*, *119*(2), 331–340.

Rogers, R. (2003). Standardizing DSM-IV diagnoses: The clinical applications of structured interviews. *Journal of Personality Assessment*, *81*(3), 220–225.

Safran, J. D., Abreu, I., Ogilvie, J., & DeMaria, A. (2011). Does psychotherapy research influence the clinical practice of researcher–clinicians? *Clinical Psychology: Science and Practice*, *18*, 357–371.

Schacter, D. L. (1987). Implicit memory: History and current status. *Journal of Experimental Psychology: Learning, Memory, and Cognition*, *13*, 501–518.

Shea, M. T., & Yen, S. (2005). Personality traits/disorders and depression: A summary of conceptual and empirical findings. In M. Rosenbluth, S. H. Kennedy, & R.

M. Bagby (Eds.), *Depression and personality: Conceptual and clinical challenges* (pp. 43–64). Washington, DC: American Psychiatric Press.

Shedler, J., Mayman, M., & Manis, M. (1993). The illusion of mental health. *American Psychologist, 48,* 1117–1131.

Smith, T. W., Uchino, B., Berg., C., Florsheim, P., Pearce, G., Hawkin, M., et al. (2008). Associations of self reports versus spouse ratings of negative affectivity, dominance, and affiliation with coronary artery disease: Where should we look and who should we ask when studying personality and health? *Health Psychology, 27,* 676–684.

Spain, J. S., Eaton, L. G., & Funder, D. C. (2000). Perspectives on personality: The relative accuracy of self versus others for the prediction of emotion and behavior. *Journal of Personality, 68*(5), 837–867.

Srivastava, S., Guglielmo, S., & Beer, J. S. (2010). Perceiving others' personalities: Examining the dimensionality, assumed similarity to the self, and stability of perceiver effects. *Journal of Personality and Social Psychology, 98*(3), 520–534.

Stepp, S. D., Trull, T. J., Burr, R. M., Wolfenstein, M., & Vieth, A. Z. (2005). Incremental validity of the Structured Interview for the Five-Factor Model of personality (SIFFM). *European Journal of Personality, 19,* 343–357.

Swann, W. B., Jr. (1997). The trouble with change: Self-verification and allegiance to the self. *Psychological Science, 8*(3), 177–180.

Terracciano, A., Lockenhoff, C. E., Zonderman, A. B., Ferrucci, L., & Costa, P. T. (2008). Personality predictors of longevity: Activity, emotional stability, and conscientiousness. *Psychosomatic Medicine, 70*(6), 621–627.

Trull, T. J., & Durrett, C. A. (2005). Categorical and dimensional models of personality disorder. *Annual Review of Clinical Psychology, 1,* 355–380.

Vazire, S. & Mehl, M. R. (2008). Knowing me, knowing you: Accuracy and unique predictive validity of self-ratings and other ratings of daily behavior. *Personality Processes and Individual Differences, 95,* 1202–1216.

Wagerman, S. A., & Funder, D. C. (2007). Acquaintance reports of personality and academic achievement: A case for conscientiousness. *Journal of Research in Personality, 41,* 221–229.

Watkins, C. E., Campbell, V. L., Nieberding, R., & Hallmark, R. (1995). Contemporary practice of psychological assessment by clinical psychologists. *Professional Psychology: Research and Practice, 26,* 54–60.

Watson, D., & Clark, L. A. (1991). Self- versus peer ratings of specific emotional traits: Evidence of convergent and discriminant validity. *Journal of Personality and Social Psychology, 60,* 927–940.

Watson, D., Hubbard, B., & Wiese, D. (2000). Self-other agreement in personality and affectivity: The role of acquaintanceship, trait visibility, and assumed similarity. *Journal of Personality and Social Psychology, 78*(3), 546–558.

Westen, D. (1997). Divergences between clinical and research methods for assessing personality disorders: Implications for research and the evolution of Axis II. *American Journal of Psychiatry, 154*(7), 895–903.

Widiger, T. A., & Samuel, D. B. (2009). Evidence-based assessment of personality disorders. *Personality Disorders: Theory, Research, and Treatment, S*(1), 3–17.

Widiger, T. A., & Simonsen, E. (2005). Alternative dimensional models of personality disorder: Finding a common ground. *Journal of Personality Disorders, 19*(2), 110–130.

Wilt, J., Cox, K. S., & McAdams, D. P. (2010). The Erikson life story: Developmental scripts and psychosocial adaptation. *Journal of Adult Development, 17,* 156–161.

Zillig, L. M. P., Hemenover, S. H., & Dienstbier, R. A. (2002). What do we assess when we assess a Big Five trait?: A content analysis of the affective, behavioral, and cognitive processes represented in Big Five personality inventories. *Personality and Social Psychology Bulletin, 28*, 847–858.

Zimmerman, M. (2003). What should the standard of care for psychiatric evaluations be? *Journal of Nervous and Mental Disease, 191*, 281–286.

Zimmerman, M., Pfohl, B., Coryell, W., Stangl, D., & Corenthal, C. (1988). Diagnosing personality disorder in depressed patients: A comparison of patient and informant interviews. *Archives of General Psychiatry, 45*, 733–737.

Zimmerman, M., Pfohl, B., Stangl, D., & Corenthal, C. (1986). Assessment of DSM-III personality disorders: The importance of interviewing an informant. *Journal of Clinical Psychiatry, 47*, 261–263.

CHAPTER 2

Multimethod Assessment of Interpersonal Dynamics

Aaron L. Pincus, Pamela Sadler, Erik Woody, Michael J. Roche, Katherine M. Thomas, and Aidan G. C. Wright

In this chapter, we describe multiple methods for conceptualizing and assessing interpersonal dynamics, review their empirical support, and demonstrate their applications in clinical assessment contexts. To present this description, we employ the interpersonal paradigm of personality assessment (Wiggins, 2003) because it provides a rich nomological net supporting multimethod approaches (Pincus & Ansell, 2013). Pincus (2010) asserted that "interpersonal assessment employs multiple models, measures, and methods at varying levels of specificity and combines these with theories of development, motivation, and regulation to examine the interpenetration of personality, psychopathology, and psychotherapy" (p. 467). These approaches include assessment of broad interpersonal motives and goals, enduring interpersonal dispositions (e.g., traits, problems, sensitivities, efficacies, and strengths), specific interpersonal behaviors, and relational patterns occurring over varying timescales. Multiple methods employed include self- and informant reports, moment-to-moment observational coding, and longitudinal ambulatory and daily diary assessment techniques. This allows for interpersonal assessment to be used in the consultation room, the laboratory, and the natural settings of daily life.

A unique strength of the interpersonal paradigm is that the organizational metaframework of agency and communion (Wiggins, 1991) provides a nomological net for defining and assessing the fundamental constructs of interpersonal functioning (Figure 2.1, top). The agency and communion

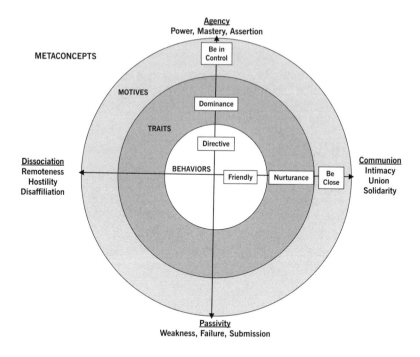

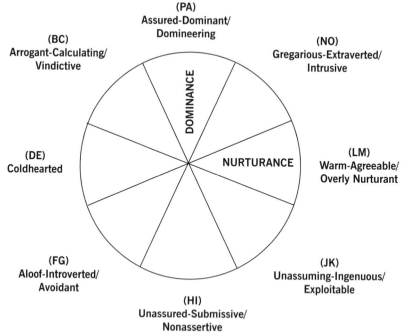

FIGURE 2.1. Agency and communion metaframework (top); interpersonal circle of traits/problems (bottom).

metaframework gives rise to the familiar interpersonal circumplex (IPC) model (Figure 2.1, bottom), which itself is conceived of in multiple forms (Locke, 2011). Employing multiple interpersonal assessment methods in clinical contexts serves to provide an *interpersonal diagnosis* to complement standard psychiatric classification. Pincus and Wright (2011) identified four elements of interpersonal diagnosis. First, interpersonal diagnosis is anchored to the agency and communion metaframework and its derivations of the interpersonal circumplex as a "key conceptual map" (Kiesler, 1996, p. 172) for an interpersonal description of psychopathology, in combination with the contemporary developmental, motivational, and regulatory assumptions of interpersonal theory for an interpersonal explanation of psychopathology (Pincus & Hopwood, 2012; Pincus, Lukowitsky, & Wright, 2010). Second, interpersonal diagnosis assumes that normality and abnormality can be conceptualized with the same dimensions, implying that (1) interpersonal descriptions of normality and abnormality should be based on the same interpersonal models, constructs, and processes; and (2) abnormality is considered to be a distortion or disturbance of normal interpersonal functioning. Third, interpersonal diagnosis assumes that psychopathology and personality are inextricably linked. Although this is most notable in the conceptualization of personality disorders, interpersonal diagnosis also views most psychiatric symptoms as embedded within the context of personality and interpersonal functioning. Fourth, interpersonal diagnosis recognizes that personality assessment and psychotherapy most commonly take place within an interpersonal context—the relationship between patient and clinician—and this highlights the need to help clinicians identify and organize the salient interpersonal data regarding patients' typical ways of seeing themselves and others, patients' typical ways of relating and reacting to others in the moment, and patients' maladaptive interpersonal patterns emerging over time and across the natural settings of daily life.

Interpersonal Dynamics

One important meaning of *dynamics*, stemming originally from Freud and having a rich history in psychoanalysis, is the "play of forces in the mind" (Erdelyi, 1985, p. 212). This kind of dynamical interplay is conceptualized *structurally*, in terms of the conflict and balance between different levels or processes in the mind. Another important meaning of dynamics, stemming from systems theory, is the unfolding of behavior over time. This kind of dynamic interplay is conceptualized *temporally*: "A phenomenon is dynamic if, in order to understand it, one has to take the temporal dimension into account" (Salvatore & Tschacher, 2012, p. 4). This chapter extensively addresses both of these meanings of the term *dynamics*. For this reason, it is important to understand that the structural and temporal realms are, in principle, closely interrelated. In other words, it is the organization of dimensions within the individual that, at least in part, underlies oscillations and other patterns of variation over time in the person's behavior (McWilliams, 2012). The underlying mental structures help to make temporal variation intelligible. Thus, although much work remains to be done to integrate the structural and temporal approaches to dynamics, both offer multiple methods to assess a crucial, common underlying feature of interpersonal behavior, namely, lawful within-person variation.

Structural Dynamics

Our structural approach to interpersonal dynamics makes use of concepts originally stemming from Leary (1957) on the interplay of different *interpersonal levels* of personality. Leary suggested that interpersonal theory should encompass the relations between types of interpersonal functioning at five levels: Level I is public communication, consisting of one's overt behavior; Level II reflects conscious descriptions of one's own and others' behavior; Level III captures private symbolization, or the unconscious symbolic themes expressed; Level IV is the unexpressed unconscious, containing those behaviors that an individual unconsciously avoids; finally, Level V refers to values or ego ideal and reflects the way an individual is motivated (consciously or unconsciously) to function interpersonally. Leary saw these relations as important in that they allow for a consistent structure (the IPC) at all levels of functioning and point to the possibility of assessing coherence and conflict across all levels of functioning. Accordingly, in this chapter we present a framework for examining the structural dynamics of personality by assessing a contemporary set of interpersonal "levels" within the person.

Temporal Dynamics

Our temporal approach to interpersonal dynamics makes use of variation at two quite different timescales. First, any social interaction is a prototypical case of an event that needs to be understood as a process unfolding over time. During an interaction, the partners' interpersonal behaviors become intertwined in fascinating ways, yielding a rich array of patterns, such as entrained oscillations (e.g., Sadler, Ethier, Gunn, Duong, & Woody, 2009). We present a framework for assessing these *moment-to-moment patterns within social interactions*. Second, at a larger timescale, people engage in many distinct interactions over the course of days, weeks, and months, and each individual's interpersonal behavior varies in important ways across these interactions (e.g., Moskowitz, 2009). Accordingly, we also present a framework for assessing this *across-occasions level of interpersonal variability* that characterizes daily life.

Organization of the Chapter

In the sections that follow, we present methods to assess the interpersonal dynamics of personality, social interaction, and daily life. This sequence begins with methods to assess the structural interplay of interpersonal levels of functioning within the person. Next we discuss reciprocal interpersonal patterns of behavior and introduce the principles of interpersonal complementarity. The subsequent section broadens the scope of assessment to the moment-to-moment temporal interplay of reciprocal interpersonal patterns in dyads. The final section further extends the scope of assessment to the reciprocal interpersonal patterns enacted across relationships and contexts. The results of such assessments complement standard psychiatric diagnosis by providing clinically relevant information beyond symptomatology alone (e.g., Cain et al., 2012; Przeworski et al., 2011) and even identifying specific targets for intervention (e.g., Cain & Pincus, in press). In each section we illustrate how the assessment of interpersonal dynamics can enhance case conceptualization and contribute to treatment planning. We then conclude with a call for further integration of these multimethod approaches in research and practice as the interpersonal dynamics of personality, social interaction, and daily life can also complement each other in clinical assessments.

Interpersonal Dynamics of Personality

Structural dynamics, by definition, imply movement. In the context of personality, these movements are comprised of a swirling composite of motivations, cognitions, and behaviors, all occurring in transaction with each other and the environment over time. However, clinical assessment that relies solely on self-report or interview measures to generate cross-sectional dispositional profiles would seem to have a long way to go toward fulfilling the promise of capturing the dynamics of personality. In this approach, understanding how a patient generally behaves, in a probabilistic sense, has become the goal. As such, most modern personality instruments focus on content domains (e.g., impulsivity), generating summary scores from groups of heterogeneous items that decontextualize functioning. Yet, by removing context, personality is rendered static.

At the same time, the benefits of cross-sectional assessment of dispositions are undeniable. For one, it is an economical enterprise. Having an individual, couple, or even a group complete a battery of questionnaires does not generally tax the practitioner's time; protocols can be completed in the office or at home, via paper and pencil or computer. Modern computing allows for efficient and accurate scoring of protocols. Furthermore, they are a familiar format to most patients, and their psychometrics and interpretation are a part of the required graduate curriculum of clinical psychology. The question then becomes, how can the standard assessment approach be applied so as to measure structural dynamics?

Although interpersonal theory is often equated with psychometric models of interpersonal variables and associated measures, this neglects the additional aspects of what is a comprehensive and dynamic theory of personality. To be certain, Leary's (1957) most well-known contribution to the field has been the IPC and its primary dimensions of dominance and affiliation, which serve to map the structural relations among interpersonal variables. However, his other major contribution was the concept of explicit "levels" of personality, which drew distinctions between various conscious and unconscious manifestations of interpersonal functioning when defining these levels. From this concept it followed that key dynamics of personality involve the interplay between levels of functioning. That is to say, what gives rise to the dynamic phenomena of clinical interest are the patterns of coherence and conflict in interpersonal functioning across levels. For example, it would likely be of clinical interest if an individual's overt behavior (i.e., public communication) were at odds with either his or her internal description of that behavior (i.e., the understanding of that behavior), or his or her "ego ideal" (i.e., valued behavior). Leary made it abundantly clear that any system of levels was arbitrary, allowing for future refinements or alternatives. What we present here is not a faithful application of Leary's highly elaborated system of levels, discrepancies, and their assessment techniques, but rather an application of this fundamental proposition using modern IPC inventories in a flexible battery approach.

Selecting, Scoring, and Interpreting Interpersonal Inventories

Modern interpersonal assessment offers a number of empirically derived and psychometrically sound measures for targeting a variety of functional domains or levels within the IPC framework (Locke, 2011). General interpersonal behavior can be captured using trait measures such as the Interpersonal Adjective Scales (IAS; Wiggins, 1995) or the newer International Personality Item Pool—IPC (IPIP-IPC; Markey & Markey, 2009). Among the most popular clinical measures is the Inventory of Interpersonal Problems—Circumplex (IIP-C; Alden, Wiggins, & Pincus, 1990), which assesses the distress associated with problematic behavior. Additional measures exist to assess the types of adaptive interpersonal behaviors that characterize the respondent (Interpersonal Strengths Inventory [ISI]; Hatcher & Rogers, 2009), those domains for which they feel competent (Circumplex Scales of Interpersonal Efficacy [CSIE]; Locke & Sadler, 2007), and the behaviors they value or the impression that is important for them to make on others (Circumplex Scales of Interpersonal Values [CSIV]; Locke, 2000). Other measures capture the manner in which the individual responds to others. For example, the Interpersonal Sensitivities Circumplex (ISC; Hopwood et al., 2011) assesses the behaviors of others that an individual finds bothersome, and the Impact Message Inventory (IMI; Kiesler & Schmidt, 1993) assesses covert reactions to others' behavior. A number of other inventories and checklists may also be chosen for specific purposes. The above list contains many of the popular measures available that use the same basic IPC structure, but differ in their focus of assessment through use of different item stems and targets (e.g., self vs. other).

In addition to using different measures, two complementary approaches serve to augment the available "levels" of data. First, it is advisable to gather data from informants who know the patient well. There is a vibrant literature that examines the utility of self–other agreement and disagreement in assessment of personality generally (see Galione & Oltmanns, Chapter 1, this volume) and the IIP-C specifically (Clifton, Turkheimer, & Oltmanns, 2005). Second, given the relative brevity of most of these measures, an individual can be asked to complete IPC measures across interpersonal contexts (e.g., How do you generally behave at work? With your wife? With your father?). (See also Benjamin, 1984)

As we mentioned earlier, using the same structure across levels allows for cross-level comparisons to identify areas of convergence and divergence. A number of approaches exist to summarize a profile of IPC scales. Most modern IPC measures use the same, eight-scale, or octant structure (see the divisions in Figure 2.1, bottom). Once scale scores have been standardized, they can be examined at the octant level, or dimensional "axis" scores can be calculated using basic geometric principles (see Wiggins, Phillips, & Trapnell, 1989). Scores on the primary dimensions can in turn be used to locate an individual in the Cartesian plane of the IPC. Although these approaches are useful, we advocate use of the circumplex structural summary approach for individual data (Gurtman & Balakrishnan, 1998). This approach, also based on the geometry of the circle, decomposes an IPC profile into three structural parameters: *elevation, angular displacement,* and *amplitude.* These parameters reduce the complexity of eight scales down to three parameters with substantive interpretations. Elevation captures the average scale score for a profile, and for many measures this has a substantive interpretation (e.g., IIP-C elevation is generalized interpersonal distress; ISC elevation is generalized interpersonal sensitivity). Angular displacement indicates the principal interpersonal theme or style of the profile, and amplitude indicates the degree of differentiation or distinctiveness of the theme. Finally, a measure of the degree to which a profile matches the predicted circular pattern, or the level of *prototypicality* of the profile, is available in the form of an R^2 statistic. We adopt the structural summary approach in conjunction with specific octant interpretations in the following case example.

Case Example: Coherence and Conflict across Interpersonal Levels of Personality

To illustrate how a contemporary multilevel interpersonal assessment might proceed, we offer the case of Mr. S, who was enrolled in a prestigious and competitive graduate engineering program. To those who knew him, and by his own admission, he was bright and had various intellectual interests, but he was socially awkward, with few close friendships. However, he had been dating a younger undergraduate woman for approximately one year, his first serious relationship. Diagnostically, the majority of his complaints were well captured by the DSM-5 diagnoses of major depressive disorder, recurrent, moderate, without psychotic features, and narcissistic personality disorder (American Psychiatric Association, 2013). He was being seen for twice weekly outpatient transference-focused psychotherapy (Clarkin, Yeomans, & Kernberg, 2006), with the focus primarily being on his personality pathology. Features associated with his narcissism (e.g., overvalued ideals and expectations for himself and others; exquisitely experienced shame; ruminative focus on how others had wronged him and accompanying rage; devaluation; protective withdrawal) left him vulnerable to experiencing intense bouts of suicidal depression. Although he had been in psychotherapy for over two years, he and his new therapist had only been working together a few months at the time of this assessment.

The decision to pursue an in-depth interpersonal assessment was motivated largely by Mr. S's consistent pattern of stating that he did not feel there was anything to say in sessions. A review of case notes from the previous therapist presaged this pattern, which had previously arisen, and was successfully, but slowly, addressed by interpreting the subtle but clear devaluation of the therapy that accompanied the message (i.e., "What is the point of talking? This therapy cannot be helpful!"). As an alternative approach, meant to bypass the intense feelings of vulnerability associated with opening up in session, and to serve as a catalyst for discussion, an interpersonal assessment was suggested in line with a therapeutic assessment approach (Finn, 2007, 2011; Hopwood, 2010). Mr. S was collaboratively enlisted in the process of the assessment by explaining its purpose, and he was encouraged to generate his own questions within the domains being assessed (Finn, Fischer, & Handler, 2012). He then completed the following interpersonal measures: IAS (Traits), ISI (Strengths), CSIV (Values), ISC (Sensitivities), and IIP-C (Problems) (the scores are given in Table 2.1). The plotted structural summary profiles (Figure 2.2) along with a generic template of the IPC (Figure 2.1, bottom) were brought into the consultation room during feedback.

Table 2.1 catalogues the octant scores and structural summary parameters for each of Mr. S's interpersonal profiles. The R^2 values suggested that each profile could be reasonably summarized using the structural summary parameters, with the exception of Mr. S's interpersonal problem profile,

TABLE 2.1. IPC Measure Scale Scores and Structural Summary Parameters for Mr. S's Assessment

| | Standardized scale scores | | | | | | | | Structural summary | | | |
	PA (90°)	BC (135°)	DE (180°)	FG (225°)	HI (270°)	JK (315°)	LM (0°)	NO (45°)	ELEV	AMP	DEGREE	R^2
Traits	-0.31	-0.30	1.89	1.73	1.21	0.69	-0.15	-2.18	0.32	1.61	231°	0.83
Strengths	-1.10	-1.24	-1.38	-0.49	-0.61	-0.47	-0.90	-1.04	-0.90	0.39	294°	0.72
Values	-0.84	-0.54	-0.68	0.76	0.64	0.46	0.97	0.56	0.17	0.80	314°	0.70
Sensitivities	-1.57	0.30	1.29	0.27	-0.44	-1.05	-0.63	-1.68	-0.44	1.13	200°	0.71
Problems	1.80	1.12	1.07	3.07	0.59	2.30	2.87	1.52	1.79	0.43	335°	0.13

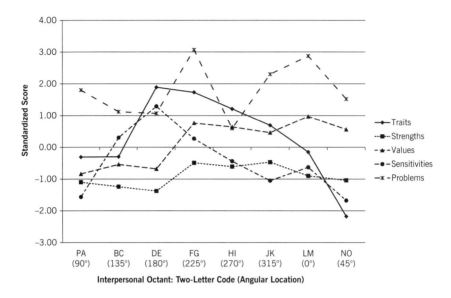

FIGURE 2.2. Interpersonal structural summary profiles for Mr. S.

which was best interpreted at the octant level due to its idiosyncratic pattern. Prior to discussing the profile with Mr. S, it was apparent that he viewed his general interpersonal behavior (Traits) as prototypically withdrawn and aloof. In terms of interpersonal strengths there were none he excelled at, and he felt generally ineffectual to some degree (low amplitude and negative elevation on the Strengths profile). Interestingly, Mr. S's sensitivities profile suggested that he was generally not bothered by the behavior of others, with the exception of when others maintained a distance from him (Sensitivities profile with negative elevation, but positive peak in cold octant). In terms of valued interpersonal behavior, Mr. S generally valued being warm and agreeable, decidedly in contrast to his characteristically aloof behavior. Finally, the interpersonal problems profile was markedly elevated, suggestive of considerable generalized interpersonal distress. Moreover, the pattern was nonprototypical (low R^2), but not flat, exhibiting peaks in the avoidant (FG) and overly nurturant (LM) octants—noteworthy due to their contrasting interpersonal content. Without pointing out specifics, on the whole there are a number of discrepancies in elevation and themes in these profiles that begin to portray the dynamic nature of Mr. S's personality, even though these are but static and dispositional self-report measures of interpersonal functioning.

We recommend that the clinician first examine the results and then develop hypotheses about potentially interesting discrepancies between levels, which can then be offered up for discussion and confirmed with the patient in a collaborative fashion (see, e.g., Finn, 2007; Hopwood, 2010).

For example, note the high degree of discrepancy in scores for the LM/NO octants, and similarly high but distinct discrepancies for the DE/FG octants. These immediately call to mind potential conflicts related to interpersonal closeness and attachment and potential difficulties in the way these issues are navigated with others. The IPC model and logic behind the assessment approach were transparently explained to Mr. S, including how to read the plots of his interpersonal profiles. Given Mr. S's engineering background and the features of his character, the full technical and quantitative details of the structural summary method were explained. This ensured maximal engagement, both by providing Mr. S with the tools for nuanced interpretation of the profiles and by ensuring that Mr. S felt respected, included, and treated as an equal. We recommend tailoring the description of the method to a patient's abilities and interest level. Subsequently, the practitioner offered general impressions about each profile, and Mr. S was invited to share his own reactions (e.g., "What do you make of these?" or "How do you see these two scores fitting together?"). The discussion focused on the primary theme of Mr. S's difficulty in effectively negotiating interpersonal closeness, despite a deep yearning for meaningful relationships and his elevated distress over repeated failures to connect.

As can be seen in Figure 2.2, Mr. S neither values nor feels he is effectively interpersonally cold (DE), yet he views many of his behaviors this way and is distressed by it. Similarly, he views himself as aloof–introverted (FG) and is highly distressed by his avoidant behavior, even though he values this interpersonal behavior more as a core coping strategy. With regard to warm–extraverted behavior (LM/NO), he values these behaviors, but he sees himself as only average in warmth and markedly introverted, and neither quality is a recognized strength. Enacting warm behaviors is also highly distressing to him. The additional result of being sensitive to others' cold behavior ties together the picture of a man who desires connection, feels incapable of it, and is attuned to others' withdrawal. Yet he is often withdrawn and cold himself, contributing to others finding him stand-offish and difficult to get to know, leading them to either pull away or not engage him. Of additional interest was the dominant octant (PA), which showed that although his traits, strengths, and values were relatively in line, he was distressed by being assertive and concerned that others found him to be domineering. Professionally, this led to him being ineffective at being assertive when necessary, and instead he would adopt a "helping" stance when he wanted someone to do something, claiming he was just watching out for them so that they could avoid mistakes. His colleagues would often find this attitude disingenuous and would react negatively, leaving Mr. S feeling puzzled, misunderstood, distant, and frustrated.

This brief case example is meant to illustrate the power of using these various measures in concert. Even though they are dispositional in nature and all at the level of conscious self-description, they have immense power to faithfully represent interpersonal personality dynamics. For Mr. S, this structural approach made tangible the very issues he found difficult to express with words in session. The data from this assessment became a touchstone that was often referred back to in therapy, and served to catalyze Mr. S's ability to recognize his own dynamics and begin to address them in and out of session.

Reciprocal Interpersonal Patterns

The interplay of different levels within the individual, as discussed in the previous section, represents the interpersonal dynamics of personality and its consequences. Additional important interpersonal dynamics are revealed in the interplay between individuals over time. In the next two sections, we examine temporal dynamics at two timescales—within an interaction and across many interactions. Interpersonal theory provides a rich theoretical foundation for understanding variations in interpersonal behavior over time as *reciprocal interpersonal patterns*. These patterns are socially reinforced through various transactional influences impacting self and other as they resolve, negotiate, or exacerbate the interpersonal situation. Interpersonal behaviors tend to pull, elicit, invite, or evoke restricted classes of responses from the other in a continual, dynamic transactional process. Carson (1991) referred to this as an interbehavioral contingency process where "there is a tendency for a given individual's interpersonal behavior to be constrained or controlled in more or less predictable ways by the behavior received from an interaction partner" (p. 191). Thus reciprocal interpersonal patterns are the consistent agentic and communal behavioral responses to the perceived agentic and communal characteristics of others in an interpersonal situation (Pincus et al., 2010).

The IPC provides conceptual anchors and a lexicon to systematically describe reciprocal interpersonal patterns. The most basic of these patterns is referred to as interpersonal *complementarity* (Carson, 1969; Kiesler, 1983). Interpersonal complementarity occurs when the agentic and communal needs of both persons are met in the interpersonal situation, leading to stability and likely recurrence of the pattern. Complementarity is defined via the IPC based on the social exchange of status (agency) and love (communion) as reflected in oppositeness (also referred to as reciprocity) for the vertical dimension (i.e., dominance pulls for submission; submission pulls for dominance) and sameness (also referred to as correspondence) for the horizontal dimension (friendliness pulls for friendliness; hostility pulls for hostility). Although complementarity is neither the only reciprocal interpersonal pattern that can be described by the IPC nor a proposed universal law of interaction, empirical studies consistently find support for its probabilistic predictions (Sadler, Ethier, & Woody, 2011). Complementarity should be considered a common baseline for the reciprocal influence of interpersonal behavior associated with healthy socialization. Deviations from complementary interpersonal signatures are more likely to disrupt interpersonal relations and may be indicative of pathological functioning (Hopwood, Wright, Ansell, & Pincus, 2013; Roche, Pincus, Conroy, Hyde, & Ram, 2013).

Complementarity should not be conceived of as simply a behavioral stimulus–response chain of events. Rather, mediating internal psychological processes (e.g., each interactant's self–other schemas, the motives and needs embedded in these schemas, and their effects on subjective experience) influence the likelihood of complementary interpersonal patterns. Chronic deviations from complementary reciprocal patterns of social behavior are indicative of psychopathology in part because they suggest impairments in: (1) recognizing the consensual understanding of interpersonal situations, (2) adaptively communicating one's own interpersonal needs and motives, and (3) comprehending the needs of others and the intent of their interpersonal behavior (Cain & Pincus, in press). In such cases, the individual may react chaotically, self-protectively, or rigidly pull for responses that complement his or her own interpersonal behavior, but has significant difficulty replying with responses complementary to others' behavior. This reduces the likelihood that the agentic and communal needs of both persons will be satisfied in the interpersonal situation, creating disturbed interpersonal relations (Hopwood et al., 2013; Pincus & Hopwood, 2012).

Interpersonal Dynamics of Social Interaction

Important interpersonal dynamics are revealed in the interplay between individuals over the course of a social interaction. Consider a clinical supervisor observing a psychotherapy session and attending to the interpersonal dynamics of the client and the therapist. The supervisor watches the choreography, so to speak, of interrelated interpersonal movements. As the interaction unfolds over time, the observer perceives various ebbs and flows, rhythms and entrainments, and other temporal patterns, all of which crucially interlink the two parties.

Capturing these rich perceptions from expert observers for purposes of scientific inquiry is a considerable challenge. Indeed, to make observer perceptions more tractable scientifically, researchers usually recast the role of the observer in either of two ways. In one commonly used approach, we ask observers, in effect, to *zoom out*, so that the details recede and the general picture remains. For example, we may ask the observer to use an inventory to rate the extent to which a client engaged in each of various dominant or submissive behaviors, and then we can aggregate by taking a sum or average to get the overall picture. This approach has many important uses. Such an aggregate indexes a person's interpersonal dispositions, and these dispositions have many very interesting applications, as the previous section of the chapter illustrates. However, in this approach, the observer's knowledge of the timing of moment-to-moment behaviors and how they were linked to surrounding behaviors, including those of the other person in the interaction, are lost. Because social interactions involve inherently dynamic phenomena, this lost information may be quite important. It is somewhat akin to characterizing a passage of music in terms of its average pitch, or characterizing a dance in terms of the average position of the two dancers. That is, without the temporal dimension, some of the sense of the activity—namely, its pattern in time—cannot be captured.

Alternatively, researchers often recast the role of the observer in an opposite way. They ask observers, in effect, to *zoom in*, so that just one detail at a time is considered and rated. For example, the client's behavior during an interaction can be segmented into discrete acts, and then we may ask observers to rate each separate act for whether it is dominant, submissive, or neutral. Although this approach, too, has many important uses, the huge collection of discrete acts that it produces also has some major limitations. The sense of a social interaction as a continual flow is lost, and the acts tend to become decontextualized because we, in effect, isolate them from the communicational flow. In other words, when we ask observers to rate each act separately, we do not make use of their knowledge of the context for the behavior. In addition, once a social interaction is deconstructed in this way, it is a great challenge to put the pieces back together in an illuminating way. It is akin to decomposing a passage of music into individual notes or a dance into discrete physical positions. That is, the temporal dimension needs to be reintroduced to bring the assessment data back to life.

The technique introduced in this section uses the expertise of observers in a way that is fundamentally different from both of these commonly used approaches. It does not ask them to zoom in or zoom out. Instead, the technique allows observers to follow the unfolding interaction in the same way as they normally do, and to record their moment-to-moment impression of a target person's interpersonal stance. Rather than recollecting and aggregating behaviors, the observer simply rates what is happening at the moment of observation. And rather than ignoring context, the observer's ratings are free to be informed by the ways in which whatever came before in a social interaction affects the interpersonal construal of an observed behavior. Moreover, with this technique the temporal dimension, rather than being ignored or temporarily set aside, is a fully integral aspect of the assessment data obtained.

A Computer Joystick Method for Observational Assessment of Interpersonal Behavior

The structural model of the IPC—a Cartesian plane defined by the orthogonal axes of agency and communion—provides a parsimonious framework in which dynamic changes in interpersonal behavior can be represented as trajectories. The problem, then, is how to translate the observer's moment-to-moment perceptions into such trajectories. The technique involves the use of a computer joystick and a joystick monitoring program. The observer watches a video of a social interaction on a computer monitor, focuses attention on one person, and uses the joystick position to indicate the moment-to-moment rating of that person's social behavior. The various possible positions of the joystick comprise a Cartesian plane, with degree of dominance versus submissiveness as the vertical axis and degree of friendliness to hostility as the horizontal axis. Each axis ranges from –1,000 (minimum possible friendliness; dominance) to 1,000 (maximum possible friendliness; dominance). Thus, the radial position of the joystick relative to the origin captures the target person's momentary interpersonal stance on the IPC, and the distance from the origin captures the momentary intensity of that interpersonal stance. As the observer indicates moment-to-moment changes in interpersonal behavior, the computer records the joystick position frequently (e.g., every half-second). Therefore, the resulting data provide a dense sampling of the reasonably continuous trajectory of the target person's behavior over time on the IPC. Later, the observer watches the video again, focusing on the other person in the interaction, and provides a trajectory of that person's interpersonal behavior over the course of the interaction. Because the two trajectories are exactly coordinated in time, they can be combined to represent and study the various patterns of entrainment that interlink the interpersonal behavior of the two parties.

There are two kinds of continuous feedback that help correctly orient observers as they use this joystick setup. The joystick program (Lizdek, Sadler, Woody, Ethier, & Malet, 2012) produces a small plot in the lower right corner of the screen that shows, using a red dot, where the current position of the joystick falls on the interpersonal plane (indicated by the orthogonal axes of dominant versus submissive and friendly versus unfriendly). In addition, if the joystick has a "force feedback" feature, it provides more resistance against the observer's hand as it moves farther from the origin, thus supplying tactile feedback about the degree of extremity of the current joystick position. Additional options are available. For example, one important option is that the joystick's "firing" button can be used to indicate a unique event or transition point during an interaction.

The Nature of the Data Obtained

The assessment of interpersonal dynamics that this technique affords is inherently dyadic, with the interpersonal behavior of each person in the interaction providing an inseparable context for the interpersonal behavior of the other. Although we may choose to focus mainly on one person for some purposes, it is well to keep in mind that interpersonal dynamics of social interaction always take place between people, and so what is being assessed is really the dyad, rather than the individual. The joystick technique generates a large volume of data. For example, the interpersonal trajectories of two people in a 10-minute interaction, sampled every half-second, yield 4,800 numbers. At first blush, then, we seem to be faced with an overwhelming explosion of data. However, the data are of a kind that has been widely studied in dynamical systems. Hence they are amenable to a variety of inventive graphical representations that visually reveal underlying structure (e.g., Boker, Xu, Rotondo, & King, 2002; Tufte, 2006) and cutting-edge data-analytic procedures that extract the main dynamical features (e.g., Boker, 2002; Boker & Wenger, 2007; Salvatore & Tschacher, 2012; Warner, 1998).

The interpersonal dimensions of affiliation and dominance define the *x*- and *y*-axes, respectively, of a plane that is called a *state space* in dynamical systems. The momentary interpersonal positions of the two people may be plotted as two points on this plane. The dimension of time constitutes a third, *z*-axis, which captures changes in the two people's interpersonal positions over the course of the interaction. Thus, the joystick technique generates a three-dimensional (3-D) structure for each interaction, in which two lines representing the partners in the interaction curve and swoop across the state space as we trace along the time dimension. This three-dimensional structure can be manipulated (e.g., rotated in various ways) and examined on a computer screen using 3-D graphing software. These 3-D structures are visually arresting and quite intriguing; however, it is not possible to show this on the static page of a book. A brief demonstration of the 3-D structures generated by two different dyads is available at *www.wlu.ca/science/psadler*.

Somewhat more prosaically, two-dimensional snapshots of the 3-D structure can be used to convey the main dynamic patterns. Two such graphs are particularly useful. One is a graph with affiliation on the *y*-axis and time on the *x*-axis, which shows how both parties' levels of affiliation changed and covaried over the course of the interaction. Another is the corresponding graph with dominance on the *y*-axis and time on the *x*-axis, which shows the interrelated dynamics of partners' levels of dominance during the interaction. To illustrate, Figure 2.3 presents such a pair of graphs for one interacting dyad. Dynamic features are not only evident from inspecting such graphs; they can also be quantified in various ways. We have found two types of descriptive statistics to be particularly helpful.

First, the linear slope for each party over the duration of the interaction provides a useful summary of the overall shifts. For example, in the graph for affiliation, both partners show a gradual, descending slope, such that the female has a linear slope of –95 and the male a slope of –107 over the duration of the interaction. Second, an index of the degree of entrainment between the parties is useful for capturing how much people's changes are correlated with each other. One way to do this is to remove the linear trend from each person's data and then compute the correlation over time across the two partners' data, which is called a *cross correlation*. For example, in

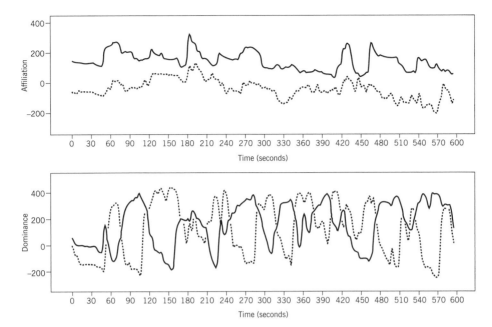

FIGURE 2.3. Affiliation behavior (top graph) and dominance behavior (bottom graph) over time for female (solid line) and male (dashed line) partners in an interacting dyad.

the graph for dominance the cross correlation is −0.57, which quantifies the moderately strong tendency for the partners' levels of dominance to vary inversely from moment to moment. In contrast, the corresponding cross-correlation for affiliation is 0.31, indexing a more modest, positive relation. Note that both of these moment-to-moment relations are consistent with interpersonal complementarity. A similar index, called *coherence*, can be calculated from a type of time-series analysis of the partners' data, called *cross-spectral analysis*. Coherence measures the degree to which partners' behaviors vary together in attuned cyclical (sine-wave-like) patterns. The tendency of these particular partners to be entrained in a rhythmically recurring way is especially evident visually in the graph for dominance in Figure 2.3. The numerical index of coherence is akin to a squared correlation and does not have a sign. Consistent with the magnitudes of the cross correlations, the average weighted coherence for dominance is 0.55 and for affiliation 0.31. Although the cross correlation and the coherence are based on very different statistical models, their application to interpersonal data typically yields consistent results. For more information about these and other indices and their interpretations, see Sadler et al. (2009, 2011).

The joystick technique also provides an excellent way to code more conventional, nondynamic aspects of interpersonal style. The average of the stream of ratings (e.g., on affiliation) is a highly reliable and valid measure of the person's interpersonal style in the interaction, and the standard deviation provides a useful index of the person's variability on that dimension. Indeed, use of the joystick for rating overall interpersonal style is consistent with the well-established recommendation of decision researchers to avoid having judges mentally aggregate ratings themselves (e.g., through recollection), because doing so tends to degrade the quality of the data (e.g., raters' overall impressions tend to be unduly influenced by the highest peak observed and the last thing observed; Kahneman, 2011).

Empirical Review

A number of studies demonstrate the promising nature of applying this joystick approach to the assessment of people's social behavior. In initial work (Sadler et al., 2009), observers recorded the moment-to-moment levels of dominance and affiliation for 50 previously unacquainted mixed-sex dyads working on a collaborative task. Results revealed that many dyads developed intriguing rhythmic patterns that were distinguishable from overall shifts in interpersonal behavior. Dyad members' shared behavior cycles had roughly the same frequency, with strongly correlated moment-to-moment variations in extremity. Moreover, their affiliation cycles tended to be strongly in phase (with peaks and troughs occurring simultaneously), and their dominance cycles tended to be strongly out of phase (with peaks of one person coinciding with troughs of the other). Furthermore, such entrainment on affiliation was uncorrelated with entrainment on dominance. Of particular relevance, dyads varied considerably in their degree of entrainment, ranging from virtually none to virtually the maximum possible.

Indeed, there is great potential for investigating meaningful individual differences of this sort. For example, the joystick approach revealed that female dyads with higher affiliative entrainment tended to complete collaborative tasks faster and with better quality (Markey, Lowmaster, & Eichler, 2010). It has also been applied to the study of parallel processes in supervision, revealing not only evidence of these processes, but also an inverted-U pattern of similarity (high–low–high) of client-to-therapist behavior that is associated with positive client outcome (Tracey, Bludworth, & Glidden-Tracey, 2012).

In addition, very recently published work shows other ways that this approach can be applied to help clarify the study of interpersonal processes in psychotherapy (Thomas, Hopwood, Woody, Ethier, & Sadler, 2014), and how these types of processes relate to cognitive-emotional processing and the therapeutic alliance in psychotherapy for depression (Altenstein, Kreiger, & Grosse Holtforth, 2013). Furthermore, the joystick approach has been applied to better understand how children evoke responses from mothers during their interactions (Klahr, Thomas, Hopwood, Klump, & Burt, 2013), and how interpersonal processes discriminate important student–teacher relationships (Pennings et al., 2014).

Ongoing and future work reveals the considerable potential of the joystick approach to assessing people's social behavior to help better understand both normal and psychopathological processes that occur during social interactions. For example, researchers are currently investigating how processes involving dominance and affiliation differ in same-sex versus mixed-sex unacquainted dyads (Sadler, Lizdek, Hunt, & Woody, 2011), how romantic couples' neutral and conflict interactions differ (Hunt, Sadler, & Zuroff, 2012), how depression affects social behavior during couples' conflicts (Lizdek, Woody, Sadler, & Rehman, 2012), how borderline women interact differently during first meetings with another person (Thomas, Hopwood, & Morey, 2012), and how the dynamics of parent–child interactions vary (Ansell, Thomas, Hopwood, & Chaplin, 2012).

Challenges

Here we briefly review three issues about the joystick technique that have not yet been fully resolved. Each of these issues points to interesting variants or extensions of how the technique may be used in the future. First, use of the joystick as a coding technique reflects an at least implicit assumption that interaction dynamics consist of reasonably continuous ebbs and flows, which include rhythmic regularities persisting long enough that cyclical patterns such as entrainment between partners can be discerned. To the extent that interactions are characterized instead by sudden discontinuities that occur at irregular intervals, the technique is arguably less applicable. However, as mentioned earlier, the joystick's "firing" button (as well as other buttons) can be used to mark unique events or transition points in the record—for example, the abrupt introduction of an important new topic, a particular type of therapist intervention, or a dramatic affective shift in a psychotherapy session. These transition points can be used to distinguish different contexts that may affect the flow of interpersonal dynamics. In addition, if one wishes to avoid assuming that the same rhythmic patterns and entrainments characterize the entire duration of an interaction (an assumption called *stationarity*), there are methods for searching out shorter periods of stable dynamic patterns within the interaction, such as the graphical technique of *windowed cross correlation* (Boker et al., 2002).

Second, in our research using the joystick technique, we take considerable pains to avoid the possible impact of biases and misperceptions of individual observers. We carefully train new joystick coders by comparing their time-series data to those from more experienced, established coders (Lizdek et al., 2012). In addition, we use multiple independent raters (typically four) and then average the data from these raters at each point in time. This yields a composite, consensual time series that attenuates the idiosyncratic perceptions of any particular individual observer. The interrater reliabilities of these consensual time series tend to be quite good (Sadler et al., 2009). However, rather than avoiding individual biases and idiosyncratic perceptions, we might also use the joystick technique to examine these biases and patterns of misperception. For example, to study the perceptions of the interacting participants themselves, we may have them watch a video of their interaction and use the joystick to rate self and other. This could provide a unique window on the interpersonal perceptions of the interactants. Another possible example would be having a student psychotherapist and her supervisor independently rate a psychotherapy session, and then compare the respective times series to look for divergent perceptions.

Third, because use of the joystick technique requires observers to simultaneously and continuously code, in effect, two orthogonal dimensions, it is interesting to reflect on the attentional demands entailed. On one hand, Wiggins (1982, 2003) argued that the IPC represents the actual circular structure that underlies people's intuitive interpersonal perceptions (see also Tracey & Rolfing, 2010). Thus, use of the Cartesian plane, involving both major dimensions at the same time, ought to provide a natural and intuitively straightforward way to organize and record interpersonal perceptions. On the other hand, it is conceivable that the attentional demands of the task would be reduced considerably by having observers rate dominance alone on one pass through the interaction video and affiliation alone on another pass. This approach might increase the quality of the resulting data and help to ensure that all observers devote equal attention to the two basic interpersonal dimensions. There is an option in the joystick-monitoring program that allows just one dimension to be rated at a time (e.g., along the horizontal axis), and the separately coded dominance and affiliation data streams can later easily be combined for graphing and data analysis. The impact of this alternative procedure on the quality of resulting data is currently being studied.

Case Examples: Moment-to-Moment Interpersonal Dynamics

The joystick method, together with appropriate graphics, may have intriguing uses for clinical training and understanding psychotherapy processes. Tracey (2004) has drawn important attention to the fact that much of complementarity lies in the inner details of an interaction—what he calls the *behavioral interchange level*. In contrast to some very labor-intensive, act-by-act rating methods for tracking these details, the joystick method may provide a fully practical way to track the inner details of an interaction. For example, a clinical student could watch a video of a substantial segment of his or her psychotherapy session twice, once to rate the client's behavior and once to rate his or her own behavior. While using the joystick, the student could use its firing button to mark any instances of what he or she perceives to be critical incidents, for later annotation of the time series.

Once the joystick coding is done, the challenge is to get all this information into a form that would facilitate thought and insight, and might be a useful adjunct for clinical supervision or therapeutic intervention. But such information processing could easily be done in less than a second with a computer program. What should the resulting output look like? For this purpose, we have adapted some ideas by Tufte (2006), specifically what he calls *sparklines*. What we want is a compact, high-resolution graphic that presents the trends and variations in an accessible way, in which all prominent visual elements convey relevant information that can be readily embedded into a narrative context such as assessment reports, therapy notes, treatment summaries, and client feedback.

Figure 2.4 shows such a graphic, based on an actual therapy session. At the top, we have the combined time series for affiliation, and at the right numbers show the average level of affiliation for each person (the client in black and the therapist in gray). An important attribute of sparklines is that they do not unnecessarily complicate and wall off the graphic with a network of axes. Below, we have the combined time series for dominance, again with numbers at the right providing the average level of dominance for the client and therapist. Note that the time-series supplements the average information in important ways. For example, although the averages indicate that overall the therapist is more dominant than the client, the plot shows that there are a number of time points when this pattern reverses.

The black vertical lines indicate critical incidents recorded by the student. We would add a brief annotation of the nature of each of these events, as they are potentially of great interest for identifying the ways in which critical incidents may change (or temporarily disrupt) the ongoing series. For example, Event A appears to bring about a striking change in the time series for affiliation—high-amplitude cycles give way to a slow drift downward—and Event B precedes the lowest troughs in the client's level of dominance. The clinical supervisor could sometimes use the joystick to

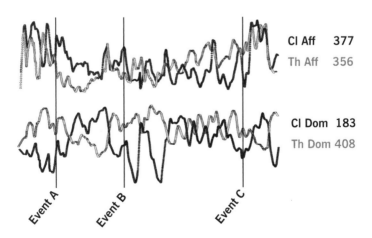

FIGURE 2.4. Sparklines for a therapy session showing affiliation (top graph) and dominance (bottom graph) over time for the client (dark) and therapist (light). The numbers at the right provide the average value across the session (Cl Aff, client affiliation; Th Aff, therapist affiliation; Cl Dom, client dominance; Th Dom, therapist dominance).

code a segment as well, to provide calibration and possibly a different point of view. However, one well-trained rater (typically the clinical trainee) appears to be sufficient for obtaining meaningful, useful output.

Several benefits for clinical supervision might come out of this approach. First, it makes the student mindful of variation in behavior and its cyclical nature. Second, to the extent that therapeutic interventions are designed to alter interaction patterns, it provides a window of evidence about whether they are having the desired effect. Third, it provides a framework for examining how critical incidents may alter ongoing interpersonal processes. Fourth, it shows how the therapist's interpersonal behavior is intertwined with the client's behavior, in ways that may shed light on the therapist's inadvertent contribution to the process. Finally, over multiple therapy sessions, it provides a detailed record of how interpersonal behavior may be changing.

More generally, the joystick method has wide applicability for studying psychotherapy processes and dynamics. Such research is consistent with broader calls to examine data from psychotherapy sessions, which provide a "natural laboratory" for psychotherapy process research (Borckardt et al., 2008). To illustrate, we briefly summarize the results of a study by Thomas et al. (2014), which applied the joystick method to the psychotherapy sessions in Shostrom's (1966) well-known films involving the client, Gloria. The films record three psychotherapy sessions with Gloria, one with each of three prominent therapists, Albert Ellis, Frederick Perls, and Carl Rogers, as they demonstrated their respective rational-emotive, gestalt, and client-centered approaches to psychotherapy. These sessions offer the opportunity to compare the interpersonal processes that unfolded with one client across sessions with three therapists whose theoretical orientations were quite distinct.

Gloria's moment-to-moment interpersonal behaviors differed across each session in ways that were, in part, predictable based on each therapist's moment-to-moment behavior. For instance, affiliative and controlling behaviors were complementary in each session, indicating a sameness between Gloria's and the therapists' affiliative behaviors and an oppositeness between their controlling and submissive behaviors. Ellis was the most controlling therapist, and, consistent with interpersonal complementarity, Gloria was more submissive in her session with Ellis than in her other sessions. In contrast, Gloria tended to be controlling in her session with Rogers, who tended to behave submissively.

These findings are consistent with the principle that clients' interpersonal behaviors are malleable and in part dependent on the behaviors of their therapists. They illustrate how therapists can create an atmosphere that encourages clients to take agency in their treatment by listening with minimal interruption, resisting temptations to make important decisions for clients, and so on (i.e., behaving submissively). In contrast, therapists can create an atmosphere in which clients follow their lead by talking frequently, providing suggestions, controlling the flow of the conversation, and the like (i.e., behaving dominantly). Each of those goals serves therapeutic functions at various times in working with various clients, and it is useful for therapists to consider ways in which their momentary interpersonal behaviors can be used to influence the behaviors of their clients to promote change processes (see also Anchin & Pincus, 2010; Cain & Pincus, in press).

Examining overall means for the entire sessions, a global complementarity also emerged for affiliation. Overall, Rogers was warmer than Ellis, and Perls was the coldest. Consistent with the theory of interpersonal complementarity, Gloria was warmest in her session with Rogers and coldest in her session with Perls. Whereas session means indicate aggregate interpersonal behaviors, the intraindividual standard deviation (*iSD*) indicates variability within each session and provides important additional information about interpersonal process. The *iSD* for Gloria's affiliative behavior was nearly three times as large in her session with Perls as her session with Rogers, indicating that Gloria rarely deviated from her warm baseline with Rogers, whereas her behaviors with Perls ranged widely from hostile to friendly. Overall, these results indicate that Gloria was generally submissive when interacting with a dominant therapist (Ellis), generally warm and assertive when interacting with a warm and submissive therapist (Rogers), and highly reactive when interacting with a therapist who had a propensity to vary in warm and cold behavior within a session (Perls). These findings highlight predictable ways in which a client's behavior differed as a function of therapists' behaviors. This indeed supports interpersonal psychotherapy's intervention recommendations regarding strategically altering therapist behavior in session to facilitate change in clients' momentary interpersonal behaviors and ultimately long-term change via social learning in the therapeutic relationship (Anchin & Kiesler, 1982; Anchin & Pincus, 2010; Benjamin, 1996).

In addition to comparing interpersonal processes across sessions, the joystick method can be fruitfully applied to single sessions to locate important shifts in interpersonal processes within a session. For example, examination of time-series graphs of a session, such as the sparklines presented earlier, can reveal such within-session changes. To illustrate, although Gloria and Ellis demonstrated the most complementary of the three therapy sessions on average, their degree of complementarity varied over the course of the interaction. Of note, midway through the interaction they demonstrated a noncomplementary pattern of affiliation. Qualitative analysis of the transcript during this window suggests that Ellis was presuming that Gloria's problems were more severe and pervasive than she felt them to be. Notably, Ellis also interrupts her during this window and asserts his status (e.g., "my trained ears") on several occasions. Uncovering relatively discrepant episodes such as this has important applications in psychotherapy-process research, as well as in clinical supervision.

In future research, comparisons across sessions can be readily conducted to examine how the therapist's behaviors vary across several clients (as occurs routinely in practice). Such work would highlight important dyadic influences on therapists' behaviors across clients with varying demographics, personalities, and diagnoses. Being aware of such influences would permit clinicians to gain increased insight into the interplay between the therapist and client interpersonal behaviors and would thus facilitate skill in promoting behavior changes in clients. For instance, Ellis promoted learning by engaging in a didactic and leading manner toward Gloria; Perls promoted a genuine expression of negative affect in Gloria by behaving critically; and Rogers promoted agency in Gloria by refusing to give her advice on several occasions.

Interpersonal Dynamics of Daily Life

Evaluating interpersonal behavior at a moment-to-moment level confers several benefits for assessment (described above), however much a patient's interpersonal difficulties are expressed outside of session. Such moment-to-moment evaluations of interpersonal behavior are difficult to gather when the patient is not in the natural laboratory of the consulting room. The clinician interested in tracking interpersonal difficulties outside of session can rely on diary methods to systematically record many of the patient's salient life moments (Mehl & Connor, 2012). In clinical psychology this is often accomplished by responding to conveniently accessible brief questionnaires and surveys (Luxton, McCann, Bush, Mishkind, & Reger, 2011; Trull, Ebner-Priemer, Brown, Tomko, & Scheiderer, 2012). Advances in various experience sampling methods allow for repeated assessments throughout the day based on various schedules or prompts (ecological momentary assessment [EMA]; Shiffman, Stone, & Hufford, 2008), or following predetermined events (event-contingent recording [ECR]; Moskowitz & Sadikaj, 2012). Assessment in the context of daily life is distinct in that it captures an individual's experience in his or her natural setting, with data that can be analyzed over different timescales (minutes, hours, days, weeks), all the way up to an aggregated summary of the individual across the entirety of the assessment timeframe.

Assessing Interpersonal Dynamics Using Event-Contingent Recording

ECR questionnaires can be completed as paper-and-pencil diaries or as electronic diaries recorded on smartphones and other electronic mobile devices. It is useful to assess the interpersonal behavior of others (i.e., the patient's interpersonal perception) and the patient's interpersonal behaviors (Roche, Pincus, Conroy, Hyde, & Ram, 2014). Interpersonal perception can be assessed using the Interpersonal Grid (IG; Moskowitz & Zuroff, 2005a), where the horizontal dimension represents communal perception (friendly vs. unfriendly) and the vertical axis represents agentic perception (dominant vs. submissive). The patient marks an "X" on the two-dimensional grid to represent the interaction partner's levels of communion and agency during the interaction. The patient's interpersonal behavior can be assessed using the Social Behavior Inventory (SBI; Moskowitz, 1994), which includes sets of behavioral acts that the patient endorses. Alternatively, one can assess agentic and communal interpersonal perceptions and behaviors using a series of bipolar dimensional ratings. Figure 2.5 presents a screenshot of this approach, which we used for an electronic diary study (expanded upon later in the chapter in the case example), where interpersonal perceptions, behaviors, and other items are represented as a series of bipolar dimensions.

Empirical Review

A number of studies employing ECR to investigate interpersonal dynamics support the reliability and validity of the assessment methodology. These studies can be organized around the dynamics of interpersonal variability, reciprocal interpersonal patterns, and interpersonal covariation.

Interpersonal Variability

Theory and research suggest that the assessment of intraindividual variability offers unique and important new methods for the description of

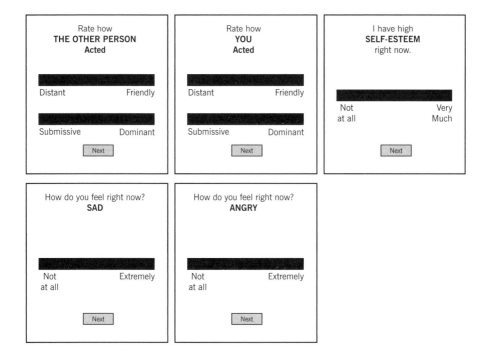

FIGURE 2.5. An event-contingent recording survey to assess interpersonal dynamics in daily life.

personality and psychopathology (Ram et al., 2013; Ram, Conroy, Pincus, Hyde, & Molloy, 2012). Different quantitative indices of variability can be derived from ECR assessments using the IPC, each based on either a linear or circular iSD around an individual's mean behavioral score (iMN). Moskowitz and Zuroff (2004, 2005b) introduced the terms *flux*, *pulse*, and *spin* to describe these different IPC-based variability indices. Consistent with the variability in moment-to-moment interactions discussed earlier, *flux* refers to the variability of agentic or communal behaviors (the iSD for the IPC dimensions or their components—dominance, submissiveness, friendliness, and quarrelsomeness). *Pulse* refers to the variability of the overall intensity of reported behavior (the iSD for all vectors from the center of the IPC). *Spin* refers to variability of the type of emitted behavior (i.e., a circular iSD based on all IPC locations of reported behaviors). For example, low flux reflects little variability on a single dimension (either agency or communion), whereas low pulse reflects little variability in global behavioral intensity. If low flux or low pulse were associated with a high mean intensity generally, it would be consistent with the chronic enactment of intense interpersonal behaviors. Low spin reflects a narrow repertoire of interpersonal behaviors enacted over time. This dynamic lexicon has important implications for the assessment of normal and abnormal behavior (Pincus et al., 2010).

In a 20-day ECR study, 38 females diagnosed with borderline personality disorder (BPD) and 44 nonclinical controls matched for gender and age reported on their social interactions (Russell, Moskowitz, Zuroff, Sookman, & Paris, 2007). Although individuals in the BPD group did not report lower average levels of friendly behavior (iMN), they did display greater variability (flux) in friendliness, suggesting acute elevations and reductions of friendly behavior. This group also exhibited increased variability (flux) in quarrelsome and dominant behaviors, consistent with clinical descriptions of BPD. The BPD group additionally exhibited higher spin, consistent with the notion of behavioral lability in patients with BPD. Patients with BPD are well known for having chaotic relationships, and interpersonal spin may be an important dynamic feature of relationship disruption. Even in community dwelling adults, higher interpersonal spin had a number of negative impacts on relationship closeness (Côté, Moskowitz, & Zuroff, 2012). Important preliminary evidence suggests that interpersonal spin is related to lower levels of serotonergic activity in the brain (Moskowitz, Zuroff, aan het Rot, & Young, 2011).

Reciprocal Interpersonal Patterns

Interpersonal behavior is not emitted in a vacuum; it must be contextualized around the influences of others (Ebner-Priemer, Eid, Kleindienst, Stabenow, & Trull, 2009; Mischel & Shoda, 2010). Assessing and identifying stable *if (situation)–then (behavior)* behavioral signatures is becoming an important area of personality and clinical research (Kammrath & Scholer,

2013; Mischel & Shoda, 2008). A key implication of situation–behavior contingencies is the need to identify the psychologically salient features of situations, and this requires an organizing psychological theory. Interpersonal theory asserts that the interpersonal features of situations are most salient (Pincus & Ansell, 2013), and we recommend that assessment of patient interpersonal behavior be contextualized by the perceived interpersonal behavior of the others with whom they interact in daily life (Roche et al., 2014). As shown in Figure 2.5, the patient's agentic and communal behaviors and perceptions of others can both be assessed with common IPC dimensions. When the perceived agentic and communal characteristics of the other person(s) in a social interaction *(ifs)* are linked with the patient's interpersonal behavior *(thens)*, we can describe a reciprocal interpersonal pattern. In addition to patient behaviors, the perceived agentic and communal characteristics of the other person(s) in a social interaction *(ifs)* can also be usefully linked with emotional or symptomatic responses *(thens)*.

The most common reciprocal interpersonal patterns examined empirically reflect the dynamics of interpersonal complementarity (i.e., sameness and oppositeness). In a 20-day ECR study (Fournier, Moskowitz, & Zuroff, 2008) of the social interactions of community-dwelling adults, the complementary themes of oppositeness along the dimension of agency (e.g., meeting dominance with submissiveness) and sameness along the dimension of communion (e.g., meeting friendliness with friendliness) were confirmed. A similar ECR study (Moskowitz, Ringo Ho, & Turcotte-Tremblay, 2007) also examined role status relative to the interaction partner and where the interaction took place (e.g., work vs. nonwork setting). The authors reported that individuals were more likely to exhibit communal complementarity when not at work and when in a high-status work role. Agentic complementarity (e.g., meeting dominance with submission or meeting submission with dominance) was only found in work settings, and this effect strengthened when the individual was in the high-status work role. In contrast, a 7-day ECR study (Roche, Pincus, Conroy, et al., 2013) examined whether noncomplementary interpersonal patterns are related to psychopathology and found that pathological narcissism moderated the relationship between interpersonal perceptions *(ifs)* and behaviors *(thens)*. Individuals high in narcissistic grandiosity tended to respond to perceiving dominance and friendliness in others with increased dominant behavior themselves (i.e., a noncomplementary pattern on dominance). However, the same individuals responded in a complementary fashion (lower dominance) when the other was perceived as dominant and unfriendly.

Research has also examined patients' emotions and symptoms *(thens)* in relation to perceptions of others' interpersonal behavior *(ifs)*. In a 20-day ECR study (Sadikaj, Russell, Moskowitz, & Paris, 2010), patients diagnosed with BPD, relative to community controls, reported a greater increase in negative affect when they perceived others as less friendly and a smaller increase in positive affect when they perceived others as more friendly. This increased negative affect contributed to increased quarrelsome behavior in patients, instigating a cycle of negative transactions (Sadikaj, Moskowitz, Russell, Zuroff, & Paris, 2013). In a similar ECR study of community-dwelling adults (Sadikaj, Moskowitz, & Zuroff, 2011), the association between perceiving others as less friendly and negative affect was stronger for individuals higher on attachment anxiety and was weaker for individuals higher on attachment avoidance. These effects were more pronounced in interactions with a romantic partner than with other persons.

Interpersonal Covariation

Researchers are also investigating how agentic and communal experiences are linked (i.e., within-person covariation) in the patient's behaviors and perceptions of others. In a 20-day ECR study (Fournier, Moskowitz, and Zuroff, 2009), investigators calculated within-person associations of agentic and communal behaviors for each participant. A tendency to concurrently behave in a dominant and friendly manner was associated with less neuroticism, less depression, and higher self-esteem. This research was extended to examine the covariation of interpersonal perceptions (Roche, Pincus, Hyde, et al., 2013). The investigators found that individuals higher in dependency, relative to those lower in dependency, exhibited a stronger tendency to concurrently perceive others' dominance as also friendly. Conversely, individuals higher in narcissistic grandiosity, relative to those lower in narcissistic grandiosity, exhibited a weaker tendency to concurrently perceive others' dominance as also friendly. This research suggests that the covariation of agentic and communal interpersonal experiences (behaviors and perceptions) in daily life is related to well-being and psychopathology.

Case Example: Occasion-to-Occasion Interpersonal Dynamics over 3 Weeks in a Patient's Life

In this section we apply the principles of variability, complementarity, and covariation to a single clinical patient participating in a 21-day diary study. He was 49 years old, married, and engaged in weekly psychotherapy at a community mental health center. The patient provided data on multiple timescales (beginning of study, end of study, end of day, event-contingent assessments throughout day), but we will only focus on his event-contingent responses (face-to-face social interactions lasting at least 5 minutes). He recorded his responses through a survey delivered on a smartphone provided to him. Dimensional ratings were indicated using a touch point continuum ranging from 0 to 100 (see Figure 2.5). Over the 21 days, he recorded 136 social interactions (75% with his spouse).

To begin, we consider his overall levels of interpersonal perception and behavior (see Table 2.2). Without sufficient normative data, it is difficult to determine whether his overall scores are high or low compared to others (e.g., is 78.79 out of 100 a high or low score for communal perception?).

Instead, we evaluate his scores across different contexts (spouse vs. others). The patient perceived his spouse as more communal compared to other interaction partners (see Table 2.2). He reported behaving in a friendlier and more dominant manner with her than with his other interaction partners. We can also consider his pattern of variability within contexts. Variability in perception and behavior was not significantly different across contexts, indicating he was as flexible when interacting with his spouse as he was with other interaction partners.

These reports also allow us to consider several important implications regarding this patient's social exchanges in daily life. For example, does he engage in communal and agentic complementarity, and with whom are those patterns strengthened or weakened? How do complementary interactions impact his well-being? Figure 2.6 plots his interactions over his 21 days. In the top series, the darker line representing communal perception tends to move together with the lighter line representing communal behavior, consistent with the principle of communal complementarity ($r =$ .71, $p < .05$). His profile demonstrates how this association moves in both directions, including meeting the other's low communion with low communion of his own. In the bottom series, the darker line representing agentic

TABLE 2.2. Means and Variability for ECR Interpersonal Assessment

	Total	Spouse	Other
Summary of perceptions			
Communal mean	78.79	81.65[a]	72.60[b]
Agentic mean	55.54	55.09	56.51
Communal flux	18.03	17.69	17.39
Agentic flux	15.52	16.85	12.26
Pulse	10.50	9.26	10.30
Spin	0.69	0.62	0.81
Summary of behaviors			
Communal mean	71.88	75.60[a]	63.84[b]
Agentic mean	54.04	56.04[a]	49.70[b]
Communal flux	21.17	20.82	19.84
Agentic flux	15.89	15.31	16.44
Pulse	13.38	12.36	13.59
Spin	0.93	0.78	1.24

Note. $N_{total} = 136$, $N_{spouse} = 87$, $N_{other} = 18$. Mean scores compared using independent t-test. Flux scores are linear standard deviations and are direct transformations (square root) of the variances for the variables. Therefore, we calculated differences in flux by examining equality of variances contained within the t-test (Levene's test). To examine pulse, we calculated vector length for each interaction and subjected these scores to an independent t-test, examining equality of variance to determine significant differences in pulse. Since spin is a circular standard deviation, the same method could not be applied, so we did not evaluate significant differences of spin across interaction context. Significant differences ($p < .05$) denoted where $a > b$.

perception moves in an opposite direction from the lighter line representing agentic behaviors, indicating agentic complementarity ($r = -.54$, $p < .05$). Although we do not present examinations of temporal interrelations in the present case, it is possible to do so employing the methods described earlier in the chapter, modified to address the fact that the time series is irregularly sampled (Stoica & Sandgren, 2006). At a molar level, adherence to complementarity may be indicative of normal interpersonal functioning. Zooming in on particular interaction patterns that deviate from this may help us to better understand the source of the patient's unique interpersonal difficulties.

We next consider whether different contexts impact the patient's complementarity. Communal complementarity was significantly stronger for interactions with his spouse ($r = .78$, $p < .05$), compared to others ($r = .50$, $r_{diff} = .28$, $z = 2.61$, $p < .05$). Agentic complementarity was also significantly stronger for interactions with his spouse ($r = -.64$, $p < .05$), compared to others ($r = -.29$, $r_{diff} = .35$, $z = 2.42$, $p < .05$). This finding might indicate a greater responsiveness to perceptions and behaviors toward his wife compared to others in his life.

However, we further investigated the patient's agentic behavior by distinguishing interactions where he perceived himself to be in a dominant position (i.e., his agentic behavior score was greater than his perception of

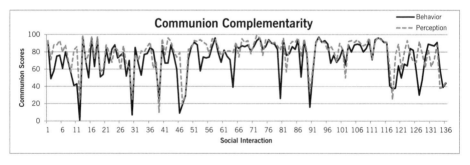

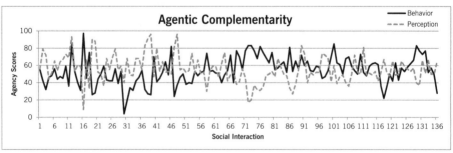

FIGURE 2.6. Interpersonal complementarity across the events reported during the patient's 21-day study.

his partner's agency, $n = 62$) or in a submissive position (n = 71). We then recalculated his agentic complementarity correlations in these two subsets of interactions, and compared the correlation coefficients. When he was in the more dominant position, agentic complementarity remained ($r = -.46$, $p < .05$), but when he was in the less dominant position, agentic complementarity was not found ($r = .02$, $p > .05$, $r_{diff} = .48$, $z = 2.94$, $p < .05$). In other words, he was much more likely to engage in agentic complementarity when he was in the dominant role; this finding might point to difficulties or conflicts with relying on, deferring to, or cooperating with others.

We then explored how complementarity concurrently impacted the patient's well-being. We created regression models in which his agentic behavior was predicted by his agentic perceptions (i.e., agentic complementarity), a functioning variable (functioning variables are self-esteem, angry, and sad, all entered into separate models), and the interaction (i.e. moderating effect) of that functioning variable with agentic perception (see Table 2.3). We found significant interactions, indicating that when agentic complementarity was weaker (e.g., weaker negative association between his agentic perception and behavior), he tended to concurrently report experiencing lower self-esteem and more sadness. We conducted similar analyses for communal complementarity (replacing agentic behavior and perceptions with communal behavior and perceptions; see Table 2.3) but found that the functioning variables did not moderate the strength of communal complementarity.

The patient's interpersonal experiences were graphed as polar plots of interpersonal perception and behavior (Figure 2.7). The plot on the left indicated that he perceived others' agency as also unfriendly ($r = -.51$, $p < .05$), and this effect was strengthened during interactions with his spouse ($r = -.67$, $p < .05$), compared to others ($r = -.06$, $p > .05$, $r_{diff} = .61$, $z = 3.95$, $p < .05$). The plot on the right indicated that he reported his own agentic behavior as also friendly, and this effect did not differ among interaction partners ($z = 1.91$, $p > .05$). These analyses suggest that he does not have a core schema that links others' dominance with coldness but instead a contextualized (wife's dominance) *if–then* pattern of interpersonal perception. Perhaps this partially explains his low likelihood of exhibiting complementarity by submitting to others.

We then explored how covariation concurrently impacted his well-being. We created regression models in which his agentic perception was predicted by his communal perception (i.e., perception covariation), as well as functioning variables and the interaction of each functioning variable with communal perception (see Table 2.3). We constructed similar regression models, replacing perceptions with behaviors to evaluate behavior covariation. The strength of perception covariation was not moderated by any of the functioning variables, but the strength of behavior covariation was moderated by all three functioning variables (see Table 2.3 and Figure 2.7). During interactions where he linked dominant and friendly behavior,

TABLE 2.3. Functioning Variables Moderating Agentic and Communal Complementarity

Models	Functioning variables (standardized betas)		
	Self-esteem	Angry	Sad
Associations of agentic behavior	Agentic complementarity		
Time	0.44*	0.44*	0.44*
Agentic perception	−0.46*	−0.46*	−0.46*
Functioning variable	0.11	0.35*	0.09
Agentic perception × functioning variable	−0.29*	0.06	0.26*
Adjusted $R^2/\Delta R^2$	.47*/.09*	.49*/< .01	−.44*/.06*
Associations of communal behavior	Communal complementarity		
Time	0.40*	0.40*	0.40*
Communal perception	0.65*	0.65*	0.65*
Functioning variable	0.39*	−0.30*	−0.19*
Communal perception × functioning variable	−0.01	−0.13	−0.01
Adjusted $R^2/\Delta R^2$	.65*/< .01	.64*/.01	.58*/< .01
Associations of agentic perception	Perception covariation		
Time	−0.24*	−0.24*	−0.24*
Communal perception	−0.48*	−0.48*	−0.48*
Functioning variable	−0.24*	0.25*	0.18*
Communal perception × functioning variable	−0.11	−0.03	−0.14
Adjusted $R^2/\Delta R^2$	.30*/.01	.31*/< .01	−.30*/.02
Associations of agentic behavior	Behavior covariation		
Time	0.44*	0.44*	0.44*
Communal behavior	0.23*	0.23*	0.23*
Functioning variable	0.27*	0.31*	0.02
Communal behavior × functioning variable	0.25*	−0.57*	−0.30*
Adjusted $R^2/\Delta R^2$	.30*/.04*	.37*/.08*	−.30*/.08*

Note. n = 136 observations for 1 individual. ΔR^2 refers to the change in variance explained after including interactions in model. Time = covariate controlling for the order in which the interactions were reported. Columns denote which functioning variable was included in the model (separately). *p < .05.

he tended to concurrently report higher self-esteem, lower anger, and lower sadness. Notably, the distinct moderation of interpersonal behavior and not interpersonal perception suggests that the way the patient views his own behaviors is more strongly linked to his current state of well-being than how he sees others in his daily life.

The interpersonal story the patient tells through his diary records is predominantly one of agency. In his daily life he engages in agentic complementarity, especially with his wife, but he is much less likely to do this by assuming a submissive position relative to others. These noncomplementary

Plots of Interpersonal Covariation

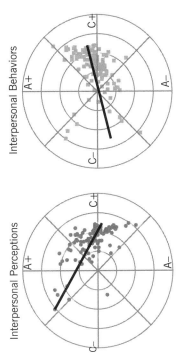

Interpersonal Perceptions   Interpersonal Behaviors

Moderators of Agentic and Communal Behavior Covariation

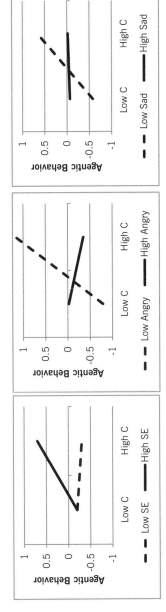

FIGURE 2.7. Plots of interpersonal covariation and moderators of interpersonal covariation. Top: Agency (A) and communion (C) scores are converted into polar coordinates, then plotted. Bottom: Low and high values are plotted ± 1 SD from the sample-centered average. C, communal behavior. SE, self-esteem.

interactions negatively impact his well-being. He perceives his wife's dominance as also unfriendly, but this does not appear to impact his well-being, and neither does communal complementarity. In contrast, he perceives his own dominance as friendly, and deviating from this self-view negatively impacts his well being. Given his profile, it is likely he has more difficulty interacting with individuals he sees as dominant, as he may be less willing to exhibit complementary oppositeness in relating to them, and leaves the interaction feeling poorly. Together, it appears that in the patient's daily life, he is minimally influenced by communion in general or his perceptions of others. Instead, his well-being depends almost entirely on his ability to engage in agentic complementarity (especially when he is in the dominant role) and to feel that his dominance is being enacted in a friendly way.

This type of analysis allows clinicians to see how the dynamics of interpersonal dysfunction occur naturally in their client's daily life. It can uncover whether the client generally engages in normative social exchanges (e.g., complementarity), and it can zoom in to uncover the particular contexts (or people) in which this pattern deviates. This is clinically quite useful for identifying focal problems and targeting therapeutic interventions. It can further help the clinician understand how these interpersonal exchanges and experiences impact the client's self-concept, emotions, and symptoms. This type of assessment may be particularly useful to uncover experiences that the client cannot identify retrospectively (e.g., realizing that he tends to see his wife's dominance as unfriendly, but he does not see others in this way). Assessments occur repeatedly and intensively every time the contingent event is experienced, and this can be flexibly determined by the clinician and patient. In conducting an ECR assessment, the clinician must be careful to select the right variables (e.g., anger, urges to self-harm, use of substances) to address the questions of importance for both patient and clinician. It is also important to balance the specificity regarding contextual categories (e.g., can family members be combined into one category, or should they be distinct given the presenting problems?). Assessments must be designed to yield more than a few reportable events for each category in order for it to be usefully analyzed and interpreted. Previous research empirically evaluating this method has typically defined the contingent event as a face-to-face social interaction lasting at least 5 minutes (Moskowitz, 2009). However, this is an arbitrary decision. For example, emerging technologies have greatly increased the frequency of real-time social interactions that are not face to face (e.g., texting, mobile phone calls, Facebook). In addition, many important social interactions, such as those involving unfriendly behaviors and unpleasant feelings, may not last 5 minutes (Roche, Pincus, Conroy, et al., 2013). Therefore, assessors should thoughtfully consider the operationalization of contingent events. This method of interpersonal assessment, though new, holds potential in helping the clinician see a larger scope of the patient's social world (Roche et al., 2014).

Conclusions

The assessment of the interpersonal dynamics of personality, social interactions, and daily life is truly a multimethod approach, with a broad range of foci for clinical research, training, and practice. In our view, assessing interpersonal dynamics supplies value-added information beyond psychiatric diagnosis by providing an important context for understanding the patient's symptoms and functioning, and for enhancing case conceptualization, treatment planning, and outcome assessment. Assessing interpersonal dynamics also has potential to directly enhance clinical training by providing detailed and tailored feedback to trainees regarding differences in relational functioning across patients, as well as shifts in relational functioning within specific sessions or in response to critical therapeutic events.

Multimethod assessment of interpersonal dynamics provides new interpretative approaches to familiar self- and informant reports, as well as newly emerging assessment techniques that are rapidly evolving with technological advances. Many of the methods for collecting, managing, scoring, and graphing the assessment data are modularized and adaptable. Continuing technological developments will help clinicians, patients, supervisors, and trainees employ these methods easily (e.g., on the patient's own mobile device and on the trainee's laptop computer) and understand assessment results quickly and collaboratively through automated scoring/graphing routines. Advances in 3-D graphics and time-series analyses will help identify moment-to-moment and occasion-to-occasion dynamic patterns of clinical interest. This is particularly exciting because new technologies allow for concurrent assessment and integration of self-report, contextual (e.g., audio, video), and physiological data in the laboratory, the consulting room, and the natural settings of daily life. Importantly, all the methods presented here are based on sound psychometric principles and have empirical support for their reliability and validity. They could be used together in assessing an individual case, and ultimately, we would like to develop guidelines for multimethod assessment of interpersonal dynamics. Although we expect structural and temporal dynamics at various timescales to be meaningfully related, empirical investigations that concurrently employ these multiple methods are a necessary next step.

REFERENCES

Alden, L. E., Wiggins, J. S., & Pincus, A. L. (1990). Construction of circumplex scales of the Inventory of Interpersonal Problems. *Journal of Personality Assessment, 55,* 521–536.

Altenstein, D., Kreiger, T., & Grosse Holtforth, M. (2013). Interpersonal microprocesses predict cognitive-emotional processing and the therapeutic alliance in psychotherapy for depression. *Journal of Counseling Psychology, 60,* 445–452.

American Psychiatric Association. (2013). *Diagnostic and statistical manual of mental disorders* (5th ed.). Arlington, VA: Author.

Anchin, J. C., & Kiesler, D. J. (1982). *Handbook of interpersonal psychotherapy*. New York: Pergamon Press.

Anchin, J. C., & Pincus, A. L. (2010). Evidence-based interpersonal psychotherapy with personality disorders: theory, components, and strategies. In J. J. Magnavita (Ed.), *Evidence-based treatment of personality dysfunction: Principles, methods, and processes* (pp. 113–166). Washington, DC: American Psychological Association.

Ansell, E. B., Thomas, K. M., Hopwood, C. J., & Chaplin, T. M. (2012). *Interpersonal complementarity and stress in a parent–adolescent interaction task*. Paper presented at the annual meeting of the Society for Personality Assessment, Chicago, IL.

Benjamin, L. S. (1984). Principles of prediction using Structural Analysis of Social Behavior. In A. Zucker, J. Aronoff, & J. Rubin (Eds.), *Personality and the prediction of behavior* (pp. 121–173). New York: Academic Press.

Benjamin, L. S. (1996). *Interpersonal diagnosis and treatment of personality disorders* (2nd ed.). New York: Guilford Press.

Boker, S. M. (2002). Consequences of continuity: The hunt for intrinsic properties within parameters of dynamics in psychological processes. *Multivariate Behavioral Research, 37*, 405–422.

Boker, S. M., & Wenger, M. J. (2007). *Data analytic techniques for dynamical systems*. Mahwah, NJ: Erlbaum.

Boker, S. M., Xu, M., Rotondo, J. L., & King, K. (2002) Windowed cross-correlation and peak picking for the analysis of variability in the association between behavioral time series. *Psychological Methods, 7*, 338–355.

Borckardt, J. J., Nash, M. R., Murphy, M. D., Moore, M., Shaw, D., & O'Neil, P. (2008). Clinical practice as natural laboratory for psychotherapy research: A guide to case-based time-series analysis. *American Psychologist, 63(2)*, 77–95.

Cain, N. M., Ansell, E. B., Wright, A. G. C., Hopwood, C. J., Thomas, K. M., Pinto, A., et al. (2012). Interpersonal pathoplasticity in the course of major depression, *Journal of Consulting and Clinical Psychology, 80*, 78–86.

Cain, N. M., & Pincus, A. L. (in press). Treating maladaptive interpersonal signatures. In W. J. Livesley, G. S. Dimaggio, & J. F. Clarkin (Eds.), *Integrated treatment for personality disorder*. New York: Guilford Press.

Carson, R. C. (1969). *Interaction concepts of personality*. Chicago: Aldine.

Carson, R. C. (1991). The social-interactional viewpoint. In M. Hersen, A. Kazdin, & A. Bellack (Eds.), *The clinical psychology handbook* (2nd ed., pp. 185–199). New York: Pergamon Press.

Clarkin, J. F., Yeomans, F. E., & Kernberg, O. F. (2006). *Psychotherapy for borderline personality: Focusing on object relations*. Washington, DC: American Psychiatric Publishing.

Clifton, A., Turkheimer, E., & Oltmanns, T. F. (2005). Self- and peer perspectives on pathological personality traits and interpersonal problems. *Psychological Assessment, 14*, 123–131.

Côté, S., Moskowitz, D. S., & Zuroff, D. C. (2012). Social relationships and intraindividual variability in interpersonal behavior: Correlates of interpersonal spin. *Journal of Personality and Social Psychology, 102*, 646–659.

Ebner-Priemer, U. W., Eid, M., Kleindienst, N., Stabenow, S., & Trull, T. J. (2009). Analytic strategies for understanding affective (in)stability and other dynamic processes in psychopathology. *Journal of Abnormal Psychology, 118*, 195–202.

Erdelyi, M. H. (1985). *Psychoanalysis: Freud's cognitive psychology*. New York: Freeman.

Finn, S. E. (2007). *In our clients' shoes: Theory and techniques of therapeutic assessment*. Mahwah, NJ: Erlbaum.

Finn, S. E. (2011). Journeys through the valley of death: Multimethod psychological assessment and personality transformation in long-term psychotherapy. *Journal of Personality Assessment, 93,* 123–141.

Finn, S. E., Fischer, C. T., & Handler, L. (2012). Collaborative/therapeutic assessment: Basic concepts, history, and research. In S. E. Finn, C. T. Fischer, & L. Handler (Eds.), *Collaborative/therapeutic assessment: A casebook and guide* (pp. 1–24). Hoboken, NJ: Wiley.

Fournier, M. A., Moskowitz, D. S., & Zuroff, D. C. (2008). Integrating dispositions, signatures, and the interpersonal domain. *Journal of Personality and Social Psychology, 94,* 531–545.

Fournier, M. A., Moskowitz, D. S., & Zuroff, D. C. (2009). The interpersonal signature. *Journal of Research in Personality, 43,* 155–162.

Gurtman, M. B., & Balakrishnan, J. D. (1998). Circular measurement redux: The analysis and interpretation of interpersonal circle profiles. *Clinical Psychology: Science and Practice, 5,* 344–360.

Hatcher, R., & Rogers, D. (2009). Development and validation of a measure of interpersonal strengths: The Inventory of Interpersonal Strengths. *Psychological Assessment, 21,* 554–569.

Hopwood, C. J. (2010). An interpersonal perspective on the personality assessment process. *Journal of Personality Assessment, 92,* 471–479.

Hopwood, C. J., Ansell, E. B., Pincus, A. L., Wright, A. G. C., Lukowitsky, M. R., & Roche, M. J. (2011). The circumplex structure of interpersonal sensitivities. *Journal of Personality, 79,* 708–740.

Hopwood, C. J., Wright, A. G. C., Ansell, E. B., & Pincus, A. L. (2013). The interpersonal core of personality pathology. *Journal of Personality Disorders, 27,* 270–295.

Hunt, R., Sadler, P., & Zuroff, D. C. (2012, May). *Is romantic conflict a process of complementarity or accommodation?* Paper presented at the annual meeting of the Society for Interpersonal Theory and Research, Montreal, Quebec.

Kahneman, D. (2011). *Thinking, fast and slow*. Toronto: Doubleday/Random House.

Kammrath, L. K., & Scholer, A. A. (2013). The cognitive-affective processing system. In H. A. Tennen & J. M. Suls (Eds.), *Handbook of psychology: Vol. 5. Personality and social psychology* (pp. 161–182). Hoboken, NJ: Wiley.

Kiesler, D. J. (1983). The 1982 interpersonal circle: A taxonomy for complementarity in human transactions. *Psychological Review, 90,* 185–214.

Kiesler, D. J. (1996). *Contemporary interpersonal theory and research: Personality, psychopathology, and psychotherapy*. Hoboken, NJ: Wiley.

Kiesler, D. J., & Schmidt, J. A. (1993). *The Impact Message Inventory: Form HA Octant Scale version*. Palo Alto, CA: Mind Garden.

Klahr, A. M., Thomas, K. M., Hopwood, C. J., Klump, K. L., & Burt, S. A. (2013). Evocative gene–environment correlation in the mother–child relationship: A twin study of interpersonal processes. *Development and Psychopathology, 25,* 105–118.

Leary, T. (1957). *Interpersonal diagnosis of personality*. New York: Ronald Press.

Lizdek, I., Sadler, P., Woody, E., Ethier, N., & Malet, G. (2012). Capturing the stream of behavior: A computer-joystick method for coding interpersonal behavior continuously over time. *Social Sciences Computer Review, 30,* 512–521.

Lizdek, I., Woody, E., Sadler, P., & Rehman, U. (2012). *Effects of depression on the dynamics of interpersonal complementarity.* Paper presented at the annual meeting of the Society for Interpersonal Theory and Research, Montreal, Quebec.

Locke, K. D. (2000). Circumplex scales of interpersonal values: Reliability, validity, and applicability to interpersonal problems and personality disorders. *Journal of Personality Assessment, 75,* 249–267.

Locke, K. D. (2011). Circumplex measures of interpersonal constructs. In L. M. Horowitz & S. Strack (Eds.), *Handbook of interpersonal psychology: Theory, research, assessment, and therapeutic interventions* (pp. 313–324). Hoboken, NJ: Wiley.

Locke, K. D., & Sadler, P. (2007). Self-efficacy, values, and complementarity in dyadic interactions: Integrating interpersonal and social-cognitive theory. *Personality and Social Psychology Bulletin, 33,* 94–109.

Luxton, D. D., McCann, R. A., Bush, N. E., Mishkind, M. C., & Reger, G. M. (2011). mHealth for mental health: Integrating smartphone technology in behavioral healthcare. *Professional Psychology: Research and Practice, 42,* 505–512.

Markey, P., Lowmaster, S., & Eichler, W. (2010). A real-time assessment of interpersonal complementarity. *Personal Relationships, 17,* 13–25.

Markey, P. M., & Markey, C. N. (2009). A brief assessment of the interpersonal circumplex: The IPIP-IPC. *Assessment, 16,* 352–361.

McWilliams, N. (2012). Beyond traits: Personality as intersubjective themes. *Journal of Personality Assessment, 94,* 563–570.

Mehl, M. R., & Connor, T. S. (2012). *Handbook of research methods for studying daily life.* New York: Guilford Press.

Mischel, W., & Shoda, Y. (2008). Toward a unified theory of personality: Integrating dispositions and processing dynamics within the cognitive–affective personality system. In O. John, R. Robbins & L. Pervin (Eds.), *Handbook of personality: Theory and research* (3rd ed., pp. 208–241). New York: Guilford Press.

Mischel, W., & Shoda, Y. (2010). The situated person. In B. Mesquita, L. Feldman-Barrett, & E. R. Smith (Eds.), *The mind in context* (pp. 149–173). New York: Guilford Press.

Molenaar, P. C. M., & Campbell, C. G. (2009). The new person-specific paradigm in psychology. *Current Directions in Psychological Science, 18,* 112–117.

Moskowitz, D. S. (1994). Cross-situational generality and the interpersonal circumplex. *Journal of Personality and Social Psychology, 66,* 921–933.

Moskowitz, D. S. (2009). Coming full circle: Conceptualizing the study of interpersonal behavior. *Canadian Psychology/Psychologie Canadienne, 50,* 33–41.

Moskowitz, D. S., Ringo Ho, M., & Turcotte-Tremblay, A. (2007). Contextual influences on interpersonal complementarity. *Personality and Social Psychology Bulletin, 33,* 1051–1063.

Moskowitz, D. S., & Sadikaj, G. (2012). Event-contingent recording. In M. R. Mehl & T. S. Connor (Eds.), *Handbook of research methods for studying daily life* (pp. 160–175). New York: Guilford Press.

Moskowitz, D. S., & Zuroff, D. C. (2004). Flux, pulse, and spin: Dynamic additions to the personality lexicon. *Journal of Personality and Social Psychology, 86,* 880–893.

Moskowitz, D. S., & Zuroff, D. C. (2005a). Assessing interpersonal perceptions using the interpersonal grid. *Psychological Assessment, 17,* 218–230.

Moskowitz, D. S., & Zuroff, D. C. (2005b). Robust predictors of flux, pulse, and spin. *Journal of Research in Personality, 39,* 130–147.

Moskowitz, D. S., Zuroff, D. C., aan het Rot, M., & Young, S. N. (2011). Tryptophan and interpersonal spin. *Journal of Research in Personality, 45,* 692–696.

Pennings, H. J. M., van Tartwijk, J., Wubbels, T., Claessens, L. C. A., van der Want, A. C., & Brekelmans, M. (2014). Real-time teacher–student interactions: A Dynamic Systems approach. *Teaching and Teacher Education, 37,* 183–193.

Pincus, A. L. (2010). Introduction to the Special Series on integrating personality, psychopathology, and psychotherapy using interpersonal assessment. *Journal of Personality Assessment, 92,* 467–470.

Pincus, A. L., & Ansell, E. B. (2013). Interpersonal theory of personality. In J. Suls & H. Tennen (Eds.), *Handbook of psychology: Vol. 5. Personality and social psychology* (2nd ed., pp. 141–159). Hoboken, NJ: Wiley.

Pincus, A. L., & Hopwood, C. J. (2012). A contemporary interpersonal model of personality pathology and personality disorder. In T. A. Widiger (Ed.), *Oxford handbook of personality disorders* (pp. 372–398). New York: Oxford University Press.

Pincus, A. L., Lukowitsky, M. R., & Wright, A. G. C. (2010). The interpersonal nexus of personality and psychopathology. In T. Millon, R. Kreuger, & E. Simonsen (Eds.), *Contemporary directions in psychopathology: Scientific foundations for DSM-V and ICD-11* (pp. 523–552). New York: Guilford Press.

Pincus, A. L., & Wright, A. G. C. (2011). Interpersonal diagnosis of psychopathology. In L. M. Horowitz & S. Strack (Eds.), *Handbook of interpersonal psychology: Theory, research, assessment, and therapeutic interventions* (pp. 359–381). Hoboken, NJ: Wiley.

Przeworski, A., Newman, M. G., Pincus, A. L., Kasoff, M., Yamasaki, A. S., & Castonguay, L. G. (2011). Interpersonal pathoplasticity in individuals with generalized anxiety disorder. *Journal of Abnormal Psychology, 120,* 286–298.

Pytlik Zillig, L. M., Hemenover, S. H., & Dienstbier, R. A. (2002). What do we assess when we assess a big 5 trait? A content analysis of the affective, behavioral and cognitive processes represented in the big 5 personality inventories. *Personality and Social Psychology Bulletin, 28,* 847–858.

Ram, N., Coccia, M., Conroy, D. E., Lorek Dattilo, A., Orland, B., Pincus, A. L., et al. (2013). Behavioral landscapes and change in behavioral landscapes: A multiple time-scale density distribution approach. *Research in Human Development, 10,* 88–110.

Ram, N., Conroy, D. E., Pincus, A. L., Hyde, A. L., & Molloy, L. (2012). Tethering theory to method: Using measures of intraindividual variability to operationalize individuals' dynamic characteristics. In G. Hancock & J. Harring (Eds.), *Advances in longitudinal modeling in the social and behavioral sciences* (pp. 81–110). Charlotte, NC: Information Age Publishing.

Roche, M. J., Pincus, A. L., Conroy, D. E., Hyde, A. L., & Ram, N. (2013). Pathological narcissism and interpersonal behavior in daily life. *Personality Disorders: Theory, Research, and Treatment, 4,* 315–323.

Roche, M. J., Pincus, A. L., Hyde, A. L., Conroy, D. E., & Ram, N. (2013). Within-person co-variation of agentic and communal perceptions: Implications for interpersonal theory and assessment. *Journal of Research in Personality, 47,* 445–552.

Roche, M. J., Pincus, A. L., Hyde, A. L., Conroy, D. E., & Ram, N. (2014). *Enriching psychological assessment using a person-specific analysis of interpersonal processes in daily life.* Manuscript submitted for publication.

Russell, J. J., Moskowitz, D. S., Zuroff, D. C., Sookman, D., & Paris, J. (2007). Stability and variability of affective experience and interpersonal behavior in borderline personality disorder. *Journal of Abnormal Psychology, 116,* 578–588.

Sadikaj, G., Moskowitz, D. S., Russell, J. J., Zuroff, D. C., & Paris, J. (2013). Quarrelsome behavior in borderline personality disorder: Influence of behavioral and affective reactivity to perceptions of others. *Journal of Abnormal Psychology, 122*, 195–207.

Sadikaj, G., Moskowitz, D. S., & Zuroff, D. C. (2011). Attachment-related affective dynamics: Differential reactivity to others' interpersonal behavior. *Journal of Personality and Social Psychology, 100*, 905–917.

Sadikaj, G., Russell, J. J., Moskowitz, D. S., & Paris, J. (2010). Affect dysregulation in individuals with borderline personality disorder: Persistence and interpersonal triggers. *Journal of Personality Assessment, 92*, 490–500.

Sadler, P., Ethier, N., Gunn, G. R., Duong, D., & Woody, E. (2009). Are we on the same wavelength? Interpersonal complementarity as shared cyclical patterns during interactions. *Journal of Personality and Social Psychology, 97*, 1005–1020.

Sadler, P., Ethier, N., & Woody, E. (2011). Interpersonal complementarity. In L. M. Horowitz & S. N. Strack (Eds.), *Handbook of interpersonal psychology: Theory, research, assessment, and therapeutic interventions* (pp. 123–142). Hoboken, NJ: Wiley.

Sadler, P., Lizdek, I., Hunt, R., & Woody, E. (2011). *The across-time dynamics of agency and communion: Do same-sex and opposite-sex dyadic interactions differ?* Paper presented at the annual meeting of the Society for Interpersonal Theory and Research, Zurich, Switzerland.

Salvatore, S., & Tschacher, W. (2012). Time dependency of psychotherapeutic exchanges: The contribution of the Theory of Dynamic Systems in analyzing process. *Frontiers in Psychology, 3*, 1–14.

Shiffman, S., Stone, A. A., & Hufford, M. R. (2008). Ecological momentary assessment. *Annual Review of Clinical Psychology, 4*, 1–32.

Shostrom, E. L. (Producer). (1966). *Three approaches to psychotherapy* [Film]. Santa Ana, CA: Psychological Films.

Stoica, P., & Sandgren, N. (2006). Spectral analysis of irregularly-sampled data: Paralleling the regularly-sampled data approaches. *Digital Signal Processing, 16*, 712–734.

Thomas, K. M., Hopwood, C. J., Woody, E., Ethier, N., & Sadler, P. (2014). Momentary assessment of interpersonal process in psychotherapy. *Journal of Counseling Psychology, 61*, 1–14.

Thomas, K. M., Hopwood, C. J., & Morey, L. C. (2012). *Evaluating the momentary interpersonal dynamics of borderline personality.* Presented at the annual meeting for the Society for Personality Assessment, Chicago, IL.

Tracey, T. J. (2004). Levels of interpersonal complementarity: A simplex representation. *Personality and Social Psychology Bulletin, 30*, 1211–1225.

Tracey, T. J. G., Bludworth, J., & Glidden-Tracey, C. E. (2012). Are there parallel processes in psychotherapy supervision? An empirical examination. *Psychotherapy: Theory, Research, Practice, Training, 49*, 330–343.

Tracey, T. J. G., & Rolfing, J. E. (2010). Variations in the understanding of interpersonal behavior: Adherence to the interpersonal circle as a moderator of the rigidity–psychological well-being relation. *Journal of Personality, 78*, 711–746.

Trull, T. J., Ebner-Priemer, U. W., Brown, W. C., Tomko, R. L., & Scheiderer, E. M. (2012). Clinical psychology. In M. R. Mehl & T. S. Connor (Eds.), *Handbook of research methods for studying daily life* (pp. 620–635). New York: Guilford Press.

Tufte, E. (2006). *Beautiful evidence.* Cheshire, CT: Graphics Press

Warner, R. M. (1998). *Spectral analysis of time-series data.* New York: Guilford Press.

Wiggins, J. S. (1982). Circumplex models of interpersonal behavior in clinical psychology. In P. C. Kendall & J. N. Butcher (Eds.), *Handbook of research methods in clinical psychology* (pp. 183–221). Hoboken, NJ: Wiley.

Wiggins, J. S. (1991). Agency and communion as conceptual coordinates for the understanding and measurement of interpersonal behavior. In D. Cicchetti & W. M. Grove (Eds.), *Thinking clearly about psychology: Essays in honor of Paul E. Meehl: Vol. 2. Personality and psychopathology* (pp. 89–113). Minneapolis: University of Minnesota Press.

Wiggins, J. S. (1995). *Interpersonal Adjective Scales: Professional manual.* Odessa, FL: Psychological Assessment Resources.

Wiggins, J. S. (2003). *Paradigms of personality assessment.* New York: Guilford Press.

Wiggins, J. S., Phillips, N., & Trapnell, P. (1989). Circular reasoning about interpersonal behavior: Evidence concerning some untested assumptions underlying diagnostic classification. *Journal of Personality and Social Psychology, 56,* 296–305.

Wright, A. G. C., & Pincus, A. L. (2010). *Cross-sectional intraindividual variability in interpersonal functioning.* Paper presented at the annual meeting of the Society for Interpersonal Theory and Research, Philadelphia.

Wright, A. G. C., & Pincus, A. L. (2011). The interpersonal profiles of narcissism. In M. R. Lukowitsky (Chair), *Further advances in the assessment of pathological narcissism.* Symposium conducted at the annual meeting of the Society for Personality Assessment, Cambridge, MA.

CHAPTER 3

Multimethod Assessment of Affective Processes

Rachel L. Tomko and Timothy J. Trull

Tara enrolled in our clinic's dialetical behavior therapy program after she was released from the hospital following her second suicide attempt in the last 12 months. She reported that her emotions were out of control, no one wanted to be her friend, and she was close to giving up on the idea that things might change for the better. Tara reported that she often became intensely sad, irritable, or anxious and that these episodes were often triggered by setbacks or arguments. In particular, her anger was unpredictable and intense. Tara reported that she felt angry almost all the time, and it seemed like she took her anger out on anyone whom she was around (often for no clear reason). Not surprisingly, her relationships with her friends, romantic partners, and parents were intense and unstable as well. As part of our intake assessment, Tara completed several questionnaires that targeted her current mood states, as well as her typical emotional experiences, urges, thoughts, and behaviors that may have proved problematic for her. In addition, Tara completed several diagnostic interviews that provided information used to establish the presence of mood, anxiety, substance use, eating, and personality disorders. During the course of treatment, Tara completed daily assessments of her mood states, her urges, her impulsive behaviors, and her attempts to cope with these emotional experiences. In this way, we were able to obtain a comprehensive picture of Tara's sense of her emotional experience, from a perspective of both her typical emotional patterns and her current emotional state. Furthermore, the daily assessments of her mood states provided the treatment team with a better sense of Tara's emotions as they unfurled in daily life, as well as the stressors and triggers related to changes in her emotional states.

The assessment of affect and affective processes presents many challenges to the clinician and to the clinical researcher. In psychological and psychiatric research, the term *affect* is used broadly to refer to emotions, feelings, and mood states.[1] Affective processes may include the subjective experience of affect, regulation of affect, expression of affect, identifying and labeling emotional states, and cognitive aspects of emotion, to name a few of the possibilities (Barrett, 2012). In other words, affect is a complex, multifaceted construct that includes subjective, cognitive, physiological, social, and cultural components (Barrett, 2012; Spielberger, 1966). To illustrate, consider the conceptual act theory of emotion (e.g., Barrett, 2006, 2009, 2011; Barrett & Kensinger, 2010; Lindquist & Barrett, 2008), a leading psychological constructionist theory of emotion. This theory proposes that emotions become real and are experienced through a complex interplay between sensations from the outside world, sensations from within the body, categorization based on context and culture, and individual differences among perceivers. Therefore, to best understand emotion and affective processes, it is necessary to consider multiple components that constitute the experience. Focusing on only one of these components (subjective report, bodily sensations, or context) will not fully explain how affective experience and expression come into being.

Similarly, due to the limitations of any single methodology, a complete understanding of affective processes cannot be gained through reliance on any single assessment tool or method. Often, multimethod assessment is used as a means of construct validation (Campbell & Fiske, 1959). In the creation of a new assessment tool, researchers want to verify that their measure relates to existing measures of similar constructs. However, there are other uses of multimethod assessment that are of particular importance for emotion research and in clinical settings. First, the strengths of one method may address the limitations of a second method, reducing measurement error and increasing the predictive power of the latent construct. Second, discrepant findings between methods may provide important information that is unattainable using either method alone. Third, in the context of the assessment of emotional experience, theories such as the conceptual act theory of emotion suggest that different components of affective experience are not necessarily uniquely related to affects such that specific features of neural functioning or physiological functioning determine specific emotional states. Rather, in a sense the perceiver constructs emotions and affects to create meaning, to regulate action, to communicate, and to influence the actions of others (Barrett, 2012). By implication, we will not fully understand emotional experience unless multiple components of affective processes are investigated within individuals.

---

[1]Despite differences in connotation, we use these terms interchangeably throughout the chapter for simplicity.

How Often Are Multiple Methods Used in Emotion Research?

Despite the value of multimethod assessment of affective processes, the majority of published emotion research still employs a single method. For example, in their review of emotion regulation assessment in children, Adrian, Zeman, and Veits (2011) reported that *only 38.9% of the reviewed literature utilized a multimethod approach.* Notably, the nature of research with children often requires parent reports or observational techniques to assess affective processes, as young children may not be developmentally able to report accurately on their mood states. So, in general, developmental researchers are less likely to rely on self-report alone.

It seems likely that multimethod assessment of affective processes is used even *less frequently* in research with adults. To further explore how frequently multiple methods are used in the assessment of emotion and affective processes, we reviewed recent assessment trends in *Emotion*, a journal dedicated specifically to research on emotional processes. *Emotion* was selected because of its specificity to the topic of this review and because of its high-impact factor (3.875; American Psychological Association, 2012). Articles published in 2002 (Issues 1–4) and 2012 (Issues 1–5)[2] were reviewed. Given the increase in publications from 2002 to 2012, a random sample of approximately half of all 2012 articles was evaluated. To be included, the research had to focus on the personally relevant affective processes of the human participant. In other words, studies focusing on recognition of the emotions of others that did not also assess trait or state affect of the participants were excluded. An article was considered to have a multimethod approach if (1) two or more measures from two or more domains (i.e., self-report, observation, informant-report, psychophysiology/biology) were used, and (2) these measures were indicators of similar affective constructs. Two measures from the same domain (i.e., two self-report measures) assessing the same or similar constructs were not sufficient for inclusion in this review.

Of the 95 (2002: $n = 27$; 2012: $n = 68$) empirical articles reviewed for this chapter, 26 were excluded because the focus was on recognition of emotions in others and on memory for emotional events; the authors purportedly induced an emotion state but did not conduct manipulation checks using one of the above domains; or the population of interest was nonhuman primates. Results indicate that of the 69 (2002: $n = 18$; 2012: $n = 51$) remaining empirical articles sampled from *Emotion* in the designated years, 30.4% (2002: 33.3%; 2012: 29.4%) used multiple methods to assess an affective process characteristic of the sample. This estimate is slightly lower than that obtained by Adrian et al. (2011) among youth. Notably, 90.5% of the *Emotion* articles in our review focused on adult

---

[2]At the time of the review, the last published issue was Volume 12, Issue 5 (October 2012).

populations. Of the multimethod articles, 90.5% used self-report, 9.5% used informant or peer reports, 23.8% used observational techniques, and 81.0% used psychophysiological or biological measures. In sum, when multiple methods were used to study emotions among adult populations, generally a self-report and psychophysiology combination was employed.

Patterns of multimethod assessment in *Emotion* do not necessarily generalize to all peer-reviewed journals. First, Adrian and colleagues (2011) demonstrated that journals with higher impact factors publish more multimethod research and more psychophysiological research. Second, the content of a single journal relies heavily on the editor's intended purpose for the journal. Thus, some journals may be more inclined to accept an empirical manuscript with a certain methodology than other journals. Consequently, in addition to changes in general prevalence of multimethod use, editorial board changes may impact the trends in publication within a single journal. Despite these limitations in our review, these results suggest that only a minority of studies targeting affective processes use multimethod assessment. We suspect that multimethod assessment of emotion is used even less frequently in clinical settings.

The remainder of this chapter will discuss the major assessment approaches used to characterize emotional experience. First, we review different methodologies used to assess affective processes and the advantages and limitations of each approach. Then, we argue for the importance of using multiple methodologies while acknowledging the difficulties involved in multimethod assessment. Finally, we conclude with examples of multimethod research on emotion dysregulation in borderline personality disorder (BPD), a disorder characterized by affective instability and intense negative affects.

Measurement of Emotion and Affective Processes

Clinicians and researchers have used diverse methodologies to study affect and related processes. Primary assessment modes include *self-report* of affective experiences (e.g., Positive and Negative Affect Schedule; Watson, Clark, & Tellegen, 1988; Watson & Clark, 1994), *informant or "other" report* (e.g., Colorado Temperament Inventory; Rowe & Plomin, 1977), *observational techniques* (e.g., Emotion Facial Action Coding System; Ekman & Friesen, 1978), and *psychophysiological recording* (e.g., electrocardiogram, electrodermal activity, respiratory sinus arrhythmia).[3] Each

---

[3] A number of methods not described in this chapter may also provide clinical information regarding affective states. For example, Mihura, Meyer, Dumitrascu, and Bombel (2013) recently reported the utility of one such method, the Rorschach Inkblot Test, in detecting negative emotionality, emotional reactivity, hopelessness, anger, and emotional suppression.

approach has unique characteristics that add to our overall understanding of affective processes. For example, informant reports and observational assessments rely heavily on the external expression of emotion out of necessity. In contrast, self-report and psychophysiological assessments rely on internal processes. Only self-report captures the subjective, self-experience of emotion. However, the other techniques may capture aspects of affect that may not be conscious processes, thus limiting clients' and participants' ability to report on them. These four assessment methodologies are discussed here, and current examples from the literature illustrate the knowledge to be gained from each method.

Self-Report

The simplest and most efficient way to gather information about someone's affect or mood state is to ask how he or she is feeling. For example, paper-and-pencil measures are extremely easy to administer, do not often require elaborate coding systems, and scores can be standardized across participants. Self-report methods are versatile, and questions or items can be administered via paper and pencil, interviewer, computer, or even handheld devices. Self-report also can capture internal cognitive processes that influence emotion and the individual's own subjective description of how he or she feels.

One of the most widely used self-report measures of affective states is the Positive and Negative Affect Schedule (PANAS; Watson, Clark, & Tellegen, 1988; Watson & Clark, 1994). The PANAS consists of two 10-item scales that measure positive and negative affect, respectively. Positive affect (PA) includes items measuring alertness, activity, and enthusiasm. Negative affect (NA) includes anger, fear, guilt, disgust, and other aversive mood states. Watson and colleagues (1988) reported that these two scales are largely orthogonal and that the PANAS has high internal consistency and good convergent and discriminant reliability. In addition, a number of time frames for ratings are available (e.g., "right now," "today," "past week," "past month," and "in general").

Despite its popularity, several critiques of the PANAS have been raised. For example, Diener, Smith, and Fujita (1995) argued that some items (e.g., alert, active, strong) used in the PA scale of the PANAS are not true emotional states. Furthermore, research has suggested that joy, interest, and activation (positive affect items on PANAS) are separate facets that should be differentiated (Egloff, Schmukla, & Burns, 2003). Additionally, it has been debated whether PA and NA are truly independent constructs. Egloff (1998) shows that the independence of PA and NA depends on the measure used and that the PANAS generally produces uncorrelated PA and NA scales. However, Diener and Emmons (1985) demonstrated that the independence of PA and NA appears to be related to the intensity of the emotional state (with more intense states showing greater negative correlations between PA and NA) and the timeframe for which the affect is assessed (longer time periods show greater independence). More recent research has not definitively shown whether PA and NA are independent, as results continue to be mixed (Crawford & Henry, 2004; Tuccitto, Giacobbi, & Leite, 2010; Watson & Clark, 1997). Despite critiques, the PANAS remains one of the most widely used measures of affect. However, future research could improve upon the PANAS by attending to the content domain and by further examining the structural validity of the measure (Tuccitto et al., 2010).

Two other commonly used affect self-report measures are the Profile of Mood States (POMS; McNair, Lorr, & Droppleman, 1971) and the Circumplex Model of Affect (Russell, 1980). The original version (McNair et al., 1971) of the POMS included a list of 65 emotion states that participants rate on a 5-point Likert scale. Spielberger (1972) provides a thorough review of the measure. The scales resulting from factor-analytic studies include tension–anxiety, depression–dejection, anger–hostility, vigor–activity, fatigue–inertia, and confusion–bewilderment; however, Spielberger (1972) argues that the iterative test construction process was implemented in a manner that would support this factor structure. Internal consistency of the POMS is high, as are stability estimates across a 20-day period. This suggests that the POMS may not pick up on subtle fluctuations in mood (Spielberger, 1972). Because of the length of the scale, a number of short forms have been developed. An independent investigator developed the Profile of Mood States—Short Form (POMS-SF; Shacham, 1983). The POMS-SF contains 37 emotion states. Correlations between the original measure and the POMS-SF were high, and internal consistencies of the POMS-SF subscales were comparable to the estimates for the full version (Curran, Andrykowski, & Studts, 1995). Additionally, the original authors created a 30-item version of the measure, which also maintains the original factor structure (Profile of Mood States—Brief; POMS-B; McNair, Lorr, & Droppleman, 1992).

The PANAS and POMS both measure each emotional state on a separate dimension. Russell's circumplex model of affect (1980) differs in that it employs a spatial approach in which each emotional state lies on a circular plane, with the x-axis representing misery (negative) to pleasure (positive) and the y-axis representing fatigue or "sleepiness" (negative) to arousal (positive). Russell (1980) argued that all affective states lie somewhere within this plane. For example, "distress" is characterized by high misery and arousal, "depression" is characterized by high misery and low arousal, "contentment" by high pleasure and low arousal, and "excitement" by high pleasure and arousal (Russell, 1980). This model is based on the theory that affect is a result of cognitive interpretations of internal, physiological sensations. Both the fatigue–arousal continuum and misery–pleasantness continuum are associated with neurophysiological systems. Russell and colleagues have argued that it is difficult for people to report on discrete emotions because the experience of emotions is not discrete, but lies on two continuums (Russell; 1980; Posner, Russell, & Peterson, 2005). Self-reported affect can be obtained by providing individuals with word pairs that represent dimensions that lie within the circumplex. Individuals rate themselves on each of the word pairs (Mehrabian & Russell, 1974; Russell & Mehrabian, 1974). It has been argued that this framework best represents patterns of findings in neurophysiological data (Posner et al., 2005).

Clinically, the PANAS, POMS, and circumplex model of affect can each be administered quickly before or after each therapy session in order to gather information about changes in affect over time. Cumulatively, this information may help the treating clinician determine consistencies (i.e., "My client chronically endorses high levels of shame.") and inconsistencies (i.e., "My client's mood is unpredictable and frequently changing.") in affective presentation, aiding in case conceptualization. Furthermore, this information may provide some sense of the effect of the treatment on the client's mood. Additionally, clinicians may wish to administer a self-report affect measure to their client both before and after each the session to evaluate the within-session effects on mood. Similarly, affective experiences during discussions of certain topics may be clinically informative.

Despite its simplicity, self-report of affective processes has a number of limitations. First, self-report is limited by the participants' awareness of their own mood states (Nisbett & Wilson, 1977; Wilson & Dunn, 2004). Notably, populations with mood dysregulation may have particular difficulty identifying and labeling their own emotions (Taylor, Bagby, & Parker, 1997) or may show greater distortions when recalling previous mood states (e.g., Safer & Keuler, 2002). For example, Solhan, Trull, Jahng, and Wood (2009) had individuals with a diagnosis of borderline personality disorder or a depressive disorder carry an electronic diary for 28 days, reporting on their mood up to six times per day. Following the 28-day protocol, participants were asked to recall days on which they had experienced shifts in mood. Although participants were high in specificity for both positive and negative affect episodes (0.90–0.95), they were extremely low in sensitivity (0.05–0.07), resulting in overall hit rate of 0.63 for positive affect and 0.64 for negative affect.

Additionally, a number of systematic retrospective recall biases affect even healthy adults. Participants' self-reported mood is subject to mood-congruent responding (i.e., reports of past mood are influenced by one's current mood state), peak-end biases (i.e., individuals more readily recall the most intense and most recent aspects of their emotional experiences), and normative memory decay. Among children, awareness of certain emotion states may be too cognitively advanced for them at their developmental stage. Lastly, among individuals with severe intellectual or developmental disabilities, self-report may not be an option (e.g., Vos et al., 2012). Thus, among certain populations, self-report may be particularly unreliable or even not feasible. Given the limitations in self-awareness and retrospective recall biases, other measures of affective processes are essential.

Informant Report

By asking individuals who frequently interact with the target participant to report on the target's mood, researchers are able to gather important information about emotional expression in interpersonal situations. Friends, romantic partners, family members, colleagues, peers, teachers, and therapists may detect subtle changes in body language, facial expressions, and voice tone of which the target herself is unaware. Typically, informant-report measures are the same or similar to self-report measures of affect. As one example, Lucas, Diener, and Suh (1996) asked parents and friends of participants to fill out the PANAS on behalf of the target participant and to respond in terms of how often the target would experience each emotion. Thus, instructions for traditional self-report measures can be modified for informant reports.

Informants may be less influenced by social desirability given that they are reporting on someone else's expression of emotion. However, the validity of informant reports is limited to the context in which the informant knows the target individual (Achenbach, Krukowski, Dumenci, & Ivanova, 2005; de Los Reyes & Kazdin, 2005). For example, a mother reporting on her teenage child who is irritable in their shared home may report different affective states than a friend of the teenager who only sees the target in other contexts. Additionally, informant reports are influenced by the psychopathology of the reporter (de Los Reyes & Kazdin, 2005; Sher & Trull, 1996). For example, depressed mothers show less agreement with their children than nondepressed mothers on constructs such as problematic behaviors (de Los Reyes & Kazdin, 2005). Research using informant reports has provided valuable information about patterns of emotional expression. Okazaki (2002) found that peer informants underestimated the depression and anxiety symptoms of Asian Americans more so than those of white Americans, offering further support for cultural differences in emotional expression and control.

The informant report is invaluable to the treating clinician. Because clinicians generally hold therapy sessions in an office or a clinic, they do not see their clients in the clients' natural environment. Additionally, as mentioned above, the client's own self-report is subjective and limited by her own self-awareness. To fully understand the clinical picture, efforts should be made to obtain informant reports, with the client's permission. Child therapists will often consult parents and teachers of the target child. However, the informant report is less regularly utilized among adult therapy clients. A family member, partner, or close friend may be able to provide valuable information about the client's affective processes, which can help the therapist understand how the client engages interpersonally or is perceived by others.

Observational Studies

Like informant reports, observation of affect and related processes provides information regarding expression of emotions. Unlike informant reports, the "observer" is generally a research assistant or even an advanced computer program utilizing a standardized coding system. Results of observational studies are limited to the context within which an individual is observed. However, observers can be trained to attend to particular details, such as body posture, eye contact, and word selection in speech. For example, observational studies have contributed greatly to our understanding of healthy marital interactions. Studies have indicated that a couple's expression of positive affect during their early years indicates the happiness and stability of the relationship (Gottman, Coan, Carrere, & Swanson, 1998) and that interactions of older couples were characterized by less anger and disgust than interactions of younger couples (Carstensen, Gottman, & Levenson, 1995).

One of the most popular observation coding systems is the Facial Action Coding System (FACS; Ekman & Friesen, 1978). The original FACS was designed to capture facial movements, including but not limited to those that may be indicative of emotion (Ekman & Friesen, 1978). Typically, participants' facial expressions are video recorded. Then, research staff views the recordings in slow motion to identify the presence or absence of 44 facial action units. Research has suggested that specific action units are related to unique affective states (e.g., Ekman, 2003; Ekman, Friesen, & Ancoli, 1980; Tracy, Robins, & Schriber, 2009). Sayette, Cohn, Wertz, Perrott, and Parrott (2001) provided evidence of interrater reliability for the FACS. A certification process for FACS coders demonstrates that they are able to reliably code action units compared to standards. Sayette et al. (2001) further demonstrated that all but two action units have good to excellent interrater reliability, but even these two had fair reliabilities. Sayette and colleagues (2001) also demonstrated that reliability differed as a function of the speed of the video display. With modern technology, automated, computerized FACS coders have also been developed that can detect action (Kaiser & Wehrle, 1992).

Other existing observational tools focus on auditory information, such as voice tone and content of speech, in order to identify emotions. A novel observational device, the electronically activated recorder (EAR; Mehl, Pennebaker, Crow, Dabbs, & Price, 2001), is an ambulatory audio recorder that participants can wear in their daily lives. The EAR is unobtrusive and captures snippets of conversations and ambient sounds in the participants' environments. The resulting sound clips can be coded and transcribed by research staff. Transcriptions are often subjected to linguistic analysis (e.g., patterns in word choice). The EAR has been used to study affect and related processes in a variety of ways. For example, Mehl (2006) demonstrated that coders could reliably identify participants with depressive symptoms (as measured by self-report) by listening to EAR audio recordings from the participants' daily lives. Other research using the EAR has examined emotions more directly. For example, Tomko and colleagues (in press) showed that coders can reliably rate anger from EAR sound clips and that the EAR can be used in clinical populations. Finally, Slatcher and Trentacosta (2012) demonstrated that with modifications to the EAR device (i.e., a smaller recording device embedded in a special shirt), this methodology can reliably be used with children. Their study examined negative emotionality in children as expressed by crying, fighting, or arguing with others, whining, and using negative emotion words. The authors found that parent self-reported negative emotionality was related to child negative emotion word use.

In clinical settings, most clinicians make informal observations about a client's affective state, using both verbal and nonverbal cues. However, with the increasing availability of technology, it could be useful for clinicians to use the FACS or other empirically supported method to analyze videotaped sessions. It is highly possible that information will be gained that the clinician missed during session, as the clinician is forced to attend to body language, voice tone, facial expression, content of speech, and his or her own responses simultaneously.

Psychophysiological Indicators

Biological or physiological indicators can provide information about affective states without requiring an individual to have insight into his or her own emotions or to show any outward displays of emotion. In this way, physiological indicators offer a unique advantage over other forms of assessment. In traditional emotion research, researchers define constructs of emotion and develop questionnaires or observational coding schemes to reflect these constructs. This does not apply to psychophysiology. Thus, in order to use psychophysiological assessment tools as measures of emotion, the field first needs to relate psychophysiological processes to existing self-reported, informant-reported, and observed affect, and determine where these processes fall within nomological networks of affective processes.

Two commonly used psychophysiological indicators of emotion regulation, respiratory sinus arrhythmia (RSA) and electrodermal activity (EDA), are reviewed here. RSA and EDA are both measures of autonomic nervous system functioning: RSA is a measure of parasympathetic activity, and EDA is an indicator of sympathetic activity. RSA is "the degree of ebbing and flowing of heart rate during the respiratory cycle" (Beauchaine, 2001) and represents vagal control of the heart. Two measures of RSA are typically studied: resting RSA and reactivity to stimuli. Differences in baseline RSA are thought to be attributable to individual differences in emotion regulation, with low resting RSA being indicative of specific difficulties with emotion regulation (Beauchaine, 2001). In particular, Thayer and Lane (2000) have proposed that low resting RSA is indicative of emotional inflexibility, or "rigidity." In contrast, a high resting RSA can also be related to emotional difficulties, and it may be expected that individuals exhibiting a high baseline are more emotionally reactive (Butler, Wilhelm, & Gross, 2006). However, this interpretation has complicated and diverse origins (Berntson, Cacioppo, & Quigley, 1993), and a number of studies have been done that have inadequately controlled for factors such as respiration and physical activity when assessing RSA (Butler et al., 2006; Grossman & Taylor, 2007). Grossman and Taylor (2007) also argue that there are greater associations between cardiac vagal tone and RSA within-person than there are between-person. They suggest that within-person changes in RSA may be largely attributable to changes in respiration rather than heart rate.

EDA is a measure of sweat gland activity underneath the skin (see Dawson, Schell, & Filion, 2007, for a review). Skin conductance (EDA) increases with an increase of eccrine sweat gland activity, which occurs when an individual is exposed to novel or significant stimuli, is concentrating or attending to stimuli, is physically active, or is experiencing psychological stress (Boucsein et al., 2012; Dawson et al., 2007). The eccrine sweat glands, which are involved in thermoregulation and emotional responding, are most prominent in the palmar and plantar surfaces (Dawson et al., 2007). Therefore, these are the best areas to obtain EDA measurements from. EDA is thought to be related to anxiety and the avoidance of negative emotional states (Fowles, 1980). With the threat of punishment, EDA should increase, according to Fowles's theory. The EDA literature is largely consistent with this view. For example, individuals thought to have decreased anxiety, such as those with psychopathy, show reduced baseline EDA (Fowles, 1980).

There are a number of other useful psychophysiological indicators of emotion and emotion regulation. Activity in the brain can be monitored using electroencephalography (EEG) or functional magnetic resonance imaging (fMRI). Muscle activity is frequently measured using electromyography (EMG). Finally, biological samples can provide information regarding hormonal functioning. Cortisol release is controlled by the hypothalamus, and it is a frequently used indicator of stress response. Further research is needed to establish links between psychophysiological measures and affective processes.

Physiological and biological assessment approaches of emotion and affective processes are not without some limitations. First, there is no one-to-one correspondence between biological markers or psychophysiological signatures and individual emotional states. For example, reduced heart rate variability (HRV) is associated with anger, anxiety, fear, noncrying sadness, and even happiness; in addition to anxiety and fear, increased EDA is associated with anger, disgust, sadness, and amusement (Kriebig, 2010). Second, most of the research linking biological and physiological features to emotional states has been conducted in the laboratory and often with standardized stimuli to elicit emotional states (e.g., pictures, film clips, music, and imagery). This limits the ecological validity of the emotional experiences, and it is an open question as to how close the emotional experiences in the laboratory reflect emotions as they are experienced in daily life. Finally, the cost and complexity of using these indices in the assessment and study or affective processes may be prohibitive to many clinical researchers and clinicians. However, biofeedback is one example of how physiological processes may be used clinically. As physiological measurement continues to become easier to use and reduced in cost, the opportunity for incorporating it into clinical settings becomes greater.

Up to this point, this chapter has focused on different modes of assessment. However, in addition to the four general modes of assessment reviewed above (e.g., self-report, observation), assessment methodology can also differ in terms of time frame assessed (e.g., state vs. trait measure) or context (e.g., laboratory, real world).

Assessment of State versus Trait Affect

It is useful to distinguish between state affect or emotion and trait affect or emotion. Briefly, state affect refers to momentary or potentially short-lived emotional states that may show different dynamic patterns across time and across contexts. In contrast, trait affect refers to composite emotional experience (i.e., aggregated across periods of time and situations) and may be used as a verbal short-hand for what is typical for each individual. This distinction has implications for both assessment and prediction of future affect and emotional experience. State affect measures target momentary or near-momentary experiences, whereas trait affect measures the attempt to aggregate affective experience over longer periods of time and to describe individuals as they typically are. State measures of affect better reflect the "experiencing self," which can then in turn be linked to autonomic and biological systems (Conner & Barrett, 2012). Therefore, if the goal is to identify biological and physiological features or systems that are associated with one's immediate experience, state affective measures provide data that are most proximal in time to the biological and physiological underpinnings of experience. On the other hand, trait affective measures will provide data most relevant to the dispositional self, and these data seem more adept at predicting future behavior and decision making (Conner & Barrett, 2012). Multiple assessments of state affect can also be converted to traitlike assessments (through aggregation or latent modeling), whereas the reverse is not possible. Depending on the research question, situation, and participants' emotional triggers, we may not expect a trait self-report measure of affect to correlate with a state psychophysiological measure, for example.

To illustrate how these different time frames (state versus trait) used to evaluate affective experience may not agree and may have different implications for prediction, we briefly discuss a recent study on the affective experience of self-injurers. Bresin, Carter, and Gordon (2013) investigated the relationship between trait impulsivity, negative affective states, and the urge to commit nonsuicidal self-injury (NSSI) in a sample of young adults with a history of self-injury over the last year. Previous research has found that although trait measures of impulsivity typically are significantly associated with NSSI, laboratory behavioral measures of impulsivity are not. In fact, the relationship between trait measures of impulsivity and laboratory (state) measures is modest at best. Furthermore, correlations between state and trait self-report measures of affect *at the same administration* are often less than 0.50 (Spielberger & Reheiser, 2009).

Bresin et al. (2013) sought to test several hypotheses about what affective states are associated with urges for NSSI (and NSSI acts, by implication) by using a daily diary method that assessed state negative affective experiences and NSSI urges. First, all participants completed a trait measure of impulsivity that reflected the propensity to act rashly *when experiencing high levels of negative affect* (i.e., the Negative Urgency scale). Over a 14-day period, participants used end-of-day reports to rate daily levels of negative affect (and sadness and guilt, specifically) as well as daily levels of urges to commit NSSI. Using multilevel modeling, Bresin et al. (2013) were able to examine the relations between trait impulsivity and daily urges for NSSI as well as interactions between trait impulsivity and state measures of negative affect in predicting urges for NSSI. Consistent with previous research, trait levels of negative-affect-driven impulsivity (i.e., negative urgency) was significantly related to reports of urges for NSSI, as was state negative affect. However, Bresin et al. found different patterns of results when examining different state negative affect scales as moderators in the model. Specifically, only state levels of sadness moderated the relations between trait impulsivity and urge for NSSI, such that daily sadness ratings were significantly correlated with urge for NSSI only for those high in trait impulsivity. This result was not found for either state NA overall or state guilt. In summary, a trait measure of impulsivity in the context of negative affect was related to urges for NSSI, but the only state measure of negative affect that moderated this effect was sadness (not state NA or state guilt). These results remind us that trait and state measures of the same or similar constructs may not predict relevant outcomes in the same way. Theory should guide investigators in deciding whether trait or state measures are most appropriate for the prediction situation at hand.

Context of Assessment

Context of assessment can refer to situational or temporal features. Most generally, the ideal assessment of affect can be generalized to an individual's real-life experience. Unfortunately, most assessments of emotional experience take place in the clinic, in the laboratory, or in unusual situations that do not mimic real life (e.g., eliciting affective states from International Affective Picture System [IAPS] pictures). Second, the timing of the assessment is rarely coordinated with naturally occurring periods of affective experience; rather, individuals are asked to retrospect about their emotional states and experience while in the lab or clinic (e.g., how anxious are you during a panic attack?). Finally, it is often of interest to assess emotional states during interpersonal encounters with certain individuals, or in certain settings, to name a few of the possibilities. However, typical assessment approaches do not ask for this contextual specificity, and, if they do, it requires retrospection and accurate recall. For these and other reasons, many social scientists (including psychologists) endorse context-sensitive assessment of emotions, behaviors, and cognitions. Such an approach necessitates a fairly novel, perhaps even radical, new approach to assessing individuals in their daily life: ambulatory assessment.

Ambulatory assessment (Trull & Ebner-Priemer, 2013), which includes ecological momentary assessment (EMA; Stone & Shiffman, 1994) and experience sampling (Csikszentmihalyhi & Larson, 1987) methods, is a methodology designed to maintain ecological validity by assessing individuals frequently over time within their own natural environments. Ambulatory assessment is a broad term that can include ambulatory self-report (e.g., Solhan et al., 2009), informant report (e.g., Gump, Polk, Kamarck, & Shiffman, 2001), observation (e.g., Mehl et al., 2001), or psychophysiology (e.g., Gump et al., 2001; Poh, Swenson, & Picard, 2010). Studies examining the correspondence between ambulatory assessment and traditional assessment methods reveal that results from these methods do not always converge (Trull & Ebner-Priemer, 2013).

Because of repeated measurements over time in patients' natural environment, ambulatory assessment methods may be more adept in informing etiological theories of affective processes and psychological problems. For example, a meta-analysis of ambulatory assessment studies tested an affect regulation model of binge eating in bulimia nervosa and binge eating disorder (Haedt-Matt & Keel, 2011). Specifically, they examined whether high negative affect precedes a binge episode (which has received support from cross-sectional studies) and decreased negative affect follows an episode (mixed support). They found that high negative affect precedes binge eating, and, in addition, negative affect continues to increase following a binge. So, it does not appear that most individuals experience relief from negative affect following bingeing behavior in real life. Future studies that integrate laboratory or cross-sectional designs with EMA methodology can also examine within-person discrepancies between these methodologies. If individuals with binge eating disorder recall that binge episodes decrease negative affect when in the moment they actually feel intensified negative affect, this has important implications for clinical intervention.

Clinically, as in the case example of Tara presented earlier, ambulatory assessment can provide vital information about within-person changes in affect over time. Because Tara reported on her mood, impulsive behaviors, and attempts to cope with her mood states on a daily basis, the treating clinician was able to provide feedback to Tara regarding how her alcohol use and self-harm behaviors (which she saw as a means of coping with negative affect) may have temporarily reduced her negative mood states, but she often felt guilty and more depressed following a drinking or self-harm episode. The clinician was also able to show Tara that her adaptive coping mechanisms were just as effective in reducing her negative moods and were not followed by increased negative mood states.

Value of Multimethod Assessment of Affect

It is well known that method bias can be a significant source of error variance in psychological research (e.g., Campbell & Fiske, 1959; Podsakoff, MacKenzie, Podsakoff, & Lee, 2003). Thus, one way to minimize method variance is to collect information on the same construct using multiple methodologies. For example, Lischetzke and Eid (2003) used both self- and peer reports to assess a number of affective processes, such as attention to emotions, clarity of feelings, emotion regulation, and general affective well-being. Self- and peer reports were used as two indicators of each latent affect construct. Specifically, they used peer reports as a means of estimating method variance (see Eid, Lischetzke, Nussbeck, & Trierweiler, 2003, for more details regarding this approach). The correlation between self- and peer reports ranged from 0.30 to 0.34, illustrating modest agreement between self- and other reports, which is fairly typical for affective processes (e.g., Stanton, Kirk, Cameron, & Danoff-Burg, 2000; Watson & Clark, 1991; Watson, Hubbard, & Wiese, 2000). Lischetzke and Eid (2003) hypothesized that attention to and clarity of emotions is predictive of overall well-being (i.e., higher positive and lower negative affect). However, they found that greater attention to feelings was unrelated to emotional well-being, but emotional clarity was predictive of better emotional well-being. This provides one example of how multiple methods can be used to mitigate potential method bias due to using a single method.

As mentioned above, it is also possible to gain valuable information from the discrepancy between two types of methodologies. Because informant-report and observational techniques rely on the expression of emotion, discrepancies between these methods and internal states provide important information about *emotional expression or suppression*. For example, in the Okazaki (2002) study referenced earlier, Asian Americans self-reported higher depression and social anxiety than white Americans. Peers also rated Asian Americans as higher on depression and social anxiety. Had these findings been published in separate studies with different samples, we may only conclude that Asian Americans suffer from more depression and social anxiety than white Americans. However, given that Okazaki used a multimethod approach, we can further determine that a greater discrepancy exists between the self- and other reports of Asian Americans than of white Americans, thus providing information regarding cultural differences in emotional expression. In a second example, Rottenberg, Kasch, Gross, and Gotlib (2002) used an observational technique to study emotional expressivity among individuals with major depressive disorder (MDD). In particular, depressed and nondepressed participants watched a series of standardized emotional film clips, and trained research staff rated the participants' facial expressions using the Emotional Behavior Coding System (Gross & Levenson, 1993). While the authors found some differences in self-reported sadness between the depressed and nondepressed groups, they did not find differences in observed sadness across groups, possibly indicating low expressivity in MDD.

Application of Multimethod Research: Emotion Dysregulation in BPD

In this section, we review several studies that have used a multimethod assessment strategy to examine affect and affective processes in borderline personality disorder (BPD). In particular, we want to illustrate the use of ambulatory assessment in studying emotion and affective processes in BPD because ambulatory assessment can incorporate self-report, observational, and psychophysiological assessment strategies. The application to BPD is instructive because this disorder is characterized by high levels of multiple affects (e.g., anxiety, depression, hostility) as well as instability in these affects.

For readers not familiar with BPD, it is a severe condition associated with extreme emotional, behavioral, and interpersonal dysfunction (American Psychiatric Association, 2013). The clinical vignette at the beginning of this chapter (Tara) describes a representative emotional profile of a client with the BPD diagnosis. Affective instability, sometimes labeled emotional dysregulation, is a core feature of BPD (American Psychiatric Association, 2013; Linehan, 1993). Affective instability refers to the highly reactive affective states of individuals with BPD; those with BPD typically shift between different varieties (e.g., anger, depression, anxiety) and degrees (e.g., moderate to extreme) of negative affect. These shifts among negative affects distinguish BPD from disorders such as bipolar disorder, in which a person may shift between both positive and negative affect (e.g., from depression to elation). Furthermore, as was true in Tara's case, in BPD affective shifts tend to occur in response to external stimuli in the person's environment (Cowdry, Gardner, O'Leary, Leibenluft, & Rubinow, 1991; Trull et al., 2008). These extreme shifts in affect typically last a few hours to a few days and may occur as a result of factors such as interpersonal stressors, perceived rejections, or events prompting identity crises. The triggers for affective shifts in BPD tend to differ from those seen in other disorders. In contrast to BPD, individuals with major depression are more likely to experience affective shifts resulting from internal cues (e.g., self-critical thinking, pessimism about the future).

Specific BPD criteria that appear to arise directly from negative emotion dysregulation include affective instability, extreme anger, and emptiness. Negative emotion dysregulation may be the driving force behind many additional behaviors seen in the disorder (Linehan, 1993). Traditionally, researchers and clinicians have used both interviews and questionnaires to assess affective instability in BPD. However, both of these measures require accurate retrospection and insight into the dynamic nature of affective changes and fluctuations (Solhan et al., 2009). The measurement of affective instability in BPD requires a more nuanced assessment approach because it is a dynamic, time-dependent process (Ebner-Priemer, Eid, Kleindienst, Stabenow, & Trull, 2009). There is a need for methods such as ecological momentary assessment (Stone & Shiffman, 1994), experience sampling (Csikszentmihalyi & Larson, 1987), and ambulatory assessment (Trull & Ebner-Priemer, 2013) that provide multiple assessments of affect and its indicators every day and over many days. This is the only way to precisely assess the ebb and flow of mood, extreme changes in affective state, and environmental triggers for these changes.

To take one example, although clearly a relationship exists between trait neuroticism and the propensity for affective instability (Miller & Pilkonis, 2006), the same score on a neuroticism measure may indicate either chronic negative affect (e.g., like that seen in major depression) or extreme fluctuations in negative affect (e.g., like that seen in BPD). Therefore, neuroticism overlaps with but is not synonymous with affective instability. More frequent assessments of mood are needed to reveal the acute increases in negative affect from one moment or occasion to the next (Trull et al., 2008). This high-frequency assessment approach yields "intensive longitudinal data" (Walls & Schafer, 2006). An added advantage of momentary assessments collected using EMA or ESM methods is that mood states are assessed in the person's natural habitat. In other words, we are able to obtain a more ecologically valid assessment of a person's mood in his or her daily life (Shiffman, Stone, & Hufford, 2008), while at the same time sampling experiences and events that may serve as antecedents, covariates, or consequences of mood changes (Ebner-Priemer, et al., 2009; Trull & Ebner-Priemer, 2013). So, as described in Tara's case, daily assessments of mood states, mood changes, and the circumstances surrounding these changes can provide rich clinical information about a client's daily life in his or her natural environment.

How Do Traditional Reports of Affective Instability Compare to Those Derived from Ambulatory Assessment?

As mentioned above, Solhan et al. (2009) examined the concordance of retrospective self-report questionnaires on affective instability with momentary assessments in psychiatric outpatients with BPD ($n = 58$) or depressive disorder ($n = 42$). Regarding the momentary assessments, the authors used repeated assessments of affect collected via electronic diaries at six random times per day over a 28-day period. For comparison, three trait measures of affective instability, the Affective Instability subscale of the Personality Assessment Inventory—Borderline Features Scale (Morey, 1991), the Affect Lability Scales (Harvey, Greenberg, & Serper, 1989), and the Affect Intensity Measure (Larsen, Diener, & Emmons, 1986) were administered immediately following the 28-day ESM assessment period. Results revealed that there was almost no relationship between questionnaire trait measures and ambulatory assessment indices of affective instability. In addition, Solhan et al. (2009) examined whether patients with BPD could recall their most pronounced affect changes. From a memory heuristic perspective, single important events (i.e., peaks) should be remembered more easily (a phenomenon referred to as the peak–end rule; Kahneman, Fredrickson, Schreiber, & Redelmeier, 1993). However, retrospective reports of extreme mood changes were largely unrelated to ambulatory assessment (AA) indices of acute affect changes, regardless of whether the previous month or the immediately preceding seven days were the time reference.

Affective Reactivity in Interpersonal Interactions

Recently, we used a combined self-report and observational strategy to examine affective reactivity within interpersonal relationships (Brown, Tragesser, Tomko, Mehl, & Trull, 2014). Specifically, clinical participants with BPD or with a history of depressive disorder (DD) wore the EAR (Mehl et al., 2001) for 3 days. The EAR device unobtrusively records ambient sounds in the participants' immediate environment. Ambient sounds recorded by the EAR can be coded for affect, behavior, and characteristics of the environment (e.g., Hasler, Mehl, Bootzin, & Vazire, 2008; Mehl, Gosling, & Pennebaker, 2006; Tomko et al., in press). In this study (Brown et al., 2014), we focused on participants' emotional experiences in interpersonal encounters as they occur in daily life.

The EAR is a digital voice recorder that captures brief intervals of sound in participants' environments. Participants received a Dell Axim 50 PDA loaded with EAR software and an attached microphone (OPTIMUS

Tie-Clip Microphone) that clipped onto their clothing. In this study, the EAR recorded approximately 47 times a day between the hours of 9:00 A.M. and 11:00 P.M., recording every 18 minutes for 50 seconds in duration. The 27 participants had a mean of 114 valid/audible waking soundfiles (SD = 32.4) out of 140 possible sound clips per participant (an average of 90% per participant). Recordings were coded for expressed positive and negative affect, and coder ratings were compared to participants' reports about their positive and negative affect (PA, NA) during interpersonal events. Affect was coded using descriptors from the Positive and Negative Affect Schedule (PANAS; Watson, Clark, & Tellegen, 1988). Positive affect items (happy, proud) and negative affect items (afraid, sad, guilty, angry) were rated on a scale ranging from 1 (not at all) to 5 (extremely). Raters were instructed to use this scale to indicate how the participants appeared to feel in any given sound file. Any audible information from the participant (e.g., voice tone, nonverbal utterances, crying) was used to inform coders' ratings.

At the end of the study period, the participants returned the EAR device and were interviewed by research staff about their most positive and most negative interpersonal interaction for each day of the study period (Thursday–Saturday), resulting in a maximum of six interpersonal events per participant. The participants were asked to provide a brief description of the event and describe those who were part of the interaction, time of day, duration of the interaction, and nature of the interaction (e.g., leisure activity). The participants also rated their own level of positive and negative affect during these events, using terms consistent with the PANAS. Recalled affect was rated on a 1 (not at all) to 5 (very much) scale. Positive recalled affect included the items happy/excited and confident/determined, while negative recalled affect included the items ashamed/guilty, nervous/ill at ease/tense, hostile/irritated, and sad/upset. Recalled PA and NA scores were calculated by taking the mean score for the items on each respective scale (range = 1.0 to 5.0).

Results indicated that participants with BPD recalled feeling more NA and less PA during negative interpersonal events compared to those in the DD group. More discrepancies between recalled and observed levels of NA and PA were found for participants with BPD, regardless of the type of interpersonal event. In particular, this discrepancy was found for all affects within both types of interpersonal events for our participants with BPD. Individuals with emotion dysregulation problems may feel misunderstood by others in their daily lives if they have difficulty expressing the intensity of the emotions or feelings as they occur or if they do not appear to react emotionally to negative interpersonal events (Butler et al., 2003; Rottenberg, Gross, & Gotlib, 2005). In particular, individuals with BPD have reported lack of clarity regarding emotional experiences as well as emotional suppression (Lynch, Robins, Morse, & Krause, 2001; Suvak et al.,

2011). This pattern of expressed emotion may be experienced as confusing or erratic to an observer, given that the display of emotion may not always match the internal intensity that a person reports feeling.

This also may be some evidence for an invalidating environment, one that is crucial to Linehan's (1993) theory of BPD. In particular, emotional invalidation occurs when one's emotional states or feelings are ignored, discounted, minimized, or punished. Results from this study suggest that observers rate the intensity of affect lower than do those who experienced it. This mismatch could potentially be the basis for the experience of emotional invalidation, to the extent that observers (e.g., the partner in the interpersonal interaction) underestimate the intensity of the feelings of the person with BPD and then engage in interpersonal behaviors that are experienced as minimizing or punishing (e.g., ignoring, belittling, or minimizing). To date, few studies have been done on emotional invalidation, and almost all have involved retrospective reports of childhood experiences with caregivers. Thus, the EAR methodology used here may be a fruitful way to characterize and explore emotional invalidation as it occurs in daily life.

Emotional Arousal, Drinking, and Consequences

A major theory of substance use and abuse focuses on the use of alcohol and other drugs as a (maladaptive) attempt to regulate one's mood state. Therefore, individuals with emotion dysregulation problems would seem to be particularly vulnerable to the development of alcohol and drug use disorders. Interestingly, however, the most consistent findings from research studies support the use of alcohol to regulate positive but not negative affect. However, most of the existing studies have used nonclinical samples, especially college students, and these samples may be more likely to engage in celebratory drinking rather than drinking in response to changes in negative affect. Conceivably, a different pattern of findings might emerge from a clinical sample, especially one characterized by higher levels of negative affect and affective instability.

In a study that used electronic diaries to assess momentary levels of affect and alcohol use, Jahng et al. (2011) found that those alcohol drinkers with BPD were more likely to drink on days characterized by higher levels of negative affect variability. However, one limitation of this study is that it still relied solely on the self-report of participants. In a follow-up pilot study targeting emotional dysregulation, arousal, and drinking in patients with BPD, we collected data that combine two forms of AA: electronic diary data on affect and drinking and EDA data to index emotional arousal (Tomko & Trull, 2012). Here we present data from one participant in order to illustrate the utility of combining AA methods of assessment in order to study alcohol use–affect relations.

Patients with BPD and community controls in this study carried an electronic diary for one week and answered up to six surveys a day that were randomly prompted during waking hours. Of most interest here, the surveys asked about affective states and alcohol use. In addition, each patient wore an AA device that recorded EDA continuously to assess emotional arousal. Specifically, patients wore a sensor worn on the inner side of the wrist (Q sensor, Affectiva). The Q Sensor is designed to measure arousal, temperature, and 3-axis movement. Using the Q Sensor, EDA is measured by passing a small current through two electrodes on the surface of the skin. This measures tonic skin conductance, and more informatively, changes in skin conductance across different states of emotion, attention, and arousal. In addition, participants pressed a button on the Q Sensor once to indicate each time they began drinking alcohol.

By combining the Q sensor and electronic diary data, we were able to graphically display patterns of emotional arousal, see the affects that were endorsed by participants, and examine how drinking behavior was related to these patterns. To illustrate, two drinking episodes are presented in Figures 3.1a and 3.1b for the same individual. In both cases, the EDA data are presented for the 2 hours before first drink (shaded in light gray, and marked at the top), and for the drinking episode (shaded in dark gray, and marked at the top). Furthermore, affect ratings for predrink baseline, first drink, during episode, and at final drink are presented for each episode. In the first episode (Figure 3.1a), arousal is initially increasing in the 2 hours before drink, but then declines closer to the first drink. Affect ratings during this period (logged on an electronic diary) indicate moderate levels of positive (but not negative affect), and these levels remain constant throughout the episode. Based on the EDA and self-report data, it appears that the participant was at least partially motivated to drink to increase positive affect. Indeed, this participant rated the drinking episode as not at all relieving. In contrast, Figure 3.1b depicts a drinking episode that seems more consistent with an attempt to relieve negative affect. In this case, arousal level was increasing dramatically before the first drink, electronic diary positive affect ratings remained fairly constant throughout the episode, and electronic diary negative affect ratings were initially moderate but then decreased by the last drink. In this case, the participant rated the drinking episode as moderately relieving.

By combining two forms of AA, we were able to collect relevant data in real time that suggested different affective motivations for drinking in this participant. Thus, this individual provided data suggesting that she is not always motivated to drink in order to relieve or regulate negative affect, but sometimes to increase positive affect. Clinically, this information could be used as a starting point for exploring other influences on drinking behavior, including expectancies, contexts, and outcomes later that night or the next day.

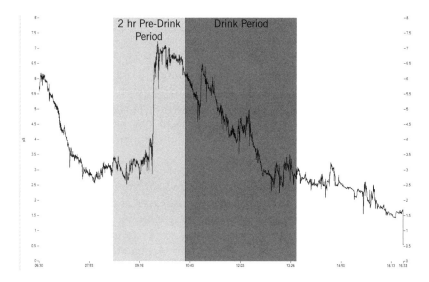

FIGURE 3.1a. For this participant, EDA is initially increasing in the 2 hours before drink, but then declines closer to the first drink. Participant reported moderate positive affect and low negative affect. The drinking episode was reported to be "not at all relieving."

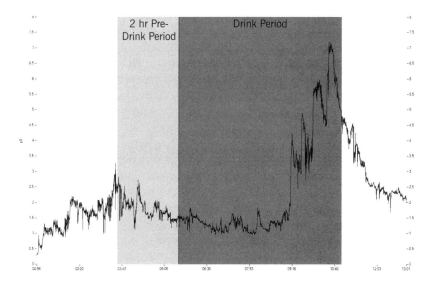

FIGURE 3.1b. This graph shows a different drinking episode for the same person as shown in 3.1a. In this case, arousal level was increasing dramatically before the first drink. Negative affect ratings were moderate, but decreased over the course of the drinking episode. The participant reported that the drinking episode was relieving.

Conclusions and Future Directions

In this chapter, we have argued for using multiple methods of assessment both in the clinic and as part of clinical research in order to best describe, characterize, and investigate emotion and affective processes. Emotion is the result of a complex interplay between subjective, cognitive, physiological, social, and cultural components. Therefore, measurement of only one of these components does not present the complete picture of how emotions become real (Barrett, 2012).

The question then becomes, what is the most promising way to conduct multimethod assessment of emotion and affective processes? As we have discussed, it is possible to use multiple assessment methods in the laboratory or the clinic, but these assessments have limited ecological validity and generalizability. A new approach, ambulatory assessment, shows much more promise (Trull & Ebner-Priemer, 2013). Ambulatory assessment can incorporate subjective, observational, and physiological measures and evaluate these indices as individuals go about their daily lives. Although self-reports collected using ambulatory assessment methods appear to be more reliable and valid than reports relying on retrospection, these latter reports are still a subjective evaluation by the patient. Therefore, it is desirable to supplement these psychological measures with objective measurements of physiological and/or behavioral data. Since the advent of mobile high-capacity micro sensors, ambulatory assessment comprises the assessment of not only psychological, but also physiological and behavioral data.

Today's biosensor technology offers compact, portable, and unobtrusive recording systems that allow assessment in the field (see Ebner-Priemer & Kubiak, 2007, or Kubiak & Krog, 2012, for an overview). Furthermore, sophisticated computer processing enables the control of confounding variables outside the laboratory, like disentangling emotional activation from the activation of physical effort (Houtveen & de Geus, 2009; Intille, 2007). Furthermore, the seminal use of physiology-triggered sampling protocols offers the possibility to examine various new research questions. Similar to branching is physiology- or context-triggered sampling (Intille, 2007). This can be seen as a kind of intelligent sampling because a specific item or sampling protocol, that is, psychological assessments (like mood state, cognition, attitude etc.), is prompted depending on a predefined physiological event (e.g., increase in heart rate) or situational context (e.g., voice of a partner).

Despite the advantages of multimethod assessment, conducted in the clinic, laboratory, or in the field, a number of challenges remain. Challenges include additional time, expense, and participant burden, aggregation of data from different sources, and the availability of psychometrically sound assessments. Observational methods require substantial work on the part of the research team to train individuals to reliably code affective processes. These challenges, however, are not unique to the study of affect but are pertinent to all multimethod research questions. In the end, however, our evaluation of emotion and affective processes will be incomplete if we do not tackle these issues. Fortunately, new technologies (notably, mobile phones, wireless sensors, and recognition software) will allow us to study multiple components of emotion as it is expressed and experienced in daily life.

ACKNOWLEDGMENTS

We would like to thank Jonathan W. Nauser, Madison O'Meara, and Amy C. Veith for their assistance in reviewing the relevant literature.

REFERENCES

Achenbach, T. M., Krukowski, R. A., Dumenci, L., & Ivanova, M. Y. (2005). Assessment of adult psychopathology: Meta-analyses and implications of cross-informant correlations. *Psychological Bulletin, 131,* 361–382.

Adrian, M., Zeman, J., & Veits, G. (2011). Methodological implications of the affect revolution: A 35-year review of emotion regulation assessment in children. *Journal of Experimental Child Psychology, 110,* 171–197.

American Psychiatric Association. (2013). *Diagnostic and statistical manual of mental disorders* (5th ed). Arlington, VA: Author.

American Psychological Association. (2012). Retrieved September 5, 2012, from *www. apa.org/pubs/journals/emo/index.aspx.*

Barrett, L. F. (2006). Solving the emotion paradox: Categorization and the experience of emotion. *Personality and Social Psychology Review, 10,* 20–46.

Barrett, L. F. (2009). The future of psychology: Connecting mind to brain. *Perspectives on Psychological Science, 4,* 326–339.

Barrett, L. F. (2011). Constructing emotion. *Psychological Topics, 20,* 359–380.

Barrett, L. F. (2012). Emotions are real. *Emotion, 12,* 413–429.

Barrett, L. F., & Kensinger, E. A. (2010). Context is routinely encoded during emotion perception. *Psychological Science, 21,* 595–599.

Beauchaine, T. (2001). Vagal tone, development, and Gray's motivational theory: Toward an integrated model of autonomic nervous system functioning in psychopathology. *Development and Psychopathology, 13,* 183–214.

Berntson, G. G., Cacioppo, J. T., & Quigley, K. S. (1993). Respiratory sinus arrhythmia: Autonomic origins, physiological mechanisms, and psychophysiological implications. *Psychophysiology, 30,* 183–196.

Boucsein, W., Fowles, D. C., Grimnes, S., Ben-Shakhar, G., Roth, W. T., Dawson, M. E., et al. (2012). Publication recommendations for electrodermal measurements. *Psychophysiology, 49,* 1017–1034.

Bresin, K., Carter, D. L., & Gordon, K. H. (2013). The relationship between trait impulsivity, negative affective states, and urge for nonsuicidal self-injury: A daily diary study. *Psychiatry Research, 205*(3), 227–231.

Brown, W. C., Tragesser, S. L., Tomko, R. L., Mehl, M. R., & Trull, T. J. (2014). Recall of expressed affect during naturalistically observed interpersonal events in those with borderline personality disorder or depressive disorder. *Assessment, 21,* 73–81.

Butler, E. A., Egloff, B., Wilhelm, F. H., Smith, N. C., Erickson, E. A., & Gross, J. J. (2003). The social consequences of expressive suppression. *Emotion , 3,* 48–67.

Butler, E. A., Wilhelm, F. H., & Gross, J. J. (2006). Respiratory sinus arrhythmia, emotion, and emotion regulation during social interaction. *Psychophysiology, 43,* 612–622.

Campbell, D. T., & Fiske, D. W. (1959). Convergent and discriminant validation by the multitrait-multimethod matrix. *Psychological Bulletin, 56,* 81–105.

Carstensen, L. L., Gottman, J. M., & Levenson, R. W. (1995). Emotional behavior in long-term marriage. *Psychology and Aging, 10,* 140–149.

Conner, T., & Barrett, L. F. (2012). Trends in ambulatory self-report: Understanding the utility of momentary experiences, memories, and beliefs. *Psychosomatic Medicine, 74,* 327–337.

Cowdry, R. W., Gardner, D. L., O'Leary, K. M., Leibenluft, E., & Rubinow, D. R. (1991). Mood variability: A study of four groups. *American Journal of Psychiatry, 148,* 1505–1511.

Crawford, J. R., & Henry, J. D. (2004). The Positive and Negative Affect Schedule (PANAS): Construct validity, measurement properties and normative data in a large non-clinical sample. *British Journal of Clinical Psychology, 43,* 245–265.

Curran, S. L., Andrykowski, M. A., & Studts, J. L. (1995). Short form of the Profile of Mood States (POMS-SF): Psychometric information. *Psychological Assessment, 7,* 80–83.

Csikszentmihalyi, M., & Larson, R. (1987). Validity and reliability of the experience-sampling method. *Journal of Nervous and Mental Disease, 175,* 526–536.

Davis, M. (2000). The role of the amygdala in conditioned and unconditioned fear and anxiety. In J. P. Aggleton (Ed.), *The amygdala* (Vol. 2, pp. 213–287). Oxford, UK: Oxford University Press.

Dawson, M. E., Schell, A. M., & Filion, D. L. (2007). The electrodermal system. In J. Cacioppo, L. G. Tassinary, & G. G. Berntson (Eds.), *Handbook of psychophysiology* (pp. 159–181). Cambridge, UK: Cambridge University Press.

de Los Reyes, A., & Kazdin, A. E. (2005). Informant discrepancies in the assessment of childhood psychopathology: A critical review, theoretical framework, and recommendations for further study. *Psychological Bulletin, 131,* 483–509.

Diener, E., & Emmons, R. A. (1985). The independence of positive and negative affect. *Journal of Personality and Social Psychology, 47,* 1105–1117.

Diener, E., Smith, H., & Fujita, F. (1995). The personality structure of affect. *Journal of Personality and Social Psychology, 69,* 130–141.

Ebner-Priemer, U. W., Eid, M., Kleindienst, N., Stabenow, S., & Trull, T. (2009). Analytic strategies for understanding affective (in)stability and other dynamic processes in psychopathology. *Journal of Abnormal Psychology, 118,* 195–202.

Ebner-Priemer, U. W., & Kubiak, T. (2007). Psychological and psychophysiological ambulatory monitoring: A review of hardware and software solutions. *European Journal of Psychological Assessment, 23,* 214–226.

Egloff, B. (1998). The independence of positive and negative affect depends on the affect measure. *Personality and Individual Differences, 25,* 1101–1109.

Egloff, B., Schmukle, S. C., & Burns, L. R. (2003). Facets of dynamic positive affect: Differentiating joy, interest, and activation in the Positive and Negative Affect Schedule (PANAS). *Journal of Personality and Social Psychology, 85,* 528–540.

Eid, M., Lischetzke, T., Nussbeck, F. W., & Trierweiler, L. I. (2003). Separating trait effects from trait-specific method effects in multitrait–multimethod models: A multiple-indicator CT-C(M–1) model. *Psychological Methods, 8,* 38–60.

Ekman, P. (2003). *Emotions revealed.* New York: Times Books.

Ekman, P., & Friesen, W. V. (1978). *Manual for the Facial Action Coding System.* Palo Alto, CA: Consulting Psychologist Press.

Ekman, P., Friesen, W. V., & Ancoli, S. (1980). Facial signs of emotional experience. *Journal of Personality and Social Psychology, 39*, 1125–1134.

Fowles, D. C. (1980). The three arousal model: Implications of Gray's two-factor learning theory for heart rate, electrodermal activity, and psychopathy. *Psychophysiology, 17*, 87–104.

Glenn, C. R., Blumenthal, T. D., Klonsky, E. D., & Hajcak, G. (2011). Emotional reactivity in nonsuicidal self-injury: Divergence between self-report and startle measures. *International Journal of Psychophysiology, 80*, 166–170.

Gottman, J. M., Coan, J., Carrere, S., & Swanson, C. (1998). Predicting marital happiness and stability from newlywed interactions. *Journal of Marriage and the Family, 60*, 5–22.

Gross, J. J., & Levenson, R. W. (1993). Emotional suppression: Physiology, self-report, and expressive behavior. *Journal of Personality and Social Psychology, 64*, 970–986.

Grossman, P., & Taylor, E. W. (2007). Toward understanding respiratory sinus arrhythmia: Relations to cardiac vagal tone, evolution and biobehavioral functions. *Biological Psychology, 74*, 263–285.

Gump, B. B., Polk, D. E., Kamarck, T. W., & Shiffman, S. (2001). Partner interactions are associated with reduced blood pressure in the natural environment: Ambulatory monitoring evidence from a healthy, multiethnic adult sample. *Psychosomatic Medicine, 63*, 423–433.

Haedt-Matt, A. A., & Keel, P. K. (2011). Revisiting the affect regulation model of binge eating: A meta-analysis of studies using ecological momentary assessment. *Psychological Bulletin, 137*, 660–681.

Harvey, P. D., Greenberg, B. R., & Serper, M. R. (1989). The affective lability scales: Development, reliability, and validity. *Journal of Clinical Psychology, 45*, 786–793.

Hasler, B. P., Mehl, M. R., Bootzin, R. R., & Vazire, S. (2008). Preliminary evidence of diurnal rhythms in everyday behaviors associated with positive affect. *Journal of Research in Personality, 42*, 1537–1546.

Houtveen, J. H., & de Geus, E. J. C. (2009). Noninvasive psychophysiological ambulatory recordings. *European Psychologist, 14*, 132–141.

Intille, S. S. (2007). Technological innovations enabling automatic, context-sensitive ecological momentary assessment. In A. A. Stone, S. Shiffman, A. A. Atienza, & L. Nebeling (Eds.), *The science of real-time data capture*. New York: Oxford University Press.

Jahng, S., Solhan, M. B., Tomko, R. L., Wood, P. K., Piasecki, T. M., & Trull, T. J. (2011). Affect and alcohol use: An ecological momentary assessment study of outpatients with borderline personality disorder. *Journal of Abnormal Psychology, 120*, 572–584.

Kahneman, D., Fredrickson, B. L., Schreiber, C. A., & Redelmeier, D. A. (1993). When more pain is preferred to less: Adding a better end. *Psychological Science, 4*, 401–405.

Kaiser, S., & Wehrle, T. (1992). Automated coding of facial behavior in human–computer interactions with FACS. *Journal of Nonverbal Behavior, 16*, 67–84.

Kreibig, S. D. (2010). Autonomic nervous system activity in emotion: A review. *Biological Psychiatry, 84*, 394–421.

Kubiak, T., & Krog, K. (2012). Computerized sampling of experiences and behavior. In M. R. Mehl & T. S. Conner (Eds.), *Handbook of research methods for studying daily life* (pp. 124–143). New York: Guilford Press.

Lang, P. J., Bradley, M. M., & Cuthbert, B. N. (2005). *International affective picture system (IAPS): Instruction manual and affective ratings* (Technical Report A-6). Center for Research in Psychophysiology, University of Florida.

Larsen, R. J., Diener, E., & Emmons, R. A. (1986). Affect intensity and reactions to daily life events. *Journal of Personality and Social Psychology, 51*, 803–815.

Lindquist, K. A., & Barrett, L. F. (2008). Constructing emotion: The experience of fear as a conceptual act. *Psychological Science, 19*, 898–903.

Linehan, M. M. (1993). *Cognitive-behavioral treatment of borderline personality disorder*. New York: Guilford Press.

Lischetzke, T., & Eid, M. (2003). Is attention to feelings beneficial or detrimental to affective well-being?: Mood regulation as a moderator variable. *Emotion, 3*, 361–377.

Lucas, R. E., Diener, E., & Suh, E. (1996). Discriminant validity of well-being measures. *Journal of Personality and Social Psychology, 71*, 616–628.

Lynch, T. R., Robins, C. J., Morse, J. Q., & Krause, E. D. (2001). A mediational model relating affect intensity, emotion inhibition, and psychological distress. *Behavior Therapy, 32*, 519–536.

McNair, D., Lorr, M., & Droppleman, L. (1971). *Manual for the Profile of Mood States*. San Diego, CA: Educational and Industrial Testing Service.

McNair, D. M., Lorr, M., & Droppleman, L. F. (1992). *Manual for the Profile of Mood States*. San Diego, CA: Educational and Industrial Testing Service.

Mehl, M. (2006). The lay assessment of subclinical depression in daily life. *Psychological Assessment, 18*, 340–345.

Mehl, M. R., Gosling, S. D., & Pennebaker, J. W. (2006). Personality in its natural habitat: Manifestations and implicit folk theories of personality in daily life. *Journal of Personality and Social Psychology, 90*, 862–877.

Mehl, M. R., Pennebaker, J. W., Crow, D. M., Dabbs, J., & Price, J. H. (2001). The electronically activated recorder (EAR): A device for sampling naturalistic daily activities and conversations. *Behavior Research Methods, 33*, 517–523.

Mehrabian, A., & Russell, J. A. (1974). *An approach to environmental psychology*. Cambridge, MA: MIT Press.

Mihura, J. L., Meyer, G. J., Dumitrascu, N., & Bombel, G. (2013). The validity of individual Rorschach variables: Systematic reviews and meta-analyses of the Comprehensive System. *Psychological Bulletin, 139*, 548–605.

Miller, J. D., & Pilkonis, P. A. (2006). Neuroticism and affective instability: The same or different? *American Journal of Psychiatry, 163*, 839–845.

Morey, L. C. (1991). *Personality Assessment Inventory: Professional manual*. Odessa, FL: Psychological Assessment Resources.

Nisbett, R. E., & Wilson, T. D. (1977). Telling more than we can know: Verbal reports on mental processes. *Psychological Review, 84*, 231–259.

Nock, M. K., Wedig, M. M., Holmberg, E. B., & Hooley, J. M. (2008). The emotion reactivity scale: Development, evaluation, and relation to self-injurious thoughts and behaviors. *Behavior Therapy, 39*, 107–116.

Okazaki, S. (2002). Self–other agreement on affective distress scales in Asian Americans and white Americans. *Journal of Counseling Psychology, 49*, 428–437.

Podsakoff, P. M., MacKenzie, S. B., Podsakoff, N. P., & Lee, J. (2003). Common method biases in behavioral research: A critical review of the literature and recommended remedies. *Journal of Applied Psychology, 88*, 879–903.

Poh, M., Swenson, N. C., & Picard, R. W. (2010). A wearable sensor for unobtrusive, long-term assessment of electrodermal activity. *IEEE Transactions on Biomedical Engineering, 57*, 1243–1252.

Posner, J., Russell, J. A., & Peterson, B. S. (2005). The circumplex model of affect: An integrative approach to affective neuroscience, cognitive development, and psychopathology. *Development and Psychopathology, 17,* 715–734.

Rottenberg, J., Gross, J. J., & Gotlib, I. H. (2005). Emotion context insensitivity in major depressive disorder. *Journal of Abnormal Psychology, 114,* 627–639.

Rottenberg, J., Kasch, K. L., Gross, J. J., & Gotlib, I. H. (2002). Sadness and amusement reactivity differentially predict concurrent and prospective functioning in major depressive disorder. *Emotion, 2,* 135–146.

Rowe, D., & Plomin, R. (1977). Temperament in early childhood. *Journal of Personality Assessment, 41,* 150–156.

Russell, J. A. (1980). A circumplex model of affect. *Journal of Personality and Social Psychology, 39,* 1161–1178.

Russell, J. A., & Mehrabian, A. (1974). Distinguishing anger and anxiety in terms of emotional response factors. *Journal of Consulting and Clinical Psychology, 42,* 79–83.

Safer, M. A., & Keuler, D. J. (2002). Individual differences in misremembering prepsychotherapy distress: Personality and memory distortion. *Emotion, 2,* 162–178.

Sayette, M. A., Cohn, J. F., Wertz, J. M., Perrott, M. A., & Parrott, D. J. (2001). A psychometric evaluation of the Facial Action Coding System for assessing spontaneous expression. *Journal of Nonverbal Behavior, 25,* 167–185.

Shacham, S. (1983). A shortened version of the Profile of Mood States. *Journal of Personality Assessment, 47,* 305–306.

Sher, K. J., & Trull, T. J. (1996). Methodological issues in psychopathology research. *Annual Review of Psychology, 47,* 371–400.

Shiffman, S., Stone, A. A., & Hufford, M. (2008). Ecological momentary assessment. *Annual Review of Clinical Psychology, 4,* 1–32.

Slatcher, R. B., & Trentacosta, C. J. (2012). Influences of parent and child negative emotionality on young children's everyday behaviors. *Emotion, 21,* 932–942.

Solhan, M. B., Trull, T. J., Jahng, S., & Wood, P. K. (2009). Clinical assessment of affective instability: Comparing EMA indices, questionnaire reports, and retrospective recall. *Psychological Assessment, 21,* 425–436.

Spielberger, C. D. (1966). Theory and research on anxiety. In C. D. Spielberger (Ed.), *Anxiety and behavior* (pp. 3–20). New York: Academic Press.

Spielberger, C. D. (1972). Profile of Mood States. *Professional Psychology, 3,* 387–388.

Spielberger, C. D., & Reheiser, E. C. (2009). Assessment of emotions: Anxiety, anger, depression, and curiosity. *Applied Psychology: Health and Well-Being, 1,* 271–302.

Stanton, A. L., Kirk, S. B., Cameron, C. L., & Danoff-Burg, S. (2000). Coping through emotional approach: Scale construction and validation. *Journal of Personality and Social Psychology, 78,* 1150–1169.

Stone, A. A., & Shiffman, S. (1994). Ecological momentary assessment (EMA) in behavioral medicine. *Annals of Behavioral Medicine, 16,* 199–202.

Suvak, M. K., Litz, B. T., Sloan, D. M., Zanarini, M. C., Feldman Barrett, L., & Hofmann, S. G. (2011). Emotional granularity and borderline personality disorder. *Journal of Abnormal Psychology, 120,* 414–426.

Taylor, G. J., Bagby, R. M., & Parker, J. D. A. (1997) *Disorders of affect regulation: Alexithymia in medical and psychiatric illness.* Cambridge, UK: Cambridge University Press.

Thayer, J. F., & Lane, R. D. (2000). A model of neurovisceral integration in emotion regulation and dysregulation. *Journal of Affective Disorders, 61,* 201–216.

Tomko, R. L., Brown, W. C., Tragesser, S. L., Wood, P. K., Mehl, M. R., et al. (in press). Social context of anger in borderline personality disorder and depressive disorders: Findings from a naturalistic observation study. *Journal of Personality Disorders, 26.*

Tomko, R. L., & Trull, T. J. (2012). *Case presentation of real-time emotion and skin conductance during alcohol curve.* Unpublished data.

Tracy, J. L., Robins, R. W., & Schriber, R. A. (2009). Development of a FACS-verified set of basic and self-conscious emotion expressions. *Emotion, 9,* 554–559.

Trull, T. J., & Ebner-Priemer, U. (2013). Ambulatory assessment. *Annual Review of Clinical Psychology, 9,* 151–176.

Trull, T. J., Solhan, M. B., Tragesser, S. L., Jahng, S., Wood, P. K., Piasecki, T. M., et al. (2008). Affective instability: Measuring a core feature of borderline personality disorder with ecological momentary assessment. *Journal of Abnormal Psychology, 117,* 647–661.

Tuccitto, D. E., Giacobbi, P. R., & Leite, W. L. (2010). The internal structure of positive and negative affect: A confirmatory factor analysis of the PANAS. *Education and Psychological Measurement, 70,* 125–141.

Vos, P., de Cock, P., Munde, V., Petry, K., Van Den Noortgate, W., & Maes, B. (2012). The tell-tale: What do heart rate; skin temperature and skin conductance reveal about emotions of people with severe and profound intellectual disabilities? *Research in Developmental Disabilities, 33,* 1117–1127.

Walls, T. A., & Schafer, J. L. (2006). *Models for intensive longitudinal data.* New York: Oxford University Press.

Watson, D., & Clark, L. A. (1991). Self- versus peer ratings of specific emotional traits: Evidence of convergent and discriminant validity. *Journal of Personality and Social Psychology, 60,* 927–940.

Watson, D., & Clark, L. A. (1994). *The PANAS-X: Manual for the Positive and Negative Affect Schedule—Expanded Form.* Unpublished manuscript, University of Iowa, Iowa City.

Watson, D., & Clark, L. A. (1997). Measurement and mismeasurement of mood: Recurrent and emergent issues. *Journal of Personality Assessment, 68,* 267–296.

Watson, D., Clark, L. A., & Tellegen, A. (1988). Development and validation of brief measures of positive and negative affect: The PANAS scales. *Journal of Personality and Social Psychology, 54,* 1063–1070.

Watson, D., Hubbard, B., & Wiese, D. (2000). Self–other agreement in personality and affectivity: The role of acquaintanceship, trait visibility, and assumed similarity. *Journal of Personality and Social Psychology, 78,* 546–558.

Wilson, T. D., & Dunn, E. W. (2004). Self-knowledge: Its limits, value, and potential for improvement. *Annual Review of Psychology, 55,* 493–518.

CHAPTER 4

Multimethod Assessment of Existential Concerns

A Terror Management Perspective

Spee Kosloff, Molly Maxfield, and Sheldon Solomon

Scientific principles and laws do not lie on the surface of nature. They are hidden, and must be wrested from nature by an active and elaborate technique of inquiry.
—JOHN DEWEY, *Reconstruction in Philosophy* (1920, p. 32)

Either because of extraordinary stress or because of an inadequacy of available defensive strategies, the individual who enters the realm called "patienthood" has found insufficient the universal modes of dealing with death fear and has been driven to extreme modes of defense.
—IRVING YALOM, *Existential Psychotherapy* (1980, p. 111)

Among the many challenges faced by social scientists, perhaps none is greater than the task of translating basic experimental findings into practically applicable approaches that foster physical and psychological welfare. Although both social psychology and clinical psychology share a common interest in delineating conditions that help or hinder human well-being, we perceive a gaping chasm between these fields that can only be bridged through shared, integrative focus on what it means to be human. This chapter represents an initial step toward such an undertaking.

Our aim is to take a burgeoning body of basic research on terror management theory (TMT; Greenberg, Pyszczynski, & Solomon, 1986; Greenberg, Solomon & Arndt, 2008)—a theory about the impact of death-related anxiety on human behavior—and distill from it a set of techniques that have potential clinical utility for assessing existential distress and dysfunctional coping methods. What originated as a hodgepodge of cognitive, affective, and behavioral measures and manipulations has become a clearly organized, well-validated set of procedures for determining vulnerability to existential concerns.

Central to this discussion is an experimental manipulation called mortality salience that entails reminding people that they are going to die someday. Time and again, this induction has been shown to elicit a cascade of "normal" defensive processes among individuals varying widely in age, race, socioeconomic status, culture, intelligence and profession. Simply put, when reminded of death, people typically respond by clinging to a sense that life is meaningful and that they themselves are agents of value in the world. Yet some individuals struggle to find purpose in the world and themselves, and others are so intensely embedded in rigid beliefs and a fragile ego as to evince profound reactivity to the thought of their death. Our primary focus in this chapter is to identify these instances of terror *mis*management by documenting personality and clinical variables that predict especially intense or otherwise dysfunctional responses to mortality salience.

We hope that summarizing the role of personality and clinical factors in terror management processes—and concretely defining how they and the defenses they produce are measured—provides the basis for viable approaches that clinicians may adopt when assessing and addressing their clients' existential concerns. With this aim in mind, the final portion of this chapter is devoted to a preliminary attempt at modeling a multimethod clinical assessment strategy that integrates the diverse assessment tools herein described.

Terror Management Theory

Terror management theory (TMT) (Greenberg et al., 1986, 2008) was derived from cultural anthropologist Ernest Becker's (1973) ideas concerning the impact of death awareness on human behavior. Becker proposed that human beings, like other life-forms, possess instinctive motivations that facilitate survival in the service of genetic propagation. Yet humans alone naturally represent the world symbolically, as a network of abstractions that permits thought to extend far beyond the bounds of immediate circumstances. Such representation enables people to become conscious of themselves, their past and their future, and thus to realize that, inevitably, they will die. This unwelcome news, when juxtaposed with basic animal drives to survive, produces a potential for paralyzing anxiety that could undermine capacities for effective behavior. Yet, in Becker's view, humans developed mechanisms that mitigate death-related anxiety, thereby sustaining psychological equanimity.

TMT identifies these protective psychological mechanisms as comprising a *dual-component anxiety buffer*. The first component is faith in a *cultural worldview*: a socially constructed set of beliefs about the nature of reality that enables individuals to construe the world in a meaningful, orderly manner. Through the lens of one's worldview, otherwise emotionless objects and events in the threatening, indifferent physical environment are transformed into seemingly significant and enduring elements of an ongoing story (answering questions such as "Where did I come from?," "Where am I going?," "What makes life meaningful?"). A piece of fabric becomes a flag; a slobbering canine becomes a lovable pet; a vicious slaughter becomes a patriotic endeavor. Most importantly, worldviews prescribe standards of valued conduct that dictate how individuals can lead a worthwhile life. This sets the stage for the second component, a sense of *self-esteem*: the perception that one is meeting or exceeding value standards espoused by one's cultural worldview. When I look good through the lens of my worldview, I can feel heroic, like I am a valued entity in a meaningful universe—rather than a nameless finite animal that will die, decay, and dissipate into oblivion like any other piece of moldering meat.

Maintaining this dual-component anxiety buffer allows individuals to transcend their mortality, becoming "immortal"—psychologically speaking—in one of two ways. *Literal immortality* is attained by firmly committing to religious or spiritual practices that bolster belief in a part of the self (e.g., a soul) which, after the body dies, literally ascends to a great heavenly realm beyond the physical world. Alternatively, *symbolic immortality* is attained when culturally valued action confers belief that one's achievements will leave an indelible imprint on the world—one that cries out, "I was here and I mattered!" This may be achieved in myriad ways: from delivering the mail on time day after day to passing on an immense financial legacy; from being the first in one's family to graduate college to compiling an epic edited volume on multimethod assessment.

In sum, TMT posits that the uniquely human awareness of death engenders potentially paralyzing terror. Faith in cultural worldviews (meaning) and a sense of self-esteem (value) function to manage this potential anxiety by conferring belief in one's literal or symbolic immortality.

Empirical Assessment of TMT

More than 500 experiments in over 20 countries over the past two decades have tested a variety of hypotheses derived from TMT (for review, see Greenberg et al., 2008). Most commonly examined is the *mortality salience hypothesis*, which states that: if faith in a cultural worldview and a sense of self-esteem function to buffer death-related anxiety, then reminders of mortality (mortality salience) should intensify efforts to fortify faith in one's worldview and gain self-esteem. Tests of this hypothesis entail manipulating whether subjects are induced to think about death or a control topic, and then measuring reliance on components of the theorized anxiety buffer.

Mortality salience (MS) has been operationalized in various ways: watching gory footage (e.g., an autopsy scene from *Faces of Death, Volume 1*, vs. a neutral scene from the same film); proximity to a funeral home (directly in front vs. 100 meters away); completing a word search task with embedded death-related terms (vs. aversive but non-death-related terms); being subliminally primed with the word *death* or *dead* (vs. length- and frequency-matched neutral or aversive but non-death-related terms). Comparable effects are obtained across operationalizations of MS, establishing the convergent validity of this manipulation.

Most commonly, participants complete two open-ended questions as part of what is described as a projective personality assessment: "Please briefly describe the emotions that the thought of your own death arouses in you" and "Jot down, as specifically as you can, what you think will happen to you as you physically die and once you are physically dead." Control participants answer parallel questions pertaining either to a neutral topic (e.g., shelving books, engaging in leisure activities) or to one of a diverse array of topics that, while highly aversive, do not overtly prime death-related thoughts (e.g., pain, taking an exam, embarrassment, failure, uncertainty, meaninglessness). MS consistently produces effects relative to these control conditions, demonstrating the discriminant validity of this manipulation (for an alternative account which challenges this claim, see, e.g., McGregor, 2004).[1]

One body of inquiry supporting the mortality salience hypothesis has shown that MS causes *cultural worldview defense*: heightened favorability toward those who support one's worldview and intensified negativity toward those who adhere to a different worldview. This work illustrates that reminders of death motivate individuals to defend meaningful social identities linked to specific groups and moral standards. For instance, MS has been found to heighten Americans' positive attitudes toward pro-U.S. targets and intensify negative attitudes toward anti-U.S. targets, to increase the amount of painfully spicy hot-sauce allocated to a person who derogated participants' political beliefs, and to exacerbate negative evaluations of moral transgressors while amplifying positive responses to heroes and famous people.

Additional research has shown that MS motivates efforts to procure meaning even in basic structured perceptions of one's own life, others' actions, and inanimate objects. For instance, MS has been found to increase perceived structural bonds between one's present actions and future goals, to heighten reliance on heuristics in making social judgments, and to diminish liking for abstract art in the absence of clarifying information (e.g., a meaningful title).

MS also motivates a quest for personal value, in a process termed *self-esteem striving*: intensified goal-pursuit in behavioral domains on which

---

[1] Various TMT research materials (e.g., MS manipulation, DTA measures, pro/anti-U.S. essays, five-item Likert-type target evaluation) can be freely obtained at *www.tmt.missouri.edu/materials.html*.

one's self-esteem depends. For example, among Israeli soldiers with strong self-esteem contingencies for driving ability, MS increased showy driving tendencies on a driving simulator; among individuals whose self-esteem depended on strength-training, MS increased the pressure with which they squeezed a hand dynamometer in front of an experimenter; and among women primed to associate tanned skin with an attractive appearance, MS decreased interest in sun-protective skin care and increased interest in tanning products and services.

Related work has shown that, after MS, people prefer to think of humans as special creatures rather than finite animals. For instance, MS has intensified disgust with feces and disdain for physical processes like breast feeding, and increased preferences for descriptions of the special status of human beings in the animal kingdom and of human dominion over nature.

Another source of meaning and value derives from close interpersonal relationships, which provide essential psychological comfort throughout the life span. The affection we get from others is a source of self-esteem, and the certainty of any belief is strengthened when close others share it. Consequently, MS amplifies motivation to form and maintain close relationships. For instance, MS has been found to heighten desires for romantic intimacy and willingness to initiate social interaction, and to elevate attraction-based commitment to a current romantic partner.

Mechanisms Underlying Effective Terror Management

The mechanisms underlying MS effects have been studied extensively in the context of a dual-process model (for review, see Hayes, Schimel, Arndt, & Faucher, 2010). This model specifies cognitive and behavioral processes by which death-related concerns are quelled after MS, among normally functioning individuals (see Figure 4.1). It is based on the operation of two forms of defense: proximal and distal.

Proximal defenses are direct efforts to push the thought of death out of one's mind and deny one's vulnerability to mortality. They occur immediately after MS, while death-related thought is active in people's current focal attention. For instance, immediately after MS, individuals seek to escape self-focused states and rate themselves high in traits associated with extended longevity. By contrast, distal defenses occur when a delay is interposed between MS and dependent measures. Rather than entailing distraction or denial of physical vulnerability, distal defenses focus on strengthening the aforementioned dual-component anxiety buffer via cultural worldview defense and self-esteem striving.

These overt processes coincide with a dynamic set of covert processes. These revolve around the suppression, activation, and deactivation of implicit death-related cognitions—termed *death thought accessibility*, or

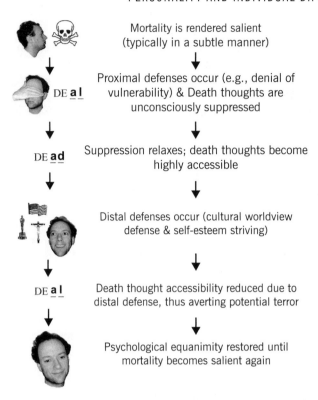

FIGURE 4.1. The dual-process model of TMT (for a review, see Hayes et al., 2010).

DTA. Researchers measure DTA in one of two ways. One method involves having participants complete word fragments (e.g., DE _ _ , SK _ _ L) that may yield death-related words (*dead, skull*) or non-death-related words (*deal, skill*). DTA is operationalized as the total number of death-related completions. The second method involves having participants perform a lexical decision task, making rapid decisions regarding whether letter strings presented on computer constitute words or nonwords. Included among the words are death-related terms, and DTA is operationalized as reaction times in identifying those terms (with faster reaction times indexing higher DTA).

The primary function of proximal and distal responses is to regulate levels of DTA and ultimately reduce them. Here is how it works. Immediately after MS, mortality salient participants do not show higher DTA than control participants. This is owing to an active suppression of death-related cognitions (an implicit counterpart to the active avoidance of self-focusing stimuli known to occur at the proximal stage). The "active" nature of this suppression is supported by findings that, when participants are put under high cognitive load (such that cognitive resources are unavailable for suppression), DTA does indeed increase immediately among mortality salient participants. Similarly, subliminal *death* primes bypass the suppression, producing immediate DTA increases.

Over time, the initial active suppression relaxes, such that death-related thoughts become highly active at the fringes of consciousness, or "accessible." When a delay period follows MS manipulations—such that participants enter the distal defense mode—mortality salient participants exhibit higher DTA than control participants. It is at this point that individuals typically employ distal defenses in order to deactivate DTA, reducing it to baseline (i.e., pre-MS) levels. A meta-analysis of 277 MS studies showed that longer delays between MS and dependent measures produce stronger distal effects, reflecting strengthened motivation to reduce DTA over time (one delay task ~1–2 minutes, $r = .34$; two delay tasks ~3–6 minutes, $r = .41$; three delay tasks ~7–12 minutes, $r = .47$; Burke, Martens, & Faucher, 2010).

Distal defenses truly deactivate DTA, rather than just re-suppressing it; cognitive load does not influence DTA levels after distal defense has occurred. And once this point of deactivation is reached, mortality salient participants no longer exhibit evidence of distal defense compared to controls. That is, among normally functioning individuals, engaging in distal defense after MS deactivates DTA, quelling existential concerns and thus allaying the need for further worldview defense or self-esteem striving.

Additional research verifies that TMT's dual-component anxiety buffer protects against DTA, and not simply against any type of aversive thought. Research using the lexical decision DTA assessment has shown that threatening a person's worldview or self-esteem quickens reaction times to death-related terms but not to frequency-matched aversive yet non-death-related terms, nor to affectively neutral terms. This supports the discriminative validity of DTA assessment. Furthermore, it is highly unlikely that DTA simply indexes a state of heightened negative affect. Whereas MS reliably elevates DTA, it typically does not influence self-report or physiological indices of affect or arousal.

DTA is most likely a cognitive "warning signal" of the potential to become anxious. Among normal functioning individuals, terror management processes operate effectively first to limit consciousness of this warning signal, then to let it ring at the unconscious level as attention focuses on opportunities for immortality, and finally—by exploiting such opportunities—to turn the warning signal off.

But what of individuals with ineffective terror management: those with tenuous or otherwise unstable senses of meaning and value, or those who struggle to effectively regulate DTA? How might such individuals be identified, and how do they respond to MS? Examining this topic reveals diverse assessment tools in the existential domain.

Terror Mismanagement: Assessing Weaknesses in the Anxiety Buffer

As a protégé of Thomas Szasz and professor in the Department of Psychiatry at the Upstate Medical Center in Syracuse, Becker was profoundly concerned with clinical issues. Yet only recently have TMT researchers begun examining implications of the theory for psychological dysfunction. A point of emphasis in this work is terror *mis*management: operations of the anxiety-buffer that result in extreme defensiveness, ineffective defensiveness, and/or failure to regulate DTA. First, this takes form as individual difference variables, with certain standard personality types showing pronounced reactivity to reminders of mortality. Second, clinical categories predict abnormal responses to MS. We consider each of these manifestations in turn (Table 4.1 summarizes the assessment tools described in the following sections).

Individual-Difference Moderators of MS Effects

Following in the psychoanalytic tradition and psychiatric perspectives of Szasz and R. D. Laing, TMT implies that mental health falls along a continuum: that no human is perfectly "healthy" because all are burdened by the potential for paralyzing existential terror. In our view, then, personality measures that predict extreme defensive reactivity to existential concerns may be interpreted as indices of terror *mis*management, even if such measures are not technically used for clinical diagnosis. The goal of this section is thus to summarize research on standard personality variables that predict abnormal responses to MS.

We begin by grouping relevant assessments into three categories: meaning rigidity, value fragility, and relational insecurity. Dispositional variables in these categories reliably moderate the nature of responses to MS. It is important to acknowledge that, in the context of MS effects, the statistical independence of these categories and of the measures in each has not been established. Research on interactions and intercorrelations among these assessments as they moderate MS effects is greatly needed in order to verify their effectiveness in quantifying distinct forms of terror *mis*management.

Yet some findings support the discrimination of these three categories (for review, see Greenberg et al., 2008). Research explicitly pitting meaning, value, and relational concerns against one another has revealed that sometimes MS motivates the pursuit of one at the expense of the others. For instance, MS-induced self-esteem striving is eliminated when positive performance entails surpassing admired qualities of a worldview representative (a political leader) or a close other (a parent). And whereas MS heightens preference for self-enhancing trophy partners in short-term dating contexts, it heightens preference for worldview-reinforcing partners

TABLE 4.1. Summary of Individual-Difference Moderators of Mortality Salience Effects, and Relevant Outcome Variables

Source article	Moderator that interacted with mortality salience	Dependent variable
Meaning rigidity		
Greenberg et al. (1990)	F-scale (Adorno et al., 1950)	Interpersonal Judgment Scale (Byrne, 1971)
Weise et al. (2012)	Right-Wing Authoritarianism (Altemeyer, 1998)	Five-item Likert-type target evaluation
Weise et al. (2012)	Belief in a Dangerous World (Altemeyer, 1998)	Five-item Likert-type target evaluation
Cozzolino et al. (2004)	Aspirations Index (Kasser & Ryan, 1996)	Number of raffle tickets taken for oneself
Jonas & Fischer (2006)	Intrinsic Religious Orientation (Feagin, 1964)	Five-item Likert-type target evaluation
Landau et al. (2004)	Personal Need for Structure (Thompson et al., 2001)	Three-item Likert-type target evaluation; Number of disparaging information items chosen re: a victim of a senseless tragedy
Value fragility		
Harmon-Jones et al. (1997)	Rosenberg Self-Esteem Scale (1965)	Five-item Likert-type target evaluation
Schmeichel et al. (2009)	Rosenberg Self-Esteem Scale (1965) & Self-Evaluative Implicit Associations Test (Jordan et al., 2003)	Three-item Likert-type rating of the extent to which a flattering personality description applies to oneself
Florian et al. (2001)	Third Generation Hardiness Scale (Maddi, 1987)	Multidimensional Social Transgression Scale (Florian & Mikulincer, 1997)
Goldenberg et al. (1999)	Eysenck Personality Inventory (Eysenck & Eysenck, 1967)	Physical Sex subscale of Goldenberg et al.'s (1999) Appeal of Sex Scale
Goldenberg et al. (2006)	Eysenck Personality Inventory (Eysenck & Eysenck, 1967)	Cold-pressor duration; duration of foot massager usage
Relational insecurity		
Mikulincer et al. (2002)	Experience in Close Relationships Scale (Brennan et al., 1998)	DTA word fragment measure
Mikulincer & Florian (2000)	Experience in Close Relationships Scale (Brennan et al., 1998) and self-classification assessment (Hazan & Shaver, 1987)	DTA word fragment measure; Multidimensional Social Transgression Scale (Florian & Mikulincer, 1997); Symbolic Immortality Scale (Mathews & Kling, 1988); Sharabany's Intimacy Scale (1994)

(continued)

TABLE 4.1. *(continued)*

Source article	Moderator that interacted with mortality salience	Dependent variable
<td colspan="3" align="center">Psychopathology</td>
Simon et al. (1996)	Beck Depression Inventory (1967)	Five-item Likert-type target evaluation
Simon et al. (1998)	Beck Depression Inventory (1967)	Kunzendorf's No Meaning Scale (1995–1996)
Strachan et al. (2007)	Specific phobia portion of the Structured Clinical Interview for DSM-IV	Time spent looking at pictures of spiders; Likert-type ratings of how threatening the spider images were
Strachan et al. (2007)	Contamination Obsessions and Washing Compulsions subscale of the Padua Inventory—Washington State University Revision (Burns et al., 1996)	Time spent washing hands
Strachan et al. (2007)	Social Interaction Anxiety Scale (Mattick & Clarke, 1998)	Time waiting in cubicle in order to avoid social interaction
Abdollahi et al. (2012)	Dissociative Experiences Scale II (Carlson & Putnam, 1993) and meeting DSM-IV criterion of a Class A1 trauma	Posttraumatic Stress Diagnostic Scale (Foa, 1995); Five-item Likert-type target evaluation
Kesebir et al. (2011)	Posttraumatic Stress Diagnostic Scale (Foa, 1995)	Multidimensional Social Transgression Scale (Florian & Mikulincer, 1997)
Chatard et al. (2012)	Post-Traumatic Stress Checklist—Civilian Version (Weathers et al., 1994)	DTA word fragment measure (French version)
Edmondson et al. (2011)	Post-Traumatic Stress Checklist—Civilian Version (Weathers et al., 1994)	DTA word fragment measure; excerpts from Multidimensional Social Transgression Scale (Florian & Mikulincer, 1997)

Note. Ordered according to when mentioned in this chapter. List includes representative variables assessed often in TMT research, but is not exhaustive and is restricted to moderators of MS manipulations. Source articles are designated by an asterisk (*) in the reference section. See Greenberg et al. (2008) for a full review of the TMT literature, and see *www.tmt.missouri.edu/materials.html* for free access to related research materials (e.g., MS manipulation, DTA measures, Pro/Anti-U.S. Essays, five-item Likert-type target evaluation).

in long-term dating contexts. Further, sometimes MS heightens desire for relational intimacy even when doing so might harm self-esteem; and MS can motivate physical proximity seeking even toward those who do not share one's worldview.

Recently, findings such as these have led researchers to propose a revision to TMT's anxiety buffer, advancing a model of a tripartite security system consisting of dynamically interrelated worldview, self-esteem, and relational processes (Hart, Shaver, & Goldenberg, 2005). We thus proceed with a similar three-pronged classification system for the assessment of vulnerability to existential concerns.

Measures of Meaning Rigidity

TMT suggests that individuals require a well-defined worldview in order to effectively manage their death anxiety. Yet certain worldviews and ways of maintaining them focus on rigid parameters of meaning that, due to their inflexibility and external dependence, are particularly sensitive to the threat of falsification. Reliance on them thus entails particularly vigorous ingroup favoritism and social stratification, and highly regimented, routinized ways of interpreting and controlling events and people. Accordingly, this first set of measures assesses the extent to which an individual's worldview inflexibly defines clear differences between groups, emphasizes external contingencies over internal fulfillments, and firmly structures perception of the physical and social world.

In this vein, one important moderator of MS effects is authoritarian personality: a pattern of traits or generalized behavioral style characterized by high regard for authority, conventionality, and contempt for those who are worse off (Adorno, Frenkel-Brunswick, Levinson, & Sanford, 1950). In a study by Greenberg and colleagues (1990), participants were told they would complete questionnaires and then engage in a problem-solving task with another person. Participants completed 12 attitude ratings concerning a variety of issues and then the F-scale measure of authoritarianism (Adorno et al., 1950). As subjects filled out the F-scale, the experimenter surreptitiously used the participant's 12 attitude responses as a basis for fabricating those of a supposed target person, such that the target's ratings were either similar to (75% agreement) or dissimilar from (25% agreement) the participant's own.

MS was then manipulated, and participants next reviewed the target's supposed responses "because people usually know a little about the people with whom they expect to interact." Finally, participants completed the Interpersonal Judgment Scale (IJS; Byrne, 1971), which asked them to rate the target's intelligence, knowledge of current events, morality, adjustment, and the extent to which they would like and enjoy working with the target. Results showed that highly authoritarian people responded to

MS with pronounced negative IJS ratings of the dissimilar target. Analogously, Weise and colleagues (Weise, Arciszewski, Verlhiac, Pyszczynski, & Greenberg, 2012) recently observed that MS caused pronounced negative evaluations of immigrants among individuals rating high in Right-Wing Authoritarianism (RWA), who also tended to be high in Belief in a Dangerous World (BDW) (Altemeyer, 1988). Together, these findings suggest that rigid meaning systems focused on defining clear group differences tend to be paired with a sense of vulnerability, and thus promote particularly rabid defensive responses to reminders of death.

Another assessment of rigid meaning focuses on the extent to which a person's worldview prioritizes external contingencies over internal fulfillments. It is common for individuals to maintain standards of valued conduct based on the pursuit of externalities (e.g., money, fame, beauty). Though defined in objective, concrete terms, the meaning afforded by such worldviews is tenuous and insecure because it is heavily dependent on continual validation from others. Indeed, research suggests that commitment to extrinsic goals is associated with diminished vitality, lower self-actualization and well-being, and elevated anxiety, depression and physical symptoms of distress (e.g., Kasser & Ryan, 1996).

Researchers have thus examined whether individuals whose worldviews prioritize external foci are less secure and more reactive to MS. For instance, Cozzolino and colleagues (Cozzolino, Staples, Meyers, & Samboceti, 2004; Study 3) used Kasser and Ryan's (1996) 30-item Aspirations Index to identify levels of extrinsic value orientation (EVO). In the study, participants had an opportunity to selfishly take more than their fair share of raffle tickets. After MS, greater EVO was associated with taking more tickets.

Similarly, Jonas and Fischer (2006) found that individuals lacking an intrinsic basis for their religious faith are particularly prone to worldview defense after MS *and* gain less security from their worldview. People high in intrinsic religiosity integrate religion into their subjective experience, private thoughts, and meditative practices, rather than emphasizing religion's objective social context as a clique to belong to. To assess this factor, participants completed the Intrinsic Religious Orientation Scale (IRO; Feagin, 1964). MS was manipulated and participants were presented with two essays, one lauding positive aspects of the participants' current city of residence (Munich, Germany) and the other lambasting it as a horrible place in which to live. Composite ratings of responses to the two essays, respectively, were computed from five evaluative items that have been used in many TMT studies and reliably register worldview defense effects: "How much do you like the author?"; "How intelligent do you think the author is?"; "How knowledgeable do you think the author is?"; "How much do you agree with the author's opinion?"; and "How true do you think the author's opinion is?"

Several interesting effects emerged. The researchers had also manipulated whether the IRO was administered before or after the worldview
defense assessment. If it came after, all participants showed pronounced
worldview defense (i.e., greater relative preference for the pro-Munich
author over the anti-Munich author). Yet if the IRO came before, only participants low in IRO exhibited worldview defense. Thus, affirming a high
IRO worldview buffered individuals from the need for worldview defense,
whereas no such security was afforded by affirming a low IRO worldview.
Analogous results occurred on a measure of DTA. Whereas affirming a
high IRO worldview functioned to eliminate the effect of MS on DTA,
affirming a low IRO worldview did not have this securing effect.

A final index of meaning rigidity is the tendency to impose and prefer structure and closure, as assessed by the Personal Need for Structure
Scale (PNS; Thompson, Naccarato, Parker & Moskowitz, 2001). Because
of intense reliance on clear and consistent knowledge, high-PNS people
respond to MS by seizing upon simplified social information and derogating people and objects that do not conform to rigid bases of comprehension and perception. Extensive research spearheaded by Mark Landau (e.g.,
Landau et al., 2004) has illustrated this in diverse ways.

In one study, participants read a transcript of people discussing a
mutual acquaintance ("Don"). Don was either consistently described
as extroverted, consistently described as introverted, or inconsistently
described (as being extroverted sometimes, introverted at other times).
Participants then evaluated Don on three items, later combined to form a
composite liking score: "How much do you like the person being spoken
about?"; "How much could you see yourself being close, personal friends
with this person?"; "How interested would you be in hearing more about
this person?" Among high-PNS people, MS led to more negative evaluation
of the inconsistent target person.

Another study examined the possibility that high-PNS individuals
would, after MS, try to make sense of a senseless tragedy by derogating
the victim (to fit the events into a simple vision of a "just world" in which
people deserve what they get and get what they deserve). Participants read
about the tragic misfortune of "Jeff Tremlet," who was shot three times
during a home invasion and sustained irremediable facial disfigurement
and cognitive deficits. Participants then had the opportunity to learn more
about the victim, including statements describing him in generally negative
terms (e.g., "Jeff often had mean things to say about others") or positive
terms (e.g., "Tremlet was actively involved in community service"). Participants were asked to choose five statements that appealed to them most and
that they would be interested in reading more about. Results showed that,
after MS, high-PNS participants exhibited a marked tendency to choose
negative statements – those implying that the tragedy happened to a bad
person, and thus protecting a simplified "just world" vision of things.

Measures of Value Fragility

TMT posits that self-esteem functions to buffer death-related anxiety. The first studies directly testing this claim showed that situationally boosting self-esteem via bogus positive personality feedback lessened reported anxiety in response to a video about death and attenuated physiological arousal in response to the threat of shock (Greenberg et al., 1992). Building upon these findings, later research demonstrated that individual difference markers of deficits in self-worth moderate MS effects. These indices of value fragility assess the extent to which individuals experience diminished and unstable self-esteem, and struggle to view themselves as more than finite physical creatures.

The role of diminished and unstable self-esteem has been assessed in several ways. In work by Harmon-Jones and colleagues (1997), the Rosenberg Self-Esteem Scale (1965) was administered to American college students twice (once at the start of the semester and again several weeks later). The researchers ensured that one-half of recruited participants exhibited stable high self-esteem across assessments (above the 75th percentile), while the other half exhibited stable moderate-to-low self-esteem (between the 50th and 25th percentile). MS was manipulated and worldview defense was measured using the five-item assessment of participants' attitudes toward the authors of pro-U.S. and anti-U.S. essays. Consistent with the idea that deficits in stable self-worth increase reactivity to existential concerns, individuals in the moderate-to-low self-esteem group responded to MS with pronounced pro-U.S. bias.

Other researchers assessed similar processes with a different methodology. Schmeichel and colleagues (2009) reasoned that self-esteem is at its most fragile—and thus most in need of defense—when a person's relatively conscious and reflective sense of self-worth ("explicit") is at odds with his or her deep-seated, relatively unconscious and spontaneous ("implicit") sense of self-worth. This idea harkens to Carl Jung's archetype called The Shadow—the negative side of ourselves about which we have doubts and fears and spend a great deal of energy working to deny and control.

To test this idea, Schmeichel et al. measured explicit self-esteem with the Rosenberg Self-Esteem Scale and measured implicit self-esteem with an Implicit Association Test (IAT; adapted by Jordan, Spencer, Zanna, Hoshino-Browne, & Correll, 2003). In the IAT, participants rapidly categorized words as either being related to or not being related to the self and as being either pleasant or unpleasant by pressing one of two computer keys. Higher implicit self-esteem was indicated by faster categorizations when self was paired with pleasant rather than when self was paired with unpleasant. The explicit self-esteem and implicit self-esteem measures were uncorrelated.

Next, MS was manipulated, and a measure of defensive self-enhancement was administered. Participants were presented with two personality profiles, one glowingly positive and the other quite negative. Participants rated each description on the extent to which it was accurate, relevant, and complete in describing their own personality. Results showed that MS heightened the perceived self-descriptiveness of the positive personality profile, but only among individuals with fragile self-esteem—those with a combined profile of high explicit self-esteem and low implicit self-esteem. Such findings converge with those of Harmon-Jones et al. (1997) and reveal additional measurement tools for assessing self-esteem fragility and defensiveness.

Another index of value fragility is hardiness, defined as "a constellation of personality characteristics that function as a resistance resource in the encounter with stressful life events" (Kobasa, Maddi, & Kahn, 1982, p. 169). To lack hardiness is to lack a commitment to one's actions, belief in control over one's life, and the ability to cope with stress. Hardiness scales correlate positively with physical and mental health and negatively with measures of anxiety and depression, and moderate the association between war-related trauma and development and severity of posttraumatic stress disorder. Although hardiness and neuroticism are highly correlated, they tap distinct constructs (see evidence reviewed by Florian, Mikulincer, & Hirschberger, 2001).

Research by Florian, Mikulincer, and Hirschberger (2001) suggests that, without the inner resources afforded by hardiness, individuals are less able to deal with death in a manner that transforms existential anxiety into a benign experience; they are too fragile to cope. The researchers administered the Third Generation Hardiness Scale (Maddi, 1987), manipulated MS, and then administered the Multidimensional Social Transgression Scale (MSTS; Florian & Mikulincer, 1997). The MSTS has proven reliably responsive to MS manipulations. It presents a variety of vignettes describing various social transgressions, including traffic offense, burglary, forgery, fraud, and medical malpractice, each varying in their intrapersonal and interpersonal consequences. For each story, participants evaluate the severity of the transgression and the punishment that should be administered to the particular transgressor. Results showed that MS heightened severity and punishment ratings on the MSTS, but only among individuals low in self-reported hardiness. Thus, low hardiness represents another index of value fragility that renders individuals vulnerable to the effects of MS, and prone to lashing out with pronounced worldview defensive tendencies.

A final domain—one in which the human sense of personal value is arguably at its most fragile—revolves around the recognition that one is a finite physical body. Jamie Goldenberg's research has shown myriad ways in which death reminders motivate people to deny their corporeal nature (for a review, see Goldenberg, 2012). This work has revealed neuroticism as a key personality moderator of the relationship between MS and the denial of human creatureliness. As reflected in Woody Allen's oeuvre, the emotional instability characteristic of neuroticism renders it difficult to accept the illusion that the body may be more than just a body—that it could possibly house a valued and potentially immortal self. Indeed, neuroticism correlates negatively with self-esteem, positively with death anxiety, and positively with disgust over one's physical nature.

To assess neuroticism, Goldenberg uses the Eysenck Personality Inventory (Eysenck & Eysenck, 1967). Her research has shown that, after MS, neurotics exhibit heightened disgust with the physical aspects of sexual experience as measured by the Physical Sex subscale of Goldenberg and colleagues' (Goldenberg, Pyszczynski, McCoy, Greenberg, & Solomon, 1999) Appeal of Sex Scale. In fact, even without MS, simply thinking about sex increases DTA among neurotics! Two other clever experiments have demonstrated that highly neurotic people avoid physical stimulation after MS. In one study, participants performed the painful task of submerging their forearm to the elbow in a cooler containing 15 liters of cold water, ranging from 1° to 4° Celsius (a "cold-pressor" task). In the other study, participants experienced pleasurable stimulation from a vibrating foot massager turned on high intensity. In both cases, highly neurotic individuals responded to MS by engaging in the behavior for a briefer duration.

Measures of Relational Insecurity

The attachment security we acquire as children models the manner in which, later as adults, we attain existential security. Our early beliefs and values are those displayed or advocated by our caregivers, and our first inklings of self-esteem derive from parental love and the conditional dispensation of their affections. As Hart, Shaver, and Goldenberg (2005) proposed, secure attachment, faith in a worldview, and a sense of self-esteem "are so intertwined developmentally as to be almost functionally indistinguishable with regard to the regulation of anxiety" (p. 1001). And just as deficits in meaning and value render an individual prone to terror *mis*management, so too do insecure interpersonal ties leave a person with an unreliable existential security net.

Led by Mario Mikulincer, researchers have extensively examined the role of attachment insecurity in terror management processes (for review, see Mikulincer, Florian, & Hirschberger, 2003). One series of studies examined whether insecure attachment renders individuals prone to disruption in the anxiety buffer. To do so, researchers assessed general level of attachment anxiety with Brennan, Clark, and Shaver's (1998) Experience in Close Relationships Scale (ECR). Participants were asked either to imagine experiencing a separation from a close relationship partner or (in the control condition) to imagine a television program they typically watched. Subsequently, participants completed the word-fragment assessment of DTA. Results showed that imagining separation caused higher DTA, but only among individuals high in attachment anxiety. Insecure attachment thus indexes proneness to terror *mis*management.

Other work has examined how people with various attachment styles respond to MS (e.g., Mikulincer & Florian, 2000). In this vein, researchers measure attachment style using a self-classification assessment from Hazan and Shaver (1987) along with the ECR, thereby distinguishing secure, avoidant, and anxious–ambivalent subjects. Effects of MS vary substantially across attachment type.

Anxious–ambivalent individuals—those characterized by a desire for enmeshed relationships and fear of rejection—exhibit particularly tenuous protection from existential concerns. In addition to a fragile sense of self-worth, self-defeating tendencies, and depressive affect, anxious–ambivalent people show a tendency toward hyperactivation and rumination on distressing thoughts (Mikulincer, Orbach, & Iavnieli, 1998). Accordingly, anxious–ambivalent participants do not suppress DTA immediately after MS. At both proximal and distal phases (i.e., with or without a delay after an MS induction), anxious–ambivalent individuals respond to MS with high DTA levels. This precipitates a sustained tendency toward defensiveness. At both proximal and distal phases, anxious–ambivalent people respond to MS with heightened worldview defense (as measured by the MSTS). Moreover, engaging in worldview defense after MS fails to reduce DTA to baseline levels among anxious–ambivalent people.

Avoidant individuals—characterized by preference for emotional distance—show a different pattern. Avoidant people exhibit pronounced mental suppression of distressing thoughts and defensive distortions of appraisals of the self and the world (e.g., Mikulincer et al., 1998). Consequently, avoidant people exhibit a seemingly "normal" pattern of terror management responses: suppressing DTA immediately after MS, activating DTA in the distal phase only, exhibiting worldview defense only in the distal phase, and reducing DTA following worldview defense.

So do avoidant people not suffer terror *mis*management? Other work suggests that they do—specifically, that avoidant attachment is associated with pronounced attachment-related defensive responses. In Hart et al. (2005), attachment style was assessed on the ECR. Participants were then asked to find a set of words embedded in a matrix of letters. For one-half of participants (in a control condition), the words could easily be found. For the other half of participants (in a self-esteem threat condition), no words from the set were actually in the matrix, and instructions stated that most participants are able to find four words in a 2-minute period. Participants then completed a Desire for Closeness in Romantic Relationships Scale, which asked them to imagine their ideal romantic relationship and provide scaled ratings of how much closeness, intimacy, sharing, and reliance there would be in the relationship. Compared to nonavoidant people, avoidantly attached participants reported significantly less desire for closeness in the self-esteem threat condition. This suggests that when the anxiety buffer of avoidantly attached individuals is threatened (in this case, their self-esteem), they flee from contact with others.

Studies have also examined how MS affects securely attached individuals—those characterized by confidence in others' availability in times of need, comfort with closeness, and positive attachment history. Securely attached people's pattern of DTA suppression–activation–deactivation appears normal. However, among securely attached individuals, MS does not alter MSTS ratings. Instead of gaining security by punishing moral violators, securely attached people respond to MS with an increased sense of symbolic immortality and increased desire for relational intimacy. Sense of symbolic immortality has been assessed using Mathews and Kling's (1988) Symbolic Immortality Scale (e.g., "I would do almost anything to ensure the future of my children"; "It is important for me to write, create, or build something that will exist after my death"). Relational intimacy has been assessed by having participants rate whether their idealized romantic relationship would have desirable levels of frankness, spontaneity, and closeness (using Sharabany's Intimacy Scale, 1994).

Psychopathology Constructs that Predict Abnormal Responses to MS

From a TMT perspective, psychological disorders may in part reflect deficiencies in mechanisms that mitigate death-related concerns. This is consistent with the view shared by personality theorists and mental health professionals that many psychological problems emanate from inabilities to successfully cope with anxiety (e.g., Horney, 1937; May, 1950/1970; Yalom, 1980). Relevant TMT research with clinical populations is scant, but emerging. Extant findings suggest that individuals fitting certain clinical categories respond to MS in ways that do not effectively procure meaning and value, nor regulate DTA well. Research has pinpointed three ways in which such difficulties manifest.

Extreme Defense among the Mildly Depressed

First, this can present as *extreme defense*, with clinical categories predicting pronounced distal responses to MS. Work in this vein has focused on existential concerns among mildly depressed people. From a TMT perspective, the perception of oneself as worthless and lacking enjoyable engagement with the world heightens vulnerability to death-related anxiety. Indeed, depression correlates positively with overarching belief that life is meaningless, and frequent thoughts about death are a depressive symptom (Simon, Arndt, Greenberg, Solomon, & Pyszczynski, 1998).

Experiments by Simon, Harmon-Jones, Greenberg, Solomon, & Pyszczynski (1996) suggest that such vulnerability creates a penchant for extreme defensive responses to MS. The researchers administered the Beck

Depression Inventory (Beck, 1967) to American participants, categorizing them as either mildly depressed or nondepressed. In control conditions, mildly depressed participants exhibited *lower* levels of worldview defense than nondepressed individuals. That is, at baseline, mildly depressed people hesitated to affirm a worldview relative to nondepressed people. Yet after MS, all participants exhibited worldview defense—and mildly depressed subjects did so at significantly *higher* levels than their nondepressed counterparts.

This extreme defense appears insufficient to quell DTA and the need for meaning. Simon et al. (1998) found that after extreme MS-induced worldview defense, mildly depressed participants went on to defensively inflate their perceptions of life's meaningfulness on Kunzendorf's No Meaning Scale (Kunzendorf, Moran, & Gray, 1995–1996). No such effect occurred among nondepressed participants. This suggests that mildly depressed people react to their mortality by persistently grasping for significance in a manner that does not restore equanimity—like an existential Sisyphus.

Terror Focalization among the Phobic, Compulsive, and Socially Anxious

Because some individuals cannot rely on a worldview and self-esteem to manage existential concerns, they may attempt to localize the nebulous fear of death in concrete, controllable objects (a process termed *terror focalization*). By exerting control over such stimuli, individuals may partly manage death-related anxiety. Yet such efforts do not afford culturally rooted inroads to immortality; consequently, terror focalization presents among people with clinical problems.

Strachan et al. (2007) assessed this process among individuals with phobic, compulsive, and socially anxious tendencies. One study involved spider phobics. Participants were screened using the specific phobia portion of the Structured Clinical Interview for DSM-IV. Those who met full diagnosis were included, along with a comparison group of nonphobics who expressed neither fear nor ambivalence toward spiders. Following an MS manipulation, participants viewed a series of images on computer, including six pictures of spiders. Participants proceeded at their own pace, and for each image rated how threatening it was. Results showed that MS caused spider phobics (but not nonphobics) to spend less time viewing the spider pictures and to rate them as more threatening. Thus, among the phobics, thoughts of mortality were focalized onto a concrete, controllable stimulus that could be identified and avoided.

Another study had participants first complete the Contamination Obsessions and Washing Compulsions (COWC) subscale of the Padua Inventory–Washington State University Revision (PI-WSUR; Burns, Keortge, Formea, & Sternberger, 1996). Recruited participants had scored in the top third or lower third of the COWC distribution. In session, MS was manipulated, and then a bogus psychophysiological assessment was implemented in order to get participants' fingers coated with sticky electrode gel. Afterward, participants' hand-washing behaviors were surreptitiously assessed. Results showed that MS caused high-COWC participants (but not low-COWC participants) to spend significantly more time washing their hands.

In a final study, participants completed the Social Interaction Anxiety Scale (SIAS; Mattick & Clarke, 1998). Those scoring in the upper or lower third of the SIAS distribution participated. In separate cubicles, subjects completed a packet of personality questionnaires with an embedded MS manipulation. Before administering the packet, the experimenter informed each participant that the study would conclude with a group discussion and that they could join the conversation at any point, but that the session would end at 15 minutes to the hour. A dependent measure of social interaction avoidance was computed as the session time remaining when participants chose to exit their cubicle. Results showed that MS caused high-SIAS people (but not low-SIAS people) to wait significantly longer in their cubicle, thus reducing the amount of anticipated time engaged in social interaction.

In sum, Strachan et al.'s (2007) work suggests that phobic, compulsive, and socially anxious individuals respond to thoughts of mortality with behaviors indicative of intensified pathology. Such outcomes may reflect efforts to mitigate death-related anxiety through actions which, though discrete and controllable, do not afford reliable bases of faith in a worldview or self-esteem.

Anxiety-Buffer Disruption among the Traumatized

Traumatic events awaken the terror of mortality in brutally direct ways. In the aftermath of a trauma, not all individuals have the psychological resources to hit the "reset" button, resiliently returning to a normal life wherein available senses of meaning and value keep death-related anxiety at bay. Studies assessing *anxiety-buffer disruption* have revealed that severely traumatized populations show unusual responses to MS, including diminished reliance on worldviews and self-esteem and dysregulation of DTA. A key factor in this process is peritraumatic dissociation: psychological disengagement during trauma that anticipates the delayed onset of anxiety-related pathology, including posttraumatic stress disorder (PTSD; Ozer, Best, Lipsey, & Weiss, 2003).

Abdolhossein Abdollahi leads this research program (Abdollahi, Pyszczynski, Maxfield, & Luszczynska, 2012). One set of experiments examined residents of Zarand, Iran, during the month following a devastating 2005 earthquake (6.4 on the Richter scale) that killed over 1,500 persons and forced over 6,700 persons to evacuate their homes. Participants were prescreened using the Dissociative Experiences Scale II (DES-II; Carlson &

Putnam, 1993), and recruited if they scored high or low. All high DES-II participants met the DSM-IV criterion of a Class A1 trauma within the month before the study.

In session, MS was manipulated and worldview defense was assessed on five Likert-type items regarding the perception that Western foreign aid would be suspiciously conditional and insubstantial. Results showed that, among low dissociators, MS provoked a typical worldview defensive response (more negative attitudes toward Western foreign aid) and MS did not influence self-reported affect (as is typical; see "Mechanisms Underlying Effective Terror Management" section above). By contrast, high dissociators did not exhibit worldview defense after MS, and instead responded to MS with an atypical increase in negative affect. This suggests that dissociation disrupts the buffering function typically served by faith in a worldview.

These abnormal responses persisted over time. Two years after the earthquake, the aforementioned DES-II scores (assessed in the month after the earthquake) positively predicted PTSD symptoms, as measured with Foa's (1995) Posttraumatic Stress Diagnostic Scale. In session, MS was manipulated, and worldview defense was assessed using the attitudes toward foreign aid items. Whereas low-PTSD participants responded to MS with heightened worldview defense, high-PTSD participants did not. Moreover, the lack of worldview defense observed among high-PTSD participants partly explained the relationship between dissociation and PTSD symptoms. Specifically, the association between DES-II scores at Time 1 and PTSD symptoms at Time 2 was partially mediated by lower worldview defense levels. These results suggest that dissociative responses to trauma disrupt the terror management anxiety buffer, rendering individuals prone to long-term psychological distress. (In 2011, Kesebir, Luszczynska, Pyszczynski, & Benight obtained analogous results among Polish survivors of domestic violence, using the MSTS to assess worldview defense.)

Research has also demonstrated that terror *mis*management among traumatized people presents as dysregulation of DTA. Chatard and colleagues (2012) examined citizens of the Ivory Coast following a vicious civil war. Whereas individuals low in PTSD symptoms exhibited the usual suppression of death-related thoughts immediately after MS, those with more severe symptoms did not display such suppression. Edmondson and colleagues (2011) obtained similar results among college students with varied levels of trauma symptoms. Those low in trauma symptoms suppressed DTA right after MS; those high in trauma symptoms instead showed high DTA right after MS. Moreover, despite elevated DTA, high trauma symptom participants did not engage in worldview defense and did not show reduced DTA following a situationally induced boost to self-esteem.

Together, these results suggest that traumatized people exhibit evidence of intense terror *mis*management. They respond to MS with low worldview defense and high negative affect, do not suppress DTA, and do not exhibit deactivation of DTA when components of the terror management anxiety-buffer are reinforced.

Notable Divergences of Cognitive and Behavioral Outcomes

As mentioned earlier (see "Mechanisms Underlying Effective Terror Management" section and Figure 4.1), the TMT research literature documents a normal cascade of processes triggered by MS: death is rendered salient → DTA is suppressed and proximal defenses occur → DTA increases over time and distal defenses occur → engaging in distal defense reduces DTA to baseline levels. We have identified a host of moderators that predict abnormally strong versions of these otherwise normal responses to MS (e.g., extreme worldview defense among authoritarians).

Yet the results just reviewed suggest that some constructs predict breakdowns in basic terror management mechanisms rather than exacerbation of normal responses. Specifically, anxious–ambivalent individuals (Mikulincer & Florian, 2000) and people who dissociate strongly in response to traumatic events (e.g., Edmonson et al., 2011) exhibit a notably disrupted pattern of responses to MS, wherein DTA is sustained at a high level across both proximal and distal phases and is not successfully reduced by worldview defense and/or self-esteem striving. How can such discontinuities between the cognitive and behavioral elements of terror management processes be explained?

One common feature of these two instances is abnormal strain on compensatory systems. In the case of ambivalent attachment, an individual bears the stress of desiring closeness with others but also desiring to push them away. In the case of dissociation, thoughts and emotions pertaining to a prior trauma are displaced from consciousness and remain as unresolved issues requiring continual suppression. Perhaps these forms of intense cognitive and emotional taxation diminish people's regulatory capacities, analogous to the burdensome effects of allostatic load on cardiovascular reactivity or of repeated blood sugar spikes on cellular response to insulin. Individuals who chronically rely on regulatory mechanisms to the point of wearing them down may lose the ability to effectively manage DTA via proximal suppression and subsequent worldview defense.

How might this issue be addressed clinically? We doubt that encouraging such individuals to adopt conventional sources of meaning (e.g., religion, nationalism) would suffice to address their existential quandaries—at least, no more than a piece of tape would render a stretched out rubber band sufficiently taut. Sustained relational ambivalence and the psychological ravages of trauma are difficult challenges that pierce through symbolic worldviews to the heart of one's animal nature, revealing fundamental helplessness, dependency, and vulnerability.

It may be useful instead to focus on an aspect of affective experience that characterizes traumatized individuals' responses to MS: negative affect. As mentioned earlier (see "Mechanisms Underlying Effective Terror Management" section), MS normally does not heighten negative affect; yet high dissociators do show heightened negative affect following MS (Abdollahi et al., 2012). Perhaps, then, interventions geared toward the regulation of negative affect will prove effective among people whose perseverative thoughts of death cannot be managed successfully by typical distal defenses. We will revisit this possibility later in the next section.

Using Multiple Methods to Assess and Treat Terror Mismanagement

We have identified cognitive, affective, and behavioral indices of pronounced and/or atypical responses to the thought of mortality. How might this host of measures and manipulations be integrated into a multimethod assessment technique that serves people? We conclude by speculating on this matter, with an eye on difficulties inherent in transitioning from the cross-sectional between-subject experimental designs employed in TMT research, to longitudinal case study approaches commonly used in clinical assessment and treatment.

One strategy could involve monitoring levels of meaning rigidity, value fragility, and relational instability over the course of treatment. As earlier reviewed, these indices predict pronounced reactivity to MS and would likely be useful for detecting vulnerability to existential concerns among clinical populations. Assessments in these categories may initially be administered in order to diagnose the sort of anxiety-buffer deficits a person is prone to experiencing. Therapeutic intervention may then target the particular anxiety-buffer deficits evinced by these assessments, and repeated measurement over time may detect improvements along the relevant dimension(s). In parallel with this strategy, it will be useful to examine behaviors characteristic of extreme distal defensiveness (e.g., pronounced worldview defense). We reviewed a variety of procedures that reliably detect such reactivity and that could be implemented repeatedly to detect reduced defensiveness over time. We would expect that, as indices of meaning rigidity, value fragility, and relational insecurity improve, behavioral indices of distal defense will decrease.

Yet will meaningful results be obtained using one distal defense measure multiple times for a single person? If not, distinct measures will be needed at distinct time points. Yet little is known about how the various distal defense measures used in TMT research relate to one another. And though different operationalizations of MS produce convergent results, will the strength of such effects vary with repeated assessment? And what if participants become aware that effects of mortality primes are being assessed, thereby interfering with the procedure of provoking existential concerns outside of focal attention? Can therapy be ethically and effectively performed in the context of an elaborate cover story that keeps participants blind to the assessment of MS's effects on them? These issues reflect the difficulty, alluded to in the Introduction, of merging basic social psychology research with practices in clinical psychology. Clearly, research and debate are needed to address these critical questions.

It is clear, however, that treatment conditions which strengthen components of the terror management anxiety-buffer can mitigate MS effects. For instance, Schmeichel and Martens (2005) found that having participants affirm values central to their worldview eliminated MS-induced worldview defense and DTA. (Recall, though, Jonas and Fischer's [2006] findings that less intrinsically oriented worldviews are less likely to serve this buffering function, suggesting that the type of worldview affirmed matters.) Similarly, Harmon-Jones et al. (1997) found that worldview defense and DTA were reduced if participants first received a self-esteem boost, in the form of bogus positive personality feedback. Further, other work has shown that, after MS, creative behavior makes people feel guilty (presumably over the disruption to social connection associated with individual expression). Yet feedback reinforcing participants' closeness and similarity to others eliminates this guilt response, replacing it instead with a sense of positive engagement and readiness to explore alternative worldviews (Arndt, Routledge, Greenberg, & Sheldon, 2005; Routledge & Arndt, 2009). Researchers should endeavor to translate analog interventions such as these into actual interventions that can be used in clinical contexts.

A model for this translational approach can be found in William Breitbart's research on meaning-centered group psychotherapy (MCGP; Breitbart, 2002; Breitbart et al., 2010). Building from the insights of Viktor Frankl, MCGP research shows that fostering a meaningful interpretation of life contributes to psychological improvement among dying individuals. In one study, cancer patients with stage III or IV solid tumors received an 8-week therapeutic intervention. Some patients received MCGP, which employs instruction, discussion, and experiential exercises that explore and cultivate a sense of historical and family legacy, acceptance of life's limitations, satisfaction with nature, art, and humor, and hope for the future. Other patients instead received supportive group psychotherapy (SPG), which focuses directly on coping with and understanding experiences and emotions surrounding cancer diagnosis and treatment. Results showed that, relative to SGP recipients, MCGP recipients experienced higher spiritual well-being and sense of significance, as well as reduced anxiety—effects that were most pronounced two months after treatment. We are hopeful that appropriating TMT research findings to the realm of clinical care will yield similar positive treatment outcomes.

Finally, in parallel with assessment of anxiety-buffer deficits and distal defense levels, it may be useful to assess how DTA regulation stabilizes over the course of treatment. We have described evidence that both clinical groups (e.g., traumatized people) and nonclinical groups (e.g., the anxious-ambivalently attached) exhibit severe dysregulation in their management of DTA. Although we think that the maintenance of meaning, value, and relationships should take priority in developing clinical treatment for patients with existential concerns, people may also benefit from interventions aimed at directly regularizing the suppression–activation–deactivation process or at least coping with consequences of its chronic dysregulation.

For individuals struggling to suppress death-related thoughts (e.g., traumatized people), it may be appropriate to encourage *mindfulness*: receptive attention to present experience. Research suggests that highly mindful people (as assessed with the Mindful Attention Awareness Scale; Brown & Ryan, 2003) show minimal suppression of DTA after MS, yet also exhibit low distal defense levels, even when defending beliefs about mindfulness itself (Niemiec et al., 2010). Thus, if individuals have difficulty using DTA suppression to initiate the process of effective DTA regulation, aversive consequences of sustained high DTA may be avoided by cultivating capacities for mindful reflection. For instance, therapeutic techniques that incorporate mindfulness techniques might allay traumatized individuals' negative affective responses to MS. Even if typical distal defenses ineffectively regulate DTA among such people, perhaps more experiential awareness could yield some peace of mind.

For individuals who can suppress and activate DTA, but then struggle to deactivate it via distal defense, a rather counterintuitive procedure may be useful: Have them imagine that they are *flying*. Fantasies of flight imply movement away from that which is earthly, limited, and vulnerable and toward that which is divine, transcendent, free, and immortal. Consequently, Cohen, Sullivan, Solomon, Greenberg, and Ogilvie (2011) found that fantasizing about flight (but not about other supernatural acts lacking vertical ascension) attenuated the effect of MS on DTA. Accordingly, therapeutic procedures that encourage flight-related ideation may help exercise and strengthen the cognitive mechanisms that quell death-related concerns.

Conclusion

Despite the psychological burden of death awareness, human beings have emerged as the dominant species on the planet. And despite our means of managing death anxiety, humans remain the most violent animal in existence and prone to intense dysfunction. A prodigious and perhaps impossible task for social science is to unite its respective disciplinary enterprises in the service of understanding this dilemma and facilitating the well-being of our fellow humans. We hope that by describing the tools and techniques associated with research on terror management—and its perilous counterpart, terror *mis*management—this chapter encourages clinical practitioners to assess, and attend to, humans' existential concerns. It is in this sense that we share Ernest Becker's (1975) aspiration to "introduce just that minute measure of reason to balance destruction" (p. 170).

REFERENCES

Source articles listed in Table 4.1 are designated by an asterisk (*).

Abdollahi, A., Pyszczynski, T., Maxfield, M., & Luszczynska, A. (2012). Posttraumatic stress reactions as a disruption in anxiety-buffer functioning: Dissociation and responses to mortality salience as predictors of severity of posttraumatic symptoms. *Psychological Trauma: Theory, Research, Practice, and Policy, 3,* 329–341. (*)

Adorno, T., Frenkel-Brunswick, E., Levinson, D., & Sanford, R. N. (1950). *The authoritarian personality.* New York: Harper.

Altemeyer, B. (1988). *Enemies of freedom: Understanding right-wing authoritarianism.* San Francisco: Jossey-Bass/Pfeiffer.

Arndt, J., Routledge, C., Greenberg, J., & Sheldon, K. M. (2005). Illuminating the dark side of creative expression: Assimilation needs and the consequences of creative action following mortality salience. *Personality and Social Psychology Bulletin, 31,* 1327–1339.

Beck, A. T. (1967). *Depression: Clinical, experimental, and theoretical aspects.* New York: Harper & Row.

Becker, E. (1973). *The denial of death.* New York: Free Press.

Becker, E. (1975). *Escape from evil.* New York: Free Press.

Breitbart, W. (2002). Spirituality and meaning in supportive care: Spirituality and meaning-centered group psychotherapy intervention in advanced cancer. *Support Cancer Care, 10,* 272–280.

Breitbart, W., Rosenfeld, B., Gibson, C., Pessin, H., Poppito, S., Nelson, C., et al. (2010). Meaning-centered group psychotherapy for patients with advanced cancer: A pilot randomized controlled trial. *Psycho-Oncology, 19,* 21–28.

Brennan, K. A., Clark, C. L., & Shaver, P. R. (1998). Self-report measurement of adult attachment: An integrative overview. In J. A. Simpson & W. S. Rholes (Eds.), *Attachment theory and close relationships* (pp. 46–76). New York: Guilford Press.

Brown, K. W., & Ryan, R. M. (2003). The benefits of being present: Mindfulness and its role in psychological well-being. *Journal of Personality and Social Psychology, 84,* 822–848.

Burke, B. L., Martens, A., & Faucher, E. H. (2010). Two decades of terror management theory: A meta-analysis of mortality salience research. *Personality and Social Psychology Review, 14,* 155–195.

Burns, G. L., Keortge, S. G., Formea, G. M., & Sternberger, L. G. (1996). Revision of the Padua Inventory of obsessive compulsive disorder symptoms: Distinctions between worry obsessions, and compulsions. *Behaviour Research and Therapy, 34,* 163–173.

Byrne, D. (1971). *The attraction paradigm.* New York: Academic Press.

Carlson, E. B., & Putnam, F. W. (1993). An update on the Dissociative Experiences Scale. *Dissociation: Progress in the Dissociative Disorders, 6,* 16–27.

Chatard, A., Pyszczynski, T., Arndt, J., Selimbegović, L., Konan, P. N., & Van der Linden, M. (2012). Extent of trauma exposure and PTSD symptom severity as predictors of anxiety-buffer functioning. *Psychological Trauma: Theory, Practice, Research, and Policy, 4,* 47–55. (*)

Cohen, F., Sullivan, D., Solomon, S., Greenberg, J., & Ogilvie, D. M. (2011). Finding everland: Flight fantasies and the desire to transcend mortality. *Journal of Experimental Social Psychology, 47,* 88–102.

Cozzolino, P. J., Staples, A. D., Meyers, L. S., & Samboceti, J. (2004). Greed, death, and values: From terror management to transcendence management theory. *Personality and Social Psychology Bulletin, 30,* 278–292. (*)

Dewey, J. (1920). *Reconstruction in philosophy.* New York: Henry Holt.

Edmondson, D., Chaudoir, S. R., Mills, M. A., Park, C. L., Holub, J., & Bartkowiak, J. M (2011). From shattered assumptions to weakened worldviews: Trauma symptoms signal anxiety buffer disruption. *Journal of Loss and Trauma, 16,* 358–385. (*)

Eysenck, H. J., & Eysenck, S. B. G. (1967). *Personality structure and measurement.* London: Routledge & Kegan Paul.

Feagin, J. R. (1964). Prejudice and religious types: A focused study of Southern fundamentalists. *Journal for the Scientific Study of Religion, 4,* 3–13.

Florian, V., & Mikulincer, M. (1997). Fear of death and the judgment of social transgressions: A multidimensional of terror management theory. *Journal of Personality and Social Psychology, 73,* 369–380.

Florian, V., Mikulincer, M., & Hirschberger, G. (2001). An existentialist view on mortality salience effects: Personal hardiness, death-thought accessibility, and cultural worldview defenses. *British Journal of Social Psychology, 40,* 437–453. (*)

Foa, E. B. (1995). *Posttraumatic Stress Diagnostic Scale (PDS) manual.* Minneapolis, MN: National Computer Systems.

Goldenberg, J. L. (2012). A body of terror: Denial of death and the creaturely body. In P. R. Shaver, & M. Mikulincer (Eds.), *Meaning, mortality, and choice: The social psychology of existential concerns* (pp. 93–110). Washington, DC: American Psychological Association.

Goldenberg, J. L., Hart, J., Pyszczynski, T., Warnica, G. W., Landau, M. J., & Thomas, L. (2006). Ambivalence towards the body: Death, neuroticism, and the flight from physical sensation. *Personality and Social Psychology Bulletin, 32,* 1264–1277. (*)

Goldenberg, J. L., Pyszczynski, T., Greenberg, J., Solomon, S., Kluck, B., & Cornwell, R. (2001). I am not an animal: Mortality salience, disgust, and the denial of human creatureliness. *Journal of Experimental Psychology: General, 130,* 427–435.

Goldenberg, J. L., Pyszczynski, T., McCoy, S. K., Greenberg, J., & Solomon, S. (1999). Death, sex, love, and neuroticism: Why is sex such a problem? *Journal of Personality and Social Psychology, 77,* 1173–1187. (*)

Greenberg, J., Pyszczynski, T., & Solomon, S. (1986). The causes and consequences of a need for self-esteem: A terror management theory. In R. F. Baumeister (Ed.), *Public self and private self* (pp. 189–212). New York: Springer-Verlag. (*)

Greenberg, J., Pyszczynski, T., Solomon, S., Rosenblatt, A., Veeder, M., Kirkland, S., et al. (1990). Evidence for terror management II: The effects of mortality salience on reactions to those who threaten or bolster the cultural worldview. *Journal of Personality and Social Psychology, 58,* 308–318.

Greenberg, J., Solomon, S., & Arndt, J. (2008). A basic but uniquely human motivation: Terror management. In J. Y. Shah & W. L. Gardner (Eds.), *Handbook of motivation science* (pp. 114–134). New York: Guilford Press.

Greenberg, J., Solomon, S., Pyszczynski, T., Rosenblatt, A., Burling, J., Lyon, D., et al. (1992). Assessing the terror management analysis of self-esteem: Converging evidence of an anxiety-buffering function. *Journal of Personality and Social Psychology, 63,* 913–922.

Harmon-Jones, E., Simon, L., Greenberg, J., Pyszczynski, T., Solomon, S., & McGregor, H. (1997). Terror management theory and self-esteem: Evidence that increased self-esteem reduces mortality salience effects. *Journal of Personality and Social Psychology, 72,* 24–36. (*)

Hart, J., Shaver, P. R., & Goldenberg, J. L. (2005). Attachment, self-esteem, worldviews, and terror management: Evidence for a tripartite security system. *Journal of Personality and Social Psychology, 88,* 999–1013.

Hayes, J., Schimel, J., Arndt, J., & Faucher, E. H. (2010) A theoretical and empirical review of the death-thought accessibility concept in terror management research. *Psychological Bulletin, 136,* 699–739.

Hazan, C., & Shaver, P. R. (1987). Romantic love conceptualized as an attachment process. *Journal of Personality and Social Psychology, 52,* 511–524.

Horney, K. (1937). *The neurotic personality of our time.* New York: Norton.

Jonas, E., & Fischer, P. (2006). Terror management and religion—Evidence that intrinsic religiousness mitigates worldview defense following mortality salience. *Journal of Personality and Social Psychology, 91,* 553–567. (*)

Jordan, C. H., Spencer, S. J., Zanna, M. P., Hoshino-Browne, E., & Correll, J. (2003). Secure and defensive self-esteem. *Journal of Personality and Social Psychology, 85,* 969–978.

Kasser, T., & Ryan, R. M. (1996). Further examining the American dream: Differential correlates of intrinsic and extrinsic goals. *Personality and Social Psychology Bulletin, 22,* 280–287.

Kesebir, P., Luszczynska, A., Pyszczynski, T., & Benight, C. C. (2011). Posttraumatic stress disorder involves disrupted anxiety-buffer mechanisms. *Journal of Social and Clinical Psychology, 30,* 819–841. (*)

Kobasa, S. C., Maddi, S. R., & Kahn, S. (1982). Hardiness and health: A prospective study. *Journal of Personality and Social Psychology, 42,* 168–177.

Kunzendorf, R. G., Moran, C., & Gray, R. (1995–1996). Personality traits and reality testing abilities, controlling for vividness of imagery. *Imagination, Cognition, and Personality, 105,* 113–131.

Landau, M. J., Johns, M., Greenberg, J., Pyszczynski, T., Solomon, S., & Martens, A. (2004). A function of form: Terror management and structuring of the social world. *Journal of Personality and Social Psychology, 87,* 190–210. (*)

Maddi, S. R. (1987). Hardiness training at Bell Telephone. In J. Opatz (Ed.), *Health promotion evaluation* (pp. 121–158). Stephen's Point, WI: Natural Wellness.

Mathews, R. C., & Kling, K. J. (1988). Self-transcendence, time perspective, and prosocial behavior. *Journal of Voluntary Action Research, 71,* 4–24.

Mattick, R. P., & Clarke, J. C. (1998). Development and validation of measures of social phobia scrutiny fear and social interaction anxiety. *Behavior Research and Therapy, 36,* 455–470.

May, R. (1970). *The meaning of anxiety.* New York: Washington Square. (Original work published 1950)

McGregor, I. (2004). Zeal, identity, and meaning: Going to extremes to be one self. In J. Greenberg, S. L. Koole, & T. Pyszczynski (Eds.), *Handbook of experimental existential psychology* (pp. 182–199). New York: Guilford Press.

Mikulincer, M., & Florian, V. (2000). Exploring individual differences in reactions to mortality salience: Does attachment style regulate terror management mechanisms? *Journal of Personality and Social Psychology, 79,* 260–273. (*)

Mikulincer, M., Florian, V., Birnbaum, G., & Malishkevich, S. (2002). The death-anxiety buffering function of close relationships: Exploring the effects of separation reminders on death-thought accessibility. *Personality and Social Psychology Bulletin, 28,* 287–299. (*)

Mikulincer, M., Florian, V., & Hirschberger, G. (2003). The existential function of close relationships: Introducing death into the science of love. *Personality and Social Psychology Review, 7*, 20–40.

Mikulincer, M., Orbach, I., & Iavnieli, D. (1998). Adult attachment style and affect regulation: Strategic variations in subjective self-other similarity. *Journal of Personality and Social Psychology, 75*, 436–448.

Niemiec, C. P., Brown, K. W., Kashdan, T. B., Cozzolino, P. J., Breen, W. E., Levesque-Bristol, C., et al. (2010). Being present in the face of existential threat: The role of trait mindfulness in reducing defensive responses to mortality salience. *Journal of Personality and Social Psychology, 99*, 344–365.

Ozer, E. J., Best, S. R., Lipsey, T. L., & Weiss, D. S. (2003). Predictors of posttraumatic stress disorder and symptoms in adults: A meta-analysis. *Psychological Bulletin, 129*, 52–73.

Rosenberg, M. (1965). *Society and the adolescent self image*. Princeton, NJ: Princeton University Press.

Routledge, C., & Arndt, J. (2009). Creative terror management: Creativity as a facilitator of cultural exploration after mortality salience. *Personality and Social Psychology Bulletin, 35*, 493–505.

Schmeichel, B. J., Gailliot, M. T., Filardo, E., McGregor, I., Gitter, S., & Baumeister, R. F. (2009). Terror management theory and self-esteem revisited: The roles of implicit and explicit self-esteem in mortality salience effects. *Journal of Personality and Social Psychology, 96*, 1077–1087. (*)

Schmeichel, B. J., & Martens, A. (2005). Self-affirmation and mortality salience: Affirming values reduces worldview defense and death-thought accessibility. *Personality and Social Psychology Bulletin, 31*, 658–667.

Sharabany, R. (1994). Intimacy Friendship Scale: Conceptual underpinnings, psychometric properties, and construct validity. *Journal of Social and Personal Relationships, 11*, 449–469.

Simon, L., Arndt, J., Greenberg, J., Solomon, S., & Pyszczynski, T. (1998). Terror management and meaning: Evidence that the opportunity to defend the worldview in response to mortality salience increases the meaningfulness of life in the mildly depressed. *Journal of Personality, 66*, 359–382. (*)

Simon, L., Harmon-Jones, E., Greenberg, J., Solomon, S., & Pyszczynski, T. (1996). The effects of mortality salience on depressed and nondepressed individuals to those who violate or uphold cultural values. *Personality and Social Psychology Bulletin, 22*, 81–90. (*)

Strachan, E., Schimel, J., Arndt, J., Williams, T., Solomon, S., Pyszczynski, T., et al. (2007). Terror mismanagement: Evidence that mortality salience exacerbates phobic and compulsive behaviors. *Personality and Social Psychology Bulletin, 33*, 1137–1151. (*)

Thompson, M. M., Naccarato, M. E., Parker, K. C. H., & Moskowitz, G. B. (2001). The personal need for structure and personal fear of invalidity measures: Historical perspectives, current applications, and future directions. In G. B. Moskowitz (Ed.), *Cognitive social psychology: The Princeton Symposium on the Legacy and Future of Social Cognition* (pp. 19–39). Mahwah, NJ: Erlbaum.

Weathers, F. W., Litz, B. T., Huska, J. A., & Keane, T. M. (1994). *The PTSD Checklist–Civilian Version (PCL-C)*. Boston: National Center for PTSD.

Weise, D. R., Arciszewski, T., Verlhiac, J., Pyszczynski, T., & Greenberg, J. (2012). Terror management and attitudes toward immigrants: Differential effects of mortality salience for low and high right-wing authoritarians. *European Psychologist, 17*, 63–72. (*)

Yalom, I. D. (1980). *Existential psychotherapy*. New York: Basic Books.

CHAPTER 5

Multimethod Assessment
of Implicit and Explicit Processes

Alex Cogswell and Natalie Emmert

Psychologists have always been interested in the determinants of behavior, although they have only intermittently noted the distinction between those determinants that are more controlled and those that are more automatic. For some time, it has been recognized that item transparency in assessment is not necessarily desirable, which has led in part to the growth in popularity of more indirect approaches to assessment (Hartshorne & May, 1928). Further, with the primacy of psychoanalytic theory, in the mid-20th century interest boomed in assessing internal, unobservable phenomena such as wishes and conflicts, which further contributed to the development of indirect, performance-based instruments such as the Rorschach and the Thematic Apperception Test (TAT; Morgan & Murray, 1935), as well as other measures as varied as figure drawings and sentence completion tasks. The clinical personality literature and its emphasis on unconscious or automatic processes, despite its origins largely in psychodynamic thought, has become increasingly palatable and remarkably prescient in more modern experimental psychology (Shevrin & Dickman, 1980). Indeed, over the last 25 years, social psychologists in particular have taken to arms in the study of so-called *implicit* phenomena of all stripes and have generated a vast, rich literature that is gradually being extended into other subareas of psychology. A trend that began with an exclusive focus on implicit attitudes has grown to encompass the study of topics ranging from motivation to self-esteem to emotion regulation. And as with any new trend in research, the rapidly expanding literature and the excitement that feeds its growth have invited as many questions as have been answered. In this chapter, we will discuss how the implicit wave has impacted the study of personality and its assessment, what is known about the role of implicit processes in personality, and what remains unknown about implicit processes and their assessment in general, with a specific emphasis on how these unknowns are relevant for future personality research. In short, we will cover how behavior may be predicted through the joint assessment of two unique, but related, types of processes, one being more controlled (explicit) and the other more automatic (implicit).

Before moving forward, some work with definitions is in order. Historically, the term *implicit* has referred, often too casually, to a class of phenomena (e.g., attitudes) that are hypothesized to operate outside of conscious awareness. Likely because of the exciting pace with which this endeavor moved forward, a basic definition of *implicit* was not firmly established. This made it quite difficult to articulate clearly what an *implicit measure* was, let alone what it measured and how such measurement might be useful. Several investigators have attempted to remedy this problem, and perhaps the most notable example is the work of Jan De Houwer and his colleagues. His group (De Houwer, Teige-Mocigemba, Spruyt, & Moors, 2009) conducted a thorough conceptual analysis, which led to two primary clarifications in how terms should be used (further discussed in Moors, Spruyt, & De Houwer, 2010). First, they recommended that *implicit* be essentially equated with the term *automatic*, which itself refers to the unconscious, unintentional, efficient, and/or uncontrollable qualities of the attribute or construct of interest. Conversely, *explicit* then refers to more controllable, deliberative, intentional, and conscious qualities of a construct. Second, they suggested that implicit and explicit should be used to describe constructs, or elements of constructs, that are being measured, rather than procedures that characterize a particular assessment instrument. Procedures, however, should be described as more direct or indirect. Of course, it is true that the procedures of choice often map predictably on to the attribute being measured, such that more indirect procedures are typically used to assess implicit constructs. In sum, an implicit measure, according to this analysis, is defined as a "measurement outcome that is causally produced by the to-be-measured attribute in the absence of certain goals, awareness, substantial cognitive resources, or substantial time" (De Houwer et al., 2009, p. 350). For the purposes of this chapter, then, implicit measures of personality or self-concept will refer to assessment outcomes that spring automatically from personality characteristics of interest. It is important to note, however, that the measures most frequently used and discussed in the literature, and therefore those that will be discussed here, have not been vetted adequately with regard to how well they fit the definition provided above. Thus, although the term *implicit measure* will be used throughout this chapter for convenience's sake, it should not be assumed that the implicitness or automaticity of the constructs have been determined empirically. Nor should it be assumed that the causal relation between personality characteristic and measurement outcome has been established. Until definitive evidence exists to establish these qualities, our terms will unfortunately remain controversial and will represent more of an "ideal" being sought than agreed-upon descriptors of our assessment tools.

Before reviewing the rationale for developing and using implicit measures, we will describe the more conventional approach of assessing explicit attributes, and briefly review the empirical support for use of such (typically self-report) instruments, as well as the potential drawbacks. We will then describe how some of the drawbacks of this approach contributed to the growing emphasis on implicit assessment and will similarly review the evidence that substantiates the continued measurement of implicit processes. A selection of the most commonly used implicit measures will be described to provide a general overview, followed by a more focused discussion of the most popular implicit measure at present (the Implicit Association Test [IAT]; Greenwald, McGhee, & Schwartz, 1998).

Next, we will discuss findings pertaining to the modest convergence, or concordance, between implicit and explicit measures. In this section, some of the most noteworthy dual-process models proposed for understanding how and why implicit and explicit measures (and more importantly the processes they measure) converge or diverge will be described. Subsequently, we will review some of the more established moderators of implicit–explicit agreement, with an eye on what these moderators tell us about implicit processes.

The latter portion of the chapter will focus on some of the more intriguing and promising, and least well-understood issues pertaining to implicit processes. We will discuss the growing, though still relatively small, literature that speaks to potential implications of the concordance or discordance between implicit and explicit measures of purportedly the same construct. This will lead into a consideration of the clinical utility of implicit measures and how using both implicit and explicit measures jointly will likely provide a richer assessment than relying solely on one class of measure versus the other. We will also discuss some of the challenges associated with using implicit measures for clinical purposes, and will provide case examples that hopefully illustrate more concretely the role of implicit assessment in clinical scenarios. In concluding, we will provide a highlighted reel of unanswered questions and suggested future directions that we hope will help push our understanding further along.

Explicit Measures

There is a long and successful history of using relatively direct procedures to assess what are assumed to be explicit processes of interest. For the sake of simplicity, self-report paper-and-pencil measures will be used as the exemplar methodology in this category. However, it is worth recalling that other types of measures may also be direct (e.g., structured diagnostic interview) and may be similarly designed to measure more controllable, intentional (explicit) processes. Further, not all self-report instruments are entirely direct. For example, although the Minnesota Multiphasic Personality Inventory (MMPI; Hathaway & McKinley, 1943) is clearly a paper-and-pencil self-report instrument, it has been labeled as "indirect" by some scholars (e.g., De Houwer, 2006) based on its relative lack of face validity.

Self-report, explicit instruments tend to rely on the assumption that the attributes of interest are accessible to introspection and that respondents will thus be willing and able to report those attributes with some degree of accuracy (see Cogswell, 2008). These measures tend to maintain objective, unambiguous scoring systems, are highly reliable, and are typically quite efficient and painless to administer (Cogswell, 2008), in both research and clinical settings. Perhaps most importantly, self-report assessments are robust predictors of external criteria, such as corresponding behaviors of interest. A recent meta-analysis demonstrated reasonable predictive validity of self-reports (N = 184 independent samples, average r = .36) across a wide range of predictor/outcome pairings (Greenwald, Poehlman, Uhlmann, & Banaji, 2009). Similarly, each of the Big Five personality dimensions, as measured by self-report, was found to have meaningful predictive utility for actual behavior aggregates conceptually related to the target dimensions (Back, Schmukle, & Egloff, 2009).

Despite widespread use, ease of administration for both evaluators and respondents, and an impressive literature demonstrating the empirical support for self-report instruments, two major concerns about these measures remain. First, based on their fundamental assumption that respondents have access to and willingness to report what the examiner is interested in, it is impossible for these measures to reveal unconscious, inaccessible influences on responses. Moreover, it is well-known that individuals have quite limited abilities to engage in accurate introspection (Nisbett & Wilson, 1977), and thus even when asked to report on explicit processes may not be terribly reliable. Along these same lines, even though self-reported and actual behavior are empirically related to each other (Back et al., 2009), they are far from identical. Thus, researchers interested in personality's prediction of relevant outcomes are right to be cautious in overly relying on self-report instruments with such known limitations.

Second, due to the greater tendency toward face validity of self-report measures, they become more susceptible to influences of both impression management and self-deception (Greenwald et al., 2002). That is, the more clearly respondents can identify what attribute is being measured by a particular instrument, the more potential there is for their responses to be biased either intentionally or unintentionally. Some of the more widely used, respected broadband personality instruments, such as the MMPI and the Personality Assessment Inventory (PAI; Morey, 1991), have incorporated validity scales to partially address this problem, and these scales have met largely with success. For example, the validity scales of the MMPI have demonstrated the ability to identify both faking good (Baer, Wetter, & Berry, 1992) and faking bad (Berry, Baer, & Harris, 1991), as well as recognizing inconsistent patterns of responding (Gallen & Berry, 1996). Unfortunately, however, despite these successes many narrower instruments (such as measures of single personality characteristics or symptom checklists, such as depression and anxiety inventories) do not include validity scales and are thus subject to the kinds of biases known to be problematic in self-report assessment (Shedler, Mayman, & Manis, 1993).

The limitations inherent in self-report instruments were recognized long ago, although it seems that the increasing impetus to address those limitations has dovetailed with the growing interest in studying implicit processes. As researchers began investigating constructs such as implicit memory (Schacter, 1987) and implicit self-concept (Greenwald et al., 2002), sole reliance on self-reports was simply no longer tenable. Thus, a whole new wave of instruments were developed with goals aiming to: (1) study phenomena that were not accessible to introspection and thus unsuitable for self-report assessment; and (2) respond to the problems of bias and faking that correlate with the higher face validity of self-reports. Of course, indirect, performance-based instruments are not new and arguably maintain some of the desirable qualities of the newer implicit measures (such as providing access to unconscious material and less susceptibility to response biases). It remains an open empirical question how much overlap, conceptually and practically, exists between the historically psychoanalytic performance-based instruments and the more social cognitive implicit measures. Leaving that question to the side at present, we will now discuss the newer measures designed to assess implicit processes.

Implicit Measures

As mentioned earlier, personality researchers have long wanted to reliably assess unobservable phenomena that individuals cannot access through introspection. As such, indirect assessment systems such as the Rorschach Inkblot Method, most commonly scored using the Comprehensive System (Exner, 1991), and the TAT (Morgan & Murray, 1935) generated quite a bit of interest, both clinically and academically. These methods were grounded in the notion that individuals had limited, if any, access to the inner states in which assessors were interested, and thus methods were required to circumvent both the intentional and unintentional (defensive) barriers to reliable assessment. Although both of these instruments, as well as others developed in the same tradition, have received notable empirical support for several indices (see Meyer & Archer, 2001), they have also been roundly criticized. Both measurements, the Rorschach in particular, have been criticized for involving too much investigator inference, interpretation, and subjectivity, thus being limited both in terms of their reliability and validity (Garb, 1999; Wood, Lilienfeld, Garb, & Nezworski, 2000). Also, the historically psychoanalytic origin of this approach to assessment has not been terribly palatable to researchers and clinicians of other theoretical orientations, which has further reduced the reliance on these instruments in the broader psychological literature.

Interestingly, many scholars and clinicians who have largely rejected the use of instruments such as the Rorschach and the TAT have in recent years given increasing notice to unconscious, unobservable phenomena, albeit with those phenomena conceptualized in a different manner. As cognitive science moved forward through the study of such things as associative priming (Bower, Montiero, & Gilligan, 1978) and implicit memory (Schacter, 1987), it became more acceptable and more desirable to pay closer attention to processes previously assumed to be outside the realm of rigorous science. This shift permitted a rapidly growing interest among social psychologists to study what became known as implicit social cognition, or processes that operated outside of conscious awareness while having predictable impacts on observable behaviors (for two sophisticated discussions of this issue, see Fazio & Olson, 2003; Wilson, Lindsey, & Schooler, 2000). Some of the most pioneering work toward this end was conducted by John Bargh, who has demonstrated convincingly the importance of automatic processing (for classic review, see Bargh & Chartrand, 1999). Bargh's work made clear the widespread role of automaticity in the activation of attitudes (Bargh, Chaiken, Govender, & Pratto, 1992), social behavior and complex social judgments (Bargh, Chen, & Burrows, 1996), and most recently choices about health behavior (Sheeran, Gollwitzer, & Bargh, 2013). Despite these social cognitive underpinnings of implicit measures such as the IAT, and the psychoanalytic origin of the Rorschach, some researchers have noted that they bear remarkable similarity with regard to their measurement outcomes of interest and their typical relations with more deliberative self-report instruments (e.g., McGrath, 2008). Indeed, research has been encouraged to explore how the more traditionally psychodynamic implicit measures like the Rorschach or TAT may function similarly to the newer social cognitive instruments such as the IAT (Cogswell, 2008; McGrath, 2008). We remain hopeful that this work will be carried out.

The study of implicit processes among social cognition scholars gained tremendous traction in attitude research, where newly developed instruments promised access to biases and preferences that may be masked when individuals respond to conventional, face-valid self-report questionnaires. The most successful of these instruments is undoubtedly the IAT (Greenwald et al., 1998), a computer-based measure of associative strength between an attitude target and an evaluative dimension. For example, to measure evaluative preferences of the Democratic versus Republican parties, subjects would first categorize Democratic words (e.g., blue, donkey) and unpleasant words on one key, and Republican words (e.g., red, elephant) and pleasant words on another. In a later phase of the task, the same subjects would categorize Democratic and pleasant words together, and Republican and unpleasant words on the same key. The IAT assumes that people can more quickly associate concepts that are more closely associated in memory, and thus the test functions by computing differences in response times between the two stages of the task.

In addition to the IAT, there are a multitude of other implicit instruments that operate on similar theoretical ground. For example, semantic and affective priming tasks assume that responses to targets of interest will be influenced by previous exposure to a prime stimulus. These tasks have shown considerable promise in assessing attitudes (e.g., Murphy, Monahan, & Zajonc, 1995; Wittenbrink, Judd, & Park, 2001). A related task is the affect misattribution procedure, which is based on the observation that individuals have substantial trouble distinguishing their emotional responses to different events happening in close proximity. When this confusion arises, priming effects can reliably impact how affect is misattributed, and thus automatic evaluations of the prime may be inferred (Payne, Cheng, Govorun, & Stewart, 2005). One additional example of a commonly used implicit measure is the class of name–letter preference tasks. These instruments have been used as simple implicit measures of self-esteem (attitudes toward self), and operate on the assumption that people prefer the letters in their own names (e.g., Pelham, Mirenberg, & Jones, 2002). Although this is just a small sampling of the ever-expanding range of implicit measures, the bulk of the remainder of this chapter will focus on findings regarding the IAT. This decision is twofold: (1) the IAT is the most widely used implicit measure at present, and thus has generated the greatest of amount of data, both favorable and unfavorable; and (2) the measure has expanded most broadly beyond attitude research into the study of personality.

Subsequent to the IAT's usage in famously assessing implicit or automatic racial attitudes (e.g., Greenwald et al., 1998), as well as attitudes toward a wide variety of other targets, its use extended into assessing many other domains of interest, including self-esteem and self-concept. Greenwald and Farnham (2000) developed an adapted IAT to measure implicit self-esteem, which has become a very widely studied construct (measured both by the IAT and other implicit measures, such as the name–letter task as noted above). A recent review of these measures called into question their validity as true measures of implicit self-esteem but provided encouragement for ongoing pursuit of reliable, valid instruments to tap this important construct (Buhrmester, Blanton, & Swann, 2011). The IAT has also been adapted successfully for measuring other implicit domains of interest, including shyness (Asendorpf, Banse, & Mucke, 2002), anxiety (Egloff & Schmukle, 2002), depression-relevant cognitions (Phillips,

Hine, & Thorsteinsson, 2010), suicidal ideation (Nock et al., 2010), moral self-concept (Perugini & Leone, 2009), relational anxiety and attachment (Dewitte, De Houwer, & Buysse, 2008), youth aggression (Grumm, Hein, & Fingerle, 2011), and emotion regulation (Koole & Rothermund, 2011).

A newer, fascinating application of the IAT's utility in measuring implicit self-concept has been the examination of how the IAT compares to self-report personality instruments in terms of the structure of personality. It is well known that the five-factor (so-called Big Five) model of personality (McCrae & Costa, 1987) is the most common and robust taxonomy of personality traits, although evidence for this model has accumulated exclusively through the administration of self-report personality inventories. Recent work has reproduced this Big Five structure using IAT-derived indices of the five factors, indicating that the implicit self-concept is similarly structured to the self-concept revealed through more deliberative self-report responses (Schmukle, Back, & Egloff, 2008). Although the correlations between implicit and self-report factors were small, the patterns of inter-correlations and the relative levels of each of the factors were quite similar between the two classes of measures.

Despite some serious criticisms of the implicit measures, including the IAT, substantial data have been collected that attest to the reliability and predictive utility of the instruments. With regard to reliability, the IAT has demonstrated consistently acceptable levels of internal consistency, with Cronbach's alphas typically ranging from .70 to .90 (Nosek, Greenwald, & Banaji, 2007). Test–retest reliabilities have commonly been somewhat lower and more variable, with a median estimate of approximately .50 (Lane, Banaji, Nosek, & Greenwald, 2007), leading to concerns about what might account for this less acceptable reliability criterion.

In addition to the selection of studies cited above, which demonstrate successful adaptations for the IAT to measure a host of constructs, there are more general pieces of evidence that support the predictive and incremental validity of the instrument. First, IAT-derived indices of the five-factor model were recently compared against self-reported personality factors with regard to how well they predicted actual, observed behavior that theoretically followed from those factors. While self-reported personality, as expected, predicted actual behavior in each of the five dimensions, IAT-assessed neuroticism and extraversion predicted observed behavior meaningfully related to those factors (Back et al., 2009). What was especially noteworthy in this study was that the implicit measures of neuroticism and extraversion provided incrementally greater utility in predicting behavior, above and beyond the variance accounted for by self-report.

Second, a recent and widely cited meta-analysis revealed high indices of predictive validity for both self-report and IAT-derived measures (Greenwald et al., 2009). In this paper, IAT instruments demonstrated an average effect size of $r = .27$ for a variety of behavioral and physiological outcome measures, while self-report scales had a slightly higher average $r = .36$.

Despite this higher value, the authors note that the range of effect sizes was larger for the self-reports and that the self-reports did not predict as well as the IAT measures for more sensitive topics, presumably due to the role played by impression management in modifying self-reported responses (Greenwald et al., 2009). Moreover, both the self-reports and IAT measures provided incremental validity, each accounting for variance above and beyond that of the other class of measures.

One additional rationale for the wide use of implicit measures is to mitigate against the influence of self-presentation effects known to impact responses to more face-valid self-report measures. With the more indirect approach to measurement that characterizes most implicit measures, respondents cannot determine as easily which construct(s) the investigators are interested in measuring. Thus, the claim has been made that implicit instruments are "immune" to faking or to the effects of impression management. The evidence has generally supported these notions, but as with much of the implicit measurement data, it is not clear-cut.

With regard to implicit measures not being susceptible to the problem of socially desirable responding, the evidence is rather mixed. In the next section, we will explore more deeply the common finding that self-report and implicit measures are only modestly correlated, but for now, it will suffice to say that if social desirability effects are not relevant to implicit measurement, then correlations between implicit and self-report measures should be higher when social desirability is low. The data that speak to this point, again, are rather contradictory. For example, Nosek (2005) found support for this predicted pattern, but other studies have either not found the same pattern or have found its opposite (e.g., Hofmann, Gawronski, Gschwendner, Le, & Schmitt, 2005). With regard to faking, the evidence is somewhat clearer: It indicates that individuals instructed to engage in faking can influence their responses to implicit measures to some extent, but that these effects are much less pronounced than on self-report instruments (Degner, 2009; Klauer & Teige-Mocigemba, 2007; Payne, 2005; Schnabel, Banse, & Asendorpf, 2006). The IAT findings regarding self-presentation effects bear some similarity to those of the "original" implicit instruments, such as the Rorschach, which likewise is assumed to be relatively immune to faking/impression management due to its ambiguous stimuli. Interestingly, the empirical data for the Rorschach in relation to faking are similar to those of the IAT—that is, promising, but somewhat inconsistent and in need of further examination (Perry & Kinder, 1990).

Now that we have briefly covered more conventional, self-report explicit measures, as well as the explosion of implicit measures and the research they have generated, we will move to discuss how explicit and implicit instruments tend to converge. We will also identify some of the moderators that have been shown to influence indices of concordance. During the course of this discussion, we will review some of the more prominent models that have been developed to explain the relative convergence or divergence of implicit and explicit measures and their associated processes.

Concordance of Explicit and Implicit Measures

Implicit measures and self-reports correlate modestly at best, a finding that was initially surprising given the hypothesis that the two approaches to measurement assessed the same construct using different means. As this finding became more consistent, and as it was continually paired with indicators that both types of measures were reliably predicting behaviors of interest, some researchers shifted their assumptions and began seeing explicit and implicit processes as unique, though related processes. Empirically, two large-scale investigations have estimated the average concordance between explicit and implicit measures. One of these examinations was a meta-analysis that summarized data from 126 studies and determined a mean effect size of $r = .24$ for the relation between explicit and implicit measures (Hofmann, Gawronski, et al., 2005). A somewhat higher estimate was found in a large analysis of Internet-based IAT data, where Nosek (2005) found a mean implicit–explicit correlation of $r = .36$. Regardless of the discrepancy between these two analyses and the potential explanations for the difference, it is clear that correlations between explicit and implicit measures are not very substantial.

Interestingly, despite the generally modest implicit–explicit correlations, there is remarkable variability in concordance indices from study to study. This has allowed other rich avenues of research, both to uncover explanations for the variability and to determine the potential implications of this variability for outcomes of interest. For example, one study is beginning to identify how implicit assessment can contribute to the understanding and prediction of psychopathology, and how it even may be useful in guiding treatment (Roefs et al., 2011). This use of implicit assessment is only possible due to the divergence between explicit and implicit instruments, and raises additional questions about how the relative concordance between explicit and implicit measures may itself be of clinical utility. This new development in studying social cognitive implicit instruments such as the IAT in some ways mirrors the longer tradition within clinical assessment of using both the MMPI and the Rorschach. For example, quite modest MMPI–Rorschach concordance has been identified in a number of studies, which has prompted the suggestion that each may provide incremental predictive utility in the clinical setting (Archer & Krishnamurthy, 1993; Finn, 1996; Meyer, 1996, 1997). The typical divergence between implicit and explicit measures, as well as how their interrelations may be clinically useful, will be discussed in further detail below in the context of clinical cases.

One further recent example, which is particularly striking, is a study that found an average relation of .00 between explicit and implicit measures of preferences for physical attractiveness in a romantic partner (Eastwick, Eagly, Finkel, & Johnson, 2011). The fascinating aspect of this finding is not just the absence of a relation between measures, but the ability of each measure to predict something meaningful about how people act on their romantic preferences. The explicit measure predicted romantic interest in photographs of potential partners, whereas the implicit measure was more closely related to romantic interest expressed toward potential real-life partners. This brings us to a discussion of moderators of the implicit–explicit correlation and to a broader consideration of how to understand the mutual ability of two different types of measures, which are modestly intercorrelated, to predict different kinds of relevant outcomes.

Moderators of Implicit–Explicit Concordance

Both of the large-scale studies (Hofmann, Gawronski, et al., 2005; Nosek, 2005) reviewed above that quantified mean explicit–implicit correlations made the further observation that much of the variability between studies with regard to these correlations was due to the presence of moderating variables. It is crucial to consider what these moderators are, as a methodological exercise for one, but more importantly as a way to understand how and when explicit and implicit processes tend to converge or diverge. In his 2005 paper, Nosek identifies four moderators of the implicit–explicit relationship, each of which will be briefly considered here. First, he found that when concerns about self-presentation are high (due to socially sensitive material, for example), implicit–explicit concordance tends to be lower. As discussed earlier, this makes sense given the greater susceptibility of explicit measures to both intentional and unintentional self-presentation motivations. Second, as evaluative strength increases, so does the degree of concordance between implicit and explicit measures. That is, there is greater concordance in the domains of more personal importance and familiarity. Third, greater concordance between implicit and explicit evaluations is found when the target of the evaluation has more of a bipolar than unipolar structure. Bipolar structures allow for greater efficiency and simplicity cognitively and thus can be activated more consistently across time and context. Finally, the more an individual views his or her evaluations as distinct, or unique relative to social norms, the greater the correspondence tends to be between explicit and implicit evaluations (Nosek, 2005).

Another well-established factor that moderates the relation between explicit and implicit instruments is structural fit. That is, as the instruments' formats become more similar, the correlations between the instruments correspondingly increase. This finding indicates that in addition to explicit and implicit processes themselves being relatively independent, the measures used to assess those processes add a layer of method variance that can artificially inflate the processes' apparent independence (Payne, Burkley, & Stokes, 2008). Another feature that likely moderates concordance is attention to content domain and cognitive elaboration. For example, greater concordance between explicit and implicit anxiety measures was found when participants were instructed to think about anxiety-provoking scenarios, relative to a condition when they thought about extraversion-relevant scenarios (Egloff, Weck, & Schmukle, 2008).

Other factors have been identified, albeit often preliminarily, that serve to increase or decrease the concordance between implicit and explicit measures. Following the presumption that implicit processes are more closely related to emotion than to cognition (e.g., see Spence & Townsend, 2008), when the participants' focus was affective as opposed to cognitive, concordance between implicit and explicit evaluations increased (Smith & Nosek, 2011). Other findings indicate that a dismissing attachment style in a sample of university students decreased the concordance between implicit and explicit self-esteem (Dentale, Vecchione, De Coro, & Barbaranelli, 2012). The proposed mechanism to explain this finding has to do with the hypothesized lack of emotional awareness associated with dismissive attachment and the previously suggested link between a lack of emotional awareness and reduced implicit-explicit concordance (Hofmann, Gschwendner, Nosek, & Schmitt, 2005). Along similar lines, alexithymia—defined as an inability to identify and process emotions in an explicit fashion—was predictive of reduced correlations between implicit and explicit self-esteem (Dentale, San Martini, De Coro, & Di Pomponio, 2010). Finally, and also similarly, individuals assigned to a meditation condition revealed greater concordance between self-reported and implicit self-esteem than individuals in a control condition (Koole, Govorun, Cheng, & Gallucci, 2009). Again, this experiment provides further evidence that greater emotional focus and awareness are related to increased correspondence between explicit and implicit processes.

Conceptual Models of Implicit and Explicit Processes

All models that attempt to conceptualize the relation between explicit and implicit processes rest on the assumption that two distinct but related processing systems exist. Within this family of dual-process models (see Wilson et al., 2000), each theory provides its own nuances with regard to how implicit and explicit processes are hypothesized to differ, and under what different sets of circumstances each type of process is thought to predict relevant behavior. All models share the common feature that, generally speaking, implicit processes operate with greater automaticity and less conscious awareness than do their corresponding explicit processes. Each model, however, presents unique features that help with understanding such issues as how explicit and implicit representations are acquired and altered, and how affect and cognition may mutually impact those representations. A complete and thorough treatment of each model is well beyond the scope of this chapter, so instead a broad overview of a few selected models will be provided.

The first major explanatory model to be considered is the associative–propositional evaluation (APE) model (Gawronski & Bodenhausen, 2006, 2007). In this model, two unique mental processes (associative and propositional) produce two distinct sets of behavioral or evaluative outcomes (implicit and explicit). Associative processes are those involving activation of associations in memory, where the strength of the associations is determined by the proximity of representations in an individual's associative network. Associative processes can be activated automatically and operate without regard for the validity or truth of the outcome that follows from the activation. Conversely, propositional processes are thought to organize the confirmation of the validity of information that follows from activated associations. In other words, following the automatic activation of associations, which may or may not be logically consistent or valid, propositional processes utilize logical principles to determine the validity of what has been activated. These two sets of processes, in addition to producing what we know as implicit and explicit evaluations, have been found to mutually influence one another. One example of this interplay is the potential for a "gut feeling" to be activated automatically (associative, implicit), and then a considered, deliberate effort made to override the gut feeling (propositional, explicit), possibly altering it before it is again activated (Gawronski & Bodenhausen, 2006, 2007).

A second major conceptual model, bearing some similarity to the APE model, is known as the reflective–impulsive model (Strack & Deutsch, 2004). In this model, mental associations are formed in the impulsive system and are created based on repeated pairings of stimuli, without regard to their factual or logical accuracy. The determination of validity is hypothesized to require reflective processes, which must be summoned consciously and which rely on principles of logical and cognitive consistency (see also Deutsch & Strack, 2010). The model further proposes that different types of assessment tools are needed for capturing the distinct outcomes of reflective and impulsive processes. Strack and Deutsch (2004) argue that direct measures (typically self-reports) are more revealing of reflective processes, whereas indirect (or implicit) measures better identify the outcomes of impulsive processes.

Indeed, there is evidence to support the matching of assessment methods to the processes of interest. For example, Rydell and McConnell (2006) have shown that explicit evaluations are the result of *fast learning*, which involves a higher order of cognition, including logical, verbal, and conscious processing. Moreover, explicit evaluations were more predictive of deliberative, controlled judgments, and thus they could be more sensitive to measurement by direct, reflective means (self-reports). On the other hand, implicit evaluations result from *slow learning*, involving lower-order cognition or the repeated pairing of associations over time that act to gradually strengthen in memory. These evaluations were found to be more predictive of spontaneous, subtle behaviors; thus they should be more responsive to measures designed to capture automatic outcomes (implicit instruments).

Similarly, McClelland, Koestner, and Weinberger (1989) and Bornstein (1998, 2002) have identified a kind of process dissociation with regard to how more direct and indirect measures are related to behavioral outcomes. More specifically, direct measures such as self-reports were argued to indicate *self-attributed* motives, or what now might be known as explicit motives; they are those processes that individuals have the ability and willingness to disclose. These self-attributed or explicit motivations were more predictive of controlled, conscious behaviors. Conversely, *implicit* motives were revealed through the use of indirect measures and were described as those processes that influence behavior automatically, outside of conscious awareness. Implicit motives in the studies cited above were better predictors of spontaneous, uncontrolled behaviors. These findings led to the description of a process dissociation procedure whereby implicit and explicit measures of purportedly the same construct (Bornstein, 2002) could be validated. (See Asendorpf et al., 2002, for a description of a quite similar double dissociation model involving differential prediction of controlled and spontaneous shy behavior.) In this procedure, explicit and implicit measures would reliably predict different classes of behavior (controlled vs. spontaneous, for example) or predict the same behavior under different sets of circumstances (e.g., slow vs. fast learning to draw on the later work of Rydell and McConnell discussed above). Process dissociation approaches have been used to parse the relative contribution of automatic (implicit) and controlled (explicit) processes to outcomes, with those contributions sometimes working in concert and sometimes in opposition (for two notable examples, see McCarthy & Skowronski, 2011; Payne, 2005).

Now that we have reviewed generally the most important models for understanding the interplay of implicit and explicit processes, we will examine the implications of concordance or discordance between these two types of processing. In this next section, we will consider what might be important about implicit and explicit processes operating in concert, versus scenarios where implicit and explicit processes are working in opposition.

Implications of Explicit–Implicit Concordance and Discordance

We have seen that explicit and implicit instruments tend to be modestly correlated and that they provide incremental predictive utility, each better at predicting different expressions of behavior, or predicting the same behaviors under different sets of circumstances. These findings alone would be reason enough for clinicians and researchers to consider administering implicit and explicit measures to their patients or subjects. Another, and perhaps even more interesting, reason for joint administration of implicit and explicit measures lies in the growing literature suggesting that discrepancies between measures are themselves constructs worthy of study. This parallels the developmental literature, which increasingly emphasizes the importance of studying cross-informant discrepancies in reports of the same child. This literature recognizes that the discrepancies themselves provide useful information about family functioning and communication and are related meaningfully to outcomes of interest (for an overview, see De Los Reyes, 2011). The current state of the explicit–implicit concordance literature is not nearly as advanced as the cross-informant developmental work, but nonetheless provides some encouraging avenues for further exploration.

Generally, discrepancies between implicit and explicit processes have been shown to be related to psychological ambivalence (Petty, Tormala, Briñol, & Jarvis, 2006), and a corresponding motive to reduce that conflict has been identified. More specifically, discrepant implicit and explicit attitudes produce an uncomfortable cognitive dissonance, which motivates individuals to engage in greater information processing designed to reduce the discrepancy (Rydell, McConnell, & Mackie, 2008). This pattern is fascinating in its own right and leads to other questions with regard to how discrepancies may function when a resolution cannot be had and how such discrepancies may be relevant clinically.

Discrepancies between implicit and explicit self-esteem have perhaps been studied most toward this end, with initial findings indicating that discrepancies are related to suppression of anger, increased nervousness, and a more depressive attributional style (Schröder-Abé, Rudolph, & Schüz, 2007). Further, a sample of socially anxious adolescents displayed a larger implicit–explicit self-esteem discrepancy than normal controls following a social threat manipulation (Schreiber, Bohn, Aderka, Stangier, & Steil, 2012). Another very compelling recent study found that explicit, but not implicit, self-esteem was an independent predictor of depressive symptoms and suicidal ideation. However, the magnitude of the discrepancy between implicit and explicit self-esteem was a significant predictor of both depressive symptoms and suicidal ideation (Creemers, Scholte, Engels, Prinstein, & Wiers, 2012). As valid approaches to implicit measurement continue to be pursued, it will be exciting to observe how additional research into implicit–explicit discrepancies becomes possible and what findings emerge.

Clinical Applicability

As data accumulate to aid in interpreting implicit assessment in general, and to facilitate understanding the implications of implicit–explicit concordance/discordance, the clinical utility of these measures will undoubtedly become more apparent. At present, however, enough is known that valid implicit measures of all stripes could be considered for inclusion in clinical assessment. Given the measures' ability to predict incrementally beyond explicit instruments, and the growing appreciation of identifying discrepancies between implicit and explicit measures, the potential for these measures in clinical settings is clear. Further, there is a lengthy history of research identifying the potential incremental validity in administering both a Rorschach and an MMPI to the same patient, with the expectation that the two instruments will likely produce varying results (e.g., Finn, 1996; Meyer, 1997). It will be interesting to explore how the ongoing work with applying social cognitive measures like the IAT to clinical practice bears similarity (if at all) to the tradition of using more psychodynamically rooted performance-based tasks (McGrath, 2008).

Despite the apparent relevance of implicit measures to clinical practice, there are surely barriers to their widespread usage. First and foremost, the technology that must accompany some of the implicit instruments (e.g., the IAT) is unlikely to be available for any clinician in any clinic who wishes to use the measures. Moreover, interpreting what the measures communicate is challenging even for implicit assessment researchers and thus would be am even larger task for a clinician unfamiliar with the nuances of the assessment literature. The interpretation step is even further complicated by the relatively young empirical literature regarding how to integrate implicit and explicit instruments in a single battery and how to make sense of scenarios where the measures seem to say two different things. As the research findings continue to amass, however, some of the challenges associated with interpretation and clinical applicability should become more manageable and more standardized, such that using an implicit measure should be no more complicated for a clinician than administering a self-report questionnaire. In the meantime, it is important to begin considering specific ways in which implicit measures may be utilized clinically.

One way in which the measures have already helped clinically are findings suggesting that implicit attitudes are impacted through more of a *slow learning* process and are therefore less responsive to single or a few presentations of counterattitudinal stimuli (Rydell & McConnell, 2006). When viewed from another angle, one study indicated that initial experiences tend to be encoded as context-free representations that are quite slow to respond to subsequent violations of the expectancy generated by that initial experience (Gawronski, Rydell, Vervliet, & De Houwer, 2010). In other words, these findings show that in order to change implicit evaluations, it is necessary to present repeated exposures to counterattitudinal stimuli across a variety of contexts or settings. Additionally, implicit measures have already proved valuable in psychopathology research and have demonstrated potential to contribute to diagnostics and potentially encourage revision of existing cognitive models of psychopathology (Roefs et al., 2011).

In order to illustrate more concretely how implicit measures can be useful clinically, two brief case examples will be presented. The first is an adult case and rests on more solid empirical grounds. The second case is of an adolescent and is somewhat more hypothetical given the relative lack of data that can be brought to bear. Both cases will involve the explicit and implicit measurement of self-esteem, given that this construct has received the greatest attention to date in the empirical literature.

Case 1

A 34-year-old man presents with vague complaints of general dissatisfaction in his life, along with symptoms of anxiety and depression, none of which cohere into a bona fide clinical diagnosis. The patient reports feeling like a failure to himself and his family because having been laid off from his previous job, he is unable to find employment "good enough for him." In addition, he has been experiencing financial trouble, which has created tension in his marriage. He appears to suffer from insomnia and has lost some weight. Ultimately, he expresses feelings of hopelessness and is worried about the future for his family. Given the patient's verbalized negative self-image and the recent stressors apparently feeding into such self-critical views, the clinician administers both self-report and implicit measures of self-esteem. The patient reports low self-esteem on an established self-report instrument, demonstrated by a score of 9 on the Rosenberg Self-Esteem Scale (Rosenberg, 1965), which is consistent with his report during the initial interview. However, on the self-esteem IAT, he appears to have relatively high implicit self-esteem, as shown by a response latency D score of 0.63. According to the budding literature surrounding IAT scoring, D scores capture the size of the IAT effect and can range from −2 to +2, with "strong" effects being those that approximate 0.65 (for a review of IAT scoring procedures, see Greenwald, Nosek, & Banaji, 2003; Lane et al., 2007). In the present example, the patient's score of 0.63 would represent a fairly strong IAT effect in the positive direction, or one pointing toward higher implicit self-esteem. This curious finding is interpreted in light of the literature which suggests that in depressive and anxiety disorders such a pattern is actually quite common. It may suggest a discrepancy between unrealistically high standards and one's perception of reality (Roefs et al., 2011). As such, the clinician draws the patient's attention to the discrepancy across measures and invites consideration of what the implications might be. As the patient's awareness of the discrepancy grows, a corresponding discomfort arises, along with the subsequent motivation to resolve the discrepancy. As discussion between clinician and patient ensues, the patient explains that he feels he is overqualified for any of the jobs that are available but feels as if taking a mediocre job would make him just as much of a failure to himself as would his inability to provide for his family without a job.

Recent meta-analysis suggests several examples of cognitive therapies that effectively relieve implicit–explicit discordance in the long term (Phillips et al., 2010), such as repeated exposure to positive experiences that could change feelings of continuous failure to success (Beevers, 2005). The clinician suggests that by obtaining a "mediocre" job, several positive experiences could follow, such as successful job performance, a promotion, or simply enjoying the experience of working or of being with his co-workers, while supporting his family financially. The clinician suggests that by following repeated exposure and attention paid to experiences that support the patient's high implicit self-esteem and new, positive experiences of success, he may gradually begin to reconcile the discrepant processes and achieve greater implicit–explicit integration. Without unrealistic expectations and by repeated exposure to positive experiences of success, he may begin to worry less about his future and to view himself more positively. Moreover, and perhaps more importantly, some of the tension in his marriage is likely to be relieved, which subsequently would predictably be related to improved sleep and reduced hopelessness.

Case 2

A 14-year-old girl presents with her mother, who reports that her daughter has become increasingly angry, disrespectful, and generally defiant at home. The adolescent indicates in the initial interview that she does not wish to participate in psychotherapy and believes instead that her mother is "the problem." Both mother and daughter complete standard self-report instruments that screen for a host of symptomatology as well as a measure of the daughter's self-views, including global self-esteem. In the clinician's estimate, the daughter does not engage well with the self-report instruments, hastily completing them with a look of disinterest, rapidly circling responses that indicate a denial of difficulties across the board. According to the Self-Perception Profile for Children (SPPC; Harter, 2012), the daughter scored a 3.6 on the global self-worth scale, indicating relatively high overall self-esteem. However, combined behavioral observations imply the possibility that the SPPC score is invalid. The clinician decides to administer an IAT measure of self-esteem, and the girl displays greater interest in completing a computer-based task, evidencing increased engagement. She generates a surprisingly low score on implicit self-esteem—a $D = 0.06$—which leads to a conversation with the clinician about what this might indicate, particularly in light of her denial of any difficulties during interview and the high self-esteem score measured by the SPPC. The daughter acknowledges to the clinician that she is undergoing a very difficult transition to high school and has been unable to discuss this problem with her mother, with whom she hashistorically had an antagonistic relationship. She states that she has been blaming herself for her trouble adjusting to high school and has become increasingly resentful of her mother for (1) not being supportive of her difficulties, and (2) treating her as if she is a "bad kid." The clinician, having obtained a better understanding of the girl's complaints, is able to facilitate a discussion between the child and parent and close the discrepancy gap between the two, while also encouraging and coaching ongoing communication and support.

These two brief case illustrations give just a small sampling of the clinical potential of implicit measures, particularly when used in concert with standard self-reports. Assuming clinicians are able to overcome the relatively insignificant technological barriers to administration, and provided that the literature continues to grow at its current pace, it is reasonable to assume that future use and interpretation of these measures will become more practical and more standardized. Implicit assessment provides another avenue for understanding the complaints with which our patients present. In addition, they offer the opportunity to assess discrepancies both between an individual's self-report and implicit responses, as well as responses across multiple informants, as in the case of children and adolescents in particular.

Concluding Comments

In this chapter, we have reviewed the growing literature on the assessment of implicit processes. We considered some of the assumptions underlying the traditional reliance on self-report measurement alone, and we examined some of the potential drawbacks of this method. We then introduced implicit assessment broadly and reviewed some of the more common measures currently in use. Then, based on typical findings that explicit and implicit measures tend to correlate only modestly, we covered some of the moderators of concordance that have been identified. Further, we looked at some initial data that speak to the implications of implicit–explicit discrepancies, an area in great need of future attention. And finally, we discussed how implicit assessment in conjunction with explicit tools may be applicable in clinical practice.

Despite the surge of attention surrounding implicit assessment in recent years, much remains to be learned and many avenues for future researchers to explore lie ahead. First, simply defining what is meant by implicit, and clearly defining what exactly constitutes an implicit measure or an implicit process, is of utmost importance. This crucial scholarship is well underway (De Houwer et al., 2009) but is in obvious need of ongoing clarification. Similarly, it remains unclear how the newer social cognitive implicit instruments, such as the IAT, may be related empirically to the "original" implicit measures, such as the Rorschach or the TAT. Studies should be conducted to clarify whether and how these measures, despite their differing historical and theoretical origins, may overlap with regard to their abilities to predict meaningful outcomes (Cogswell, 2008; McGrath, 2008).

Second, findings showing similar five-factor structure of the implicit and explicit self-concepts of personality are fascinating (Schmukle et al., 2008). Moreover, we have seen that implicit and self-report personality measures have incremental predictive validity, implying that both used in conjunction may yield greater precision in predicting behavioral outcomes (Back et al., 2009). As suggested by Back and colleagues (2009), future studies should explore how well self-report, other-report, and implicit personality measures hang together, as well as how they jointly or separately predict observable behaviors. Not only would this type of inquiry improve prediction of behavior, it also could contribute to richer conceptualizations of personality, including both explicit and implicit processes, as well as their integration. Although not precisely in this vein, some of the work being done to develop big-picture conceptualizations of explicit and implicit processes operating jointly in personality has already begun (for one noteworthy example, see Corr, 2010). It is our hope that this work is closely attended to and extended.

Third, as reviewed above, discrepancies between implicit and explicit instruments are likely themselves constructs worthy of study. The evidence is beginning to accumulate with regard to some of the implications of discrepancies, as well as demonstrating that increased affective awareness (Hofmann, Gschwendner, et al., 2005), or practicing meditation (Koole et al., 2009), may lead to greater implicit–explicit concordance. Additional work is clearly needed to pursue other potential predictors of concordance, as well as downstream outcomes of different levels of implicit–explicit concordance.

Finally, there has been much speculation regarding the origins of implicit as compared to explicit processes, and to date speculation is more or less where the field remains. Achieving a better understanding of the developmental roots of implicit processes is key to firming up a broader conceptualization of what implicit processes truly are, how they relate to more observable explicit phenomena, and, perhaps most importantly, how they may be changed when such change is desirable. Reaching such a developmental understanding obviously requires adapting implicit measures for use with children, and this work thankfully has begun to show promise. Indeed, the IAT has recently been shown to be useful in children as young as 4 (Cvencek, Greenwald, & Meltzoff, 2011), and it will be important to continue investigating how different adaptations for children compare. And of course, large-scale prospective studies are required to examine how implicit and explicit processes develop in children, how these processes normatively converge and diverge over time, and what predictors and implications of concordance emerge as most important over the course of development into adulthood.

REFERENCES

Archer, R. P., & Krishnamurthy, R. (1993). Combining the Rorschach and the MMPI in the assessment of adolescents. *Journal of Personality Assessment, 60*(1), 132–140.

Asendorpf, J. B., Banse, R., & Mucke, D. (2002). Double dissociation between implicit and explicit personality self-concept: The case of shy behavior. *Journal of Personality and Social Psychology, 83*, 380–393.

Back, M. D., Schmukle, S. C., & Egloff, B. (2009). Predicting actual behavior from the explicit and implicit self-concept of personality. *Journal of Personality and Social Psychology, 97*(3), 533–548.

Baer, R. A., Wetter, M. W., & Berry, D. T. (1992). Detection of underreporting of psychopathology on the MMPI: A meta-analysis. *Clinical Psychology Review, 12*, 509–525.

Bargh, J. A., Chaiken, S., Govender, R., & Pratto, F. (1992). The generality of the automatic attitude activation effect. *Journal of Personality and Social Psychology, 62*(6), 893–912.

Bargh, J. A., & Chartrand, T. L. (1999). The unbearable automaticity of being. *American Psychologist, 54*(7), 462–479.

Bargh, J. A., Chen, M., & Burrows, L. (1996). Automaticity of social behavior: Direct effects of trait construct and stereotype activation on action. *Journal of Personality and Social Psychology, 71*(2), 230–244.

Beevers, C. G. (2005). Cognitive vulnerability to depression: A dual process model. *Clinical Psychology Review, 25*(7), 975–1002.

Berry, D. T., Baer, R. A., & Harris, M. J. (1991). Detection of malingering on the MMPI: A meta-analysis. *Clinical Psychology Review, 11*, 585–598.

Bornstein, R. F. (1998). Implicit and self-attributed dependency strivings: Differential relationships to laboratory and field measures of help seeking. *Journal of Personality and Social Psychology, 75*, 778–787.

Bornstein, R. F. (2002). A process dissociation approach to objective-projective test score interrelationships. *Journal of Personality Assessment, 78*, 47–68.

Bower, G. H., Montiero, K. P., & Gilligan, S. G. (1978). Emotional mood as a context for learning and recall. *Journal of Verbal Learning and Verbal Behavior, 17*, 573–585.

Buhrmester, M. D., Blanton, H., & Swann, W. B., Jr. (2011). Implicit self-esteem: Nature, measurement, and a new way forward. *Journal of Personality and Social Psychology, 100*(2), 365–385.

Cogswell, A. (2008). Explicit rejection of an implicit dichotomy: Integrating two approaches to assessing dependency. *Journal of Personality Assessment, 90*(1), 26–35.

Corr, P. J. (2010). Automatic and controlled processes in behavioural control: Implications for personality psychology. *European Journal of Personality, 24*, 376–403.

Creemers, D. H. M., Scholte, R. H. J., Engels, R. C. M. E., Prinstein, M. J., & Wiers, R. W. (2012). Implicit and explicit self-esteem as concurrent predictors of suicidal ideation, depressive symptoms, and loneliness. *Journal of Behavior Therapy and Experimental Psychiatry, 43*(1), 638–646.

Cvencek, D., Greenwald, A. G., & Meltzoff, A. N. (2011). Measuring implicit attitudes of 4-year-olds: The Preschool Implicit Association Test. *Journal of Experimental Child Psychology, 109*(2), 187–200.

De Houwer, J. (2006). What are implicit measures and why are we using them? In R. W. Wiers & A. W. Stacy (Eds.), *Handbook of implicit cognition and addiction* (pp. 11–28). Thousand Oaks, CA: Sage.

De Houwer, J., Teige-Mocigemba, S., Spruyt, A., & Moors, A. (2009). Implicit measures: A normative analysis and review. *Psychological Bulletin, 135*(3), 347–368.

De Los Reyes, A. (2011). Introduction to the special section: More than measurement error: Discovering meaning behind informant discrepancies in clinical assessments of children and adolescents. *Journal of Clinical Child and Adolescent Psychology, 40*(1), 1–9.

Degner, J. (2009). On the (un-)controllability of affective priming: Strategic manipulation is feasible but can possibly be prevented. *Cognition and Emotion, 23*(2), 327–354.

Dentale, F., San Martini, P., De Coro, A., & Di Pomponio, I. (2010). Alexithymia increases the discordance between implicit and explicit self-esteem. *Personality and Individual Differences, 49*(7), 762–767.

Dentale, F., Vecchione, M., De Coro, A., & Barbaranelli, C. (2012). On the relationship between implicit and explicit self-esteem: The moderating role of dismissing attachment. *Personality and Individual Differences, 52*(2), 173–177.

Deutsch, R., & Strack, F. (2010). Building blocks of social behavior: Reflective and impulsive processes. In B. Gawronski & B. K. Payne (Eds.), *Handbook of implicit social cognition: Measurement, theory, and applications* (pp. 62–79). New York: Guilford Press.

Dewitte, M., De Houwer, J., & Buysse, A. (2008). On the role of the implicit self-concept in adult attachment. *European Journal of Psychological Assessment, 24*(4), 282–289.

Eastwick, P. W., Eagly, A. H., Finkel, E. J., & Johnson, S. E. (2011). Implicit and explicit preferences for physical attractiveness in a romantic partner: A double dissociation in predictive validity. *Journal of Personality and Social Psychology, 101*(5), 993–1011.

Egloff, B., & Schmukle, S. (2002). Predictive validity of an implicit association test for assessing anxiety. *Journal of Personality and Social Psychology, 83*, 1441–1455.

Egloff, B., Weck, F., & Schmukle, S. (2008). Thinking about anxiety moderates the relationship between implicit and explicit anxiety measures. *Journal of Research in Personality, 42*, 771–778.

Exner, J. E., Jr. (1991). *The Rorschach: A comprehensive system: Vol. 2. Interpretation.* New York: Wiley.

Fazio, R. H., & Olson, M. A. (2003). Implicit measures in social cognition research: Their meaning and use. *Annual Review of Psychology, 54*, 297–327.

Finn, S. E. (1996). Assessment feedback integrating MMPI–2 and Rorschach findings. *Journal of Personality Assessment, 67*(3), 543–557.

Gallen, R. T., & Berry, D. T. R. (1996). Detection of random responding in MMPI-2 protocols. *Assessment, 3*, 171–178.

Garb, H. N. (1999). Call for a moratorium on the use of the Rorschach Inkblot Test in clinical and forensic settings. *Assessment, 6*, 313–317.

Gawronski, B., & Bodenhausen, G. V. (2006). Associative and propositional processes in evaluation: An integrative review of implicit and explicit attitude change. *Psychological Bulletin, 132*(5), 692–731.

Gawronski, B., & Bodenhausen, G. V. (2007). Unraveling the processes underlying evaluation: Attitudes from the perspective of the APE model. *Social Cognition, 25*(5), 687–717.

Gawronski, B., Rydell, R. J., Vervliet, B., & De Houwer, J. (2010). Generalization versus contextualization in automatic evaluation. *Journal of Experimental Psychology: General, 139*(4), 683–701.

Greenwald, A. G., Banaji, M. R., Rudman, L. A., Farnham, S. D., Nosek, B. A., &

Mellott, D. S. (2002). A unified theory of implicit attitudes, stereotypes, self-esteem, and self-concept. *Psychological Review, 109*, 3–25.

Greenwald, A. G., & Farnham, S. (2000). Using the Implicit Association Test to measure self-esteem and self-concept. *Journal of Personality and Social Psychology, 79*, 1022–1038.

Greenwald, A. G., McGhee, D. E., & Schwartz, J. L. K. (1998). Measuring individual differences in implicit cognition: The implicit association test. *Journal of Personality and Social Psychology, 74*, 1464–1480.

Greenwald, A. G., Nosek, B. A., & Banaji, M. R. (2003). Understanding and using the Implicit Association Test: I. An improved scoring algorithm. *Journal of Personality and Social Psychology, 85*(2), 197–216.

Greenwald, A. G., Poehlman, T. A., Uhlmann, E. L., & Banaji, M. R. (2009). Understanding and using the Implicit Association Test: III. Meta-analysis of predictive validity. *Journal of Personality and Social Psychology, 97*(1), 17–41.

Grumm, M., Hein, S., & Fingerle, M. (2011). Predicting aggressive behavior in children with the help of measures of implicit and explicit aggression. *International Journal of Behavioral Development, 35*(4), 352–357.

Harter, S. (2012). *Self-Perception Profile for Children: Manual and questionnaires.* Denver, CO: University of Denver.

Hartshorne, H., & May, M. A. (1928). *Studies in deceit. Book I. General methods and results. Book II. Statistical methods and results.* Oxford, UK: Macmillan.

Hathaway, S. R., & McKinley, J. C. (1943). *The Minnesota Multiphasic Personality Inventory.* New York: Psychological Corporation.

Hofmann, W., Gawronski, B., Gschwendner, T., Le, H., & Schmitt, M. (2005). A meta-analysis on the correlation between the Implicit Association Test and explicit self-report measures. *Personality and Social Psychology Bulletin, 31*(10), 1369–1385.

Hofmann, W., Gschwendner, T., Nosek, B. A., & Schmitt, M. (2005). What moderates implicit-explicit consistency? *European Review of Social Psychology, 16*, 335–390.

Klauer, K. C., & Teige-Mocigemba, S. (2007). Controllability and resource dependence in automatic evaluation. *Journal of Experimental Social Psychology, 43*(4), 648–655.

Koole, S. L., Govorun, O., Cheng, C. M., & Gallucci, M. (2009). Pulling yourself together: Meditation promotes congruence between implicit and explicit self-esteem. *Journal of Experimental Social Psychology, 45*(6), 1220–1226.

Koole, S. L., & Rothermund, K. (2011). "I feel better but I don't know why": The psychology of implicit emotion regulation. *Cognition and Emotion, 25*(3), 389–399.

Lane, K. A., Banaji, M. R., Nosek, B. A., & Greenwald, A. G. (2007). Understanding and using the Implicit Association Test: IV. What we know (so far) about the method. In B. Wittenbrink & N. Schwarz (Eds.), *Implicit measures of attitudes* (pp. 59–102). New York: Guilford Press.

McCarthy, R. J., & Skowronski, J. J. (2011). The interplay of controlled and automatic processing in the expression of spontaneously inferred traits: A PDP analysis. *Journal of Personality and Social Psychology, 100*(2), 229–240.

McClelland, D. C., Koestner, R., & Weinberger, J. (1989). How do self attributed and implicit motives differ? *Psychological Review, 96*, 690–702.

McCrae, R. R., & Costa, P. T. (1987). Validation of the five-factor model of personality across instruments and observers. *Journal of Personality and Social Psychology, 52*(1), 81–90.

McGrath, R. E. (2008). The Rorschach in the context of performance-based personality assessment. *Journal of Personality Assessment, 90*(5), 465–475.

Meyer, G. J. (1996). The Rorschach and MMPI: Toward a more scientifically differentiated understanding of cross-method assessment. *Journal of Personality Assessment, 67*(3), 558–578.

Meyer, G. J. (1997). On the integration of personality assessment methods: The Rorschach and MMPI. *Journal of Personality Assessment, 68*(2), 297–330.

Meyer, G. J., & Archer, R. (2001). The hard science of Rorschach research: What do we know and where do we go? *Psychological Assessment, 13*(4), 486–502.

Moors, A., Spruyt, A., & De Houwer, J. (2010). In search of a measure that qualifies as implicit: Recommendations based on a decompositional view of automaticity. In B. Gawronski & B. K. Payne (Eds.), *Handbook of implicit social cognition: Measurement, theory, and applications* (pp. 19–37). New York: Guilford Press.

Morey, L. C. (1991). *Personality Assessment Inventory Professional manual.* Odessa, FL: Psychological Assessment Resources.

Morgan, C. D., & Murray, H. H. (1935). A method for investigating fantasies: The Thematic Apperception Test. *Archives of Neurology and Psychiatry, 34,* 289–306.

Murphy, S. T., Monahan, J. L., & Zajonc, R. B. (1995). Additivity of nonconscious affect: Combined effects of priming and exposure. *Journal of Personality and Social Psychology, 69*(4), 589–602.

Nisbett, R. E., & Wilson, T. D. (1977). Telling more than we can know: Verbal reports on mental processes. *Psychological Review, 84*(3), 231–259.

Nock, M. K., Park, J. M., Finn, C. T., Deliberto, T. L., Dour, H. J., & Banaji, M. R. (2010). Measuring the suicidal mind: Implicit cognition predicts suicidal behavior. *Psychological Science, 21*(4), 511–517.

Nosek, B. A. (2005). Moderators of the relationship between implicit and explicit evaluation. *Journal of Experimental Psychology: General, 134,* 565–584.

Nosek, B. A., Greenwald, A. G., & Banaji, M. R. (2007). The Implicit Association Test at Age 7: A nethodological and conceptual review. In J. A. Bargh (Ed.), *Social psychology and the unconscious: The automaticity of higher mental processes* (pp. 265–292). New York: Psychology Press.

Payne, B. K. (2005). Conceptualizing control in social cognition: How executive functioning modulates the expression of automatic stereotyping. *Journal of Personality and Social Psychology, 89*(4), 488–503.

Payne, B. K., Burkley, M. A., & Stokes, M. B. (2008). Why do implicit and explicit attitude tests diverge?: The role of structural fit. *Journal of Personality and Social Psychology, 94*(1), 16–31.

Payne, B. K., Cheng, C. M., Govorun, O., & Stewart, B. D. (2005). An inkblot for attitudes: Affect misattribution as implicit measurement. *Journal of Personality and Social Psychology, 89*(3), 277–293.

Pelham, B. W., Mirenberg, M. C., & Jones, J. T. (2002). Why Susie sells seashells by the seashore: Implicit egotism and major life decisions. *Journal of Personality and Social Psychology, 82*(4), 469–487.

Perry, G. G., & Kinder, B. N. (1990). The susceptibility of the Rorschach to malingering: A critical review. *Journal of Personality Assessment, 54*(1–2), 47–57.

Perugini, M., & Leone, L. (2009). Implicit self-concept and moral action. *Journal of Research in Personality, 43*(5), 747–754.

Petty, R. E., Tormala, Z. L., Briñol, P., & Jarvis, W. B. G. (2006). Implicit ambivalence from attitude change: An exploration of the PAST model. *Journal of Personality and Social Psychology, 90*(1), 21–41.

Phillips, W. J., Hine, D. W., & Thorsteinsson, E. B. (2010). Implicit cognition and depression: A meta-analysis. *Clinical Psychology Review, 30*(6), 691–709.

Roefs, A., Huijding, J., Smulders, F. T. Y., MacLeod, C. M., de Jong, P. J., Wiers, R.

W., et al. (2011). Implicit measures of association in psychopathology research. *Psychological Bulletin, 137*(1), 149–193.

Rosenberg, M. (1965). *Society and the adolescent selfimage.* Princeton, NJ: Princeton University Press.

Rydell, R. J., & McConnell, A. R. (2006). Understanding implicit and explicit attitude change: A systems of reasoning analysis. *Journal of Personality and Social Psychology, 91*(6), 995–1008.

Rydell, R. J., McConnell, A. R., & Mackie, D. M. (2008). Consequences of discrepant explicit and implicit attitudes: Cognitive dissonance and increased information processing. *Journal of Experimental Social Psychology, 44*(6), 1526–1532.

Schacter, D. L. (1987). Implicit memory, history and current status. *Journal of Experimental Psychology: Learning, Memory, and Cognition, 13,* 501–518.

Schmukle, S. C., Back, M. D., & Egloff, B. (2008). Validity of the five-factor model for the implicit self-concept of personality. *European Journal of Psychological Assessment, 24*(4), 263–272.

Schnabel, K., Banse, R., & Asendorpf, J. (2006). Employing automatic approach and avoidance tendencies for the assessment of implicit personality self-concept: The Implicit Association Procedure (IAP). *Experimental Psychology, 53*(1), 69–76.

Schreiber, F., Bohn, C., Aderka, I. M., Stangier, U., & Steil, R. (2012). Discrepancies between implicit and explicit self-esteem among adolescents with social anxiety disorder. *Journal of Behavior Therapy and Experimental Psychiatry, 43*(4), 1074–1081.

Schröder-Abé, M., Rudolph, A., & Schüz, A. (2007). High implicit self-esteem is not necessarily advantagous: Discrepancies between explicit and implicit self-esteem and their relationship with anger expression and psychological health. *European Journal of Personality, 21*(3), 319–339.

Shedler, J., Mayman, M., & Manis, M. (1993). The illusion of mental health. *American Psychologist, 48,* 1117–1131.

Sheeran, P., Gollwitzer, P. M., & Bargh, J. A. (2013). Nonconscious processes and health. *Health Psychology, 32,* 460–473.

Shevrin, H., & Dickman, S. (1980). The psychological unconscious: A necessary assumption for all psychological theory? *American Psychologist, 35*(5), 421–434.

Smith, C. T., & Nosek, B. A. (2011). Affective focus increases the concordance between implicit and explicit attitudes. *Social Psychology, 42*(4), 300–313.

Spence, A., & Townsend, E. (2008). Spontaneous evaluations: Similarities and differences between the affect heuristic and implicit attitudes. *Cognition and Emotion, 22*(1), 83–93.

Strack, F., & Deutsch, R. (2004). Reflective and Impulsive Determinants of Social Behavior. *Personality and Social Psychology Review, 8*(3), 220–247.

Wilson, T. D., Lindsey, S., & Schooler, T. Y. (2000). A model of dual attitudes. *Psychological Review, 107,* 101–126.

Wittenbrink, B., Judd, C. M., & Park, B. (2001). Evaluative versus conceptual judgments in automatic stereotyping and prejudice. *Journal of Experimental Social Psychology, 37*(3), 244–252.

Wood, J. M., Lilienfeld, S. O., Garb, H. N., & Nezworski, M. T. (2000). The Rorschach test in clinical diagnosis: A critical review, with a backward look at Garfield (1947). *Journal of Clinical Psychology, 56,* 395–430.

PART II

Psychopathology and Resilience

CHAPTER 6

Multimethod Assessment of Anxiety

Integrating Data from Subjective Experience, Cognitive Performance, and Neurophysiological Measures

Jason S. Moser, Amy Przeworski, Hans S. Schroder, and Kimberly Marie Dunbeck

Anxiety is a basic human experience that represents an adaptive response to threat (Marks & Nesse, 1994). At its extreme, however, disordered anxiety is the most common psychological problem reported across the life span (Beesdo, Knapp, & Pine, 2009; Kessler, Chiu, Demler, Merikangas, & Walters, 2005). In fact, roughly one in five Americans suffer from anxiety-related disorders (Kessler et al., 2005; McLean, Asnaani, Litz, & Hofmann, 2011). Moreover, maladaptive anxiety is associated with extensive societal costs in the form of billions of dollars spent each year on treatment, lost work productivity, and reduced academic performance (Beilock, 2008; Kessler et al., 2005; Rice & Miller, 1998). In order to address this public health concern, thorough assessments of anxiety are critical. Such assessments provide clarity on the nature of anxiety and the foundation for early identification and prevention and treatment efforts across research and clinical settings. In this chapter, we discuss the multimethod assessment of anxiety. In particular, we focus on the integration of information gathered from traditional self-report and diagnostic assessments with that from newer cognitive and neurophysiological methods. We focus on the inclusion of cognitive and neurophysiological measures because theory and application of these tools have seen significant advancement in recent years and provide promise for a richer understanding of anxiety-related problems and their treatment.

Background

The traditional view of assessment of anxiety is Lang's (1968) three-systems approach, which identifies the following three components of anxiety: subjective experience, behaviors, and psychophysiological response. Subjective experience is derived from self-report on questionnaires and during interviews. Behaviors are broadly construed and include overt avoidance, facial expressions, and performance biases or deficits. Psychophysiological responses were originally defined as those generated by the autonomic nervous system, such as heart rate, skin conductance, respiration, and blood pressure. Lang specified that all manifestations of anxiety are informative and no single component has priority over another in terms of indicating one's level of anxiety—that is, anxiety is a multifaceted phenomenon and could reveal itself in different ways across different response systems across different individuals. The importance of this multisystem or multimethod assessment of anxiety was further highlighted by Rachman and Hodgson (1974), who noted that desynchrony and discordance among measures could provide unique diagnostic and treatment information. Also, Wolpe's (1977) discussion of the heterogeneity of anxiety symptom presentations pointed to the need for assessing anxiety at multiple levels.

In the 1970s and 1980s, multimodal assessment of anxiety in psychopathology and intervention research was fairly common. An analysis of assessment trends in the literature, however, indicates that in recent years researchers have been relying more heavily on subjective reports of behavior and symptoms and single-response system assessment (Lawyer & Smitherman, 2004). Lawyer and Smitherman's review does not generally clarify what led to this decrease in multimethod assessment of anxiety over the years; however, concerns about the psychometric properties of physiological measures (e.g., Arena, Blanchard, Andrasik, Cotch, & Myers, 1983; Holden & Barlow, 1986) were noted. It is also likely that lack of training and access to certain technology, and the ease of collecting self-report questionnaires led to the decline in multimethod assessments. Given that multimethod assessments are uncommon in research, it should come as no surprise that few, if any, practitioners assess anxiety across these different systems and integrate information from each in their diagnostics and treatment planning. As such, most assessments of anxiety are composed almost entirely of subjective and unstructured behavioral measures.

Another potential reason for the decline of multimethod assessment of anxiety may be the reliance on diagnostic status determined by interviews based on the *Diagnostic and Statistical Manual of Mental Disorders* (DSM; American Psychiatric Association, 2013). DSM-based diagnosis is generally considered the gold standard criterion for defining clinically significant anxiety. This point is particularly well illustrated in work on posttraumatic stress disorder (PTSD). As reviewed by Steenkamp, McLean, Arditte, and Litz (2010), "psychophysiological measures may have limited use in confirming the diagnosis of PTSD when used as the sole index"

(p. 324). This conclusion was based on data from a large-scale Veterans Affairs study showing that psychophysiological markers correctly identified two-thirds of the veterans diagnosed with DSM-defined PTSD (Keane et al., 1998). That is, the psychophysiological markers were not perfect predictors of DSM-based PTSD diagnosis and thus were not considered clinically useful. Our concern with this logic is that it assumes that DSM-based diagnosis captures all of the "truth" about an individual's anxiety. It seems to us that this prioritization of DSM diagnosis runs counter to Lang's (1968) original proposal that information gathered from one particular response system—for example, a subjective report—cannot, alone, indicate one's anxiety level, but rather anxiety is a multifaceted construct that is reflected in responses across systems.

In the same vein, researchers and clinicians are apparently satisfied with considering an assessment "multimethod" if questionnaires and diagnostic/clinical interviews are used. Beyond DSM-based diagnostic interviews, researchers have developed a number of clinical interviews to capture the severity of anxiety problems (e.g., the Liebowitz Social Anxiety Scale [LSAS]; Heimberg et al., 1999). There are two problems with this approach. First, both questionnaires and clinical interviews rely on self-report and thus do not measure anxiety across different systems. Second, questionnaire and interviewer measures tend to be highly correlated/redundant. For example, the correlation between the clinician-administered LSAS and the self-report version of the LSAS is roughly 0.90 (e.g., Rytwinski et al., 2009).

Despite the decline in multimethod assessment of anxiety, limited extant data demonstrate the benefits of combining measures across systems. For instance, combining subjective report and cardiac reactivity measures, Schmidt, Forsyth, Santiago, and Trakowski (2002) identified meaningful subtypes within a group of panic patients. More impressive, Ost and colleagues (Ost, Jerremalm, & Johansson, 1981; Ost, Johansson, & Jerremalm, 1982) demonstrated that socially phobic and claustrophobic patients who were matched to either an exposure or applied relaxation treatment based on their pattern of behavioral and physiological reactions to fear-provoking situations, respectively, had better outcomes than when mismatched based on their response pattern. That is, individuals with phobias showing relatively greater behavioral than physiological reactivity did better in exposure therapy, whereas individuals with phobias showing relatively greater physiological reactivity did better with applied relaxation. It is unfortunate that such studies have fallen out of favor because they clearly indicate the clinical utility of the multimethod assessment of anxiety.

Recent Trends

Three recent trends seem to be making multimethod assessment more popular in the research literature: the rise of the cognitive bias paradigm, the growth of neuroscience research, and the focus on dimensional assessment and classification of mental disorders. We briefly introduce these trends here and elaborate on them in subsequent sections.

The cognitive bias paradigm has grown out of the information-processing tradition in cognitive science. Since the 1980s, research has increased exponentially on how anxiety relates to systematic biases in attention, memory, and interpretation (Hertel & Mathews, 2011; Mathews & MacLeod, 2005). Typically, these biases manifest as tendencies to selectively attend to and remember negative information and interpret ambiguous information in a negative light. A broader literature further suggests that anxiety has several deleterious effects on performance of affectively neutral tasks because of the distracting effects of worry (Beilock, 2008; Eysenck, Derakshan, Santos, & Calvo, 2007; Sylvester et al., 2012). The majority of this work is conducted with simple reaction time (RT) tasks, and the resulting behavioral performance is compared across anxious and nonanxious groups or correlated with anxiety symptoms. In this way, readouts from these RT tasks represent output of the behavioral system as proposed by Lang (1968) and are related to the subjective experience reports.

Clinical science is also drawing more and more from neuroscience (e.g., Sylvester et al., 2012). Considerable research has been conducted using multiple neuroimaging methods, including functional magnetic resonance imaging (fRMI), positron emission tomography (PET), and electroencephalography (EEG). Although Lang (1968) initially focused on output of the autonomic nervous system as representing the psychophysiological response of anxiety, this emphasis might have easily been just a by-product of the technology available at the time. The proliferation of neuroscience methodology since the 1990s puts central nervous system functioning more easily in play as serving as another marker of the psychophysiological response of anxiety. Again, much of this work involves relating neural activity with self-reported anxiety, whether measured by questionnaires or clinical interviews.

High comorbidity of anxiety disorders indicates that the current categorical diagnostic system (i.e., DSM) is not functioning to distinguish between emotional disorders (e.g., Andrews, 1990, 1996; Brown, 1996). Rather, it suggests that a more parsimonious structure consisting of fewer categories likely more accurately reflects the nature of anxiety-related problems (Krueger, 1999; Watson, 2005). This notion draws on decades of research from personality psychology suggesting that covariance between seemingly distinct psychological problems arises from shared underlying processes (e.g., Millon, 1969). Moreover, research has shown that anxiety is best represented as a dimensional construct that varies along a continuum from mild to extreme, with disordered patients falling at the high end of extreme (Brown & Barlow, 2009; Ruscio, Borkovec, & Ruscio, 2001; Ruscio, Ruscio, & Keane, 2002; Watson, 2005). Thus, research has begun to focus more on dimensions of anxiety that cut across traditional diagnostic lines.

Converging lines of evidence suggest that anxiety is made up of two overlapping but separable dimensions: fear/anxious arousal versus anxiety/anxious apprehension (Krueger, 1999; Nitschke, Heller, Imig, McDonald, & Miller, 2001; Watson, 2005). Fear/anxious arousal can be understood as experiences and responses associated with immediate, circumscribed threat, whereas anxiety/anxious apprehension is generally thought of as experiences and response associated with future, ambiguous threat. Somatic tension and physiological hyperarousal characterize fear/anxious arousal, whereas worry characterizes anxiety/anxious apprehension. The advantage of focusing on these dimensions is that they likely represent more viable targets for mapping out experiential, behavioral, and biological mechanisms than highly heterogeneous and overlapping diagnostic categories (Bearden & Freimer, 2006). This approach has garnered so much support in recent years that the National Institute of Mental Health has created the Research Domain Criteria (RDoC) initiative, which is tasked with funding research that will help move the field toward a classification system rooted in dimensions of behavior and neurobiological measures (e.g., Sanislow et al., 2010). Specifically, the RDoC initiative directly supports the multimethod assessment of all mental disorders by requiring the measurement of relevant dimensions across multiple units of analysis—for example, behavior, self-report, physiology, and circuits. Herein we focus on how this government directive has potentially influenced recent trajectories in anxiety research.

Building on Lang's (1968) three-systems approach to anxiety, we follow recent trends and focus the remainder of this chapter on studies examining associations between self-reported experience of anxiety and cognitive biases/deficits and neural activity. With regard to neural activity, we selectively review studies using event-related brain potentials (ERPs) and focus on a couple of specific ERP components that show significant promise for use in the multimethod assessment of anxiety. Our motivation for covering ERP studies is twofold: (1) ERPs provide more precision for identifying underlying mechanisms involved in anxiety because of their excellent temporal resolution and (2) ERPs are less expensive and invasive to record than other neuroimaging technologies such as fMRI and PET and therefore have a greater potential to be utilized in various populations and contexts.

Multimethod Assessments

Cognitive Biases/Deficits

Although anxiety has been associated with a number of biases/deficits in cognition, we focus here on attentional biases/deficits because they have been the most rigorously studied. Eysenck et al.'s (2007) attentional control theory (ACT) provides provides an elegant formulation of attentional biases/deficits in anxiety across various task conditions (i.e., those including emotional and neutral stimuli). In general, ACT suggests that anxious individuals prioritize threatening information that is either internal (i.e., worry) or external (e.g., angry face), which leads to rapid detection of threat, sometimes at the expense of affectively neutral task-related stimuli. The idea is that this bias in attention results from the bottom-up attentional selection mechanism, overpowering the volitional, top-down control system. The theory draws on decades of research suggesting that attentional selection is determined by the interaction of two attentional systems: a stimulus-driven system and a goal-driven system (Posner & Petersen, 1990; Corbetta & Shulman, 2002)—that is, by the interplay of early exogenous (e.g., stimulus saliency) and later endogenous (e.g., expectations) processes, respectively (Theeuwes & Van Der Burg, 2007; van Zoest, Donk, & Theeuwes, 2004). Much of the work in this area has focused on how externally threatening stimuli capture attention using the dot-probe task (for a review, see Bar-Haim, Lamy, Pergamin, Bakermans-Kranenburg, & van IJzendoorn, 2007), although a growing body of research is examining anxiety's effects on affectively neutral task performance that is presumably impaired by distracting worries (Eysenck & Derakshan, 2011).

In the dot probe task, task-irrelevant threatening and neutral stimuli (words or faces) are presented simultaneously on a computer screen and are followed by a target stimulus (in the classic example a dot) presented in either the location of the preceding threatening or the neutral stimulus. The typical finding is that anxious individuals are relatively faster at detecting the target when it is presented at the same location as the preceding threatening stimulus. This effect has been demonstrated across a number of anxious groups, from high trait anxious college students to patients diagnosed with a range of anxiety disorders (Bar-Haim et al., 2007). Therefore, procedures such as the dot-probe task may become useful assessment tools when screening for anxiety disorders or anxiety vulnerability (Amir, Beard, Burns, & Bomyea, 2009). However, there is currently no evidence indicating how these biases/deficits differ across anxiety disorders or relate to anxiety dimensions such as fear and anxiety. Moreover, extant data do not pinpoint the exact mechanisms at play. That is, more refined investigation of attentional bias is needed to understand what stages of information processing differ between anxious and nonanxious individuals. Further, it is currently unclear what neural substrates are associated with these biases/deficits (Bar-Haim et al., 2007). The limitations of this literature provide an excellent segue to the next section on neurophysiology.

Neurophysiology

ERPs, which are measured by averaging electroencephalographic (EEG) activity time-locked to stimuli or responses, offer exciting insights into cognitive processes such as memory, attention allocation, information processing, and cognitive control (Luck, 2005). Below, we briefly focus on anxiety assessment using two ERPs: the error-related negativity (ERN) and the late positive potential (LPP).

Error-Related Negativity

The ERN, a negative-going ERP elicited immediately following response errors in speeded-choice tasks (Gehring, Goss, Coles, Meyer, & Donchin, 1993), has garnered much attention from anxiety researchers. The ERN is typically elicited in standard affectively neutral conflict tasks such as the Eriksen flanker task (Eriksen & Eriksen, 1974) where subjects are instructed to respond to the center stimulus under congruent (e.g., HHHHH) and incongruent (SSHSS) conditions. Converging evidence from source localization (Dehaene, Posner, & Tucker, 1994; van Veen & Carter, 2002) and functional magnetic resonance imaging (fMRI; Ridderinkhof, Ullsperger, Crone, & Nieuwenhuis, 2004) suggests that the anterior cingulate cortex (ACC) is involved in the generation of the ERN. The ACC is typically considered a bridge between cognitive and emotional brain regions involved in several critical functions such as cognitive control, the generation of negative affect, and autonomic regulation (Shackman et al., 2011).

The ERN is most consistently enhanced in individuals with symptoms of generalized anxiety disorder (GAD; Moser, Moran, & Jendrusina, 2012; Weinberg, Olvet, & Hajcak, 2010) and obsessive–compulsive disorder (OCD; Gehring, Himle, & Nisenson, 2000; Hajcak & Simons, 2002). Several hypotheses have been put forward to account for enhanced ERN in anxiety. Researchers have claimed that it reflects a "comparator dysfunction" resulting in many events being incorrectly classified as wrong (Gehring et al., 2000), heightened defensive reactivity (Weinberg, Riesel, & Hajcak, 2012), or inefficient performance monitoring caused by worries (Moser et al., 2012). Nonetheless, enhanced ERN in anxiety is perhaps the most replicated finding in the neurophysiology literature. Although the ERN has not yet been systematically studied across the entire spectrum of anxiety disorders, recent work has aimed to clarify how the ERN relates to broad dimensions of anxiety per RDoC (Vaidyanathan, Nelson, & Patrick, 2012) and suggests that ERN enhancement appears to be specific to the anxious apprehension (worry) dimension (Moser et al., 2012).

Late Positive Potential

The late positive potential (LPP) is a broad positive deflection that reaches maximum amplitude 300–800 milliseconds after the onset of motivationally relevant stimuli. It can last up to several seconds. A decade of research demonstrates that the LPP reflects the arousal properties of emotional stimuli. Indeed, the magnitude of the LPP is closely coupled with subjective ratings of arousal reactions to emotional pictures, further linking the LPP to emotional experience (e.g., Cuthbert, Schupp, Bradley, Birbaumer, & Lang, 2000). Early time windows (300–1,000 milliseconds) index attention allocation, whereas later time windows (>1,000 milliseconds) index memory and meaning making stages. Both time windows are enhanced in response to arousing stimuli regardless of their valence (Olofsson, Nordin, Sequeira, & Polich, 2008) and show strong associations with visual cortex and amygdala activity measured fMRI (Liu, Huang, McGinnis-Deweese, Keil, & Ding, 2012; Sabatinelli, Lang, Keil, & Bradley, 2007), confirming its significance in emotional processing.

The LPP is also sensitive to top-down attentional control (Schienle, Kochel, & Leutgeb, 2011; Scharmuller, Leutgeb, Schafer, Kochel, & Schienle, 2011). Specifically, early and late time windows of the LPP are reliably reduced at centroparietal sites during emotion regulation indicating reductions in arousal-related attention and memory processes (Moser, Hajcak, Bukay, & Simons, 2006; Moser, Krompinger, Dietz, & Simons, 2009; Thiruchselvam, Blechert, Shepppes, Rydstrom, & Gross, 2011). Moreover, LPP decreases during emotion regulation are associated with decreases in emotional experience (Hajcak & Nieuwenhuis, 2006).

The increasing use of the LPP as an index of emotional processing and regulation (Hajcak, Dunning, & Foti, 2009; Moser et al., 2006) demonstrates its clinical potential for disorders characterized by deficits in these processes such as anxiety. Consistent with this potential application, numerous studies have found abnormal modulation of the LPP during passive viewing tasks in several anxiety disorders, including GAD (MacNamara & Hajcak, 2010), social anxiety (Moser, Huppert, Duval, & Simons, 2008), and dental phobia (Leutgeb, Schafer, & Schienle, 2011). Moreover, the LPP modulation during emotion regulation is sensitive to individual differences in trait worry (Moser, Hartwig, Moran, Jendrusina, & Kross, 2014).

However, as was the case with the ERN, the LPP has not been studied across the entire spectrum of anxiety disorders. The LPP has also been less extensively studied than the ERN in terms of its stability, reliability, and heritability. Thus, much work remains to be done to clarify the clinical utility of the LPP. Nonetheless, the LPP is a well-characterized ERP in terms of its functional significance and has already demonstrated its association with anxiety in reflecting abnormalities in emotion processing and regulation. For these reasons, we feel it has significant potential to be utilized in the multimethod assessment of anxiety.

Clinical Application

In this section, we present the results of a case study in order to demonstrate a multimethod assessment approach involving the methods described earlier. In doing so, we progress through a stepwise process of hypothesis testing, seeking confirmation of initial impressions/formulation while at the same time ruling out competing notions and diagnoses. Assessment- and treatment-related data are provided to more fully illustrate the utility of the multimethod approach. Such an intensive, single-subject analysis has the potential to not only exemplify the clinical value of multimethod assessment of anxiety but also inform basic science in this area—that is, it is an example of translational research.

Case Presentation

Sarah, a young lawyer, presented to the clinic for assessment and treatment of fear of vomiting (i.e., emetophobia). She reported struggling with emetophobia since she was 5 years old, but that these fears became most bothersome during stressful transitions (e.g., from high school to college). Her worries about vomiting caused her significant distress, almost always leading her to seek reassurance and support from friends and family members. This reassurance and support seeking became problematic, as it made her dependent on others for emotion regulation. Sarah's emetophobia also led to decreases in body weight, as she avoided eating certain foods or too much food so as to decrease the likelihood of vomiting. Sarah's symptoms also interfered with her social functioning: She avoided certain social gatherings she would have otherwise liked to attend (i.e., parties) for fear that someone would vomit, and she had not engaged in intimate relationships with members of the opposite sex because she wanted to keep her distance so as to avoid getting sick from intimate contact (e.g., kissing) and ultimately vomiting.

Sarah's presentation is typical in many respects. She presented to the clinic with complaints of anxiety at a stressful time in her life (i.e., she was just out of law school) and was already taking a selective serotonin reuptake inhibitor (SSRI) with, at best, modest relief. Less typically, however, Sarah reported suffering from emetophobia, a rarer and more understudied anxiety disorder. Emetophobia, or specific phobia of vomiting (SPOV), falls under the category of specific phobia, other type in DSM-5 (American Psychiatric Association, 2013). The prevalence of SPOV is elusive, but a recent investigation in German women indicates a lifetime prevalence of 0.2% (Becker et al., 2007), making it one of the rarest specific phobias. The fear of vomiting—not necessarily meeting DSM diagnostic criteria—may be more common, with rates as high as 7% in women (Philips, 1985; van Hout & Bouman, 2012). As is typical of the anxiety disorders, emetophobia is much more common in women than in men (Lipsitz, Fyer, Paterniti, & Klein, 2001; Philips, 1985; van Hout & Bouman, 2012).

Emetophobia appears to be more impairing than other specific phobias (Kartsounis, Mervyn-Smith, & Pickersgill, 1983). It typically has an onset in childhood, a chronic course (average of 26 years), and significant impact on functioning, including low body weight and avoidance of major life goals such as desired pregnancy (Lipsitz et al., 2001; Manassis & Kalman, 1990; Veale, 2009; Veale & Lambrou, 2006). It also commonly shows considerable overlap with other nonphobic anxiety disorders, including panic disorder (PD) and obsessive–compulsive disorder (Veale, 2009; Veale & Lambrou, 2006). Similarly, Boschen (2007) suggests that individuals with emetophobia are more vulnerable to general anxiety than individuals suffering from other phobias. Due to the common problems with maintaining a healthy body weight, some individuals with emetophobia are also misdiagnosed with anorexia nervosa (Manassis & Kalman, 1990).

Assessment

Self-Report and Clinical Interview

After a preliminary unstructured consultation session, one of us (J. S. M.) began the formal assessment of Sarah with administration of a set of syndrome-specific questionnaires, including two scales designed to detect clinical levels of emetophobia and two to capture cognitive and physiologic anxiety. Scores on these measures for the assessment period and subsequent treatment changes are presented in Figure 6.1. Sarah scored a 46 on the Vomit Phobia Inventory (VPI; Veale, Ellison, Whelen, & Henry, 2010) and an 89 on the Emetophobia Questionnaire (EmetQ; Price, Veale, & Brewin,

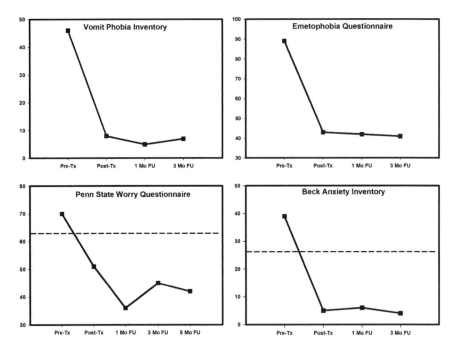

FIGURE 6.1. Self-reports across assessment and treatment phases. Questionnaires in the top panels do not have established cut scores. The range on the Vomit Phobia Inventory is 0–60. The range of the Emetophobia Questionnaire is 21–105. In the bottom panels, the dashed horizontal lines indicate typical clinical cut scores (62 for the Penn State Worry Questionnaire; 26 for the Beck Anxiety Inventory).

2012), scores that are quite similar to and somewhat higher than those reported in a recent sample of individuals with Emetophobia (*M* VPI = 33, *SD* VPI = 16; *M* EmetQ = 79, *SD* EmetQ = 13; Price et al., 2012). Her scores on the Penn State Worry Questionnaire (PSWQ; Meyer, Miller, Metzger, & Borkovec, 1990) and the Beck Anxiety Inventory (BAI; Beck, Epstein, Brown, & Steer, 1988), 70 and 39, respectively, also indicated clinical levels of anxiety-related problems. In fact, her score on the PSWQ places here above the clinical cut score (62) for a diagnosis of GAD (Behar et al., 2003). Together, Sarah's scores on these measures are consistent with research on emetophobia in that she reported extreme fears of vomiting and severe general anxiety comprised of chronic worry and physiologic anxiety.

To further evaluate the clinical significance of Sarah's anxiety problems, JSM then conducted a semistructured interview, the Mini International Neuropsychiatric Interview (MINI; Sheehan et al., 1998), to assess for DSM disorders. Consistent with the research on emetophobia, OCD and PD were considered in differential diagnosis. Indeed, Sarah demonstrated compulsive behaviors such as washing her hands excessively; however, her concerns/worries/obsessions were specific to fears about vomiting and didn't include other content areas typical of patients with OCD (e.g., concern about contracting a deadly virus). Thus, her "compulsions" could be considered safety/avoidance behaviors aimed at managing her specific fear of vomiting, which is more common among individuals with emetophobia. Although Sarah also reported physiologic anxiety, her concerns about these symptoms were always driven by a fear of vomiting, not the physiologic symptoms themselves or the consequences of going crazy, being embarrassed, or being unable to escape, typical of patients with PD (Barlow, 2002). Despite the fact that Sarah reported chronic worry on the PSWQ, her worries were mostly confined to vomiting. She reported other general worries about finances, grades, and friends, but none of these other concerns were uncontrollable or frequent enough to warrant a separate diagnosis of GAD. Sarah also denied any weight or shape concerns, ruling out anorexia. Finally, Sarah reported significant impairment associated with her emetophobia. She reported spending substantial time washing her hands, losing weight because of restricting her diet to "safe" foods, and eating small amounts. As noted earlier, she limited her social life by avoiding parties where people might vomit (from alcohol consumption) and by avoiding intimate relationships so as to decrease her likelihood of being close to someone who might be or get sick.

There was strong evidence from the self-report and interview data that Sarah was suffering from SPOV. She presented to the clinic reporting significant fears of vomiting, she scored well in the clinical range on psychometrically sound questionnaires of emetophobia, she reported significant impairment due to her emetophobia, and she complained of significant general anxiety. The level of general worry and anxiety she reported is in line with research on emetophobia, suggesting that heightened general anxiety and broad functional impairment separate it from other phobias (Boschen, 2007; Kartsounis et al., 1983). Her phobia veritably followed her wherever she went. All sorts of environmental stimuli could serve as triggers, whereas people with other phobias, such as animal phobias, can reasonably navigate most of the world without encountering feared stimuli. Triggers for individuals with vomit phobia are more generalized. Next, data from lab-based assessments are presented to further characterize Sarah's pathology.

Attention Bias

Sarah completed a standard word version of the dot-probe paradigm described above as part of her assessment. Her negative attention bias scores derived from this task across assessment and treatment phases are presented in Figure 6.2. The 0 point on the y-axis indicates no attention bias for either negative or neutral stimuli and negative scores indicate a bias toward neutral information. Her initial bias score (pretraining) was nearly 0, although she had a very slight bias for neutral information. Thus, a negative attention bias did not seem to be an important aspect of maintaining her pathology as she was quite symptomatic without one. Although seemingly inconsistent with the wealth of evidence demonstrating a negative attention bias in a range of anxious populations, the meta-analysis by Bar-Haim et al. (2007) shows that the negative attention bias effect in anxious individuals is actually small ($r = .22$; see Cohen, 1988, for standard practice of interpreting effect sizes). Therefore, it is not that surprising that Sarah did not demonstrate a negative attention bias despite her anxious presentation.

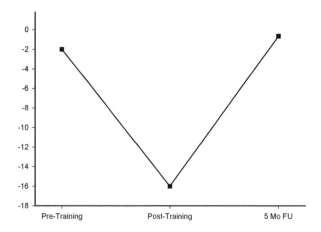

FIGURE 6.2. Negative attention bias data across assessment and treatment phases. 0 indicates no preferential bias, whereas negative scores indicate an attentional preference for neutral stimuli.

Error-Related Negativity

Sarah also completed a standard letter-version of the Eriksen flanker task. Her ERN waveforms extracted from the flanker task across assessment and treatment phases are presented in Figure 6.3. Sarah demonstrated a robust ERN of typical morphology (e.g., peaked within the first 100 milliseconds). Applying standard measurement procedures to the waveform revealed an ERN magnitude of –8.00 microvolts at pretreatment. Because we routinely measure the ERN and related anxiety problems in students around Sarah's age, we had a (local) "normative" sample with which to compare her score. Her pretreatment score placed her in the 79th percentile of other females assessed in our lab. This enhanced ERN is in line with her high worry scores on the PSWQ and diagnosis of SPOV, which is more complex than other specific phobias. Individuals with specific phobia do not demonstrate an enhanced ERN (Hajcak, McDonald, & Simons, 2003), whereas those with more generalized anxiety do (Hajcak et al., 2003; Moser et al., 2012). Thus, Sarah's ERN provided convergent evidence for her more generalized anxious presentation characteristic of those with SPOV and is consistent with the ability of the ERN to distinguish phobias from nonphobic anxiety (Vaidyanathan et al., 2012).

Late Positive Potential

Sarah's lab assessment concluded with an emotion regulation task in which she was asked to react naturally and cognitively reappraise her reactions to

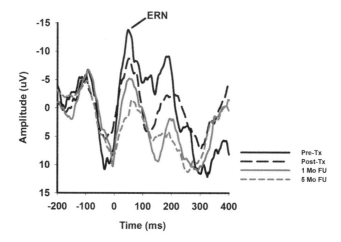

FIGURE 6.3. Error-related negativity (ERN) data across assessment and treatment phases. Negative amplitude is plotted up. Time 0 on the *x*-axis indicates response onset. The ERN is quantified as the average amplitude in the 0- to 100-millisecond postresponse time window.

negative scenes. The LPP waveforms extracted from this task across assessment and treatment phases are presented in Figure 6.4. Sarah demonstrated a typical LPP elicited in emotion and emotion regulation paradigms, which lasted for the duration of the picture presentation (i.e., 6 seconds). Inconsistent with previous research in unselected participants showing reduced LPP for reappraisal instructions (Hajcak & Nieuwenhuis, 2006; Moser et al., 2006, 2009), Sarah demonstrated a somewhat enhanced LPP for reappraise

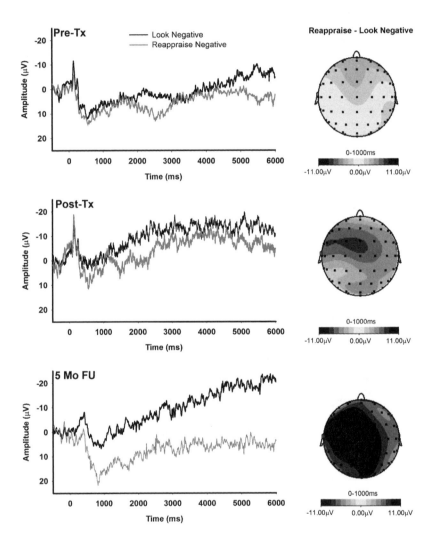

FIGURE 6.4. Late positive potential (LPP) data across assessment and treatment phases. Left: ERP waveforms. Negative amplitude is plotted up. Time 0 on the *x*-axis indicates target picture onset. Right: Scalp maps showing scalp distribution of the LPP in the 0- to 1,000-millisecond time window.

trials compared to trials in which she was asked to react naturally (look trials) at pretreatment. This finding is consistent, however, with a recent study conducted in our lab in which individuals who scored higher on chronic worry (as measured by the PSWQ) showed similarly enhanced LPP on reappraise trials (Moser et al., 2014). Recent studies using complementary psychophysiological methods also indicate that anxious-prone individuals (e.g., people who score high on trait anxiety measures, GAD patients, and social phobic patients), who are characterized by the tendency to worry excessively, have difficulty when asked to implement reappraisal in the laboratory (e.g., Campbell-Sills et al., 2011). Such findings are consistent with the notion that emotion regulation deficits characterize anxiety and other related emotional problems (Campbell-Sills & Barlow, 2007).

As with the ERN, we have a (local) "normative" sample with which to compare her pretreatment LPP scores. Measuring the LPP enhancement for reappraise compared to look trials (i.e., the reappraise LPP—the look LPP) at its peak—400–1,000 milliseconds after stimulus onset—her pretreatment score placed her in the 82nd percentile of other females assessed in our lab. Similarly, measuring the LPP enhancement for reappraise trials during the remainder of picture presentation—1–6 seconds—her pretreatment score placed her in the 96th percentile. Again, Sarah's emotion regulation LPP provided convergent evidence for her more generalized anxious presentation, involving worry, characteristic of those with SPOV and is consistent with the ability of the LPP to serve as a biomarker for negative affective psychopathology (Hajcak, MacNamara, & Olvet, 2010; Moser et al., 2014).

Treatment-Related Changes

In addition to initial assessment data, we present treatment data for the purposes of demonstrating if and how the various measures responded to a course of cognitive-behavioral therapy (CBT) for SPOV. These data further allow us to evaluate whether and how the different measures hang together as indicators of her anxiety-related problems. Changes in measures across treatment would suggest malleable maintenance markers, whereas lack of changes might indicate trait indicators or mechanisms not directly contributing to maintenance of her pathology.

Self-Reports and Clinical Interview

In Figure 6.1, the treatment data show a dramatic decrease in symptoms from pre- to posttreatment and consistent maintenance of gains at follow up across the various syndrome specific measures. Her scores were under 10 on the VPI, well below scores for individuals with emetophobia on the EmetQ (Price et al., 2012), well below the clinical cut score for GAD on the PSWQ (Behar, Alcaine, Zuelig, & Borkovec, 2003), and in the minimal anxiety range on the BAI. Together, Sarah's scores on these measures demonstrated a consistent decline in various anxiety-related problems as a result of therapy, which aligns with extant data showing reductions in a range of symptoms following CBT for different anxiety disorders (Barlow, Allen, & Choate, 2004).

With respect to diagnostics, Sarah reported that her SPOV symptoms no longer significantly interfered with daily functioning at the end of treatment and at follow-up assessments. She had gained weight, was much more socially active, and had had two romantic relationships with peers of the opposite sex. Furthermore, Sarah placed significantly less reliance on others for emotion regulation, relieving the strain on her relationships with family members and close friends.

Thus, evidence from self-report and interview data indicated that Sarah had an excellent response to CBT. Although the CBT targeted her SPOV, Sarah received benefit across a range of anxiety-related symptoms. The gains she achieved in symptom reduction were paralleled by dramatic positive changes in physical and psychosocial health.

Attention Bias

Along with receiving a course of CBT for SPOV, Sarah also completed an eight-session attention bias modification (ABM) protocol (Amir et al., 2009). This computer task procedure 'trains' the patient to pay more attention to neutral stimuli than negative stimuli by presenting target stimuli in the location of the neutral stimuli (versus the location of negative stimuli) 100% of the time. Thus, whether explicitly or implicitly, individuals' attention is drawn to the neutral stimuli because they predict the location of the target they are to detect. In doing so, the notion is that the negative attention bias characterizing anxious individuals is modified towards a more neutral/benign bias and resultant reductions in anxiety occur because negative attention bias is thought to be a significant causal and maintenance mechanism of anxiety-related problems (Mathews & MacLeod, 2005).

As can be seen in Figure 6.2, Sarah's bias score indicates that she was faster to detect targets following neutral than negative words, suggesting the development of a more neutral/benign bias. Thus, the training procedure was successful in that Sarah's attention was drawn to neutral stimuli more so than negative stimuli. However, by 5-month follow-up, Sarah's bias score returned to 0, which was her pretreatment level. Given that Sarah showed significant reductions in anxiety symptoms and significant improvements in functioning after treatment and at follow-up assessments, her attention bias data suggest that a negative attention bias was not contributing to the maintenance of her pathology. Indeed, this is consistent with her pretreatment data indicating a lack of a bias in either direction (i.e., no attention bias). Again, given the small association between anxiety and negative attention bias, this is not a surprising effect (Bar-Haim et al.,

2007) and importantly rules out the role of one particular maintenance mechanism. These findings also dovetail with a recent report showing that adding ABM to standard CBT for anxiety does not enhance outcomes regardless of pretreatment attention bias score (Rapee et al., 2013).

Error-Related Negativity

Figure 6.3 displays steady decreases in Sarah's ERN amplitudes across treatment and follow-up. Her posttreatment ERN amplitude was –5.00, nearly half the size of her pretreatment value. Comparing this score to our local normative sample, Sarah fell at the 50th percentile at posttreatment. Her ERN continued to decrease over the course of follow-up assessments, scoring in the 5th percentile (amplitude = 3.44) at 1-month follow-up and the 9th percentile (amplitude = 2.00) at 5-month follow-up. Thus, her ERN amplitude seemed to be a good indicator of her anxiety-related problems in that both decreased across treatment and follow-up. Importantly, this decrease in ERN was not accompanied by significant performance decrements in the flanker task. In fact, her error-related behavioral performance improved across treatment and follow-up. As seen in Figure 6.5, Sarah became more accurate after errors and also slowed down less after errors across treatment and follow-up assessments. This pattern of faster and more accurate responding following mistakes is considered an adaptive response to errors (Danielmeier & Ullsperger, 2011; Moser & Schroder, 2012). That is, Sarah successfully bounced back from her mistakes (Moser, Schroder,

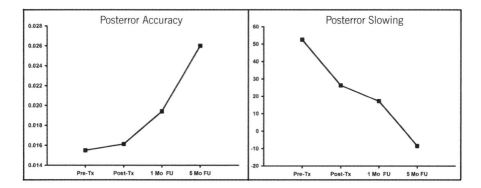

FIGURE 6.5. Posterror behavioral data across assessment and treatment phases. Left: Posterror accuracy difference scores (posterror accuracy minus postcorrect accuracy). Right: Posterror slowing (posterror reaction time minus postcorrect reaction time) in milliseconds. A positive posterror slowing value indicates reaction time was slower following an error trial relative to a correct trial; a negative posterror slowing value indicates reaction time was faster following an error trial relative to a correct trial.

Heeter, Moran, & Lee, 2011) using fewer neural resources (smaller ERN) to do so; she was more efficient and effective (Moser et al., 2012; Sylvester et al., 2012).

That Sarah's ERN decreased and posterror performance increased following therapy suggests these mechanisms were involved, or affected by, her level of symptomatology. Significant debate exists in the literature as to whether the ERN is a trait marker of anxiety or represents a malleable mechanism (Moser, Hajcak, & Simons, 2005; Olvet & Hajcak, 2008; Riesel, Endrass, Kaufman, & Kathmann, 2011). The current data support the notion that the ERN is a malleable mechanism and does not represent an endophenotype. Thus, Sarah's treatment-related ERN changes suggest that relieving her SPOV symptoms improved her cognitive functioning.

Late Positive Potential

Figure 6.4 shows that Sarah's LPP during reappraise trials increased (relative to look trials) across treatment and follow-up assessments, especially at frontal and central recording sites (see right panel head maps for scalp distributions). These findings were somewhat unexpected, as higher worry and anxiety symptoms are associated with increased neural activation, including LPP, during emotion regulation (Campbell-Sills et al., 2011; Moser et al., 2014). Our initial prediction was that as Sarah's anxiety and worry symptoms decreased over the course of treatment, her emotion regulation ability, as indexed by a smaller LPP during reappraise than during look trials, would increase. Instead, Sarah's reappraise-related LPP increased relative to her look-related LPP. Importantly, this increase in reappraise-related LPP was elicited in the presence of fewer worry and anxiety symptoms. Thus, the reappraise-related LPP appeared to reflect processes important to Sarah's pathology and, more broadly, seems to be a malleable neural marker of anxiety.

Although inconsistent with our initial prediction, the increase in reappraise-related LPP at frontal and central recording sites across treatment might reflect enhanced activation of cognitive control brain regions. This interpretation is in line with recent reports showing enhanced LPP following CBT for specific phobia (Leutgeb et al., 2009). Functional neuroimaging research also supports the conclusion that successful CBT is associated with increases in frontal control centers like the ACC and PFC in anxious and depressed patients (DeRubeis, Siegle, & Hollon, 2008; Saxena et al., 2009). Given that the LPP has distributed neural sources in cortex, it is naturally reflective of the interaction of emotional and cognitive processes. Extant literature therefore suggests that Sarah's CBT-related changes in LPP amplitude might reflect increases in cognitive control over emotion more so than decreases in emotional reactivity. This is in accord with conceptualizations of CBT as acting primarily on top-down brain mechanisms (DeRubeis et al., 2008).

Summary

The above-reviewed case study illustrates a process of integrating multimethod data to come to a richer understanding of clinical problems. Together, the data provided clarity on diagnosis, mechanisms involved in maintaining anxious pathology and successful CBT response, and the processes reflected in neural markers of cognition and emotion. This case therefore demonstrates not only the clinical utility of a multimethod approach but also how such single-subject designs can feed back on informing basic science. Moreover, our view is that the coherence of changes across multiple systems—verbal, behavioral, and physiological—provide strong evidence for a good prognosis for Sarah. It may be, then, that a coherent set of changes is most predictive of long-term maintenance of gains from therapy (cf. Rachman & Hodgson, 1974). This is an exciting avenue for future research to explore.

Practical Considerations

Although we have argued for and demonstrated the clinical utility of a multimethod approach to the assessment of anxiety using self-reports, interviews, behavioral task performances, and neurophysiology (EEG/ERP), we acknowledge the costs associated with employing such a battery of tests. In particular, the costs associated with collecting neurophysiological data include the financial costs of purchasing and maintaining the equipment and the time and financial costs for training in the appropriate use of the equipment. These costs may seem like significant barriers to administering neurophysiological assessments. However, financial costs for neurophysiological data collection systems have decreased in recent years, and these systems are readily available from several companies such as BIOPAC and Emotiv. Moreover, recent efforts have been dedicated to creating small, low-cost systems that are suitable for recording neurophysiology in various types of real-world settings, including while walking outdoors (Debener, Minow, Emkes, Gandras, & De Vos, 2012). The technology is therefore becoming more affordable and flexible for application in clinical settings.

Collecting EEG/ERP data is fairly noninvasive and generally tolerated by patients, as evidenced by the exponential increase in psychopathology studies examining EEG/ERPs over the past several decades. These attributes also make EEG/ERP data collection more feasible for clinicians. EEG is already commonly collected in hospitals for testing seizure-related conditions and may serve as a natural bridge to using such methods with mental health patients. Last, psychologists already invest significant resources in other assessment batteries such as intelligence and achievement tests. We hope that future clinicians will also have neurophysiological methods more readily at their disposal to help advance assessment and treatment of psychological problems.

Clinicians working in academic medical centers and in or around research universities will have the greatest likelihood of taking advantage of the sort of technology reviewed herein. One potentially useful approach we demonstrated here is how clinicians could compare patient-collected data to existing "local norms" generated by researchers using larger samples. Clinicians and researchers should aim to create stronger ties to one another in order to realize the translational potential of this approach. Such an approach could be used with neurophysiological data as well as with behavioral data such as that generated by negative attention bias tasks.

Finally, the methods reviewed herein and employed with the case example are also fairly easily and commonly applied across the life span. There are several anxiety questionnaires and interviews designed for use in children (e.g., the Multidimensional Anxiety Scale for Children; March 1997). In addition, attention bias tasks have been developed for use with children and have demonstrated the expected negative attention bias in anxious youth (Bar-Haim et al., 2007). As for ERPs, they can be and have been recorded in humans as young as 4 months old (e.g., Reynolds, Courage, & Richards, 2010) and as old as 80 years old (e.g., Polich, Howard, & Starr, 1985). Thus, such a multimethod approach could help illuminate anxiety-related processes in a wide range of age groups. That being said, certainly some development changes will affect the nature of the relationships between measures that should be carefully considered in clinical and research contexts (e.g., Meyer, Weinberg, Klein, & Hajcak, 2012).

Conclusion

The multimethod assessment of anxiety has a long history, dating back to Lang's (1968) original three-system approach to anxiety. Unfortunately, multimethod assessment of anxiety fell out of favor for many years and only more recently has it come back into vogue. Recent trends in cognitive science and neuroscience seem to be largely responsible for renewed interest in this area. In this chapter, we merged Lang's (1968) original multisystem conception of anxiety with recent trends in cognitive science and neuroscience to illustrate the potential of multimethod assessment of anxiety using questionnaires, clinical interview, dot-probe performance, and ERPs. Our case demonstration provided further practical evidence for merging data gathered from these methods. Future translational research will help to realize the promise of such integration of data across multiple levels of analysis. Although representing only one approach to the multimethod assessment of anxiety, we hope the current chapter can serve as a model for more fully appreciating our most common mental health problem.

REFERENCES

American Psychiatric Association. (2013). *Diagnostic and statistical manual of mental disorders* (5th ed.). Arlington, VA: Author.

Amir, N., Beard, C., Burns, M., & Bomyea, J. (2009). Attention modification program in individuals with generalized anxiety disorder. *Journal of Abnormal Psychology, 118*, 28–33.

Andrews, G. (1990). Classification of neurotic disorders. *Journal of the Royal Society of Medicine, 83*, 606–607.

Andrews, G. (1996). Comorbidity in neurotic disorders: The similarities are more important than the differences. In R. M. Rapee (Ed.), *Current controversies in the anxiety disorders.* New York: Guilford Press.

Arena, J. G., Blanchard, E. B., Andrasik, F., Cotch, P. A., & Myers, P. E. (1983). Reliability of psychophysiological assessment. *Behaviour Research and Therapy, 21*, 447–460.

Bar-Haim, Y., Lamy, D., Pergamin, L., Bakermans-Kranenburg, M. J., & van IJzendoorn, M. H. (2007). Threat-related attentional bias in anxious and nonanxious individuals: A meta-analytic study. *Psychological Bulletin, 133*, 1–24.

Barlow, D. H. (2002). *Anxiety and its disorders: The nature and treatment of anxiety and panic* (2nd ed.). New York: Guilford Press.

Barlow, D. H., Allen, L. B., & Choate, M. L. (2004). Toward a unified treatment for emotional disorders. *Behavior Therapy, 35*, 205–230.

Bearden, C. E., & Freimer, N. B. (2006). Endophenotypes for psychiatric disorders: Ready for primetime? *Trends in Genetics, 22*, 306–313.

Beck, A. T., Epstein, N., Brown, G., & Steer, R. A. (1988). An inventory for measuring clinical anxiety: Psychometric properties. *Journal of Consulting and Clinical Psychology, 56*, 893–897.

Becker, E., Rinck, M., Turke, V., Kause, P., Goodwin, R., Neumer, S., et al. (2007). Epidemiology of specific phobia subtypes: Findings from the Dresden Mental Health Study. *European Psychiatry, 22*, 69–74.

Beesdo, K., Knappe, S., & Pine, D. S. (2009). Anxiety and anxiety disorders in children and adolescents: Developmental issues and implications for DSM-V. *Psychiatric Clinics of North America, 32*, 483–524.

Behar, E., Alcaine, O., Zuelig, A. R., & Borkovec, T. D. (2003). Screening for generalized anxiety disorder using the Penn State Worry Questionnaire: A receiver operating characteristic analysis. *Journal of Behavior Therapy and Experimental Psychiatry, 34*, 25–43.

Beilock, S. L. (2008). Math performance in stressful situations. *Current Directions in Psychological Science, 17*, 339–343.

Boschen, M. J. (2007). Reconceptualizing emetophobia: A cognitive-behavioral formulation and research agenda. *Journal of Anxiety Disorders, 21*, 407–419.

Brown, T. A. (1996). Validity of the DSM-III-R and DSM-IV classification systems for anxiety disorders. In R. M. Rapee (Ed.), *Current controversies in the anxiety disorders* (pp. 21–45). New York: Guilford Press.

Brown, T. A., & Barlow, D. H. (2009). A proposal for a dimensional classification system based on the shared features of the DSM-IV anxiety and mood disorders: Implications for assessment and treatment. *Psychological Assessment, 21*, 256–271.

Campbell-Sills, L., & Barlow, D. H. (2007). Incorporating emotion regulation into conceptualizations and treatments of anxiety and mood disorders. In J. Gross (Ed.), *Handbook of emotion regulation* (pp. 542–559). New York: Guilford Press.

Campbell-Sills, L., Simmons, A. N., Lovero, K. L., Rochlin, A. A., Paulus, M. P., & Stein, M. B. (2011). Functioning of neural systems supporting emotion regulation in anxiety-prone individuals. *NeuroImage, 54,* 689–696.

Cohen, J. (1988). *Statistical power of analysis for the behavioral sciences* (2nd ed.). Hillsdale, NJ: Erlbaum.

Corbetta, M., & Shulman, G. L. (2002). Control of goal-directed and stimulus-driven attention in the brain. *Nature Reviews Neuroscience, 3,* 201–215.

Cuthbert, B. N., Schupp, H. T., Bradley, M. M., Birbaumer, N., & Lang, P. J. (2000). Brain potentials in affective picture processing: Covariation with autonomic arousal and affective report. *Biological Psychology, 52,* 95–111.

Danielmeier, C., & Ullsperger, M. (2011). Post-error adjustments. *Frontiers in Psychology, 2,* 1–10.

Debener, S., Minow, F., Emkes, R., Gandras, K., & De Vos, M. (2012). How about taking a low-cost, small, and wireless EEG for a walk? *Psychophysiology, 49,* 1449–1453.

Dehaene, S., Posner, M. I., & Tucker, D. M. (1994). Localization of a neural system for error detection and compensation. *Psychological Science, 5,* 303–305.

DeRubeis, R. J., Siegle, G. J., & Hollon, S. D. (2008). Cognitive therapy versus medication for depression: treatment outcomes and neural mechanisms. *Nature Reviews Neuroscience. 9,* 788–796.

Eriksen, B. A., & Eriksen, C. W. (1974). Effects of noise letters upon the identification of a target letter in a nonsearch task. *Perception and Psychophysics, 16,* 143–149.

Eysenck, M. W., & Derakshan, N. (2011). New perspectives in attentional control theory. *Personality and Individual Differences, 50,* 955–960.

Eysenck, M. W., Derakshan, N., Santos, R., & Calvo, M. G. (2007). Anxiety and cognitive performance: Attentional control theory. *Emotion, 7,* 336–353.

Gehring, W. J., Goss, B., Coles, M. G. H., Meyer, D. E., & Donchin, E. (1993). A neural system for error detection and compensation. *Psychological Science, 4,* 385–390.

Gehring, W. J., Himle, J., & Nisenson, L. G. (2000). Action monitoring dysfunction in obsessive–compulsive disorder. *Psychological Science, 11,* 1–6.

Hajcak, G., Dunning, J. P., & Foti, D. (2009). Motivated and controlled attention to emotion: Time-course of the late positive potential. *Clinical Neurophysiology, 120,* 505–510.

Hajcak, G., MacNamara, A., & Olvet, D. M. (2010). Event-related potentials, emotion, and emotion regulation: An integrative review. *Developmental Neuropsychology, 35,* 129–155.

Hajcak, G., McDonald, N., & Simons, R. F. (2003). To err is autonomic: Error-related brain potentials, ANS activity, and posterror compensatory behavior. *Psychophysiology, 40,* 895–903.

Hajcak, G., & Nieuwenhuis, S. T. (2006). Reappraisal modulates the electrocortical response to negative pictures. *Cognitive, Affective, and Behavioral Neuroscience, 6,* 291–297.

Hajcak, G., & Simons, R. F. (2002). Error-related brain activity in obsessive–compulsive undergraduates. *Psychiatry Research, 110,* 63–72.

Heimberg, R. G., Horner, K. J., Juster, H. R., Safren, S. A., Brown, E. J., Schneier, F. R., et al. (1999). Psychometric properties of the Liebowitz Social Anxiety Scale. *Psychological Medicine, 29,* 199–212.

Hertel, P. T., & Mathews, A. (2011). Cognitive bias modification: Past perspectives, current findings, and future applications. *Perspectives on Psychological Science, 6,* 521–536.

Holden, A. E., & Barlow, D. H. (1986). Heart rate and heart rate variability recorded *in vivo* in agoraphobics and nonphobics. *Behavior Therapy, 17,* 26–42.

Kartsounis, L. D., Mervyn-Smith, J., & Pickersgill, M. J. (1983). Factor analysis of the responses of British University students to the Fear Survey Schedule (FSS-III). *Personality and Individual Differences, 4,* 157–163.

Keane, T. M., Kolb, L. C., Kaloupek, D. G., Orr, S. P., Blanchard, E. B., Thomas, R. G., et al. (1998). Utility of psychophysiology measurement in the diagnosis of posttraumatic stress disorder: Results from the department of Veterans Affairs cooperative study. *Journal of Consulting and Clinical Psychology, 66,* 914–923.

Kessler, R. C., Berglund, P., Demler, O., Jin, R., Merikangas, K. R., & Walters, E. E. (2005). Lifetime prevalence and age-of-onset distributions of DSM-IV disorders in the National Comorbidity Survey Replication. *Archives of General Psychiatry, 62,* 593–602.

Kessler, R. C., Chiu, W. T., Demler, O., Merikangas, K. R., & Walters, E. E. (2005). Prevalence, severity, and comorbidity of 12-month DSM-IV disorders in the National Comorbidity Survey replication. *Archives of General Psychiatry, 62,* 617–627.

Krueger, R. F. (1999). The structure of common mental disorders. *Archives of General Psychiatry, 56,* 921–926.

Lang, P. J. (1968). Fear reduction and fear behavior: Problems in treating a construct. In J. Schlien (Ed.), *Research in psychotherapy* (Vol. III, pp. 90–103). Washington, DC: American Psychiatric Press.

Lawyer, S. R., & Smitherman, T. A. (2004). Trends in anxiety assessment. *Journal of Psychopathology and Behavioral Assessment, 26,* 101–106.

Leutgeb, V., Schäfer, A., & Schienle, A. (2009). An event-related potential study on exposure therapy for patients suffering from spider phobia. *Biological Psychology, 82,* 293–300.

Leutgeb, V., Schafer, A., & Schienle, A. (2011). Late cortical positivity and cardiac responsibitiyy in female dental phobics when exposed to phobia-relevant pictures. *International Journal of Psychophysiology, 79,* 410–416.

Lipsitz, J. D., Fyer, A. J., Paterniti, A., & Klein, D. F. (2001). Emetophobia: Preliminary results of an Internet survey. *Depression and Anxiety, 14,* 149–152.

Liu, Y., Huang, H., McGinnis-Deweese, M., Keil, A., & Ding, M. (2012). Neural substrates of the late positive potential in emotional processing. *Journal of Neuroscience, 32,* 14563–14572.

Luck, S. J. (2005). *An introduction to the event-related potential technique.* Cambridge, MA: MIT Press.

MacNamara, A., & Hajcak, G. (2010). Distinct electrocortical and behavioral evidence for increased attention to threat in generalized anxiety disorder. *Depression and Anxiety, 27,* 234–243.

Manassis, K., & Kalman, E. (1990). Anorexia resulting from fear of vomiting in four adolescent girls. *Canadian Journal of Psychiatry, 35,* 548–550.

March, J. S. (1997). *Manual for the Multidimensional Anxiety Scale for Children.* Toronto, Ontario: Multihealth Systems.

Marks, I. M., & Nesse, R. M. (1994). Fear and fitness: An evolutionary analysis of anxiety disorders. *Ethology and Sociobiology, 15,* 247–261.

Mathews, A., & MacLeod, C. (2005). Cognitive vulnerability to emotional disorders. *Annual Review of Clinical Psychology, 1,* 167–195.

McLean, C. P., Asnaani, A., Litz, B. T., & Hofmann, S. G. (2011). Gender differences in anxiety disorders: Prevalence, course of illness, comorbidity, and burden of illness. *Journal of Psychiatric Research, 45,* 1027–1035.

Meyer, T. J., Miller, M. L., Metzger, R. L., & Borkovec, T. D. (1990). Development and validation of the Penn State Worry Questionnaire. *Behavioral Research and Therapy, 28,* 487–495.

Meyer, A., Weinberg, A., Klein, D. N., & Hajcak, G. (2012). The development of the error-related negativity and its relationship with anxiety: Evidence from 8- to 13-year-olds. *Developmental Cognitive Neuroscience, 2*, 152–161.

Millon, T. (1969). *Modern psychopathology.* Philadelphia: Saunders.

Moser, J. S., Hajcak, G., Bukay, E., & Simons, R. F. (2006). Intentional modulation of emotional responding to unpleasant pictures: An ERP study. *Psychophysiology, 43*, 292–296.

Moser, J. S., Hajcak, G., & Simons, R. F. (2005). The effects of fear on performance monitoring and attentional allocation. *Psychophysiology, 42*, 261–268.

Moser, J. S., Hartwig, R., Moran, T. P., Jendrusina, A. A., & Kross, E. (2014). Neural markers of positive reappraisal and their associations with trait reappraisal and worry. *Journal of Abnormal Psychology, 123*, 91–105.

Moser, J. S., Huppert, J. D., Duval, E., & Simons, R. F. (2008). Face processing biases in social anxiety: An electrophysiological study. *Biological Psychology, 78*, 93–103.

Moser, J. S., Krompinger, J. W., Dietz, J., & Simons, R. F. (2009). Electrophysiological correlates of decreasing and increasing emotional responses to unpleasant pictures. *Psychophysiology, 46*, 17–27.

Moser, J. S., Moran, T. P., & Jendrusina, A. A. (2012). Parsing dimensions of anxiety and action monitoring brain potentials in female undergraduates. *Psychophysiology, 49*, 3–10.

Moser, J. S., & Schroder, H. S. (2012). Making sense of it all?: Cognitive and behavioral mechanisms needing clarification in the meaning maintenance model. *Psychological Inquiry, 23*, 367–373.

Moser, J. S., Schroder, H. S., Heeter, C., Moran, T. P., & Lee, Y.-H. (2011). Mind your errors: Evidence for a neural mechanism linking growth mind-set to adaptive post-error adjustments. *Psychological Science, 22*, 1484–1489.

Nitschke, J. B., Heller, W., Imig, J. C., McDonald, R. P., & Miller, G. A. (2001). Distinguishing dimensions of anxiety and depression. *Cognitive Therapy and Research, 25*, 1–22.

Olofsson, J. K., Nordin, S., Sequeira, H., & Polich, J. (2008). Affective picture processing: An integrative review of ERP findings. *Biological Psychology, 77*, 247–265.

Olvet, D., & Hajcak, G. (2008). The error-related negativity (ERN) and psychopathology: Toward an endophenotype. *Clinical Psychology Review, 28*, 1343–1354.

Ost, L.-G., Jerremalm, A., & Johansson, J. (1981). Individual response patterns and the effects of different behavioral methods in the treatment of social phobia. *Behaviour Research and Therapy, 19*, 1–16.

Ost, L.-G., Johansson, J., & Jerremalm, A. (1982). Individual response patterns and the effects of different behavioral methods in the treatment of claustrophobia. *Behaviour Research and Therapy, 20*, 445–460.

Philips, H. C. (1985). Return of fear in the treatment of a fear of vomiting. *Behaviour Research Therapy, 23*, 45–52.

Polich, J., Howard, L., & Starr, A. (1985). Stimulus frequency and masking as determinants of P300 latency in event-related potentials from auditory stimuli. *Biological Psychology, 21*, 309–318.

Posner, M. I., & Petersen, S. E. (1990). The attention system of the human brain. *Annual Review of Neuroscience, 13*, 25–42.

Price, K., Veale, D., & Brewin, C. R. (2012). Intrusive imagery in people with a specific phobia of vomiting. *Journal of Behavior Therapy and Experimental Psychiatry, 43*, 672–678.

Rachman, S., & Hodgson, R. (1974). I. Synchrony and desynchrony in fear and avoidance. *Behaviour Research and Therapy, 12*, 311–318.

Rapee, R. M., MacLeod, C., Carpenter, L., Gaston, J. E., Frei, J., Peters, L., et al. (2013). Integrating cognitive modification into a standard cognitive behavioural treatment package for social phobia: A randomized controlled trial. *Behaviour Research and Therapy, 15,* 207–215.

Reynolds, G. D., Courage, M. L., & Richards, J. E. (2010). Infant attention and visual preferences: Converging evidence from behavior, event-related potentials, and cortical source location. *Developmental Psychology, 46,* 886–904.

Rice, D. P., & Miller, L. S. (1998). Health economics and cost implications of anxiety and other mental disorders in the United States. *British Journal of Psychiatry, 173,* 4–9.

Ridderinkhof, K. R., Ullsperger, M., Crone, E. A., & Nieuwenhuis, S. (2004). The role of the medial frontal cortex in cognitive control. *Science, 306,* 443–447.

Riesel, A., Endrass, T., Kaufmann, C., & Kathmann, N. (2011). Overactive error-related brain activity as a candidate endophenotype for obsessive–compulsive disorder: Evidence from unaffected first-degree relatives. *American Journal of Psychiatry, 68,* 317–324.

Ruscio, A. M., Borkovec, T. D., & Ruscio, J. (2001). A taxometric investigation of the latent structure of worry. *Journal of Abnormal Psychology, 110,* 413–422.

Ruscio, A. M., Ruscio, J., & Keane, T. M. (2002). The latent structure of posttraumatic stress disorder: A taxometric investigation of reactions to extreme stress. *Journal of Abnormal Psychology, 111,* 290–301.

Rytwinski, N. K., Fresco, D. M., Heimberg, R. G., Coles, M. E., Liebowitz, M. R., Cissell, S., et al. (2009). Screening for social anxiety disorder with the self-report version of the Liebowitz Social Anxiety Scale. *Depression and Anxiety, 26,* 34–38.

Sabatinelli, D., Lang, P. J., Keil, A., & Bradley, M. M. (2007). Emotional perception: Correlation of functional MRI and event related potentials. *Cerebral Cortex, 17,* 1066–1073.

Sanislow, C. A., Pine, D. A., Quinn, K. J., Kozak, M. J., Garvey, M. A., Heinssen, R. K., et al., (2010). Developing constructs for psychopathology research: Research domain criteria. *Journal of Abnormal Psychology, 119,* 631–639.

Saxena, S., Gorbis, E., O'Neill, J., Baker, S. K., Mandelkern, M. A., Maidment, K. M., et al. (2009). Rapid effects of brief intensive cognitive-behavioral therapy on cerebral glucose metabolism in obsessive–compulsive disorder. *Molecular Psychiatry, 14,* 197–205.

Scharmuller, W., Leutgeb, V., Schafer, A., Kochel, A., & Schienle, A. (2011). Source localization of late electrocortical positivity during symptom provocation in spider phobia: An sLORETA study. *Brain Research, 1397,* 10–18.

Schienle, A., Kochel, A., & Leutgeb, V. (2011). Frontal late positivity in dental phobia: A study on gender differences. *Biological Psychology, 88,* 263–269.

Schmidt, N. B., Forsyth, J. P., Santiago, H. T., & Trakowski, J. H. (2002). Classification of panic attack subtypes in patients and normal controls in response to biological challenge: Implications for assessment and treatment. *Journal of Anxiety Disorders, 16,* 625–638.

Shackman, A. J., Salomons, T. V., Slagter, H. A., Fox, A. S., Winter, J. J., & Davidson, R. J. (2011). The integration of negative affect, pain, and cognitive control in the cingulate cortex. *Nature Reviews Neuroscience, 12,* 154–167.

Sheehan, D. V., Lecrubier, Y., Sheehan, K. H., Amorim, P., Janavs, J., Weiller, E., et al. (1998). The Mini International Neuropsychiatric Interview (M.I.N.I.): The development and validation of a structured diagnostic psychiatric interview for DSM-IV and ICD-10. *Journal of Clinical Psychiatry, 59,* 22–33.

Steenkamp, M., McLean, C. P., Arditte, K. A., & Litz, B. T. (2010). Exposure to trauma in adults. In M. M. Anthony & D. H. Barlow (Eds.), *Handbook of assessment and treatment planning for psychological disorders* (2nd ed., pp. 301–343). New York: Guilford Press.

Sylvester, C. M., Corbetta, M., Raichle, M. E., Rodebaugh, T. L., Schlagger, B. L., Sheline, Y. I., et al. (2012). Functional network dysfunction in anxiety and anxiety disorders. *Trends in Neurosciences, 35,* 527–525.

Theeuwes, J., & Van der Burg, E. (2007). The role of spatial and nonspaital information in visual selection. *Journal of Experimental Psychology: Human Perception and Performance, 33,* 1335–1351.

Thiruchselvam, R., Blechert, J., Sheppes, G., Rydstrom, A., & Gross, J. J. (2011). The temporal dynamics of emotion regulaton: An EEG study of distraction and reappraisal. *Biological Psychology, 87,* 84–92.

Vaidyanathan, U., Nelson, L. D., & Patrick, C. J. (2012). Clarifying domains of internalizing psychopathology using neurophysiology. *Psychological Medicine, 42,* 447–459.

van Hout, W. J., & Bouman, T. K. (2012). Clinical features, prevalence and psychiatric complaints in subjects with fear of vomiting. *Clinical Psychology and Psychotherapy, 19,* 531–539.

van Veen, V., & Carter, C. S. (2002). The timing of action-monitoring processes in the anterior cingulate cortex. *Journal of Cognitive Neuroscience, 14,* 593–602.

van Zoest, W., Donk, M., & Theeuwes, J. (2004). The role of stimulus-driven and goal-driven control in saccadic visual selection. *Journal of Experimental Psychology: Human Perception and Performance, 30,* 746–759.

Veale, D. (2009). Cognitive behaviour therapy for a specific phobia of vomiting. *Cognitive Behaviour Therapist, 2,* 272–288.

Veale, D., Ellison, N., Whelan, C., & Henry, K. (2010). *The specific phobia of vomiting inventory.* Poster presented at World Congress of Behavioural and Cognitive Psychotherapies CBT, Boston, MA.

Veale, D., & Lambrou, C. (2006). The psychopathology of vomit phobia. *Behavioural and Cognitive Psychotherapy, 34,* 139–150.

Watson, D. (2005). Rethinking the mood and anxiety disorders: A quantitative hierarchical model for DSM-V. *Journal of Abnormal Psychology, 114,* 522–536.

Weinberg, A., Olvet, D. M., & Hajcak, G. (2010). Increased error-related brain activity in generalized anxiety disorder. *Biological Psychology, 85,* 472–480.

Weinberg, A., Riesel, A., & Hajcak, G. (2012). Integrating multiple perspectives on error-related brain activity: The ERN as a neural indicator of trait defensive reactivity. *Motivation and Emotion, 36,* 84–100.

Wolpe, J. (1977). Inadequate behavior analysis: The Achilles heel of outcome research in behavior thearpy. *Journal of Behavior Therapy and Experimental Psychiatry, 8,* 1–3.

CHAPTER 7

Multimethod Assessment of the Adult Externalizing Spectrum

Disorders of Antisocial Behavior and Substance Use

Daniel M. Blonigen and Amy Wytiaz

Conceptual Framework of the Externalizing Spectrum

Recognition of individual differences in the tendency to inhibit rather than to express one's impulses extends back to the earliest days of psychology as an academic discipline (James, 1890/1983). Over the years, such tendencies have become instantiated within an array of psychological constructs such as impulsivity (Gray, 1981; Whiteside & Lynam, 2001), sensation-seeking (Zuckerman & Kulhman, 2000), constraint (Tellegen, 1985), and novelty-seeking (Cloninger, Svrakic, & Przybeck, 1993)—to name a few. Within the domain of psychopathology, these constructs align with the *externalizing spectrum* and are reflected in disorders of antisocial behavior (e.g., antisocial personality disorder [ASPD]) and substance use (e.g., dependence on alcohol and other drugs). These disorders are conceptualized as discrete categories and classified separately within current nosologies (e.g., the fifth edition of the *Diagnostic and Statistical Manual of Mental Disorders* [DSM-5; American Psychiatric Association, 2013]); however, they co-occur at levels well beyond chance and are conceptualized in the empirical literature as correlated indicators of a latent spectrum marked by proneness to disinhibition (Waldman & Slutske, 2000).

Goals of This Chapter

In this chapter, we provide a systematic review of methods used to assess disorders from the externalizing spectrum. From a clinical standpoint, the importance of assessing this spectrum is clear, given robust links between externalizing tendencies and a wide range of adverse outcomes and behaviors with significant cost to society—for example, suicide (Verona & Patrick, 2000); violence (Caspi et al., 1997)—as well as its deleterious impact on the course, treatment, and management of other Axis I mental health disorders (Kopta, Howard, Lowry, & Beutler, 1994; Magyar, Edens, Epstein, Stiles, & Poythress, 2012) and medical disorders (Ward, 2004). Our intention in this review is not to simply provide a list of measures that are commonly used to assess for these disorders, but rather to highlight more generally (1) the most commonly used and valid *methods* of assessment, (2) the degree of convergence across these methods, and (3) the evidence base for integrating these methods in a clinical assessment. By reviewing the empirical literature on these topics, we hope to strengthen links between evidence-based multimethod assessment and clinical practice, and provide both researchers and clinicians with an empirically supported model for incorporating diverse assessment techniques in both laboratory and real-world settings.

To help structure this chapter, we will focus on the *adult externalizing spectrum model*, which can be conceptualized as a coherent spectrum of traits and mental disorders linked by way of a shared liability for disinhibition (Krueger et al., 2002; Krueger, Markon, Patrick, Benning, & Kramer, 2007). Our focus in the first two sections will be on psychopathological indicators of externalizing—that is, disorders of antisocial behavior (i.e., ASPD and psychopathy) and disorders of substance use. For each of these sections, a number of assessment approaches will be covered, with some variability across the disorders—for example, self-report questionnaires; structured interviews; file/chart reviews; observer/collateral reports; projective (or "performance-based") testing (Mihura, Meyer, Dumitrascu, & Bombel, 2013); and biological assays. In the final section, we will briefly review a new measure—the Externalizing Spectrum Inventory (Krueger et al., 2007)—which utilizes a multifaceted approach to assess trait *and* behavioral indicators of externalizing and may serve as an integrative model for future multimethod assessment research in this area.

Disorders of Antisocial Behavior

Clinical conditions marked by antisocial behavior are the most salient markers of severity along the externalizing spectrum (Krueger, Markon, Patrick, & Iacono, 2005). In this section, we review the assessment literature on ASPD and psychopathic personality disorder (or psychopathy)—a construct related to, but conceptually distinct from, ASPD. Our review of ASPD will not be exhaustive, given that a more detailed review of the multimethod assessment literature on personality disorders, which includes ASPD and other personality disorders linked to the externalizing spectrum (e.g., borderline personality disorder; Eaton et al., 2011), can be found elsewhere in this volume. Instead, we will focus on psychopathy, which is (1) the conceptual father to the DSM-based construct of ASPD, and (2) will be represented to a greater extent in the alternative Section III diagnosis of ASPD in DSM-5 (Latzman, Lilienfeld, Latzman, & Clark, 2013).

Antisocial Personality Disorder

Derived largely from the work of Robins (1966), the diagnostic label of ASPD captures individuals who engage in "a pervasive pattern of disregard for, and violation of, the rights of others" (American Psychiatric Association, 2013; p. 659). A key feature of this diagnosis is that it is based largely on behavioral criteria reflected in the commission of criminal acts (e.g., repeated physical fights or assaults). From an assessment standpoint, this approach can facilitate diagnostic concordance across raters; however, it has been criticized as being both overinclusive and underinclusive in its representation of classic conceptions of psychopathy (Lilienfeld, 1994). Nonetheless, ASPD remains the only formal diagnosis of antisocial behavior among adults in current nosologies, and it is therefore relevant for practitioners who must work within these diagnostic systems.

Self-Report Questionnaires and Structured Interviews

By far, the most common methods of assessing ASPD are self-report (paper-and-pencil) questionnaires and structured/semistructured clinical interviews. As with most psychological constructs, neither approach can lay claim to having the "gold standard" tool for assessing antisocial behavior, as both methods certainly have their limitations. For example, interviews are often resource-intensive and require advanced clinical training to administer, whereas self-report questionnaires tend to be briefer, require minimal clinical training (aside from interpretation of the results), and can be administered to multiple individuals at once. By contrast, there are long-standing concerns that self-report questionnaires may be inherently mismatched to the assessment of an antisocial personality, given that individuals with these traits tend to lack insight into their behavior and may deny or minimize socially deviant attributes, especially if there are legal implications to reporting this information (Edens, Hart, Johnson, Johnson, & Olver, 2000).

With regard to the degree of correspondence between self-report and interview-based measures of ASPD, only two studies, to our knowledge, have investigated this issue. Among a sample of male, mentally disordered forensic patients, Blackburn, Donnelly, Logan, and Renwick (2004) examined the convergent and discriminant validity of these approaches by performing confirmatory factor analyses of a multitrait–multimethod matrix of scores from an interview—the International Personality Disorder Examination (IPDE; World Health Organization, 1995)—and two self-report measures of personality disorders—the Personality Diagnostic Question-naire (PDQ-4; Hyler & Rieder, 1994); and the Millon Clinical Multiaxial Inventory (MCMI-II; Millon, 1987). Convergence in categorical diagnoses of ASPD was in the poor range (k = .28–.36 for the IPDE in relation to the PDQ-4 and MCMI-II, respectively). However, comparison of continuous scores across measures indicated strong evidence for convergent validity across the two methods. Per the conclusions of the authors, the results did not support the alleged superiority of interviews over questionnaires in the assessment of personality disorders, including ASPD. However, measure-ment error attributable to method variance was substantial for all instru-ments and exceeded the trait variance in almost one-half of the individual measures. Thus, sole reliance on either method for the assessment of ASPD would not be advised, particularly in clinical settings where there may be direct legal implications for making such diagnoses.

Guy, Poythress, Douglas, Skeem, and Edens (2008) focused on the degree of correspondence between self-report and interview-based assess-ments of ASPD in a sample of 1,345 offenders who were court-mandated to either residential substance abuse treatment or prison. Using two self-report indices (the ASPD and Antisocial Features [ANT] scales, respectively, from the PDQ-4 and Personality Assessment Inventory [PAI]; Morey, 2007) and the Structured Clinical Interview for Axis II Personality Disorders (First, Spitzer, Gibbon, Williams, & Benjamin, 1997), the authors found poor agreement on a categorical diagnosis of ASPD across methods (k = .31 and .32 for the PDQ-4 and PAI, respectively, in relation to SCID-based diagnoses), but stronger convergence between self-reported scale scores and interview-based symptom counts (r's = .67 and 51 for the PDQ-4 and PAI, respectively). The degree of convergence for both categorical diagnoses and continuous symptom counts was invariant across gender, race, and setting. Interpretation of these findings, however, must bear in mind that (1) the PDQ (but not the PAI) was designed to correspond to the DSM, and (2) the PAI-ANT scale was designed to capture behavioral features of DSM-defined ASPD, as well as interpersonal features of psychopathy—which is not instantiated in the DSM. Thus, these two self-report indices may not be isomorphic in their assessment of ASPD.

Summary and Conclusions

Establishing concordance between self-report and interview-based meth-ods of ASPD is a necessary prerequisite to a discussion of how to utilize both assessment approaches in research and clinical practice. The avail-able work in this area indicates strong convergence across these methods of assessment when based on continuous scores. Conversely, agreement for categorical diagnoses of ASPD is generally poor, which is consistent with past reviews of the assessment of antisocial behavior in adults (Lilienfeld, Purcell, & Jones-Alexander, 1997). Depending on the goal of an assess-ment, however, lack of diagnostic concordance may not be particularly concerning, given that there is (1) limited evidence that ASPD is a taxon (Marcus, Lilienfeld, Edens, & Poythress, 2006), and (2) overwhelming evidence that the psychometrics of dimensionalized scores are superior to categorical diagnoses (Markon, Chmielewski, & Miller, 2011).

Although the convergence between continuous scores on self-report and interview-based measures of ASPD supports the integration of these methods, there are no formal guidelines for combining the two methods in a clinical setting. Further, the unique psychometric properties and conventions of each method highlight some potential challenges to this process. For example, the base rates of categorical disorders tend to be higher with paper-and-pencil questionnaires than interviews (Guthrie & Mobley, 1994), which is relevant if the primary goal of an assessment is to establish a diagnosis of ASPD. Conversely, quantifying and tracking the severity of ASPD in relation to established norms, while feasible with both questionnaires and interviews, may be more practical to do with questionnaires than with interviews, due to time and cost constraints. Best clinical practices for the assessment of ASPD need to take these issues into account when determining how self-report indices can complement information gathered via interview, and vice versa. For example, self-report indices could be used to both "screen out" those who are unlikely to have ASPD and do not require further assessment, and "screen in" for further assessment (via a structured interview) those who may have ASPD. In addition, for individuals identified as likely having ASPD, a self-report questionnaire could be used to quantify an individual's severity of antisociality relative to established norms, which in turn could help to enhance the clinical picture and guide treatment planning and clinical decision making.

Psychopathy

Current conceptualizations of psychopathy derive largely from the writings of Cleckley (1976) among others (Karpman, 1941; McCord & McCord, 1964), and emphasize traits such as egocentricity, guiltlessness, callousness, dishonesty, failure to form close emotional bonds, and propensity to externalize blame. These early clinical descriptions are often described as "personality-based" conceptualizations and are contrasted with the "behavior-based" construct of ASPD. Both constructs are linked via shared emphases on externalizing-relevant criteria. However, historic conceptions of psychopathy have emphasized the externalizing spectrum to varying degrees.

Recently, Patrick, Fowles, and Krueger (2009) proposed a Triarchic model of psychopathy to integrate these historic conceptualizations and organized them into three distinctive components:

1. *Disinhibition* reflects a general proclivity for poor impulse control and is largely synonymous with the externalizing spectrum of psychopathology. Psychopathy measures that correspond to this

component are associated with diagnoses of ASPD, substance use problems, as well as disinhibitory traits marked by impulsivity and negative affect.

2. *Meanness* reflects a callous, exploitative style in which pleasure or personal gain is sought without regard for the feelings or rights of others. Although less closely aligned to the externalizing spectrum than "disinhibition," this component is marked by aggression, which is a core subfactor of the hierarchical externalizing spectrum model of Krueger et al. (2007).

3. *Boldness* refers to a combination of social dominance, stress immunity, and thrill- and adventure-seeking. In contrast to disinhibition and meanness, boldness is largely unrelated (or in some cases inversely related) to deviant behavior, addiction, and traits of impulsivity and negative affect. Thus, indices of psychopathy that tap this domain may be less relevant to the assessment of the externalizing spectrum (e.g., Fearless Dominance; Miller & Lynam, 2012).

In the following section, we will highlight links between common methods and measures of psychopathy and components from the Triarchic model in order to clarify which of these methods and measures are most relevant to assessment of the externalizing spectrum.

Structured Interviews

The clinical interview is arguably the most commonly used method for assessing psychopathy. The principal measure of this assessment domain is Hare's Psychopathy Checklist—Revised (PCL-R; Hare, 1991, 2003), which was designed for use within forensic settings. Administration of the PCL-R entails a semistructured interview and review of collateral files to obtain information on respondents across a range of life domains (e.g., early childhood behavior, criminal history, substance use, social functioning). This information is used to rate respondents on 20 items reflecting various traits and behaviors associated with psychopathy. Each item is rated on a three-point scale (0 = *doesn't apply*; 1 = *applies somewhat*; 2 = *definitely applies*) and items are summed to yield total scores, ranging from 0 to 40, which reflect the extent to which an individual resembles the prototypical psychopath. A cutoff of 30 and higher is used to make a "diagnosis" of psychopathy. Relative to a diagnosis of ASPD, which applies to 50–80% of incarcerated offenders (Widiger & Corbitt, 1993), PCL-R-based diagnoses of psychopathy apply to approximately 15% of the prison population (Hare, 1991, 2003) and are therefore more discriminating in their classification of offenders. This notwithstanding, taxometric research of the PCL-R indicates that scores on this measure are better captured by a dimensional model (Marcus et al., 2006), which may argue for greater use of PCL-R scale scores in clinical assessments.

Although designed to assess psychopathy as a unitary construct, factor-analytic work demonstrates that the PCL-R is underpinned by at least two factors, which are moderately correlated (~0.5) and evince convergent and discriminant validity in relation to a range of external criterion variables (Harpur, Hare, & Hakstian, 1989). Factor 1 (F1) is marked by interpersonal-affective characteristics regarded by many as central to the classic clinical descriptions of the syndrome (e.g., superficial charm, grandiosity, shallow affect); Factor 2 (F2) captures a chronic, socially deviant lifestyle (e.g., impulsivity, irresponsibility, poor behavioral controls) and is more closely aligned with the behavior-based construct of ASPD. This two-factor model remains the convention in the literature and has the largest research basis on which to evaluate assessment-related questions. However, alternative three- and four-factor models have also been proposed. Specifically, Cooke and Michie (2001) parse F1 into factors labeled "arrogant and deceitful interpersonal style" and "deficient affective experience," and reduce F2 to a five-item factor labeled "impulsive and irresponsible behavioral style," which is purged of overt indicators of antisocial behavior. In Hare's (2003) PCL-R four-facet model, Interpersonal, Affective, and Lifestyle facets are proposed, which are equivalent to the respective factors of the Cooke and Michie (2001) model, and the F2 items omitted from the Cooke and Michie (2001) model are included as a distinct "Antisocial" facet.

Regarding its links to the externalizing spectrum, PCL-R total scores are largely isomorphic with a latent externalizing factor marked by child and adult antisocial behavior, alcohol, and drug problems (Patrick, Hicks, Nichol, & Krueger, 2007), which indicates that total scores from this interview are generally a good index of the disinhibition component from the Triarchic model. However, this association is accounted for almost entirely by variance unique to F2 (Patrick, Hicks, Krueger, & Lang, 2005). Accordingly, assessment of externalizing via the clinical interview method may be captured most precisely by the PCL-R items that load onto F2 and its constituent facets (i.e., Lifestyle and Antisocial).

Although the PCL-R remains one of the most commonly used and well-validated methods for assessing psychopathy, it is not without its limitations. Most notably, the administration is very time- and resource-intensive, including both a lengthy interview and comprehensive review of respondents' official records. Moreover, recommended qualifications include advanced clinical training and prior experience working with forensic populations. Consequently, administration of the PCL-R may not be appropriate or even feasible in nonincarcerated settings. See Hart, Cox, and Hare (1995), however, for discussion of the PCL-R screening version, which was designed for nonforensic settings.

Another notable issue regarding the use of the PCL-R (and one that directly applies to this chapter) is that the administration of this measure is inherently a multimethod process, requiring a face-to-face interview, as well as a review of available records to corroborate the information gathered via interview. Indeed, scoring the PCL-R on the basis of an interview alone is explicitly discouraged (Hare, 1998) and has been shown to produce lower scores than PCL-Rs completed with a file-review, thereby increasing the risk of false negatives (Alterman, Cacciola, & Rutherford, 1993). An integrated assessment combining the interview and file-review methods could, therefore, be regarded as "best clinical practices" for the assessment of psychopathy in forensic settings. That said, exclusive use of the file-review method to score the PCL-R may be permissible in two circumstances: (1) the information obtained in the official records is extensive and detailed, and (2) the specific goal of the assessment is to predict risk for recidivism. Regarding the first issue, Wong (1988) found a high degree of convergence between PCL-R ratings based on an interview + file review and a file review alone ($r = .74$, $p < .01$), and noted that the interrater reliability and mean ratings across the two approaches were not significantly different from one another ($z = 0.91$, ns). Regarding the second issue, work by Walters, Wilson, and Glover (2011) found that scoring of just the PCL-R Antisocial facet, which largely entails a review of an individual's criminal history from official records, provides incremental prediction for risk of general and violent recidivism above and beyond the other PCL-R facets. Together, these findings may be relevant for forensic clinicians who are not able to conduct a full administration of the PCL-R and/or are interested in assessing psychopathy specifically because of its relevance for recidivism risk.

Self-Report Questionnaires

Historically, the use of self-report questionnaires to assess psychopathy has been viewed with skepticism (for a review, see Lilienfeld & Fowler, 2006). Common criticisms of this method include (1) psychopathy is marked by dishonesty; therefore, psychopaths may present with distorted response styles that would be difficult to predict (e.g., depending on the context, dissimulation may take the form of either positive or negative impression management); (2) separate from a tendency toward dissimulation, psychopaths are characterized by a poverty of affect and thus may have difficulty reporting accurately on affective states they have not experienced or experienced only weakly; (3) consistent with its conception as a personality disorder, psychopaths often lack insight into their behavioral tendencies and may therefore be highly prone to "blind spots" that could be detected more easily by observers (Grove & Tellegen, 1991).

Despite these ostensible limitations, use of the self-report method has greatly expanded over the past two decades. This resurgence may be due to a number of distinct advantages of this method—for example, ease of assessing psychopathy in nonforensic settings; economical administration; ability to assess subjective cognitive styles and affective states (e.g., feelings of superiority and alienation). Further, there have been recent efforts to correct misconceptions regarding the self-report assessment of psychopathy

(Lilienfeld & Fowler, 2006). One common misconception, for example, is that the validity of the self-report method is dependent on veridical responding. However, regardless of their veracity, self-report responses can provide helpful diagnostic data by revealing an individual's perceptions of themselves and their world around them (e.g., the extent to which they feel victimized by others; see Meehl, 1945). In addition, contrary to the assumption that psychopaths are prone to impression management, scores on self-report psychopathy measures tend to correlate negligibly, or even *negatively*, with indices of social desirability (Lilienfeld & Andrews, 1996). Furthermore, in contrast with concerns that psychopaths may lack sufficient insight into their behavioral tendencies, Miller, Jones, and Lynam (2011) reported a high degree of self-informant convergence across three different measures of psychopathy (median $r = .64$) and only modest evidence that participants rated themselves as less psychopathic than informants. Thus, psychopathic individuals may be perfectly capable of reporting accurately about themselves.

Integrating Self-Reports Questionnaires with Other Methods

A limitation of the aforementioned study by Miller et al. (2011) is that it was based on a community sample and thus may only apply to situations where there are no direct consequences to reporting accurately. Indeed, several scholars have suggested that use of self-report questionnaires in clinical settings should be supplemented with information gathered from other sources, particularly in situations where motivation for either positive or negative impression management is high (Lilienfeld & Fowler, 2006; Shadish, Cook, & Campbell, 2001). However, recommendations for how to combine self-reports with other methods is complicated by the fact that relatively little research has directly examined the incremental validity of self-reports over other methods of assessing psychopathy, and what research does exist is equivocal (e.g., Edens, Poythress, & Lilienfeld, 1999). Aside from the paucity of studies, one of the primary challenges to evaluating the integration of self-report and interview-based measures of psychopathy in the prediction of externalizing criteria (e.g., violence, substance use problems) has been an inability of most studies to account for the impact of shared method variance across predictors and criteria. One would expect that an interview-based index of psychopathy would demonstrate incremental validity over a self-report index in predicting antisocial behaviors measured via interview, whereas the same self-report index should prove better at predicting scores on a self-report criterion measures of antisocial traits.

To address this issue, Blonigen et al. (2010) used a large forensic sample to examine associations between the PPI and PCL-R with both self-report and interview-based measures of externalizing in order to evaluate the correspondence between psychopathy scores and externalizing criteria from the same versus different measurement domains. Analyses focused primarily on the pattern of associations across the two factors of both the PCL-R and PPI. The PPI two-factor model is conceptually similar to the PCL-R two-factor model (Benning, Patrick, Hicks, Blonigen, & Krueger, 2003): PPI-I ("Fearless Dominance") corresponds to the "boldness" component of the Triarchic model and is marked by traits of narcissism, dominance, and stress immunity; PPI-II ("Impulsive Antisociality") corresponds to the "disinhibition" component of the Triarchic model and is marked by traits of aggression, alienation, and impulsivity. Both the zero-order and first-order relations for the PPI and PCL-R showed a clear pattern of method convergence. That is, PPI total scores and PPI-II evinced significantly higher correlations with a self-report composite of externalizing than with an interview-based composite, whereas the inverse pattern was observed for the PCL-R total scores and F2. However, the magnitude of associations for the PPI and PCL-R in relation to the externalizing composites was nearly identical when scores for each were derived from the same assessment domain, and when variance shared across the PCL-R factors was removed. PPI-II was correlated 0.69 with the self-report externalizing composite, and PCL-R F2 had a partial correlation of 0.65 with the interview-based composite, after controlling for variance shared with F1.

While acknowledging the dangers of generating too-broad conclusions based on a single study, the findings of Blonigen et al. (2010) suggest that the self-report PPI and interview-based PCL-R may be indexing nearly equivalent constructs within different assessment domains. These findings highlight the importance of accounting for method variance when comparing the validity of different assessment methods in predicting external criteria. In terms of clinical implications, it appears that either method should prove valid for the prediction of externalizing-related criteria and could be integrated in a clinical assessment using the same guidelines and recommendations for integrating self-reports and interviews in the assessment of ASPD.

Observer/Informant Reports

It has long been suggested that observers and informants can be useful for detecting "blind spots," which are ego-syntonic for a given respondent and therefore are not accessible via self-report (Grove & Tellegen, 1991). Besides the PCL-R, which utilizes raters' observations of the respondents during the interview to score select items from this inventory (e.g., glib, superficial charm), only a handful of psychopathy measures have directly tapped this assessment approach. Among these measures is the Interpersonal Measure of Psychopathy (IM-P; Kosson, Steuerwald, Forth, & Kirkhart, 1997), a standardized inventory consisting of 21 items to detect interpersonal behaviors associated with psychopathy. Kosson et al. (1997) emphasized that the IM-P was designed as "an adjunct or additional measure of psychopathy, not as a substitute for the PCL-R" (p. 90). Therefore, like the PCL-R, the IM-P is itself a multimethod assessment instrument, combining the clinical interview and observer rating methods.

Initial validation work on the IM-P in samples of federal prisoners and undergraduates reported stronger associations for this measure with PCL-R F1 than F2 (Kosson et al., 1997). In addition, there was evidence for the incremental validity of IM-P scores over PCL-R scores in the prediction of adult fighting in the prison sample and ratings of participant dominance in the undergraduate sample. Zolondek, Lilienfeld, Patrick, and Fowler (2006) also examined the construct and incremental validity of the IM-P in a sample of male prisoners and, similar to Kosson et al. (1997), found that IM-P scores related preferentially to PCL-R F1. Notably, IM-P scores exhibited incremental validity over and above PCL-R total scores in the prediction (inversely) of self-reported fear and anxiety, but not in relation to criterion measures of externalizing (e.g., child and adult antisocial behaviors).

Collectively, these studies support the validity of the IM-P as an observer-rated index of psychopathy. However, the pattern of findings for this inventory suggests greater correspondence with markers of the "boldness" component of the Triarchic model, rather than the "disinhibition" component that is more closely aligned with the externalizing spectrum. Furthermore, given that the administration of the IM-P is bound to the PCL-R, it does not permit an assessment of psychopathy via lay observers. Work by Fowler, Lilienfeld, and Patrick (2009), however, has shown that the interpersonal features of psychopathy can be assessed reliably and validly by lay observers and can be done so based on only brief samples of behavior (e.g., 20 seconds).

One standardized measure that has shown promise as an observational index of psychopathic features with lay observers is the Psychopathy Q-Sort (PQS; Reise & Oliver, 1994). The PQS was developed by asking seven judges with expertise in psychopathy to sort items from the California Q-sort into a forced-choice quasi-normal distribution based on their conceptions of this syndrome. The aggregate of these Q-sorts was used to construct the psychopathy Q-sort prototype (internal consistency = .90). A key advantage of the PQS is that it affords completion by both observers and target respondents and is therefore conducive to direct examination of convergence, as well as incremental validity, between self and observer report methods, unconfounded by measure. To our knowledge, only one study has explicitly examined self and informant (peer) reports of the PQS in relation to criterion measures (Fowler & Lilienfeld, 2007). Self- and peer-PQS ratings were moderately correlated in this study (.32); however, peer reports evinced minimal incremental validity over self-reports in prediction of the criterion measures. Some limitations of this study include an undergraduate sample, which might not be particularly high on externalizing tendencies, a small sample size ($N = 65$), and selection of criterion measures based largely on self-report questionnaires.

Only one other study, to our knowledge, has compared self-and informant reports of psychopathy in the prediction of externalizing criteria (e.g., substance use, antisocial behavior, gambling, and intimate partner violence; Jones & Miller, 2012). In contrast to the study by Fowler and Lilienfeld (2007), which examined the incremental prediction of these reports in relation to self-report criterion measures only, this study used both self- and informant-reported outcomes of externalizing behavior to address issues of method variance. Across three well-validated measures of psychopathy, self- and informant reports were consistently related to all externalizing criteria. However, the evidence for incremental validity of informant reports over self-reports was observed only in the prediction of intimate partner violence. In conjunction with the work of Fowler and Lilienfeld (2007), the findings of Jones and Miller (2012) suggest that informant ratings are a valid approach to assessing psychopathy, but their contributions over the self-report method may be limited in the prediction of externalizing per se. However, given that both studies were based on nonforensic samples, it is conceivable that informant reports may provide greater incremental validity in settings where the motivation for impression management and dissimulation is higher.

Performance-Based Testing

Due to concerns (or rather misconceptions, we would argue) of self-report methods, it has been suggested that projective tests (now commonly referred to as "performance-based" tests; Mihura et al., 2013) may help to tap implicit or unconscious processes (e.g., underlying aggression) that are otherwise not accessible to respondents using "objective" questionnaires. Indeed, such performance-based tests are commonly used by forensic clinicians; for example, 32% of forensic clinicians have reported routine use of the Rorschach inkblot test (1921) when conducting criminal responsibility assessments (Borum & Grisso, 1995). To examine the merit of this method for assessing psychopathy, Wood and colleagues (2010) conducted a meta-analysis of associations between scores on 37 variables derived from the Rorschach and scores on versions of Hare's PCL. In total, 173 validity coefficients based on Exner's (2003) Comprehensive System for the Rorschach and derived from 22 studies (a total of 780 forensic patients) were included. Mean validity coefficients ranged from –.11 to .24, with mean and median validity coefficients of .06 and .07, respectively. Out of the 37 different variables, a medium-sized association was found between PCL scores and number of aggressive potential responses (weighted mean validity = .23). Validity coefficients for the remaining Rorschach variables were either not significant or small in magnitude.

Consequently, there appears to be insufficient evidence for using the Rorschach in the assessment of ASPD or psychopathy, at least for the purposes of diagnosis. At the same time, such testing could contribute unique variance to the prediction of select psychopathic tendencies or externalizing criteria (e.g., potential for aggression). The Rorschach, properly administered and carefully scored using the Comprehensive System, may be useful in the clinical assessment of cases in which psychopathy is an issue. In this vein, a recent meta-analysis by Mihura et al. (2013) provided support for the validity of individual Rorschach variables and clarified that such validity is higher in relation to externally assessed characteristics (e.g., observer ratings) than introspectively assessed characteristics (e.g., self-report). Nevertheless, it should be noted that the Rorschach is relatively difficult to learn and administer; thus, any incremental benefit from this measure may be offset by its cost.

Summary and Conclusions

Based on our review of the literature, a number of general conclusions can be made with regard to use and integration of different methods of assessment for psychopathy. First, the interview method—as operationalized via the PCL-R—is the most commonly used and well-validated method for the assessment of psychopathy and is typically combined with the file-review approach in forensic settings. However, the file-review method may be sufficient as a standalone method if official records are detailed and risk assessment is the primary goal. Second, self-report questionnaires may have more promise than previously suggested and can serve as a viable approach to the assessment of psychopathy in nonforensic settings. Conversely, in clinical contexts where the motivation for dissimulation or impression management is high, the self-report method should be supplemented with other methods and may be better suited to "screening in" or "screening out" individuals for further assessment. Third, observer reports are a valid and reliable approach to the assessment of psychopathy and are typically integrated with a structured interview (e.g., PCL-R) in forensic settings. However, with some exceptions (e.g., intimate partner violence), this approach may be better suited to the assessment of interpersonal features of psychopathy, which tend to correspond more closely to the "boldness" component rather than the disinhibition (i.e., externalizing) component. Finally, despite its popularity in the forensic arena, there is limited evidence that performance-based testing such as the Rorschach is clinically useful for discriminating psychopaths from nonpsychopaths; however it may be useful in the prediction of select externalizing tendencies, particularly externally assessed characteristics.

Disorders of Substance Use

Abuse of and dependence on alcohol and other drugs is featured prominently within the externalizing spectrum model (Krueger et al., 2002,

2007). Such disorders are commonly comorbid with disorders of antisocial behavior (Waldman & Slutske, 2000) and are of central interest to both clinicians and researchers. In particular, accurate assessment of substance use disorders (SUDs) and substance use patterns in clinical and research settings is paramount in guiding treatment and policy decisions, and in advancing work in this area more generally. From a clinical standpoint, assessment is crucial in determining the appropriate type and level of care (e.g., residential, outpatient) and treatment interventions (e.g., motivational enhancement versus relapse prevention). In addition, inaccurate measurement may compromise the validity of research findings and, in turn, conclusions drawn with regard to treatment efficacy, prevalence rates, and generalizability, which may lead to detrimental results on a number of policy fronts (e.g., allocation of treatment funds, guidelines for best clinical practice in specialty SUD care). Clearly, the stakes are high for assessing substance use and SUDs.

A number of assessment methods have been described in the SUD literature and will be reviewed here (i.e., self-reports via questionnaires and interviews; collateral reports; and biological assays). Each method is associated with unique strengths and limitations, which should be carefully reviewed prior to selection of an assessment procedure (Babor, Stephens, & Marlatt, 1987; Carroll, 1995; Maisto, McKay, & Connors, 1990). In the following section, these assessment methods, with a focus on empirical evidence for employing a multimethod approach, are described. In addition, special considerations when selecting assessment methods are reviewed, including differences between populations and settings, the function of assessment timing, limitations of certain methods, and techniques to reduce these limitations.

Self-Report Methods of Assessment

Two methods of obtaining self-report data on substance use include paper-and-pencil questionnaires and face-to-face structured interviews. By and large, reviews support the reliability and validity of self-report methods to assess outcome data related to use of alcohol (Babor, Steinberg, Anton, & Del Boca, 2000) and illicit drugs (Darke, 1998) by demonstrating high rates of concordance with, and low rates of underreporting relative to, biological indices (e.g., urinalysis). Nevertheless, questions regarding the acceptability of relying solely on self-reported information continue to be raised, as previous research suggests that the reliability and validity of this information vary depending on how, when, where, and from whom the data are collected (Babor et al., 1987; Maisto et al., 1990).

The first factor to consider is whether or not substance abusers are willing or able to reliably recall details about their use, particularly over lengthy time frames (e.g., lifetime assessments). In general, problems with accurate retrospective recall of autobiographical information is a normative process, which has been documented in the literature with an estimated 20% of important details being forgotten within one year of an event and approximately 50% being forgotten after five years (Bradburn, Rips, & Shevell, 1987). In a study examining the consistency with which narcotics addicts retrospectively recalled behaviors across a 10-year interval, interviews detailing participants' involvement with substance use and illegal behaviors were conducted (Hser, Anglin, & Chou, 1992). Indeed, self-report data were inconsistent across assessment periods, and a higher rate of substance abuse was associated with less consistency over time.

In terms of validity, several factors appear to inhibit the accuracy with which individuals provide accounts of their patterns and problems with substances. Some of these factors include withdrawal or intoxication states during the assessment (Skinner, 1984); consequences of admitting to use, such as impact on treatment services (Magura, Goldsmith, Casriel, & Goldstein, 1987); assessment of specific versus global information (Ehrman & Robbins, 1994); assessment at treatment entry versus follow up (Sherman & Bigelow, 1992); and length of time between assessment and actual use (Hser et al., 1992).

To mitigate the impact of these limitations, Del Boca and Noll (2000) recommend several techniques: (1) ensure confidentiality of responses; (2) clearly define the assessor's role (e.g., researchers may be perceived as more neutral than clinicians and thus may obtain more accurate reports); (3) construct items with user-friendly language; and (4) attach significant events to periods of assessment. In addition, informing individuals that confirmatory data (i.e., collateral reports and/or toxicological tests) will be collected may increase the accuracy of their reporting (Colon et al., 2010). Further, in settings in which supplemental data collection is not possible, merely informing individuals that these tests may be administered may increase self-report validity—a phenomenon termed the *bogus pipeline effect* (Jones & Sigall, 1971). Finally, the application of therapeutic assessment (Finn, 2008) strategies has been shown to be useful in obtaining more accurate self-reports. Finn has described the process of intersubjectivity (i.e., clients' need to be understood by others and to understand themselves) as a motivating force, and suggests that purposefully activating clients' innate needs for such empathy and understanding will lead to more valid responses.

Aside from these recommendations, another way of analyzing data collected via self-report has been proposed which obviates the need for objectively "accurate" reporting on the part of the respondent. Specifically, Meehl (1945) suggested that verbal responses to self-report items can be viewed as surrogates for behavioral sampling and therefore can reveal unique insights into the individual's perceptions of themselves and others, regardless of their accuracy. (See the earlier discussion of this issue in the section on the use of self-report questionnaires to assess psychopathy.) Clinicians rarely consider this perspective when interpreting self-report data from substance-dependent clients. However, this data could be valuable in cases where underreporting of substance use per se is likely, but knowledge of the personality and motivation of a client is clinically useful.

Self-Report Questionnaires

The most common approach to assessing for substance use and misuse is use of self-report questionnaires, an abundance of which are available to clinicians and researchers. Examples of well-validated measures include the Drug Abuse Screening Test (DAST; Skinner, 1982), which has demonstrated strong psychometrics (Yudko, Lozhkina, & Fouts, 2007) and been found to accurately classify individuals by diagnostic status (Gavin, Ross, & Skinner, 1989); and the Alcohol Use Disorders Identification Test (AUDIT; Babor, de la Fuente, Saunders, & Grant, 1992), which displays concurrent validity with other alcohol screening measures and biological indices (Reinert & Allen, 2002) and effectively discriminates between problem and nonproblem drinkers in medical settings (Bohn, Babor, & Kranzler, 1995). In general, the plethora of self-report questionnaires in the literature varies in terms of a number of factors (e.g., assessment of quantity/frequency and diagnostic symptoms; time-frame covered; contextual factors related to use). Selection of any given measure must take these factors into consideration (Babor, Longabaugh, Zweben, & Fuller, 1994). In addition, a number of measures have also been developed to target specific substances; however, a more general assessment of substance use may be recommended due to similarities in the timing and pattern of use across individual substances (Kosten, Rounsaville, Babor, & Spitzer, 1987).

Relative to other methods, self-report questionnaires may be most practical to administer, especially in environments in which resources are limited. They are inexpensive, they can be administered quickly and easily, and they require minimal training to administer. In addition, it has been suggested that self-report questionnaires may offer some defense against social desirability biases due to the fact that clients complete them without direct interactions with assessors (Petroczi & Nepusz, 2011). Although the effects of social desirability have serious implications for assessment of substance use, the degree to which social desirability affects responses may vary, depending on the population assessed. For example, Richter and Johnson (2001) suggested that heavier drug users may be less embarrassed about their substance use than occasional users.

Structured Interviews

As previously mentioned, self-report data may be collected via structured clinical interviews. One of the most widely used interviews for the assessment of SUD is the Addiction Severity Index (ASI; McLellan, Luborsky, Woody, & O'Brien, 1980), which assesses lifetime and/or past-30-day substance use. The ASI produces composite scores representing substance use and related problems as well as severity-rating indices. The ASI has established reliability and validity (McLellan et al., 1985), and convergent validity when compared with other structured interviews (Rikoon, Cacciola, Carise, Alterman, & McLellan, 2006), urinalysis (Denis et al., 2012), and self-report questionnaires (Cacciola, Alterman, Habing, & McLellan, 2011).

Despite its popularity and validity, limitations to the ASI have been noted. In a review of 37 studies of the ASI, Makela (2004) highlighted problems with practicality (e.g., high level of training required for reliable administration), as well as weak convergence with a number of well-validated self-report indices. Another limitation is that ASI drug composite scores are based on frequency of use across a variety of substances. Thus, individuals with greater dependence on a single substance may score lower than individuals using multiple substances with less intensity (Carroll, Rounsaville, Nich, & Gordon, 1994). Furthermore, use of the ASI may not be generalizable across different substance use populations. For example, Corse, Hirschinger, and Zanis (1995) suggested that the item wording may not be appropriate for capturing substance use among individuals with co-occurring SUD and serious mental illnesses. Taken together, these findings suggest that while the ASI may be reliable and valid in some settings and populations, the addition of other methods of assessment such as self-report questionnaires may provide incremental validity to this structured interview. For example, the ASI may be useful in assessing whether or not an individual has used a particular substance in the past month, and the addition of self-report questionnaires may add value by capturing the frequency of use (Ehrman, Robbins, & Cornish, 1997).

Another popular interview is the Timeline Follow-Back (TLFB; Sobell & Sobell, 1992), a calendar-based interview in which participants are asked about use of a given substance over a discrete period of time (e.g., past 90 days). A purported strength of this inventory is that calendar formatting helps participants anchor their use with specific dates, thereby facilitating accurate recall of substance use (Del Boca & Noll, 2000). The TLFB has been shown to be a valid index of alcohol consumption (yes/no) in the past 30 days in comparison to real-time monitoring. However, similar to the ASI, it may be less sensitive to the assessment of drinking patterns— for example, quantity/frequency (Carney, Tennen, Affleck, Del Boca, & Kranzler, 1998). In terms of assessing drugs other than alcohol, a recent meta-analysis found that the TLFB exhibits high agreement with biological assays of drug use (k range across substances = .74–.94), especially among samples diagnosed with SUDs (Hjorthoj, Hjorthoj, & Nordentoft, 2012).

In sum, the TLFB may be useful in determining the presence of substance use over the past 30 days and, relative to other methods, has the advantages of being relatively inexpensive and easy to administer. However, as with the ASI, a number of factors may moderate the validity of the TLFB as an index of substance use. One such factor is the timing of the assessment relative to actual substance use. Hjorthoj et al. (2012) found that agreement rates between the TLFB and biomarkers declined as the time frame between the use and assessment of substance use decreased. One interpretation of these results may be that, as biological testing neared participants' actual use in time, biological tests may have increased in sensitivity, thus detecting use that was denied. Another factor is the length of time participants must recall, such that as the time frame assessed expands, the amount of substance use reported is reduced (Vinson, Reidinger, & Wilcosky, 2003). In other words, assessment of shorter, more manageable time frames is preferable as substance users may be better able to recall recent use in comparison to distant or historic use.

Collateral Reports

In addition to self-report methods, collateral reports from a number of informants (e.g., significant others, family, peers, clinicians) may be useful for assessing a target individual's substance use. This method can clearly obviate problems of dissimulation and social desirability biases, which plague self-report methods. However, in order for these reports to sufficiently augment self-reports, an informant should be sufficiently familiar with the habits and patterns of a target individual—an issue complicated by the fact that substance users are frequently isolated and often lack adequate social connections to nominate useful informants (Carroll, 1995). In addition, while informants may provide useful information regarding whether or not participants have used a particular substance over a given period, they (1) may not be privy to more detailed information such as patterns of use or symptoms of abuse and dependence (Rounsaville, Wilber, Rosenberger, & Kleber, 1981), and (2) could be prone to dissimulation as well.

In general, level of agreement is good between self-report assessments and collateral reports. Further, this level of agreement can be augmented in research settings by (1) informing participants that collateral information may be collected; (2) using the same interviewers across assessments; and (3) using clinically trained interviewers (Fals-Stewart, O'Farrell, Freitas, McFarlin, & Rutigliano, 2000). More generally, the extent to which collateral reports converge with and provide useful information over and above patient reports varies based on a number of factors. For example, self-collateral agreement tends to be higher with regard to a target individual's drug of choice. In a sample of opiate addicts, moderate to strong agreement was found between self- and significant others' reports of participant substance use (range .55–.83; Darke, Heather, Hall, Ward, & Wodak, 1991); however, significant others proved most useful in reporting participants' use of heroin, specifically. Another issue impacting the utility of collateral reports is the frequency of contact between the informant and the target individual. In one study of psychiatric outpatients, collateral reports of patient substance use were found to have more utility (i.e., corroborate self-reports) when the frequency of contact between informants and participants was once per week or more (Carey & Simons, 2000). Notably, this trend extended to mental health treatment staff nominated by participants, who were as informative as family and peers. Nonetheless, the authors also concluded that collateral reports rarely provided incremental prediction over and above the patient's reports. Thus, collateral reports may be useful in assessing some aspects of substance abuse, especially in circumstances where target participants are unable or unwilling to report such use; however they should not be used in isolation. Further, cross-informant agreement, in general, is modest across a range of psychological variables (Meyer et al., 2001), but is not necessarily problematic as it suggests the potential for different informants to provide unique sources of information.

Biological Methods of Assessment

In comparison to self- and collateral reports, biological samples such as urine, hair, or blood provide "objective" data that are not susceptible to the limitations of self-reports (e.g., intentional omissions, retrospective recall biases, and social desirability). Therefore, biological samples are often regarded as the "gold standard" in substance use assessment. However, biological methods themselves have several limitations. For example, biological specimens are more costly, time consuming, and invasive than other assessment methods, and have limited sensitivity—proving useful only when recent substance use is assessed (Schwartz, 1988). Perhaps most importantly, biological samples cannot provide information on patterns of use or problems due to use, which is essential to establish diagnosis of a SUD. Thus, other methods of assessment are needed to fill in the gaps regarding details of use and substance-related behaviors and problems. One approach to integrating methods is to obtain biological assessments *prior to* the administration of self-report measures (Fals-Stewart et al., 2000). In one study, for example, agreement between self-reports and urinalysis results reached 58% when urinalyses were conducted after the interviews, but increased to 93% when the urinalyses were completed first (Hamid, Deren, Beardsley, & Tortu, 1999).

Studies assessing the validity of self-report methods by using biological markers as the criterion measure have suggested that vast underreporting may exist for a wide range of clinical populations. In a meta-analytic review, Magura and Kang (1996) found significant underreporting of substance use by high-risk populations when self-reports were compared with hair and urine tests (median $k = .42$). For example, among high-risk samples, hair samples were found to detect nearly five times more substance use than self-reports (Fendrich, Johnson, Sudman, Wislar, & Spiehler, 1999). Thus, when assessing individuals at high risk for substance misuse, supplemental assessment via biological methods may prove useful.

Among individuals in SUD treatment, as well as methadone maintenance (Chermack et al., 2000), concordance rates between self-reports and biological indices tend to decrease as time spent in treatment increases (e.g., Myrick, Henderson, Dansky, Pelic, & Brady, 2002; Schuler, Lechner, Carter, & Malcolm, 2009). This temporal effect of decreasing validity in self-reports over time in SUD treatment may be the result of individuals intentionally underreporting in order to avoid negative evaluation by treatment providers, early termination from treatment, or loss of contingencies dependent on remaining abstinent (e.g., housing, employment). Conversely, when individuals enter SUD treatment they may be less concerned with consequences and/or stigma associated with reporting substance use and may be more motivated to report honestly about their use in order to secure treatment services.

Other populations that have been shown to underreport substance use via self-report methods include individuals currently and previously involved with the criminal justice system (e.g., Pluddemann & Parry, 2003; Lu, Taylor, & Riley, 2001), and individuals seeking medical services, particularly those presenting to emergency departments (Vitale, van de Mheen, van de Wiel, & Garretsen, 2006) or those seeking transplants (Webzell et al., 2011). Each of these groups is likely to underreport use for obvious motivations to avoid negative consequences. Thus, when assessing substance use or SUD in these populations, multimethod approaches that include biological testing are highly recommended.

Summary and Conclusions

As with disorders of antisocial behavior, clinicians and researchers interested in the assessment of substance use and misuse should consider the strengths and limitations of various methods available to them, particularly as they apply to their target population. In general though, the consensus in the literature is that the assessment of use and misuse of substances should involve multiple methods in order to address the complex nature of SUD and to increase the validity of data collected (Connors, Allen, Cooney, & DiClemente, 1994; Donovan, 2012).

Integrating the Assessment of the Adult Externalizing Spectrum: A Hierarchical Model of Personality and Psychopathology

Thus far, our review of the assessment literature on the adult externalizing spectrum has focused exclusively on psychopathological indicators of this spectrum. However, extant conceptualizations consistently recognize (1) the continuity, as opposed to the discreteness, between specific externalizing disorders (Krueger et al., 2005), and (2) robust correlations between these disorders and disinhibitory personality traits marked by impulsivity (e.g., sensation-seeking) and negative affectivity (e.g., aggression, alienation) (Krueger, 1999; Sher & Trull, 1994). In other words, externalizing may be conceptualized as a dimensional construct in which normal-range personality traits serve alongside "diagnosable" mental disorders as indicators of this spectrum. Accordingly, a comprehensive clinical assessment of the externalizing spectrum should entail a multifaceted approach, which comprises indicators of antisocial behavior, substance use, and disinhibitory traits within a single model. Such an approach may not only provide greater breadth of coverage of this spectrum, but also serve as an integrative model to guide future multimethod assessment research in this area.

Krueger et al. (2007) recently provided just such a model in the self-report domain. Using iterative data collection from over 1,787 adult participants (male and female prisoners and undergraduates), factor analyses and item-response theory techniques were applied to a host of self-report items targeting all known externalizing constructs in the literature. Item analyses yielded a final set of 23 unidimensional facet scales, comprising a total of 415 items to form the Externalizing Spectrum Inventory (ESI). These 23 scales index a range of distinct, yet interrelated, trait and behavioral constructs in the domains of aggression, empathy, alienation, substance use, impulsivity, theft and dishonesty, irresponsibility, and rebelliousness. Moreover, these scales are organized hierarchically and include a superordinate factor with loadings on all subscales ("general disinhibitory proneness") and two subordinate factors marked by callousness–aggression and substance abuse (Venables & Patrick, 2012). A key feature of this model is that some facets provide for a more direct index of a general externalizing vulnerability (i.e., subscales of Irresponsibility and Problematic Impulsivity), whereas other subscales capture unique, residual variance independent of the superordinate factor, thereby providing dual assessment of general risk for disinhibition and specific risk for aggression and/or substance abuse. Since the work of Krueger et al. (2007), Venables and Patrick (2012) have provided evidence of the validity of an abbreviated (159-item) version of the ESI in relation to both self-report and interview-based criterion measures of externalizing.

It should be reiterated that, at present, the ESI is operationalized within the self-report domain only. Hence, much more work is needed to extend this measurement model to other modes of assessment. Nevertheless, this model holds a number of advantages, with potential implications for assessment. For example, the domains of personality and mental illness have traditionally been assessed using distinct methods of assessment (e.g., personality via self-report questionnaires, mental disorders via structured interviews). However, the ESI integrates these domains into a single measurement model. While a multimethod approach to assessment that includes both self-reports and interviews may still be recommended for this spectrum, it is clear that such methods should not be limited to a single domain or set of constructs. In addition, the ESI measurement model may also serve as a useful referent for psychophysiological assessment of the externalizing spectrum. For example, Patrick, Durbin, and Moser (2012) argue for the use of broad dispositional constructs such as the general externalizing factor to serve as the primary targets in efforts to develop neurobiological measures of vulnerability for mental illness. This approach, termed *psychoneurometrics*, may help to integrate disparate findings with respect to observed relations between brain responses and various problems and traits associated with the externalizing spectrum. Recently, Nelson, Patrick, and Bernat (2011) created a composite of three correlated event-related potentials, which served as a direct physiological index of externalizing proneness and correlated with a number of criterion variables from this spectrum. Composites such as these, which target a general liability for externalizing rather than any one specific indicator, may produce neurobiological measures that are more robust and reliable indicators of this spectrum. In the future these composites could be integrated with more traditional psychometric approaches to the assessment of externalizing.

General Conclusions

In this chapter, we have attempted to provide a broad overview of methods of assessment for indicators of the adult externalizing spectrum, including ways of integrating these methods in clinical and research settings. In addition to the aforementioned recommendations for assessment of specific externalizing disorders, we wish to emphasize that multimethod assessment of this spectrum would likely benefit from a focus on integrative models such as the ESI, which organizes this spectrum not on the basis of surface manifestations of discrete disorders (e.g., antisocial behavior, substance abuse), but on the basis of links to common dispositional constructs that may be expressed through a wide range of trait and behavioral constructs. At present, however, such an approach may be more practical for research settings than clinical settings that must operate under a number of constraints (e.g., time, resources) and tend to have very circumscribed assessment goals (e.g., predicting risk for recidivism). Nonetheless, greater attention to the correlated nature of the indicators of the externalizing spectrum and knowledge of the unique assessment challenges for these indicators can guide future efforts to integrate and consolidate the multiple methods of assessment in this area.

ACKNOWLEDGMENTS

Daniel M. Blonigen was supported by a Career Development Award–2 from the VA Office of Research and Development (Clinical Sciences Research and Development).

REFERENCES

Alterman, A. I., Cacciola, J. S., & Rutherford, M. J. (1993). Reliability of the Revised Psychopathy Checklist in substance abuse patients. *Psychological Assessment, 5,* 442–448.

American Psychiatric Association. (2013). *Diagnostic and statistical manual of mental disorders* (5th ed.). Arlington, VA: Author.

Babor, R. F., Longabaugh, R., Zweben, A., & Fuller, R. K. (1994). Issues in the definition and measurement of drinking outcomes in alcohol treatment research. *Journal of Studies on Alcohol, Suppl. 12*, 101–111.

Babor, R. F., Steinberg, K., Anton, R., & Del Boca, F. (2000). Talk is cheap: Measuring drinking outcomes in clinical trials. *Journal of Studies on Alcohol, 61*, 55–63.

Babor, T. F., de la Fuente, J., Saunders, J., & Grant, M. (1992). *AUDIT—Alcohol Use Disorders Identification Test: Guidelines for use in primary health care.* Geneva: World Health Organization.

Babor, T. F., Stephens, R. S., & Marlatt, G. (1987). Verbal report methods in clinical research on alcoholism: Response bias and its minimization. *Journal of Studies on Alcohol, 48*, 410–424.

Benning, S. D., Patrick, C. J., Hicks, B. M., Blonigen, D. M., & Krueger, R. F. (2003). Factor structure of the Psychopathic Personality Inventory: Validity and implications for clinical assessment. *Psychological Assessment, 15*, 340–350.

Blackburn, R., Donnelly, J. P., Logan, C., & Renwick, S. J. D. (2004). Convergent and discriminative validity of interview and questionnaire measures of personality disorder in mentally disordered offenders: A multitrait–multimethod analysis using confirmatory factor analysis. *Journal of Personality Disorders, 18*, 129–150.

Blonigen, D. M., Patrick, C. J., Douglas, K. S., Poythress, N. G., Skeem, J. L., Lilienfeld, S. O., et al. (2010). Multimethod assessment of psychopathy in relation to factors of internalizing and externalizing from the Personality Assessment Inventory: The impact of method variance and suppressor effects. *Psychological Assessment, 22*, 96–107.

Bohn, M. J., Babor, T. F., & Kranzler, H. R. (1995). The Alcohol Use Disorders Identification Test (AUDIT): Validation of a screening instrument for use in medical settings. *Journal of Studies on Alcohol, 56*, 423–432.

Borum, R., & Grisso, T. (1995). Psychological test use in criminal forensic evaluations. *Professional Psychology: Research and Practice, 26*, 465–473.

Bradburn, N., Rips, L., & Shevell, S. (1987). Answering autobiographical questions: The impact of memory and inference on surveys. *Science, 236*, 157–161.

Cacciola, J., Alterman, A., Habing, B., & McLellan, A. T. (2011). Recent status scores for version 6 of the Addiction Severity Index (ASI-6). *Addiction, 106*, 1588–1602.

Carey, K. B., & Simons, J. (2000). Utility of collateral information in assessing substance use among psychiatric outpatients. *Journal of Substance Abuse, 11*, 139–147.

Carney, M., Tennen, H., Affleck, G., del Boca, F. K., & Kranzler, H. R. (1998). Levels and patterns of alcohol consumption using timeline follow-back, daily diaries and real-time "electronic interviews." *Journal of Studies on Alcohol, 59*, 447–454.

Carroll, K. M. (1995). Methodological issues and problems in the assessment of substance use. *Psychological Assessment, 7*, 349–358.

Carroll, K. M., Rounsaville, B. J., Nich, C., & Gordon, L. T. (1994). One-year follow-up of psychotherapy and pharmacotherapy for cocaine dependence: Delayed emergence of psychotherapy effects. *Archives of General Psychiatry, 51*, 989–997.

Caspi, A., Begg, D., Dickson, N., Harrington, H., Langley, J., Moffitt, T. E., et al. (1997). Personality differences predict health-risk behaviors in young adulthood: Evidence from a longitudinal study. *Journal of Personality and Social Psychology, 73*, 1052–1063.

Chermack, S. T., Roll, J., Reilly, M., Davis, L., Kilaru, U., & Grabowski, J. (2000). Comparison of patient self-reports and urinalysis results obtained under naturalistic methadone treatment condition. *Drug and Alcohol Dependence, 59*, 43–49.

Cleckley, H. (1976). *The mask of sanity* (4th ed.). St. Louis, MO: Mosby.

Cloninger, C. R., Svrakic, D. M., & Przybeck, T. R. (1993). A psychobiological model of temperament and character. *Archives of General Psychiatry, 50,* 975–990.

Colon, H. M., Perez, C. M., Melendez, M. M., Marrero, E. E., Ortiz, A. P., & Suarez, E. E. (2010). The validity of drug use responses in a household survey in Puerto Rico: Comparison of survey responses with urinalysis. *Addictive Behaviors, 35,* 667–672.

Connors, G. J., Allen, J. P., Cooney, N. L., & DiClemente, C. C. (1994). Assessment issues and strategies in alcoholism treatment matching research. *Journal of Studies on Alcohol, Suppl. 12,* 92–100.

Cooke, D. J., & Michie, C. (2001). Refining the construct of psychopathy: Towards a hierarchical model. *Psychological Assessment, 13,* 171–188.

Corse, S. J., Hirschinger, N. B., & Zanis, D. (1995). The use of the Addiction Severity Index with people with severe mental illness. *Psychiatric Rehabilitation Journal, 19,* 9–18.

Darke, S. (1998). Self-report among injecting drug users: A review. *Drug and Alcohol Dependence, 51,* 253–263.

Darke, S., Heather, N., Hall, W., Ward, J., & Wodak, A. (1991). Estimating drug consumption in opioid users: Reliability and validity of a "recent use" episodes method. *British Journal of Addiction, 86,* 1311–1316.

Del Boca, F. A., & Noll, J. A. (2000). Truth or consequences: The validity of self-report data in health services research on addictions. *Addiction, 95,* S347–S360.

Denis, C., Fatseas, M., Beltran, V., Bonnet, C., Picard, S., Combourieu, I., et al. (2012). Validity of the self-reported drug use section of the Addiction Severity Index and associated factors used under naturalistic conditions. *Substance Use and Misuse, 47,* 356–363.

Donovan, D. A. (2012). Primary outcome indices in illicit drug dependence treatment research: Systematic approach to selection and measurement of drug use endpoints in clinical trials. *Addiction, 107,* 694–708.

Eaton, N. R., Krueger, R. F., Keyes, K. M., Skodol, A. E., Markon, K. E., Grant, B. F., et al. (2011). Borderline personality disorder co-morbidity: Relationship to the internalizing-externalizing structure of common mental disorders. *Psychological Medicine, 41,* 1041–1050.

Edens, J. F., Hart, S. D., Johnson, D. W., Johnson, J. K., & Olver, M. E. (2000). Use of the Personality Assessment Inventory to assess psychopathy in forensic populations. *Psychological Assessment, 12,* 132–139.

Edens, J. F., Poythress, N. G., & Lilienfeld, S. O. (1999). Identifying inmates at risk for disciplinary infractions: A comparison of two measures of psychopathy. *Behavioral Sciences and the Law, 17,* 435–443.

Ehrman, R. N., & Robbins, S. J. (1994). Reliability and validity of 6-month timeline reports of cocaine and heroin use in a methadone population. *Journal of Consulting and Clinical Psychology, 62,* 843–850.

Ehrman, R. N., Robbins, S. J., & Cornish, J. W. (1997). Comparing self-reported cocaine use with repeated urine tests in outpatient cocaine abusers. *Experimental and Clinical Psychopharmacology, 5,* 150–156.

Exner, J. E. (2003). *The Rorschach: A comprehensive system* (4th ed.). New York: Wiley.

Fals-Stewart, W., O'Farrell, T. J., Freitas, T. T., McFarlin, S. K., & Rutigliano, P. (2000). The Timeline Followback reports of psychoactive substance use by drug-abusing patients: Psychometric properties. *Journal of Consulting and Clinical Psychology, 68,* 134–144.

Fendrich, M., Johnson, T., Sudman, S., Wislar, J., & Spiehler, V. (1999). Validity of drug use reporting in a high-risk community sample: A comparison of cocaine and heroin survey reports with hair tests. *American Journal of Epidemiology, 149*, 955–962.

Finn, S. E. (2008, March). *Empathy, intersubjectivity, and the longing to be known: Why personality assessment works.* Paper presented at the annual meeting of the Society for Personality Assessment, New Orleans, LA.

First, M. B., Spitzer, R. L., Gibbon, M., Williams, J. B. W., & Benjamin, L. S. (1997). *Structured Clinical Interview for DSM-IV Axis II Personality Disorders (SCID-II).* Washington, DC: American Psychiatric Press.

Fowler, K. A., & Lilienfeld, S. O. (2007). The Psychopathy Q-sort: Construct validity evidence in a nonclinical sample. *Assessment, 14*, 75–79.

Fowler, K. A., Lilienfeld, S. O., & Patrick, C. J. (2009). Detecting psychopathy from thin slices of behavior. *Psychological Assessment, 21*, 68–78.

Gacono, C. B., & Meloy, J. R. (2009). Assessing antisocial and psychopathic personalities. In J. N. Butcher (Ed.), *Oxford handbook of personality assessment* (pp. 567–581). New York: Oxford University Press.

Gavin, D. R., Ross, H., & Skinner, H. (1989). Diagnostic validity of the drug abuse screening test in the assessment of DSM-III drug disorders. *British Journal of Addiction, 84*(3), 301–307.

Gray, J. A. (1981). A critique of Eysenck's theory of personality. In H. J. Eysenck (Ed.), *A model of personality* (pp. 246–276). New York: Springer.

Grove, W. M., & Tellegen, A. (1991). Problems in the classification of personality disorders. *Journal of Personality Disorders, 5*, 31–42.

Guthrie, P. C., & Mobley, B. D. (1994). A comparison of the differential diagnostic efficiency of three personality disorder inventories. *Journal of Clinical Psychology, 50*, 656–665.

Guy, L. S., Poythress, N. G., Douglas, K. S., Skeem, J. L., & Edens, J. F. (2008). Correspondence between self-report and interview-based assessments of antisocial personality disorder. *Psychological Assessment, 20*, 47–54.

Hamid, R., Deren, S., Beardsley, M., & Tortu, S. (1999). Agreement between urinalysis and self-reported drug use. *Substance Use and Misuse, 34*, 1585–1592.

Hare, R. D. (1991). *The Hare Psychopathy Checklist–Revised.* Toronto, Ontario, Canada: Multi-Health Systems.

Hare, R. D. (1998). The Hare PCL-R: Some issues concerning its use and misuse. *Legal and Criminological Psychology, 3*, 101–122.

Hare, R. D. (2003). *The Hare Psychopathy Checklist—Revised* (2nd ed.). Toronto, Ontario, Canada: Multi-Health Systems.

Harpur, T. J., Hare, R. D., & Hakstian, A. R. (1989). Two-factor conceptualization of psychopathy: Construct validity and assessment implications. *Psychological Assessment, 1*, 6–17.

Hart, S. D., Cox, D. N., & Hare, R. D. (1995). *Manual for the Psychopathy Checklist: Screening version (PCL:SV).* Toronto, Ontario, Canada: Multi-Health Systems.

Hjorthoj, C., Hjorthoj, A., & Nordentoft, M. (2012). Validity of Timeline Follow-Back for self-reported use of cannabis and other illicit substances: Systematic review and meta-analysis. *Addictive Behaviors, 37*, 225–233.

Hser, Y., Anglin, M., & Chou, C. (1992). Reliability of retrospective self-report by narcotics addicts. *Psychological Assessment, 4*, 207–231.

Hyler, S. E., & Rieder, R. O. (1994). *Personality Diagnostic Questionnaire–4+.* New York: Author.

James, W. (1983). *The principles of psychology.* Cambridge, MA: Harvard University Press. (Original work published 1890)

Jones, E. E., & Sigall, H. (1971). The bogus pipeline: A new paradigm for measuring affect and attitude. *Psychological Bulletin, 76,* 349–364.

Jones, S., & Miller, J. D. (2012). Psychopathic traits and externalizing behaviors: A comparison of self- and informant reports in the statistical prediction of externalizing behaviors. *Psychological Assessment, 24,* 255–260.

Karpman, B. (1941). On the need for separating psychopathy into two distinct clinical types: Symptomatic and idiopathic. *Journal of Criminology and Psychopathology, 3,* 112–137.

Kopta, S., Howard, K., Lowry, J., & Beutler, L. (1994). Patterns of symptomatic recovery in psychotherapy. *Journal of Consulting and Clinical Psychology, 62,* 1009–1016.

Kosson, D. S., Steuerwald, B. L., Forth, A. E., & Kirkhart, K. J. (1997). A new method for assessing the interpersonal behavior of psychopathic individuals: Preliminary validation studies. *Psychological Assessment, 9,* 89–101.

Kosten, T. R., Rounsaville, B. J., Babor, T. F., & Spitzer, R. L. (1987). Substance-use disorders in DSM-III-R: Evidence for the dependence syndrome across different psychoactive substances. *British Journal of Psychiatry, 151,* 834–843.

Krueger, R. F. (1999). The structure of common mental disorders. *Archives of General Psychiatry, 56,* 921–926.

Krueger, R. F., Hicks, B. M., Patrick, C. J., Carlson, S. R., Iacono, W. G., & McGue, M. (2002). Etiologic connections among substance dependence, antisocial behavior, and personality: Modeling the externalizing spectrum. *Journal of Abnormal Psychology, 111,* 411–424.

Krueger, R. F., Markon, K. E., Patrick, C. J., Benning, S. D., & Kramer, M. D. (2007). Linking antisocial behavior, substance use, and personality: An integrative quantitative model of the adult externalizing spectrum. *Journal of Abnormal Psychology, 116,* 645–666.

Krueger, R. F., Markon, K. E., Patrick, C. J., & Iacono, W. G. (2005). Externalizing psychopathology in adulthood: A dimensional-spectrum conceptualization and its implications for DSM-V. *Journal of Abnormal Psychology, 114,* 537–550.

Latzman, R. D., Lilienfeld, S. O., Latzman, N. E., & Clark, L. A. (2013). Exploring callous and unemotional traits in youth via trait personality: An eye toward DSM-5. *Personality Disorders: Theory, Research, and Treatment, 4,* 191–202.

Lilienfeld, S. O. (1994). Conceptual problems in the assessment of psychopathy. *Clinical Psychology Review, 14,* 17–38.

Lilienfeld, S. O., & Andrews, B. P. (1996). Development and preliminary validation of a self-report measure of psychopathic personality traits in non-criminal populations. *Journal of Personality Assessment, 66,* 488–524.

Lilienfeld, S. O., & Fowler, K. A. (2006). The self-report assessment of psychopathy: Problems, pitfalls, and promises. In C. J. Patrick (Ed.), *Handbook of psychopathy* (pp. 107–132). New York: Guilford Press.

Lilienfeld, S. O., Purcell, C., & Jones-Alexander, J. (1997). Assessment of antisocial behavior in adults. In D. M. Stoff, J. Breiling, & J. Maser (Eds.), *Handbook of antisocial behavior* (pp. 60–74). Hoboken, NJ: Wiley.

Lu, N. T., Taylor, B. G., & Riley, K. J. (2001). The validity of adult arrestee self-reports of crack cocaine use. *American Journal of Drug and Alcohol Abuse, 27,* 399–420.

Magura, S., Goldsmith, D. S., Casriel, C., & Goldstein, P. J. (1987). The validity of methadone clients' self-reported drug use. *International Journal of the Addictions, 22,* 727–749.

Magura, S., & Kang, S. (1996). Validity of self-reported drug use in high risk populations: A meta-analytic review. *Substance Use and Misuse, 31,* 1131–1153.

Magyar, M. S., Edens, J. F., Epstein, M., Stiles, P. G., & Poythress, N. G. (2012).

Examining attitudes about and influences on research participation among forensic psychiatric inpatients. *Behavioral Sciences and the Law, 30*, 69–86.

Maisto, S. A., McKay, J. R., & Connors, G. J. (1990). Self-report issues in substance abuse: State of the art and future directions. *Behavioral Assessment, 12*, 117–134.

Makela, K. (2004). Studies of the reliability and validity of the Addiction Severity Index. *Addiction, 99*, 398–410.

Marcus, D. K., Lilienfeld, S. O., Edens, J. F., & Poythress, N. G. (2006). Is antisocial personality disorder continuous or categorical?: A taxometric analysis. *Psychological Medicine, 36*, 1571–1581.

Markon, K. E., Chmielewski, M., & Miller, C. J. (2011). The reliability and validity of discrete and continuous measures of psychopathology: A quantitative review. *Psychological Bulletin, 137*, 856–879.

McCord, W., & McCord, J. (1964). *The psychopath: An essay on the criminal mind.* Princeton, NJ: Van Nostrand.

McLellan, A., Luborsky, L., Cacciola, J., Griffith, J., Evans, F., Barr, H., et al. (1985). New data from the Addiction Severity Index: Reliability and validity in three centers. *Journal of Nervous and Mental Diseases, 173*, 412–423.

McLellan, A., Luborsky, L., Woody, G. E., & O'Brien, C. P. (1980). An improved diagnostic evaluation instrument for substance abuse patients: The Addiction Severity Index. *Journal of Nervous and Mental Diseases, 168*, 26–33.

Meehl, P. E. (1945). The dynamics of structured personality tests. *Journal of Clinical Psychology, 1*, 296–303.

Meyer, G. J., Finn, S. E., Eyde, L. D., Kay, G. G., Moreland, K. L., Dies, R. R., et al. (2001). Psychological testing and psychological assessment. *American Psychologist, 56*, 128–165.

Mihura, J. L., Meyer, G. J., Dumitrascu, N., & Bombel, G. (2013). The validity of individual Rorschach variables: Systematic reviews and meta-analyses of the Comprehensive System. *Psychological Bulletin, 139*, 548–605.

Miller, J. D., Jones, S. E., & Lynam, D. R. (2011). Psychopathic traits from the perspective of self and informant reports: Is there evidence for a lack of insight? *Journal of Abnormal Psychology, 120*, 758–764.

Miller, J. D., & Lynam, D. R. (2012). An examination of the Psychopathic Personality Inventory's nomological network: A meta-analytic review. *Personality Disorders: Theory, Research, and Treatment, 3*, 305–326.

Millon, T. (1987). *Millon Clinical Multiaxial Inventory II Manual.* Minneapolis, MN: National Computer Systems.

Morey, L. (2007). *Manual for the Personality Assessment Inventory.* Lutz, FL: Psychological Assessment Resources.

Myrick, H. T., Henderson, S., Dansky, B., Pelic, C., & Brady, K. T. (2002). Clinical characteristics of under-reporters on urine drug screens in a cocaine treatment study. *American Journal on Addictions, 11*, 255–261.

Nelson, L. D., Patrick, C. J., & Bernat, E. M. (2011). Operationalizing proneness to externalizing psychopathology as a multivariate psychophysiological phenotype. *Psychophysiology, 48*, 64–72.

Patrick, C. J., Durbin, C. E., & Moser, J. S. (2012). Reconceptualizing antisocial deviance in neurobehavioral terms. *Development and Psychopathology, 3*, 1047–1071.

Patrick, C. J., Fowles, D. C., & Krueger, R. F. (2009). Triarchic conceptualization of psychopathy: Developmental origins of disinhibition, boldness, and meanness. *Developmental and Psychopathology, 21*, 913–938.

Patrick, C. J., Hicks, B. M., Krueger, R. F., & Lang, A. R. (2005). Relations between psychopathy facets and externalizing in a criminal offender sample. *Journal of Personality Disorders, 19*, 339–356.

Patrick, C. J., Hicks, B. M., Nichol, P. E., & Krueger, R. F. (2007). A bifactor approach to modeling the structure of the Psychopathy Checklist–Revised. *Journal of Personality Disorders, 21*, 118–141.

Petroczi, A., & Nepusz, T. (2011). Methodological considerations regarding response bias effect in substance use research: Is correlation between the measured variables sufficient? *Substance Abuse Treatment, Prevention, and Policy, 6*, 1–11.

Pluddermann, A. H., & Parry, C. (2003). A short report: Self-reported drug use vs. urinalysis in a sample of arrestees in South Africa. *Drugs: Education, Prevention and Policy, 10*, 379–383.

Reinert, D. F., & Allen, J. P. (2002). The Alcohol Use Disorders Identification Test (AUDIT): A review of recent research. *Alcoholism: Clinical and Experimental Research, 26*, 272–279.

Reise, S. P., & Oliver, C. J. (1994). Development of a California Q-set indicator of primary psychopathy. *Journal of Personality Assessment, 62*, 130–144.

Richter, L., & Johnson, P. B. (2001). Current methods of assessing substance use: A review of strengths, problems, and developments. *Journal of Drug Issues, 31*, 809–832.

Rikoon, S. H., Cacciola, J. S., Carise, D., Alterman, A. I., & McLellan, A. (2006). Predicting DSM-IV dependence diagnoses from Addiction Severity Index composite scores. *Journal of Substance Abuse Treatment, 31*, 17–24.

Robins, L. N. (1966). *Deviant children grown up*. Baltimore, MD: Williams & Wilkins.

Rounsaville, B. J., Wilber, C. H., Rosenberger, D., & Kleber, H. D. (1981). Comparison of opiate addicts' reports of psychiatric history with reports of significant other informants. *American Journal of Drug and Alcohol Abuse, 8*, 51–69.

Schuler, M. S., Lechner, W. V., Carter, R. E., & Malcolm, R. (2009). Temporal and gender trends in concordance of urine drug screens and self-reported use in cocaine treatment studies. *Journal of Addiction Medicine, 3*(4), 211–217.

Schwartz, R. (1988). Urine testing in the detection of drugs of abuse. *Archives of Internal Medicine, 148*, 2407–2412.

Shadish, W. R., Cook, T. D., & Campbell, D. T. (2001). *Experimental and quasi-experimental designs for generalized causal inferences*. Berkeley, CA: Houghton Mifflin.

Sher, K. J., & Trull, T. J. (1994). Personality and disinhibitory psychopathology: Alcoholism and antisocial personality disorder. *Journal of Abnormal Psychology, 103*, 92–102.

Sherman, M. F., & Bigelow, G. E. (1992). Validity of patients' self-reported drug use as a function of treatment status. *Drug and Alcohol Dependence, 30*, 1–11.

Skinner, H. A. (1982). The Drug Abuse Screening Test. *Addictive Behaviors, 7*, 363–371.

Skinner, H. A. (1984). Assessing alcohol use by patient in treatment. In R. G. Smart et al. (Eds.), *Research advances in alcohol and drug problems* (pp. 183–207). New York: Plenum.

Sobell, L. C., & Sobell, M. B. (1992). Timeline follow-back: A technique for assessing self-reported alcohol consumption. In R. Z. Litten & J. P. Allen (Eds.), *Measuring alcohol consumption: Psychological and biochemical methods* (pp. 41–72). Totowa, NJ: Humana Press.

Tellegen, A. (1985). Structures of mood and personality and their relevance to assessing anxiety with an emphasis on self-report. In A. H. Tuma & J. D. Maser (Eds.), *Anxiety and the anxiety disorders* (pp. 681–706). New York: Routledge.

Venables, N. C., & Patrick, C. J. (2012). Validity of the Externalizing Spectrum Inventory in a criminal offender sample: Relations with disinhibitory psychopathology, personality, and psychopathic features. *Psychological Assessment, 84,* 88–100.

Verona, E., & Patrick, C. J. (2000). Suicide risk in externalizing syndromes: Temperamental and neurobiological underpinnings. In T. E. Joiner & D. Rudd (Eds.), *Suicide science: Expanding the boundaries* (pp. 137–173). Boston: Kluwer.

Vinson, D. C., Reidinger, C., & Wilcosky, T. (2003). Factors affecting the validity of a Timeline Follow-Back interview. *Journal of Studies on Alcohol, 64,* 733–740.

Vitale, S. G., van de Mheen, H. H., van de Wiel, A. A., & Garretsen, H. L. (2006). Substance use among emergency room patients: Is self-report preferable to biochemical markers? *Addictive Behaviors, 31,* 1661–1669.

Waldman, I. D., & Slutske, W. S. (2000). Antisocial behavior and alcoholism: A behavioral genetic perspective on comorbidity. *Clinical Psychology Review, 20,* 255–287.

Walters, G. D., Wilson, N. J., & Glover, A. J. (2011). Predicting recidivism with the Psychology Checklist: Are factor score composites really necessary? *Psychological Assessment, 23,* 552–557.

Ward, R. K. (2004). Assessment and management of personality disorders. *American Family Physician, 70,* 1505–1512.

Wezbell, I., Ball, D., Bell, J., Sherwood, R., Marsh, A., O'Grady, J., et al. (2011). Substance use by liver transplant candidates: An anonymous urinalysis study. *Liver Transplantation, 17,* 1200–1204.

Whiteside, S. P., & Lynam, D. R. (2001). The Five Factor Model and impulsivity: Using a structural model of personality to understand impulsivity. *Personality and Individual Differences, 30,* 669–689.

Widiger, T. A., & Corbitt, E. M. (1993). Antisocial personality disorder: Proposals for *DSM-IV. Journal of Personality Disorders, 7,* 63–77.

Wong, S. (1988). Is Hare's Psychopathy Checklist reliable without the interview? *Psychological Reports, 62,* 931–934.

Wood, J. M., Lilienfeld, S. O., Nezworski, M. T., Garb, H. N., Allen, K. H., & Wildermuth, J. L. (2010). Validity of Rorschach inkblot scores for discriminating psychopaths from nonpsychopaths in forensic populations: A meta-analysis. *Psychological Assessment, 22,* 336–349.

World Health Organization. (1995). *International statistical classification of diseases and health related problems.* Geneva, Switzerland: Author.

Yudko, E., Lozhkina, O., & Fouts, A. (2007). A comprehensive review of the psychometric properties of the Drug Abuse Screening Test. *Journal of Substance Abuse Treatment, 32,* 189–198.

Zolondek, S., Lilienfeld, S. O., Patrick, C. J., & Fowler, K. A. (2006). The interpersonal measure of psychopathy: Construct and incremental validity in male prisoners. *Assessment, 13,* 470–482.

Zuckerman, M., & Kulhman, D. M. (2000). Personality and risk-taking: Common biosocial factors. *Journal of Personality, 68,* 999–1029.

CHAPTER 8

Clinical Assessment of Thought Quality

A Multimethod Approach

Mark A. Blais and Iruma Bello

The knowledge that thinking has conquered for humanity is vast, yet our knowledge of thinking is scant. . . . And yet the dream-stuff out of which world-changing thought is made is present in all of us, in the sentence-fragments of the brain-injured, in the delusions of the schizophrenic, and the babbling of the child. This is its enigma.
—DAVID RAPAPORT, *Organization and Pathology of Thought* (1951, p. vii)

Thinking is a fundamental human capacity and a central feature in many models of personality (Blais & Hopwood, 2010; Freud, 1900/1959; Mayer, 2005). It is a complex phenomenon composed of a fluid, ever-changing mixture of perceptual, neurocognitive and psychological abilities. To be effective thinking must alternate in a controlled and reversible manner between being logical and illogical, cohesive and disjointed, goal directed and unfettered, spontaneous and predictable, as well as fantastic and associated with consensual reality. Yet at the same time, thinking is such a basic human process that upon casual observation there appears to be minimal individual variability at least in thinking about common everyday situations. Much of our individual behavior and collective actions as a society are based on the assumption that people tend to think about the world in a highly similar fashion. In this chapter we will present a multidimensional model for conceptualizing the thought process and review clinical instruments commonly used to assess thought quality. In addition, clinical examples and guidelines will be provided to demonstrate how multimethod assessment data can be integrated to yield a comprehensive detailed evaluation of thought quality.

Given the significant role of thinking in human experience, it is not surprising that efforts to understand thought quality have been a significant part of psychiatry and clinical psychology since their inceptions. Initial attention was directed at the most obvious form of impaired thinking, psychosis. In fact, both Kraepelin (1919) and Bleuler (1950) considered disordered thinking or "loosening of associations" to be the primary sign of schizophrenia. Years of systematic observation produced a rich descriptive lexicon for categorizing the salient features of disordered thinking that were evident in the speech of patients with schizophrenia. These categories focused on poverty of speech, tangentiality, derailment, circumstantiality, perseveration, loss of goals, thought blocking, and neolgisms (Andreasen, 1979). Categorizing a patient's speech using this lexicon became the standard method for identifying a formal thought disorder (FTD). The presence of an FTD was diagnostic of a psychotic condition. As a concept, FTD refers to a marked disruption in the logical links between thoughts and ideas. Patients with an FTD are unable to maintain a coherent or connected flow of thoughts and ideas; as a result their thinking becomes confused, illogical, or bizarre. Although the concept of FTD has increasingly been questioned because of overlapping and imprecise category definitions (Rule, 2005), it continues to be widely used in clinical assessment.

Assessment of FTD

Traditionally, the presence of an FTD was identified through clinical observation and diagnostic interviewing (Andreasen, Flaum, & Arndt, 1992). However, in general, unstructured clinical interviews produce limited diagnostic agreement (Meyer, 1996) and with regard to identifying FTD the style and focus of these diagnostic interviews tended to vary greatly from clinician to clinician (Hurt, Holzman, & Davis, 1983). Recognition of these limitations resulted in the development of standardized assessment procedures, especially structured symptom rating scales, to assess FTD (Andreasen et al., 1992; Hurt et al., 1983). The Brief Psychiatric Rating Scale (BPRS) is one of the most widely used FTD rating scales (Overall & Gorham, 1962). The BPRS assesses psychotic and affective symptoms based on the patient's report as well as the clinician's observation. Studies have repeatedly demonstrated that the BPRS has excellent interrater and retest reliability (Bell, Lysaker, Beam-Goulet, Milstein & Lindenmayer, 1993; Dingemans, Linszen, Lenior, & Smeets, 1995; Overall & Rhoades, 1982) and a four-factor structure consisting of positive symptoms, negative symptoms, depression-anxiety, and agitation (Kopelowicz, Ventura, Liberman, & Mintz, 2008; Mueser, Curran, & McHugo, 1997; Thomas, Donnell, & Young, 2004). While the BPRS continues to be widely used, Kay, Fiszbein, & Opler (1987) adapted the BPRS and other rating scales to create the Positive and Negative Syndrome Scale (PANSS). The PANSS provides a more complete and balanced assessment of the positive and negative symptoms associated with schizophrenia. The PANSS has demonstrated solid psychometric qualities and is a valid measure for identifying psychotic symptoms (Gottlieb, Fan, & Goff, 2010). Nonetheless, neither the BPRS nor the PANSS provides a comprehensive evaluation of thought quality suitable for all patients.

As clinical experience and research became more systematic, it became evident that disordered thinking was expressed on a continuum of severity (Meehl, 1990). This continuum ranges from adaptively creative and unique, to normal and conventional, to mild cognitive slippage (idiosyncratic language), to frank psychosis (disorganization and hallucinations). It is also now recognized that meaningful differences in thought quality are not limited to schizophrenic spectrum conditions but exist both across and within psychiatric disorders (Andreasen & Grove 1986). Furthermore, it is now commonly recognized that thought quality is multidimensional and that no single instrument is adequate for assessing the full range of thought quality. Rather, a multimethod assessment approach is necessary for meaningfully describing and quantifying an individual's thought quality.

Multidimensional Nature of Thinking

If thought quality is not a unitary construct, then a multidimensional model for understanding the nature of thinking becomes necessary. Weiner (1966) developed a multidimensional model for conceptualizing thought quality that has considerable relevance for utilizing multimethod psychological assessment strategies primarily because he breaks the thinking process into its component parts (Table 8.1). In Weiner's model, thinking is composed of cognitive focusing, reality testing, reasoning, and concept formation (Kleiger, 1999). Cognitive focusing entails scanning, selecting, and attending to the most relevant stimuli within the environment while being able to screen out irrelevant stimuli. This component of thinking relies on basic neurocognitive abilities such as working memory, processing speed, and cognitive flexibility. Reality testing is the capacity to perceive sensory experiences in a realistic and consensual, conventional manner. To be effective, reality testing requires the interplay of basic neurophysiological abilities (sensory perception) and psychological processes (apperception). In many ways reality testing is similar to the concept of perceptual accuracy. The components of reasoning and concept formation are highly related and in this chapter are treated as a single process. Reasoning and concept formation encompass the ability to maintain a coherent logical flow of associations and to identify an appropriate level of abstraction (generalization or categorization) needed to solve a given problem or communicate one's experience. These components of thinking, reasoning and concept formation, are generally seen as being primarily psychological in nature. Weiner's multidimensional model of thinking has a number of practical advantages, including identifying the basic components of thought quality and how they may be interrelated as well as informing the choice of assessment tools needed to adequately evaluate thought quality.

Multimethod Assessment of Thought Quality

Clinical personality assessment is most effective when clinicians use a multimethod–multitrait test battery that draws on the clinical wisdom developed out of the Rapaport–Menninger assessment tradition (Rapaport, Gill, & Schafer, 1968) and the empirical measurement tradition of Campbell and Fiske (1959). The Rapaport–Menninger full-battery approach to personality assessment emphasizes the need to employ multiple assessment tools that capture conscious (explicit) and unconscious (implicit) behavior across a range of tasks. In addition, this tradition emphasizes the need for tasks to vary in the degree of external structure or guidance they provide for the subject. The multimethod approach to clinical assessment also reflects the psychometric insights of Campbell and Fiske regarding the importance of incremental validity (Campbell & Fiske, 1959). Using their multitrait and multimethod approach to construct validation, Campbell and Fiske demonstrated that while different assessment methods measuring the same psychological construct had limited correlations, they could be combined to enhance predictive power. This finding has been repeatedly replicated (Meyer, 1996) and reinforces the importance of method variance in both research and clinical assessment.

The multimethod personality assessment approach outlined in this chapter is based on the clinical experience and research findings from our assessment group, the Psychological Evaluation and Research Laboratory (PEaRL). The PEaRL is an active clinical service and research unit that provides psychological evaluations to adult psychiatric patients. Data from these evaluations (inpatient and outpatient) along with demographic information are entered into an IRB-approved deidentified database. (See Stein, Slavin-Mulford, Sinclair, Siefert, & Blais, 2012, and Slavin-Mulford et al., 2012 for a detailed overview of our clinic procedures.) At present this database contains over 700 cases. The PEaRL assessment battery consists of a core group of multimethod instruments, including the Wechsler Abbreviated Scale of Intelligence–II (WASI-II; Wechsler, 2011), Digit Symbol Coding Subtest of the Wechsler Adult Intelligence Scale–IV (WAIS-IV; Wechsler, 2008); Trail Making Test: Parts A and B (Reitan & Wolfson, 2004), Stroop Color–Word Test (Trenerry, Crosson, Deboe, & Leber, 1989), the Personality Assessment Inventory (PAI; Morey, 1991, 2007), the NEO–Five-Factor Inventory (NEO-FFI; Costa & McCrae, 1992), the Rorschach Inkblot Test (Rorschach, 1921/1942), and/or the Thematic Apperception Test (TAT; Murray, 1943). This core battery is supplemented with additional tests as indicated and is modified or shortened for inpatients. This battery provides both implicit (performance-based) and explicit (self-reported) data on a wide range of psychopathology, personality, and neurocognitive functioning constructs that are relevant for assessing thought quality. Table 8.1 presents the *PEaRL* battery measures that are primarily related to thought quality and their association to Weiner's model.

We will use the following case example to highlight our approach to the multimethod assessment of thought quality:

> Ms. Jones is a 46-year-old divorced woman. She is a college graduate and successful self-employed software engineer. She is currently between jobs and "living off of personal savings." She has had one prior manic episode, approximately 20 years ago, "triggered by an antidepressant." She has no chronic or acute medical problems. She has never been hospitalized for psychiatric reasons and has never attempted suicide. She reported suffering a possible head injury with brief loss of consciousness from a motor vehicle accident during her early 20s for which she did not receive any medical treatment. She recently consulted a psychiatrist to resume pharmacotherapy and was referred for a comprehensive psychological assessment for diagnostic

TABLE 8.1. Conceptual Organization of Weiner's Model of Thought Quality and Select Multimethod Assessment Measures

Multimethod measures	Cognitive focus	Reality contact	Reasoning and concept formation
Ability measures: processing speed	Digit Symbol Coding Trails A		
Ability measures: flexibility	Trails B Stroop		
Implicit measures		RIM XA% RIM X–% RIM *Populars*	RIM *WSum6* RIM LvL 2 SS
Explicit measures	NEO–Openness NEO–Conscientiousness		NEO–Openness NEO–Conscientiousness PAI SCZ
		PAI-SCZ-P	PAI PAR PAI SCZ-T PAI ARD-T PAI MAN-A PAI ARD-O

Note. RIM, Rorschach Inkblot Method; PAI, Personality Assessment Inventory; and NEO, NEO–Five-Factor Inventory.

clarity and treatment planning. At the time of her evaluation she was on no psychiatric medication.

Measurement of Cognitive Focusing

Neuropsychological instruments are used to assess the basic neurocognitive abilities related to thinking. These instruments are standardized and therefore allow an individual's score to be interpreted based on normative data. Results on these tests can also detect mild or relative impairment when compared to the respondent's estimated premorbid level of functioning (Howieson & Lezak, 1992). The neurocognitive instruments used in our battery are designed to measure fluid cognitive abilities such as processing speed and cognitive flexibility. Fluid cognitive abilities are required for on-the-spot problem solving and adaptive functioning (Carroll, 1993; Cattell, 1971). These abilities are broad, moderately complex, and govern or influence a great variety of behaviors (Carroll, 1993). Fluid neurocognitive abilities are dependent on neural circuitry associated with the prefrontal cortex (PFC), a brain area that has also been associated with personality and psychopathology (DeYoung & Gray, 2009). Furthermore, fluid cognitive abilities are commonly impaired in psychiatric patients (Putnam & Blais, 2010), especially those with schizophrenia (Palmer et al., 1997) and these abilities are strong predictors of functional life impairment (Harvey, Keefe, Patterson, Heaton, & Bowie, 2009). A developing body of research suggests that these neurocognitive abilities may be more related to communication failures, such as the loss of meaning and information in speech, than to specific signs of thought disorder (Docherty, 2005). This more general association would be consistent with Weiner's model of thought quality in which cognitive focus represents a basic neural foundation or network that helps shape thought quality. It is also consistent with findings from neuroimaging studies suggesting that deficits in attention and information-processing systems may in part cause disordered thinking rather than be an expression of thought disorder (Kuperberg, Deckersbach, Holt, Goff, & West, 2007).

Processing speed refers to the speed with which different cognitive operations can be executed (Dickinson, Ramsey, & Gold, 2007). Two commonly used tests of processing speed are the Digit Symbol Coding subtest of the WAIS-IV, (Wechsler, 2008) and the Trail Making Test: Part A (Reitan & Wolfson, 1985). Dickinson and colleagues (2007) performed a meta-analysis to compare the magnitude of impairment in processing speed tasks to that of other traditional neurocognitive tasks in schizophrenia. Results of the meta-analysis demonstrated that digit symbol coding obtained the greatest effect size (–1.57) from all of the neurocognitive tests and therefore is most sensitive to impairment in schizophrenia. Furthermore, decreased performance on coding tasks has been found to distinguish individuals who would later develop schizophrenia from their siblings who would not develop the illness (Niendam et al., 2003). As such, deficits in processing speed might serve as a more specific, discriminant feature of thought quality than some of the more complex high-level cognitive tasks.

Two common measures of cognitive flexibility are the Trail Making Test: Part B (Reitan & Wolfson, 1985) and the Stroop Color–Word Test (Trenerry et al., 1989). The Trail Making Test: Part B is a test of visual scanning, motor speed, and mental flexibility. The validity and reliability of the Trails B has long been established (Reitan, 1992). The Stroop Color–Word Test is a standardized version of the Stroop that assesses selective attention and inhibition, a form of cognitive flexibility. The Stroop has adequate test–retest reliability (.90) and correctly differentiates 79–92% of individuals with brain damage from normal adults (Trenerry et al., 1989).

Lastly, the use of neurocognitive ability measures in the multimethod assessment of thought quality is essential given that explicit (self-report) measures of cognitive inefficiency have very limited association with ability-based measures of processing speed or working memory. For example, the Meyer et al. (2001) meta-analysis showed a correlation of just 0.06 between subjective and neurocognitive measures of inattention. Similarly, a recent meta-analysis by Beaudoin and Desrichard (2011) found only a small (but statistically significant) correlation ($r = .15$) between self-report memory problems and scores on neurocognitive memory tests. Therefore, in order to meaningfully measure the neurocognitive underpinnings of thought quality, measures of basic neurocognitive ability must be included in a test battery. Fortunately, brief low-burden instruments can be used to efficiently assess these important neurocognitive domains (Harvey, Keefe, Patterson, Heaton, & Bowie, 2009).

Clinically, we are not attempting to identify true neuropsychological impairment or use these brief measures as a substitute for a comprehensive neuropsychological evaluation. Rather, we want to identify inefficiencies or mild relative weaknesses in processing speed and cognitive flexibility. To do this, we use the WASI Vocabulary score or level of educational achievement to estimate a patient's premorbid cognitive ability. Next, we compare their mean processing speed (average of Digit Symbol Coding and Trails A) and mean cognitive flexibility (average of Trails B and Stroop) to see if these scores fall 0.75 or more standard deviations below their estimated premorbid ability level. In our clinical database, 27% of patients with a history of psychosis have processing speed weaknesses (as defined above), and 20% show cognitive flexibility weaknesses. For patients without a history of psychosis the percentages are 17 and 14, respectively.

Ms. Jones obtained a Verbal IQ of 118, consistent with her level of education. Her aggregate score on measures of possessing speed was a Standard Score (SS) of 85 (low average range), while on measures of cognitive flexibility her aggregate SS was 90 (average range). These findings provide an initial indication of a mild or relative disruption in her fluid cognitive abilities in the presence of retained higher-order intellectual capacity.

Implicit Measurement of Thinking

Subjective experience may suggest that thinking occurs largely within the conscious portion of our mind and is available to us for direct self-report. In fact, the early investigations of thought quality, reviewed above, relied on the assumption that thought quality could be readily inferred from speech and explored with the subject through a clinical interview. However, Weiner's multidimensional model suggests that many components of thought, such as focus and perception, occur outside of awareness. In recent years cognitive psychologists have proposed that perception, thinking, and behavior result from two separate but somewhat interrelated mental systems (see Pinker, 1997; Strack & Deutsch, 2004). One system operates at the explicit level and accounts for our conscious mental life, while the other system operates at an implicit level influencing our thoughts and behaviors in ways we are only dimly aware of. Multimethod assessment of thought quality requires instruments capable of tapping both implicit and explicit facets of thinking.

The Rorschach Inkblot Method (RIM; Weiner, 1996) is an excellent tool for assessing implicit factors related to thought quality. In essence, the RIM presents patients with 10 standard but ambiguous visual stimuli (the Inkblots) and requires them to tell the examiner what the inkblot "might be" and "what made it look like that." Together, these two RIM tasks allow for measuring the implicit processes that support perceptual accuracy and concept formation, the next two components of thought quality. The ability of the RIM to detect impaired thinking is well supported by research and represents one of the few things that both critics and proponents of the test agree upon (Wood, Lilienfeld, Garb, & Nezworski, 2000). O'Connell, Cooper, Perry, and Hoke (1989) found that the quality of thinking as revealed by the RIM was a better predictor of the later appearance of psychotic symptoms than a structured psychiatric interview. In a neuroimaging study, Kircher et al. (2001) showed that RIM responses were linked to the neural-anatomical correlates of disordered thinking. Hilsenroth, Eudell-Simmons, DeFife, and Charnas (2007) found that a composite RIM score, the Perceptual-Thinking Index (PTI), successfully differentiated nonpatients, personality-disordered patients, and psychotic patients. And a recent meta-analysis found substantial validity for the RIM PTI and individual variables considered to be markers of impaired thought quality (Mihura, Meyer, Dumitrascu, & Bombel, 2013). The RIM PTI may be the best single implicit measure available for assessing an individual's vulnerability to disordered thinking. However, because the PTI is a composite index that combines variables related to perceptual accuracy and associational quality (reasoning), it is best thought of as a measure of thought disorder severity and is less suited for the type of multidimensional evaluation of thought quality discussed in this chapter. Still, clinically one should always review the RIM PTI score (which can range from 0 to 5) and become concerned about the presence of a thought disorder whenever the PTI score is ≥ 3 (Hilsenroth et al., 2007). Ms. Jones's PIT score was 3, raising further concerns about a potential thought disorder.

Measurement of Reality Testing

Adequate reality testing requires an individual to form accurate impressions or interpretations of internal and external sensory experiences. They have to be able to "see" themselves, others, and the environment in a realistic or consensual manner. In completing the first part of the RIM task, determining "what" (the inkblot) "might this be," subjects must organize vague visual images into perceptions that are more or less realistic. The Comprehensive System (CS; Exner, 2003) is the most widely used and best validated method presently available for administering, scoring, and interpreting the RIM (Kleiger, 1999). The CS evaluates thought quality along two primary dimensions: perceptual accuracy and associational quality. Perceptual accuracy is conceptually similar to reality testing as it quantifies the subject's ability to perceive the Rorschach stimuli as others do (i.e., accurately). In the CS, perceptual accuracy is primarily measured by Form Quality (FQ) variables. Each RIM response is rated for how well it fits or matches the contours of the inkblot. Responses that show reasonably good fit are given an FQ rating of Ordinary (Xo), indicating the ability to see the world as others do; responses that fit the blot but are mildly idiosyncratic receive an FQ of Unusual (Xu), while poor-fitting responses receive an FQ rating of minus (X–). Given that both Xo and Xu reflect basically acceptable FQ, these scores are combined into XA% (Form Appropriate Extended). XA% is the percentage of responses in the full protocol that show relatively "good" fit to the inkblot. In the CS system, the expected value for XA% is 0.88 (standard deviation [SD] = 0.07). Research has shown XA% to be a good implicit marker of conventional perception (reality testing) and is able to successfully differentiate nonpatients from patients with significant thought impairment (Hilsenroth et al., 2007; Mihura et al., 2013).

The RIM X–% is the percentage of distorted or poorly fitting responses in a record and may be more sensitive to milder disruptions in perceptual accuracy. The X–% is more directly related to impaired reality testing and has been shown to differentiate between nonpatients, personality disordered patients, and psychotic patients (Mihura et al., 2013). In the CS system, the expected value for X– is 0.11 (SD = 0.07). When X–% exceeds .20, impaired perceptual accuracy is increasingly likely. It is important to emphasize that FQ ratings tap implicit perceptual processes. Therefore, a score reflecting excessive minus FQ responses (high X–%) suggests a perceptual disturbance and a breakdown in reality testing. When used in combination, the XA% and X–% allow for a nuanced evaluation of reality testing or conventional perception.

The RIM *Popular* score provides another useful measure of conventional perception or reality testing. In the CS, there are 13 responses that occur with sufficient frequency to be considered *Popular* responses. *Popular* responses reveal the degree to which individuals translate their experiences into socially common or conventional ways, especially when the perceptual cues for conventional responding are clearly apparent. On average nonpatients produce approximately seven (7) *Popular* responses. When individuals produce four (4) or fewer *Popular* responses, it signals either an inability or unwillingness to engage in conventional or socially expected actions. In cases where the number of *Popular* responses is low and X–% is elevated, you have a strong indication that the patient suffers from impaired reality testing. Interestingly, some thought-disordered patients produce an average number of *Popular* responses while also having an elevated X–%. Such individuals may be able to mask their impaired thinking especially during brief or highly structured interactions, such as the typical bedside interview conducted in psychiatric hospitals.

While implicit measures like the RIM offer important insights into the psychological processes underlying thought quality, self-report measures also provide valuable information on the patient's degree of reality testing. In our clinic, the Personality Assessment Inventory (PAI; Morey, 1991) is the preferred explicit measure of psychopathology and personality functioning. However, other broadband multiscaled instruments such as the Minnesota Multiphasic Personality Inventory–2 (MMPI-2; Butcher, Dahlstrom, Graham, Tellegen, & Kaemmer, 1989) or the Millon Clinical Multiaxial Inventory–III (MCMI-III; Millon, 1994) could also serve this role. For assessing thought quality, the PAI has two scales in particular, the SCZ (Schizophrenia) and PAR (Paranoia) scales, that measure a patient's self-attributed reality testing. Research findings support the utility of these PAI scales for assessing thought quality. Slavin-Mulford et al. (2012) found that both the PAI Schizophrenia (SCZ) and Paranoia (PAR) scales were meaningfully correlated with a history of psychotic experiences (hallucinations and paranoid ideation), and Klonsky (2004) demonstrated the ability of PAI-SCZ to differentiate psychotic inpatients from nonpsychotic inpatients. One of the PAI-SCZ subscales, SCZ-P (Psychotic Experiences), appears to be highly sensitive to self-reported disruptions in reality testing. Slavin-Mulford et al. (2012) found the PAI SCZ-P correlated at 0.39 with a history of hallucinations and at 0.31 with a history of paranoid ideation. Furthermore, in our clinical experience, the PAI SCZ scale tends to be moderately elevated across diagnostic groups (mean *T*-score of 60.14 for all patients in our database), while the SCZ-P subscale is more normative (mean *T*-score of 48.20 for all patients). This may provide further support for SCZ-P being more specific to primary psychotic deficits like unusual perceptions and impaired reality testing. Clinically, we typically use the criteria of PAI SCZ full scale T-score ≥ 70 and SCZ-P T-score ≥ 65 to indicate the possible presence of psychotic symptoms.

The observed correlation between self-report and implicit measures of common constructs is impacted by a host of intrapersonal, social, and situational factors (McClelland, 1980). For measures tapping reality testing, these factors include insight into one's illness, conscious motivation to present oneself in a certain manner, and the specific context of the evaluation (hospital or forensic unit). As such, correlations among implicit and explicit measures of perceptual accuracy/reality contact are expected to be minimal at best (Meyer, 1996). Interestingly, in our database the PAI SCZ correlates with the RIM variables of XA%, X–%, and *Popular* scores at –0.21, 0.16, and –0.16, respectively (only the correlation between SCZ and XA% reached statistical significance at $p < .05$); however when we limit the sample to non-defensive patients (those with PAI Positive Impression Management [PIM] scores ≤ 45) these correlations increase to –0.30, 0.22, and –0.18, respectively, with all being statistically significant. These findings are consistent with those of McClelland (1980) and Meyer (1996), suggesting that conceptually related implicit and explicit measures are only minimally associated and may offer some insight into factors that impact the relationship between implicit and explicit data, possibly defensiveness.

As noted above, Ms. Jones's RIM PTI score was 3 and suggestive of a potential thought disorder. Her RIM FQ scores were XA% of 0.77 and X–% of 0.23. Both FQ scores are in the range consistent with impaired reality testing. However, she also produced seven *Popular* responses, suggesting that when the perceptual cues are highly apparent she is able to respond conventionally. On the PAI she was somewhat defensive with a PIM T-Score $= 55$; as such she may deny or have limited insight into her psychiatric problems. Neither her PAI PAR (T-score $= 63$) nor SCZ (T-score $= 60$) scales were clinically elevated. Still, given her guarded profile, scores in this range might hint at impaired reality contact. However, her PAI SCZ-P subscales score was not elevated (T-score $= 53$), so she was not openly endorsing psychotic experiences. When combined, the implicit and explicit data regarding her quality of reality contact are somewhat discordant. These data seem to suggest a decrease in perceptual accuracy rather than psychotic level reality impairment.

Measures of Reasoning and Concept Formation

Reasoning and concept formation reflect how people understand and communicate their experiences. In Weiner's multidimensional model of thinking, this component builds on the process of reality testing (perceptual accuracy) as it taps into how subjects interpret, elaborate, and express their perceptual experiences. Adequate reasoning and concept formation allows individuals to form reasonable conclusions about the relationships that exist among their (sensory) experiences, ideas, and events. Being able to maintain a logical, coherent, and flexible understanding of the continuously flowing experience in daily life allows for adaptive, self-directed functioning. When subjects are vulnerable to illogical, incoherent, or overly personalized interpretations of their daily experience, the quality or adaptive value of their functioning will be diminished. Furthermore, when the capacity to reason logically and express one's ideas clearly becomes impaired, it leads to subjective confusion, inability to understand oneself, and bewilderment in others. A full assessment of reasoning and concept formation also relies on both implicit and explicit measures. The goal becomes that of quantifying both the processes the patient uses to reason (implicit) and how well he or she expresses his or her reasoning (explicit) to others. To assess reasoning and concept formation, we use the RIM as an implicit measure along with the PAI (Morey, 1991) and NEO-FFI (Costa & McCrae, 1992) as the main explicit measures.

The second phase of the RIM task requires subjects to tell the examiner "what made" their response "look like that" to them. To complete this task, subjects must verbally elaborate or expand on their initial visual perceptions. As a result, the verbalized RIM response is quite sensitive to fluctuations in the implicit processes that guide reasoning. Exner's CS contains six scoring categories (*Special Scores [SS]*) that measure the quality of a subject's reasoning and logic. Four of the *SS*—Incongruous Combinations (INCOM), Fabulized Combinations (FABCOM), Autistic Logic (ALOG), and Contamination (CONTAM)—measure impaired reasoning and logic. The other two *SS*—Deviant Verbalization (DV) and Deviant Responses (DR)—capture oddities in the patient's verbal response (i.e., strange, rambling, redundant, or tangential verbalizations). Together, these *SS* provide an implicit measure of the degree of cognitive slippage present in a patient's reasoning and expression.

The CS *SS* were influenced by the work of Rapaport (Rapaport, Gill, & Schafer, 1968) and have considerable conceptual overlap with the Thought Disorder Index (TDI; Johnston & Holzman, 1979). The TDI is one of the best empirically validated measures of disordered thinking for free verbal responses, but its complex scoring has limited routine clinical use (Hurt et al., 1983; Kleiger, 1999). However, Exner's *SS* are less complicated to score and can be more reliably applied in clinical assessments.

The average number of *SS* in the record of nonpatients is 2.5; personality-disordered patients tend to have 3 or 4 *SS,* while psychotic patients on average have 5 *SS.* Not all odd reasoning or peculiar speaking is considered equally impairing. To capture these distinctions, the CS assigns weighted values to each *SS.* Nonpatients have an average weighted special score value (*WSum6*) of 7, personality disorder patients typically have *WSum6* values between 10 and 17, and psychotic patients have an average *WSum6* of 44 (Exner, 2003). Consistent with these expectations, Hilsenroth et al. (2007) reported that nonpatients had an average *WSum6* of 9.4, while psychotic patients produced a *WSum6* of 40.1. CS *SS* are also classified as either level 1 (LvL1) or level 2 (LvL2), with the LvL2 scores reflecting more extreme cognitive slippage. It is extremely rare for nonpatients to give even a single LvL2 *SS*, while psychotic patients on average produce 5 LvL2 *SS*. The recent meta-analysis by Mihura et al. (2013) also provides evidence for the validity of both *WSum6* and LvL2 *SS*. In clinical work, when the *WSum6* is ≥ 17 and LvL2 SS ≥ 2, the presence of a meaningful impairment in reasoning and communicating should be considered. In our database we find that *WSum6* and LvL2 *SS* are moderately correlated with the OMNI-IV (Loranger, 2001) Paranoid Personality Disorder scale (0.38 and 0.29, respectively). Also, when we limit the sample in our database to nondefensive patients (PAI PIM ≤ 45), both *WSum6* and LvL2 *SS* show a significant association with a history of paranoia (0.27 and 0.22, respectively).

In Weiner's model of thought quality, the reasoning and concept formation component is conceptually most similar to the categories of formal thought disorder reviewed above. Therefore explicit measures may play a greater role in quantifying impairments in reasoning. In our clinic we use the PAI (Morey, 1991) and the NEO-FFI (Costa & McCrae, 1992) to assess the subjective experience of impaired reasoning. In particular, we focus on the PAI subscales of SCZ-T (Thought Disorder), PAR-P (Persecution), MAN-A (Mania Activity Level), ARD-T (Anxiety Related Disorders—Traumatic Stress), and ARD-O (Anxiety Related Disorders—Obsessive–Compulsive). When elevated (*T*-score ≥ 70), both SCZ-T and ARD-T indicate the experience of mental confusion and intrusive distracting thoughts. MAN-A suggests racing or pressured thoughts when elevated or poverty of mental activity when scores are low. The PAI ARD-O in part measures the subjective experience of mental control. A low ARD-O score (*T*-score < 40) suggests reduced ability to direct and control one's thinking, *T*-scores ≥ 70 suggest rigid and inflexible thinking. The PAR scale in general and PAR-P in particular capture misinterpretation of interpersonal interactions. When PAR-P is *T*-score ≥ 70, it suggests not only the misperception of interpersonal experiences, but also a conceptual impairment in determining cause-and-effect relationships within social interactions. Slavin-Mulford et al. (2012) found the PAR-P correlated at 0.31 with a history of paranoid ideation, and Gay and Combs (2005) found that the PAR-P subscale was elevated in patients with persecutory delusions.

It may seem unusual that we include a measure of normal personality, the NEO-FFI (Costa & McCrae, 1992), in our core assessment battery. However, the NEO-FFI's ability to capture unique explicit information (see Stein et al., 2012) combined with its brevity (60 items) make it a useful clinical assessment tool. The NEO-FFI measures the Five Big dimensions (Neuroticism, Extraversion, Openness, Agreeableness, and Conscientiousness) that organize words describing personality. While all Big Five personality domains contain information relevant to thought quality, we find two of these dimensions, Openness (NEO-O) and Conscientiousness (NEO-C), to be particularly informative regarding a patient's style and quality of thinking. NEO-O is linked to creative and divergent thinking (Costa & McCrae, 1992) and measured intelligence (DeYoung & Gray, 2009). In our database, NEO-O is one of the few self-report scales that is significantly correlated with measured intelligence and neurocognitive abilities (NEO-O with Verbal IQ [$r = .48$], Trails B [$r = .20$], and Stroop [$r = .22$]). In this way, NEO-O provides an explicit link to more basic cognitive abilities. Clinically, when other signs of thought disorder are present, elevations (*T*-score ≥ 65) on NEO-O suggest overly abstract, divergent, and poorly controlled thinking, while low scores (*T*-score < 40) point to concrete, rigid thinking. In our database, we find NEO-C to be related to measures of subjective mental confusion (NEO-C and SCZ-T [$r = -.32$] and ARD-O [$r = -.24$]). When NEO-C is low (*T*-score < 40), the patient is likely to subjectively experience confusion and difficulty, willfully directing their thoughts, even though such qualities may not be evident in their performance on the neurocognitive measures.

Ms. Jones's *WSum6* was elevated (26), and her protocol contained 2 LvL2 *SS*. These findings suggest impairment in the implicit processes that support reasoning and concept formation. In addition, the PAI subscales MAN-A, SCZ-T, and ARD-T were all elevated at a *T*-score ≥ 70. Likewise, her *T*-score on the NEO-Openness scale was a 66, and on the NEO-Conscientiousness scale her *T*-score was 40. Together, the explicit measures all point to undercontrolled, racing, confused, and inefficient thinking. When combined, all measures (implicit and explicit) of reasoning and concept formation strongly suggest a decrease in thought quality and a marked vulnerability to illogical, incoherent, or overly personalized thinking. Furthermore, the consistency and magnitude of these findings suggest that impaired reasoning is negatively impacting her daily functioning.

Social Cognition: An Emerging Focus in the Assessment of Thought Quality

Social cognition refers to the psychological operations that underlie social interactions, including perceiving, interpreting, and responding to the behaviors of others. Social cognition is increasingly of interest to researchers studying autism spectrum disorders (ASD) and psychotic disorders and as such may have important implications for the broader measurement of thought quality. Although not yet fully defined, the domain of social cognition generally includes Theory of Mind (ToM), accuracy of social perception and emotional perception, and processing (Docherty et al., 2013). There is evidence suggesting that social cognition is a uniquely human ability (Tomasello & Herrmann, 2010) and is supported by specialized neural substrates that operate somewhat independently of other more general neurocognitive networks (Uhlhaas, Phillips, Schenkel, & Silverstein, 2006). Although the National Institute of Mental Health (NIMH)-sponsored assessment battery (Measurement and Treatment Research to Improve Cognition and Schizophrenia; MATRICS) includes a measure of social cognition (Geyer, 2012), there are currently few well-validated measures of social cognition available for routine clinical application.

In our clinic we are exploring the utility of the Thematic Apperception Test (TAT; Murray, 1943) as a measure of social cognition. Westen (1991, 1995) has argued that the TAT, with its moderately ambiguous drawings of human figures in various emotional and interpersonal situations, is uniquely suited for eliciting information regarding a patient's understanding of social interactions, emotions, and intentions. Westen (1991) has developed a reliable and valid multidimensional measure of social cognition and object relations (Social Cognition and Object Relations Scale [SCORS]; Weston, 1995). The SCORS consists of eight variables that are rated on a seven-point anchored scale where lower scores (e.g., 1, 2, or 3) indicate more pathological responses and higher scores (e.g., 5, 6, or 7) indicate healthy responses. The eight variables are Complexity of Representations, Affective Quality of Representations, Emotional Investment in Relationships, Emotional Investment and Values in Moral Standards, Social Causality, Experience and Management of Aggressive Impulses, Self-Esteem and Identity, and Coherence of Self. More thorough descriptions of the SCORS variables and training examples are provided in a manual developed by Stein et al. (2011). The findings reported in Stein et al. (2012) provide preliminary evidence that SCORS domains capture implicit aspects of interpersonal perception. However, additional empirical and conceptual work is needed to clarify the clinical implications of these findings. The Rorschach minus FQ Human Movement response (M–) may also hold potential as an implicit measure of distorted interpersonal perception. However, empirical support for the validity of M– was rated as only modest by Mihura et al. (2013). Therefore, further research is also needed to clarify the potential value of Rorschach M– as an implicit measure of social misperception. Other potential measures of social cognition include the Reading the Mind in the Eyes (Baron-Cohen, Wheelwright, Hill, Raste, & Plumb, 2001), a measure of emotion recognition and more general measures of emotional intelligence (EI) (see Roberts, Schulze, & MacCann, 2008). However, at present no single test or constellation of existing routinely collected variables (test scores) can be endorsed for assessing social cognition in routine clinical practice.

The Challenge of Multimethod Assessment: Integration of Data

The primary challenge of multimethod assessment is integrating the extensive range of data generated by the test battery. For example, a battery composed of the RIM, PAI, NEO-FFI, WASI-II, and the neurocognitive measures reviewed above would yield approximately 132 scores or data points. Understanding, organizing, and integrating this amount of information represents a significant challenge for assessment psychologists. In the preceding, we have argued that a multidimensional model of thinking can be used to guide the selection and integration of a subset of multimethod variables and provide a detailed evaluation of thought quality. Using Weiner's model of thought process, we identified the specific measures of (1) processing speed (Digit Symbol Coding and Trails A) and cognitive flexibility (Trails B and Stroop Color–Word Test); (2) implicit (RIM XA%, X–%, *Popular*) and explicit (PAI SCZ, SCZ-P, and PAR) measures of reality contact; and (3) implicit (RIM *WSum6* and LvL2 *SS*) and explicit (PAI MAN-A, SCZ-T, PAR-P, ARD-O, ARD-T, NEO-O, and NEO-C) measures of reasoning and concept formation. We have also reviewed published validity data for these variables and provided additional empirical data from a large clinical database, both of which support their conceptual validity. The chapter also outlined how these variables might be combined rationally to reveal a detailed description of thinking. Still this theory/model-guided rational approach should be reinforced with empirical support.

To illustrate how these variables combine empirically, Table 8.2 presents the results of a principal components analysis (PCA) of 14 thought quality variables based on 118 subjects in our database (all subjects with complete data). A three-component solution was suggested by a parallel

TABLE 8.2. Principal Components Analysis of Select Thought Quality Variables with Varimax Rotation

Thought quality variables	Component 1 Implicit	Component 2 Neurocognitive	Component 3 Explicit
Rorschach X–%	.83		.25
Rorschach XA%	–.78		–.34
Rorschach LvL2 SS	.73		
WSum6	.75		
Digit Symbol Coding		.81	
Trails B		.77	
Stroop		.73	
Trails A		.69	
NEO–Openness	.33	.42	
NEO–Conscientiousness		–.29	–.24
PAI SCZ			.88
PAI SCZ-P			.81
PAI PAR			.78
Populars			–.38

Note. N = 108; only loadings with an absolute value ≥ .20 are included.

analysis (Horn, 1965); the components were only minimally intercorrelated (the highest correlation was Component 1 and Component 2 at $r = .16$), so a varimax rotation was employed. As Table 8.2 shows, Component 1 is primarily composed of RIM variables (X–%, XA%, *WSum6*& LvL2 *SS*) but does have a secondary loading for NEO-O. Component 2 is marked by the neurocognitive measures (Coding, Stroop, Trails A & B) but also has a primary loading for the NEO-O and NEO-C. Component 3 was marked by PAI scales (SCZ, SCZ-P, and PAR) but also has a primary loading for RIM *Populars* and secondary loadings for X– and XA%. The component loadings suggest that fairly clear and distinct dimensions underlie the thought quality measures we identified in our battery and at the same time reveal a moderate degree of cross-method overlap. Conceptually, these PCA components seem to bear some relationship to Weiner's model of thought quality: Component 2 is clearly related to cognitive focus, Component 1 is mainly related to reality testing (perceptual accuracy), and Component 3 is primarily related to reasoning and concept formations. Alternatively, the components could be conceptualized as reflecting assessment method differences: neurocognitive (Component 2), implicit (Component 1), and explicit (Component 3) dimensions of thought quality.

Next the PCA scores were saved and used in a stepwise multiple regression analysis (MRA) to predict total past psychotic symptoms (the sum of reported auditory hallucinations, visual hallucinations, and paranoid ideation). The MRA showed that all three components were independent predictors of past psychotic symptoms: Component 3 (explicit) entered at step 1 (beta = .269, $p = .004$), Component 2 (neurocognitive) entered at step 2 (beta = .252, $p = .007$), and Component 1 (implicit) entered at step 3 (beta = –.190, $p = .04$). The final multiple R was .418, and the adjusted R^2 was .15 ($df = 3, 114$). These results suggest that these empirically combined thought quality variables are related to (a history of) psychotic thinking. However, a large proportion of the variance in our proxy for thought quality remained unaccounted for.

Returning to our clinical example, we find that the data presented on Ms. Jones reveal a clear but relative disruption in the neurocognitive abilities required for adaptive thought, discrepant or equivocal findings regarding psychotic-level reality impairment, and strong consistent indications of a marked disruption in her reasoning and concept formation abilities. When combined with her history (one prior manic episode, good educational attainment, and periods of reasonably successful employment), these data would be most consistent with disordered thinking associated with an affective bipolar illness (see Kleiger, 1999, pp. 256–273). Beyond diagnostic clarification, these multimethod assessment findings can be used to identify meaningful treatment targets, serve as quantitative markers for monitoring treatment progress, and offer insights into the degree of functional impairment Ms. Jones might currently be experiencing.

Conclusion

After more than half a century, Rapaport's verdict that "our knowledge of thinking is scant" still seems to ring true. However, we hope this chapter demonstrates that the field has made important gains in understanding and measuring thought quality. Furthermore, we believe that approaches, such as the one outlined above, that integrate multimethod clinical assessment with a theory or model of thinking and rigorous empirical exploration hold the greatest promise for achieving continued progress in understanding and assessing thought quality.

REFERENCES

Andreasen, N. C. (1979). Thought, language and communication disorders. *Archive of General Psychiatry, 36*, 1315–1321.

Andreasen, N. C., Flaum, M., & Arndt, S. (1992). The comprehensive assessment of symptoms and history (CASH): An instrument for assessing diagnosis and psychopathology, *Archive of General Psychiatry, 49*, 615–623.

Andreasen, N. C., & Grove, W. (1986). Thought, language and communication in schizophrenia: Diagnosis and prognosis. *Schizophrenia Bulletin, 12*, 348–359.

Baron-Cohen, S., Wheelwright, S., Hill, J., Raste, Y., & Plumb, I. (2001). The "Reading the Mind in the Eyes" test revised version: A study with normal adults and adults with Asperger syndrome of high-functioning autism. *Journal of Psychology and Psychiatry, 42*, 241–251.

Beaudoin, M., & Desrichard, O. (2011). Are memory self-efficacy and memory performance related?: A meta-analysis. *Psychological Bulletin, 137*(2), 211–241.

Bell, M. D., Lysaker, P. H., Beam-Goulet, J. L., Mistein, R. M., & Lindenmeyer, J. P. (1993). Five-component model of schizophrenia: Assessing the factorial invariance of the positive and negative syndrome scale. *Psychiatry Research, 52*(3), 295–303.

Blais, M. A., & Hopwood, C. J. (2010). Personality focused assessment with the PAI. In M. Blais, M. Baity, & C. J. Hopwood (Eds.), *Clinical applications of the Personality Assessment Inventory* (pp. 195–209). New York: Routledge.

Bleuler, E. (1950). *Dementia praecox, or the group of schizophrenias* (J. Zinkin, Trans). New York: International Universities Press.

Butcher, J. N., Dahlstrom, W. G., Graham, J. R., Tellegen, A., & Kaemmer, B. (1989). *MMPI-2: Minnesota Multiphasic Personality Inventory: Manual for administration and scoring.* Minneapolis: University of Minnesota Press.

Campbell, D. T., & Fiske, D. W. (1959). Convergent and discriminant validation by the multitrait—multimethod matrix, *Psychological Bulletin, 56*, 81–105.

Carroll, J. B. (1993). *Human cognitive abilities: Their survey of factor-analytic studies.* Cambridge, UK: Cambridge University Press.

Cattell, R. B. (1971). *Abilities: Their structure, growth and action.* Boston: Houghton-Mifflin.

Costa, P. T., Jr., & McCrae, R. R. (1992). *NEO PI-R Professional Manual: Revised NEO Personality Inventory (NEO OI-R) and NEO Five-Factor Inventory (NEO-FFI).* Lutz, FL: Psychological Assessment Resources.

DeYoung, C. G., & Gray, J. R. (2009). Personality neuroscience: Explaining individual differences in affect, behavior and cognition. In P. J. Corr & G. Matthews (Eds.),

The Cambridge handbook of personality psychology (pp. 323–346). New York: Cambridge University Press.

Dickinson, D., Ramsey, M. E., & and Gold, J. M. (2007). Overlooking the obvious: A meta-analytic comparison of digit symbol coding tasks and other cognitive measures in schizophrenia. *Archives of General Psychiatry, 64*, 532–542.

Dingemans, P. M. A. J., Linszen, D. H., Lenior, M. E., & Smeets, R. M. W. (1995). Component structure of the expanded Brief Psychiatric Rating Scale (BPRS-E). *Psychopharmacology, 122*, 263–267.

Docherty, N. M. (2005). Cognitive impairments and disordered speech in schizophrenia: Thought disorder, disorganization, and communication failure perspectives. *Journal of Abnormal Psychology, 11*, 269–278.

Docherty, N. M., McCleery, A., Divilbiss, M, Schumann, E. B., Moe, A., & Shakeel, M. (2013). Effects of social cognitive impairment on speech disorder in schizophrenia. *Schizophrenia Bulletin, 39*(3), 608–616.

Exner, J. (2003). *The Rorschach: A comprehensive system: Vol. 1. Basic foundations* (4th ed.). New York: Wiley.

Freud, S. (1959). *The interpretation of dreams* (Standard Edition, Vols. 4 and 5). London: Hogarth Press. (Original work published 1900)

Gay, N. W., & Combs, D. R. (2005). Social behavior in persons with and without persecutory delusions. *Schizophrenia Research, 80*, 361–362.

Geyer, M. A. (2012). New opportunities in the treatment of cognitive impairments associated with schizophrenia. *Current Directions in Psychological Science, 19*, 264–269.

Gottlieb, J. D., Fan, X., & Goff, D. C. (2010). Rating scales in schizophrenia. In L. Baer & M. A. Blais (Eds.), *Handbook of clinical rating scales and assessment in psychiatry and mental health* (pp. 209–238). New York: Humana Press.

Harvey, P. D., Keefe, R. S. E., Patterson, T. L., Heaton, R. K., & Bowie, C. R. (2009). Abbreviated neuropsychological assessment in schizophrenia: Prediction of different aspects of outcome. *Journal of Clinical and Experimental Neuropsychology, 31*, 462–471.

Hilsenroth, M., Eudell-Simmons, E., DeFife, J., & Charnas, J. (2007). The Rorschach Perceptual and Thought Index (PTI): An examination of reliability, validity, and diagnostic efficiency. *International Journal of Testing, 7*, 269–291.

Horn, J. L. (1965). A rationale and test for the number of factors in factor analysis. *Psychometrika, 30*, 179–185.

Howieson, D. B., & Lezak, M. D. (1992). The neuropsychological evaluation. In S. C. Yudofsky & R. E. Hales (Eds.), *The American Psychiatric Press textbook of neuropsychiatry* (2nd ed., pp. 127–150). Washington, DC: American Psychiatric Press.

Hurt, S. W., Holzman, P. S., & Davis, J. M. (1983). Thought disorder: The measurement of its changes, *Archives of General Psychiatry, 40*, 1281–1285.

Johnston, M. H., & Holzman, P. S. (1979). *Assessing schizophrenic thinking.* San Francisco: Jossey-Bass.

Kay, S. R., Fiszbein, A., & Opler, L. A. (1987). The Positive and Negative Syndrome Scale (PANSS) for schizophrenia. *Schizophrenia Bulletin, 13*, 261–276.

Kircher, T. T. J., Liddle, F. P., Brammer, M. J., Williams, S. C. R., Murray, R. M., & McGuire, P. K. (2001). Neural correlates of formal thought disorder in schizophrenia. *Archives of General Psychiatry, 58*, 769–774.

Kleiger, J. H. (1999). *Disordered thinking and the Rorschach.* Hillsdale, NJ: Analytic Press.

Klonsky, E. D. (2004). Performance of Personality Assessment Inventory and Rorschach indices of schizophrenia in a public psychiatric hospital. *Psychological Services, 1,* 107–110.

Kopelowicz, A., Ventura, J., Liberman, R. P., & Mintz, J. (2008). Consistency of Brief Psychiatric Rating Scale factor structure across a broad spectrum of schizophrenia patients. *Psychopathology, 41*(2), 77–84.

Kraepelin, E. (1919). *Dementia praecox and paraphrenia* (R. M. Barclay, Trans). Edinburgh: E&S Livingston Co.

Kuperberg, G. R., Deckersbach, T., Holt, D. J., Goff, D., & West, W. C. (2007). Increased temporal and prefrontal activity in response to semantic associations in schizophrenia. *Archive of General Psychiatry, 64,* 138–151.

Loranger, A. W. (2001). *OMNI-IV Personality Inventories: Professional manual.* Odessa, FL: Psychological Assessment Resources.

Mayer, J. D. (2005). A tale of two visions: Can a new view of personality help integrate psychology? *American Psychologist.60,* 294–307.

McClelland, D. C. (1980). Motive dispositions: The merits of operant and respondent measures. In L. Wheeler (Ed.), *Review of personality and social psychology* (Vol. 1, pp. 10–41). Beverly Hills, CA: Sage.

Meehl, P. E. (1990). Toward an integrated theory of schizotaxia, schizotypy, and schizophrenia. *Journal of Personality Disorder, 4,* 1–99.

Meyer, G. J. (1996). The Rorschach and MMPI: Toward a more scientifically differentiated understanding of cross-method assessment, *Journal of Personality Assessment, 67,* 558–578.

Meyer, G. J., Finn, S. E., Eyde, L. D., Kay, G. G., Moreland, K. L., Dies, R. R., et al. (2001). Psychological testing and psychological assessment: A review of evidence and issues. *American Psychologist, 56,* 128–165.

Mihura, J. L., Meyer, G. J., Dumitrascu, N., & Bombel, G. (2013). The validity of individual Rorschach variables: Systematic reviews and meta-analyses of the comprehensive system. *Psychological Bulletin, 139,* 548–605.

Millon, T. (1994). *Millon Clinical Multiaxial Inventory–III: Manual.* Minneapolis, MN: Pearson Assessments.

Morey, L. C. (1991). *Personality Assessment Inventory: Professional manual.* Odessa, FL: Psychological Assessment Resources.

Morey, L. C. (2007). *Personality Assessment Inventory: Professional manual* (2nd ed.). Odessa, FL: Psychological Assessment Resources.

Mueser, K. T., Curran, P. T., & McHugo, G. J. (1997). Factor structure of the Brief Psychiatric Rating Scale in schizophrenia. *Psychological Assessment, 9,* 196–204.

Murray, H. A. (1943). *Manual for the Thematic Apperception Test.* Cambridge, MA: Harvard University Press.

Niendam, T. A., Bearden, C. E., Rosso, I. M., Sanchez, L. E., Hadley, T., Nuechterlein, K. H., et al. (2003). A prospective study of childhood neurocognitive functioning in schizophrenic patients and their siblings. *American Journal of Psychiatry, 160,* 2060–2062.

O'Connell, M., Cooper, S., Perry, J. C., & Hoke, L. (1989). The relationship between thought disorder and psychotic symptoms in borderline personality disorder. *Journal of Nervous and Mental Disease, 177,* 273–278.

Overall, J. E., & Gorham, D. R. (1962). The brief psychiatric rating scale. *Psychological Reports, 10,* 799–812.

Overall, J. E., & Rhoades, H. M. (1982). Use of Hamilton Rating Scale for classification of depressive disorders. *Comprehensive Psychiatry, 23*(4), 370–376.

Palmer, B. W., Heaton, R. K., Paulsen, J. S., Kuck, J., Braff, D., Harris M. J., et al. (1997). Is it possible to be a schizophrenic yet neuropsychologically normal? *Neuropsychology, 11*, 437–446.

Pinker, S. (1997). *How the mind works*. New York: Norton.

Putnam, M. C., & Blais, M. A. (2010). Neuropsychology in adult psychiatry. In E. A. Arzubi & E. Mambrino (Eds.), *A guide to neuropsychological testing for health care professionals* (pp. 323–342). New York: Springer.

Rapaport, D. (1951). *Organization and pathology of thought*. New York: Columbia University Press.

Rapaport, D., Gill, M., & Schafer, R. (1968*)*. Diagnostic psychological testing. In R. R. Holt (Ed.), *Diagnostic psychological testing, Vols. 1 and 2* (rev ed.). New York: International Universities Press.

Reitan, R. M. (1992). *Trail making test: Manual for administration and scoring*. Tucson, AZ: Reitan Neuropsychology Laboratory.

Reitan, R. M., & Wolfson, D. (1985). *The Halstead–Reitan Neuropsychological Test Battery: Theory and clinical interpretation*. Tucson, AZ: Neuropsychology Press.

Reitan, R. M., & Wolfson, D. (2004). Trail making test as an initial screening procedure for neuropsychological impairment in older children. *Archives of Clinical Neuropsychology, 19*, 281–288.

Roberts, R. D., Schulze, R., & MacCann, C. (2008). The measurement of emotional intelligence: A decade of progress? In G. J. Boyle, G. Matthews, & D. H. Saklofske (Eds.), *The SAGE handbook of personality theory and assessment* (Vol. 2, pp. 461–482). Thousand Oaks, CA: Sage.

Rorschach, H. (1942). *Psychodiagnostics*. Bern, Switzerland: Hans Huber. (Original work published 1921)

Rule, A. (2005). Ordered thoughts on thought disorder. *Psychairic Bulletin, 29*, 462–464.

Slavin-Mulford, J., Sinclair, S. J., Stein, M., Malone, J. C., Bello, I., & Blais, M. A. (2012). External validity of the Personality Assessment Inventory (PAI) in a clinical sample. *Journal of Personality Assessment, 94*, 593–600.

Stein, M. B., Hilsenroth, M., Slavin-Mulford, J., & Pinsker, J. (2011). Social cognition and Object Relations Scale: Global Rating Method (SCORS-G), 4th ed. Unpublished manuscript. Massachusetts General Hospital and Harvard Medical School, Boston.

Stein, M. B., Slavin-Mulford, J., Sinclair, S. J., Siefert, C. J., & Blais, M. A. (2012). Exploring the construct validity of the social cognition and object relations scale in a clinical sample. *Journal of Personality Assessment, 94*, 533–540.

Strack, F., & Deutsch, R. (2004). Reflective and impulsive determinants of social behavior. *Personality and Social Psychology Review, 8*, 220–247.

Thomas, A., Donnell, A. J., & Young, T. R. (2004). Factor structure and differential validity of the expanded Brief Psychiatric Rating Scale. *Assessment 2004, 11*, 177–187.

Tomasello, M., & Herrmann, E. (2010). Ape and human cognition: What's the difference? *Current Directions in Psychological Science, 19*, 3–8.

Trenerry, M. R., Crosson, B., Deboe, J., & Leber, W. (1989). *Stroop Neuropsychological Test (SNST)*. Odessa, FL: Psychological Resources.

Uhlhaas, P. J., Phillips, W. A., Schenkel, L. S., & Silverstein, S. M. (2006). The theory of mind perceptual cognitive processing in schizophrenia. *Cognitive Neuropsychiatry, 11*, 416–436.

Wechsler, D. (2008). *Wechsler Adult Intelligence Scale—4th Edition (WAIS-IV)*. San Antonio, TX: NCS Pearson.

Wechsler, D. (2011).*Wechsler Abbreviated Scale of Intelligence*—2nd Edition *(WASI-II)*. San Antonio, TX: NCS Pearson.

Weiner, I. B. (1966). *Psychodiagnosis in schizophrenia*. New York: Wiley.

Weiner, I. B. (1996). Some observations on the validity of the Rorschach Inkblot Method. *Psychological Assessment, 8,* 206–213.

Westen, D. (1991). Clinical assessment of object relations using the TAT. *Journal of Personality Assessment, 56*(1), 56–74.

Westen, D. (1995). *Social Cognition and Object Relations Scale: Q-sort for projective stories (SCORS–Q)*. Unpublished manuscript, Cambridge Hospital and Harvard Medical School, Department of Psychiatry, Cambridge, MA.

Wood, J. M., Lilienfeld, S. O., Garb, H. N., & Nezworski, M. T. (2000). The Rorschach test in clinical diagnosis: A critical review, with a backward look at Garfield (1947). *Journal of Clinical Psychology, 56,* 395–430.

CHAPTER 9

Multimethod Assessment of Resilience

Integration with an Individual-Differences Model

Christy A. Denckla and Anthony D. Mancini

At some point, given life's contingent nature, the perils that may lurk unseen around the next corner will be made swiftly clear to virtually everyone. We may lose a loved one, experience a serious accident or illness, be victimized by a crime, find ourselves uprooted by natural disaster, or suffer grievous injury at the hands of another human being. Most people will experience at least one such event at some point in their lives (Kessler, Sonnega, Bromet, Hughes, & Nelson, 1995). Despite the near universality of these experiences, our capacity to cope with these events has long been underestimated (Bonanno, 2004).

For example, imagine Damon, a 17-year-old African American male who has recently experienced the loss of his biological father. To an observer, he might appear neat and well dressed, make excellent eye contact, and speak in a direct, somewhat quiet voice. He tells his story with a range of affect, describing his sense of loss and some of the details surrounding his father's death, which was sudden and the result of an automobile accident. However, Damon is also demonstrating a pattern of adaptive functioning: His academic performance remains strong, he stays involved in multiple extracurricular activities, and he endorses positive relationships with peers and family members. Also, he is not endorsing clinical mental health concerns; his mood is stable, his thought content is linear and goal directed, and he reports no changes in sleep patterns or appetite. Damon states that he coped with this tragic event by "staying focused on his future" and making the best choices he could in his present. He also states that he generally opts to "put things behind him."

This brief vignette of a young man who experienced exposure to a traumatic event captures features of resilience, as we will outline further in this chapter. The definition of resilience that we present challenges the common assumption that most people will experience incapacitating distress following an acute stressor and universally require an extensive recovery period. Indeed, the absence of distress has often in itself been considered pathological and a likely harbinger of future difficulties (Middleton, Moylan, Raphael, Burnett, & Martinek, 1993), or a consequence of exceptional strength and thus is thought to be relatively rare. Although these cultural assumptions have long held sway, they have begun to give way to a very different perspective: Most people cope with even the most acute stressors adaptively and return to their former levels of functioning relatively soon after (Bonanno, 2004; Bonanno, Westphal, & Mancini, 2011; Mancini & Bonanno, 2009).

This resilient capacity has drawn increasing interest from scholars studying widely varying stressful events. Resilience has been observed as the modal response to events as diverse as breast cancer (Deshields, Tibbs, Fan, & Taylor, 2006; Lam et al., 2010), bioepidemic (Bonanno et al., 2008), terrorist attack (Bonanno, Galea, Bucciarelli, & Vlahov, 2007), bereavement (Bonanno et al., 2002; Mancini, Bonanno, & Clark, 2011), traumatic injury (deRoon-Cassini, Mancini, Rusch, & Bonanno, 2010), spinal cord injury (Bonanno, Kennedy, Galatzer-Levy, Lude, & Elfström, 2012), and military deployment (Bonanno, Mancini, et al., 2012). Among children exposed to adverse and stressful conditions in childhood, such as poverty, neglect, and abuse, a similar degree of resilience has been documented, with most children revealing adaptive developmental trajectories (Luthar & Zelazo, 2003; Masten, 2001).

These findings attest that resilience is common, the product of ordinary coping abilities. However, the key question with respect to what is meant by resilience remains. How do we know whether someone is resilient? As important are the questions, how do we assess resilience and who is most likely to possess resilience?

Most scholars define resilience as relatively stable levels of functioning following exposure to an acutely stressful event. For example, Bonanno (2004) offers this definition:

> Resilience pertains to the ability of adults in otherwise normal circumstances who are exposed to an isolated and potentially highly disruptive event, such as the death of a close relation or a violent or life-threatening situation, to maintain relatively stable, healthy levels of psychological and physical functioning. A further distinction is that resilience is more than the simple absence of psychopathology. (p. 20)

A similar definition is offered by Luthar (2006): *"positive adaptation despite experiences of significant adversity or trauma"* (p. 242; emphasis in original). Both definitions require an acutely stressful event and the ability to preserve normal functioning, and imply that resilience is a consequence of adaptation rather than a cause of it. In other words, we can only identify resilience after the fact, when a person is confronted and successfully copes with an acutely stressful event. Resilience as defined here is distinct from related constructs such as posttraumatic growth (Tedeschi & Calhoun, 2004), hardiness (Kobasa, 1979), toughness (Dienstbier, 1989), and grit (Duckworth, Peterson, Matthews, & Kelly, 2007).

In this chapter, we define resilience as an outcome or process following exposure to acute adversity. We first distinguish resilience to acute adversity from other reaction patterns. We then consider how to assess whether someone is resilient, addressing the role of psychopathological symptoms, such as posttraumatic stress disorder and depression, and the presence of positive adaptation, such as role functioning and quality of life. We then address person-centered factors that *contribute* to a resilient outcome, such as personality, positive emotions, and flexible coping strategies, as well as factors external to the person, such as social support and material resources. We address the relative advantages of a multimethod assessment approach to include self-report, clinical interviews, reports of friends and family, implicit and performance-based measures, and physiological approaches in capturing a more reliable picture of individual functioning after exposure to a potentially traumatic event (PTE).

A key point about the assessment of resilience is that it is distinct from other prototypical reaction patterns following acute stress. Bonanno and others have found evidence for four primary and encompassing response patterns following acute stress (Bonanno et al., 2011). In addition to resilience, patterns may comprise recovery, chronic distress, and delayed reactions. Recovery is distinguished from resilience by elevated symptoms and some functional impairment after the acute stressor, followed by a gradual return to normal levels of functioning. Chronic distress is characterized by a sharp elevation in symptoms and by functional impairment that may persist for years. Moderate to elevated symptoms characterize delayed reactions soon after the event and a gradual worsening across time. It is important to emphasize, however, that resilient persons do experience some upset related to an acutely adverse event. But they are able to manage these difficult experiences in such a way that they are able to maintain adaptive functioning.

Rationale for the Multimethod Approach

The importance of accurate assessment following exposure to a traumatic event has obvious public health consequences, and there is general consensus regarding the need to improve the capacity to predict elevated and persistent stress reactions (Bonanno, Brewin, Kaniasty, & Greca, 2010). Multimethod assessment is typically recommended in evaluating post-exposure adjustment owing to the many advantages associated with this approach (Barlow & Wolfe, 1981; Duckworth, Steen, & Seligman, 2005; Litz, Gray, Bryant, & Adler, 2002). Simply defined, the multimethod assessment battery integrates data from multiple sources—self-report, informant/observer, performance-based measures, and psychophysiological measures—to develop a comprehensive analysis of individual functioning (Blais, Hilsenroth, Castlebury, Fowler, & Baity, 2001; Bornstein, 2009; Campbell & Fiske, 1959; Meyer, 2000). The primary advantage of a multimethod approach is the incremental validity that multiple instruments introduce beyond what any single measurement can provide (Grilo, Masheb, & Wilson, 2001; Hopwood et al., 2008). For example, the Implicit Association Test (IAT; Greenwald & Banaji, 1995) and self-report measures typically provide incremental validity in predicting outcome, with each demonstrating predictive criterion variance over the other (Greenwald, Poehlman, Uhlmann, & Banaji, 2009). In related findings, Meyer's (2000) meta-analysis demonstrated that both the Rorschach Prognostic Rating Scale (RPRS; Klopfer, Kirkner, Wishman, & Baker, 1951) and measured IQ contributed unique variance to predicting treatment outcome, suggesting that after taking into account predictive information that can be obtained from measured IQ, the RPRS contributed unique predictive criterion variance when estimating the outcome of mental health treatment.

Because resilience is optimally measured and defined by functioning across multiple domains, a multimethod assessment is particularly well suited to assessing it. For example, resilience cannot be captured completely via self-report because subjective appraisal of internal functioning is only one aspect (though an important one) of a resilient trajectory, which by definition includes behavioral markers. Second, resilient individuals may experience some degree of internal distress as a result of exposure to a PTE, even though they are able to maintain an adaptive level of functioning. If an assessment does not incorporate observable behavior (e.g., measured by semistructured interviews or knowledgeable informant methods), then evidence of adaptive functioning could potentially go overlooked. See Table 9.1 for a complete summary of instruments used in the assessment of resilience organized by construct, discussed in the following sections.

Assessing Resilience in the Clinical Context: The Dual Role of Adaptive Functioning and Psychopathology

To be clinically useful, multimethod assessment must distinguish the target group of interest (those individuals displaying evidence of resilience) from groups similar to the target (individuals exposed to PTE and presenting with clinical symptoms) on as many dimensions as possible. Assessing

TABLE 9.1. Summary of Instruments Used in the Multimethod Assessment of Resilience, Organized by Construct

Resilience domain	Construct	Instrument	Assessment technique
Symptomatic functioning	Symptomatology	PCL (Blanchard, Jones-Alexander, Buckley, & Forneris, 1996); PAI (Morey, 2007); MMPI-2; BDI (Beck, 1961); PHQ (Spitzer, Kroenke, & Williams, 1999)	Questionnaire
	Psychopathology	CAPS (Blake et al., 1995); SCID (First, Spitzer, Gibbon, & Janet, 2002)	Clinician-administered interview
Adaptive functioning	Ego strength	Es scale of the MMPI-2 (Barron, 1953)	Questionnaire
	Quality of life	QOLS (Flanagan, 1978)	Questionnaire
	Well-being	SWLS (Diener, Emmons, Larsen, & Griffin, 1985); PWB (Ryff & Singer, 1996)	Questionnaire
	PTE adjustment trajectory	Informant-ratings (Bonanno, Rennicke, & Dekel, 2005)	Informant-rated
Contributing factors	Resiliency	ER-89 (Block & Kreman, 1996); CD-RISC (Connor & Davidson, 2003); RSA (Friborg, Hjemdal, Rosenvinge, & Martinussen, 2003); IIS-64 (Hatcher & Rogers, 2009)	Questionnaire
		IAT (Greenwald, McGhee, & Schwartz, 1998)	Implicit
	Emotion regulation	ERQ (Gross & John, 2003)	Questionnaire
	Coping	PACT (Bonanno, Pat-Horenczyk, & Noll, 2011); Repressive Coping (Weinberger, Schwartz, & Davidson, 1979)	Questionnaire

Note. The Rorschach Inkblot Method is not specifically restricted to one domain or construct (see Weiner, 1994) and is therefore not included in this table.

resilience in the clinical context presents a number of conceptual and methodological challenges (Bonanno, 2012; Luthar, Cicchetti, & Becker, 2000; Luthar & Cushing, 2002; Lyons, 1991). Clinicians and researchers recognize that discriminating between pathological and adaptive responses after a PTE is a differential diagnostic issue for which more clinical guidance is necessary (Litz et al., 2002; Litz, Miller, Ruef, & McTeague, 2011; Mancini & Bonanno, 2006).

Before we can identify factors associated with resilience, however, we have to translate our operational definition of resilience into measurement strategies. Assessing resilience in the clinical context entails a detailed appraisal of functioning in two separate but related domains. The first domain encompasses disease-related processes and includes symptomatology (posttraumatic stress disorder [PTSD], grief, and depression) and health (somatic complaints, worsened health problems, and disease). The second separate but related domain to be assessed is the presence of adaptive functioning (role functioning, positive emotions, and pleasure in life). Because adaptive functioning cannot be defined simply as the lack of symptomatic functioning, the measurement strategies and scales used to assess these two domains require different approaches (Bonanno, 2012).

Measures of Posttraumatic Functioning

First, we address measurement strategies of distress-related processes. Self-report instruments are some of the most widely used means of assessing posttraumatic functioning in the clinical context. They are relatively easy to administer, impose fewer demands on clinicians, possess good construct validity and reliability, and can be deployed rapidly following exposure to trauma. Furthermore, self-report measures are sometimes used to alert clinicians to the need for further assessment (Widiger & Samuel, 2005). They are especially useful when the primary measurement question relies on beliefs, values, and attitudes because the nature of the instrument relies on respondents' self-attributions (Lucas & Baird, 2006). Brief screening instruments may be used proximally after exposure (at least one week after) to distinguish among those who are experiencing symptoms of adjustment difficulties (Bonanno, 2012; Litz et al, 2011).

A number of well-validated self-report clinical instruments are commonly used to assess symptoms of posttraumatic adjustment difficulties; these instruments include the Posttraumatic Stress Disorder Checklist (PCL; Blanchard, Jones-Alexander, Buckley, & Forneris, 1996), the Personality Assessment Inventory (PAI; Morey, 2007), and the Minnesota Multiphasic Personality Inventory (MMPI). All three scales have been validated in the assessment of PTSD. The MMPI-2 is a widely used broad-band self-report measure of clinical psychopathology. It has been validated among PTSD samples (Keane, Malloy, & Fairbank, 1984) and shows particular utility in detecting malingering among veterans (Lyons & Wheeler-Cox, 1999; Thomas, Hopwood, Orlando, Weathers, & McDevitt-Murphy, 2012). The PAI is a 344-item measure of psychological functioning that has been validated in military populations and has demonstrated the ability to discriminate between veterans diagnosed with PTSD and combat-exposed asymptomatic individuals (Morey et al., 2011). Finally, the PCL is perhaps the most widely used checklist measure to screen for PTSD. It contains 17 items that assess symptom clusters identified in the *Diagnostic and Statistical Manual of Mental Disorders*, fourth edition, text revision (DSM-IV-TR; American Psychiatric Association, 2000), and its diagnostic accuracy is adequate (McDonald & Calhoun, 2010).

In the context of the death of a loved one, clinicians may need to assess symptoms associated with prolonged grief. Diagnostic criteria for prolonged grief can include clinical impairment following the death of someone with whom the bereaved was associated. Specific symptoms include strong yearning for the deceased; preoccupation with thoughts about the loss; recurrent regrets or self-blame about behavior toward the deceased; and marked loneliness or sense of emptiness or meaninglessness (Horowitz, Bonanno, & Holen, 1993). Diagnosis can be achieved employing consensus criteria established previously (Prigerson et al., 1999).

Major depressive disorder (MDD) is frequently comorbid with PTSD and is typically assessed using semistructured or structured clinician administered interviews (Litz et al., 2011). A frequently used brief self-report measure of depressive features includes the Beck Depression Inventory (BDI; Beck, 1961). Twenty-five years of use suggests that this brief measure is an effective tool to screen for the presence of depressive disorders (Beck, Steer, & Carbin, 1998). The Patient Health Questionnaire (PHQ) also assesses current symptoms of major depression, and it has shown good agreement with clinician-assessed ratings of depression (Spitzer, Kroenke, & Williams, 1999).

In addition to the self report measures mentioned previously, clinician administered assessments of functioning are frequently employed in the diagnosis of psychopathology. The Clinician-Administered PTSD Scale (CAPS; Blake et al., 1995) specifically assesses criteria associated with PTSD. It has been used in nearly 200 studies in the 10 years since its development (Weathers, Keane, & Davidson, 2001). The Structured Clinical Interview of DSM-IV-TR Disorders (SCID; First, Spitzer, Gibbon, & Janet, 2002) also assesses PTSD, in addition to depression and other disorders (see Litz et al., 2011), for an extensive review).

Measures of Adaptive Functioning: Self-Report

The second component of the recommended measurement strategy for assessing resilient functioning entails an evaluation of adaptive functioning. Among the factors that influence adaptive functioning after exposure to trauma are both social and personal resources (Bonanno et al., 2007; Litz & Maguen, 2010). Mounting evidence suggests that specific forms of social support promote recovery from trauma (Charuvastra & Cloitre, 2008; Pietrzak, Russo, Ling, & Southwick, 2011). However, not all forms of social support provide buffers against mental health symptoms. For example, one study found that receiving emotional support was associated with fewer depressive symptoms in women but not men. This finding suggests that assessment of social support must take into account context and gender (Fiori & Denckla, 2012). In addition to an assessment of social and personal resources, the following scales may also be useful in detecting adaptive functioning.

Quality of Life

While hundreds of scales exist that assess quality of life indicators (Berzon, Donnelly, Simpson, Simeon, & Tilson, 1995) one of the more widely used is the Quality of Life Scale (QOLS; Flanagan, 1978). It is a 16-item measure that assesses five conceptual domains of quality of life: material and physical well-being; relationships with other people; social, community, and civic activities; personal development and fulfillment; and recreation. It is therefore conceptually distinct from causal indicators of health status, instead assessing subjective functioning across a range of human experiences.

Well-Being

Two of the more widely used scales of subjective well-being include the Satisfaction with Life Scale (SWLS; Diener, Emmons, Larsen, & Griffin, 1985) and the Psychological Well-Being Scale (PWB; Ryff & Singer, 1996). The SWLS is a brief five-item measure that assesses global life satisfaction, and the PWB assesses six dimensions of well-being. These two scales assess well-being from two different philosophical traditions: the PWB scale draws from a eudaimonic tradition that includes engagement with existential challenges with life, and the SWL scale draws on a hedonic tradition that incorporates those affective states associated with life satisfaction (Joseph et al., 2011).

Factors That Contribute to Resilient Functioning: Self-Report

A measurement strategy that addresses both the functional and the adaptive components of resilience should be integrated with a third measurement strategy for assessing *factors that may contribute* to a resilient outcome. These factors, such as personality, worldviews, positive emotionality, and coping styles, may contribute to a resilient outcome but alone are not sufficient to identify a resilient trajectory. A number of self-report, observer-rated, performance-based, and implicit measures exist that assess these various factors are reviewed in the following sections.

Ego Resiliency

The construct of ego resiliency (ER) is a theoretically driven formulation of a trait view that conceptualizes resiliency as the capacity for flexible adaption to stressors (Block & Kremen, 1996; Klohnen, 1996). More specifically, ego resiliency refers to the capacity to modify self-expression based on changing contextual demands through behavioral flexibility, a broad use of problem-solving skills, and the ability to up- or down-regulate arousal to meet the immediate needs presented by a specific context (Letzring, Block, & Funder, 2005). ER encompasses principles of flexibility, resourceful adaptation to life's stressors and novel situations, and regulation of impulses, factors that are consistent with other studies demonstrating similar qualities associated with resiliency (Bonanno, Papa, Lalande, Westphal, & Coifman, 2004; Consedine, Magai, & Bonanno, 2002).

ER is commonly assessed by a 14-item measure called the Ego Resiliency Scale (ER-89; Block & Kreman, 1996). More recently, the ER-89 Scale was reduced to a 10-item scale by eliminating four items with lower reliability (ER89-R; Alessandri, Vecchione, Caprara, & Letzring, 2012). The ER-89 has been widely validated (Block & Kreman, 1996; Funder & Block, 1989), including among Kuwati Arab students six years after the Gulf War concluded (Al-Naser & Sandman, 2000) and among Spanish and Italian populations (Alessandri et al., 2012). Recent twin studies have identified a genetically determined association between ER-89 assessed resiliency and mental health outcomes among a sample of 1,394 Norwegian twin families (Waaktaar & Torgersen, 2012). Finally, emerging evidence suggests that persons who score highly on ego resiliency display less brain activity in the insula when recovering from a threat cue (Waugh, Wager, Fredrickson, Noll, & Taylor, 2008). The insula is a region in the cerebral cortex associated with sensory representations (Martin, 2003).

Ego Strength

The Ego Strength (Es) Scale is a supplementary MMPI scale that contains items originally developed on a clinical sample of patients who demonstrated response to psychotherapy (Barron, 1953). The scale was conceptualized as a measure of adaptability, personal resourcefulness, and effective interpersonal functioning. In response to concerns raised by subsequent analysis (Colligan & Offord, 1987; Colligan, Osborne, Swenson, & Offord, 1983), revisions of the scale resulted in a measure with fewer items that suggested improved psychometric properties and demonstrated expected relationships with psychological health (Schuldberg, 1992). Other studies have suggested a relationship between high Es scores, fewer reported mental health symptoms, and increased ability to cope with stress (Graham, Ben-Porath, & McNulty, 1997).

Connor–Davidson Resilience Scale

A second commonly used self-report scale of resiliency is the 25-item Connor–Davidson Resilience Scale (CD-RISC; Connor & Davidson, 2003). Items were generated atheoretically from a number of sources to include Kobasa's (1979) construct of hardiness, Rutter's theory of resilience (Rutter, 1985), and a descriptive account of Sir Edward Shackleton's 1912 Antarctic expedition (Connor & Davidson, 2003). Problematically, this scale is not theoretically generated, and it is therefore less clear exactly what construct this scale is measuring, outside of a collection of descriptive correlates of asymptomatic functioning (see Bonanno et al., 2011, and Mancini & Bonanno, 2010, for similar comments).

Despite these limitations, the CD-RISC is broadly utilized, particularly in medical settings. Campbell-Sills and Stein (2007) have modified the original 24-item scale using three undergraduate samples, resulting in a unidimensional 10-item scale that appears to display comparable internal reliability (alpha = .85) to the 24-item scale and factor loadings ranging from .44 (*able to adapt to change*) to .74 (*think of self as strong person*). In addition to the 10-item scale, a 2-item brief screening instrument was developed (CD-RISC-2; Vaishnavi, Connor, & Davidson, 2007). Connor and Davidson selected the two scale items because they "etymologically capture the essence of resilience" (*able to adapt to change*) and (*tend to bounce back after illness or hardship*) (Vaishnavi et al., 2007, p. 294).

Resilience Scale for Adults

The Resilience Scale for Adults (RSA; Friborg, Hjemdal, Rosenvinge, & Martinussen, 2003) was developed by Norwegian researchers and was designed to measure the presence of protective resources that promote adult resilience. The authors sought to assess three classes of protective features associated with the ability to sustain normal development despite the presence of stressors: psychological/dispositional attributes, family support, and external support systems (Garmezy, 1991). The scale therefore departs from personality-based scales assessing resiliency as a trait, such as the ER-89 and CD-RISC, and instead integrates assessment of features of a resilient personality with protective factors such as social and family support. The first scale contained 45 items (Friborg et al., 2003) and was later revised and validated on both a community and an outpatient sample (Hjemdal et al., 2011). The final scale consisted of 37 items and replicated the five-factor structure of the original 45-item measure.

Subsequent analyses of the psychometric properties of the RSA yielded a reliability coefficient for each subscale, with alphas ranging from .67 to .90, and 4-month test–retest reliability for each factor spanning .69 to .84 among a community sample (Friborg et al., 2003). The scale has since been validated among a Persian sample, demonstrating both the same five-factor structure originally identified in the Norwegian sample and similar reliability in addition to accurate differentiation between college students and runaway girls (Jowkar, Friborg, & Hjemdal, 2010). In an experimental laboratory procedure, high-RSA individuals reported lower subjective pain in high-stress conditions when compared to those in the low-RSA group (Friborg et al., 2006).

Five-Factor Model of Personality

Many studies have examined resilience from the perspective of the five-factor model (FFM; Costa & McCrae, 1992). Given the typically adaptive qualities associated with resiliency, it is not surprising that resilient personality profiles are characterized by higher than average scores on all five dimensions of the FFM. Converging findings generally identify a profile consistent with high scores on Agreeableness, Extraversion, Openness, and Conscientiousness, and low scores on Neuroticism (Cumberland-Li, Eisenberg, & Reiser, 2004; Davey, Eaker, & Walters, 2003; Riolli, Savicki, & Cepani, 2002; Torgersen & Vollrath, 2006). Laboratory findings offer convergence: Williams, Rau, Cribbet, and Gunn (2009) found that higher scores on Openness was associated not only with a slight increase in positive affect during a laboratory stressor, but also with reduced blood pressure reactivity and increases in respiratory sinus arrhythmia. Furthermore, participants who endorsed greater levels of Openness demonstrated reduced heart reactivity while discussing a stressful event in a laboratory condition.

Waaktaar and Torgersen (2010) conducted one of the few studies examining whether resilience scales could estimate adjustment above and beyond that predicted by the FFM Big Five traits. Specifically, the authors found that ER-89 assessed resilience contributed a significant amount of explained variance to models predicting life satisfaction, loneliness, caring relationships, meaningful opportunities, and school connectedness and satisfaction among adolescents. However, the same study reported that the Resilience Scale (RS; Wagnild & Young, 1993) did not offer incremental validity to that predicted by FFM with respect to adjustment (Waaktaar & Torgersen, 2010). Results suggest some variability in the performance of resilience scales compared to FFM traits.

Inventory of Interpersonal Strengths

Emerging evidence suggesting the importance of the protective role of social support indicates that interpersonal resources are correlates of adaptive functioning. The Inventory of Interpersonal Strengths (IIS-64; Hatcher & Rogers, 2009) is a 64-item self-report measure based on the interpersonal circle (Leary, 1957). This instrument was created by recasting the original circumplex descriptors of interpersonal functioning into positive descriptors. It has recently been revised into a briefer 34-item instrument that retains the original properties of the 64-item measure (Hatcher & Rogers, 2012). Initial validation suggested that the IIS added predictive validity over and above the relative absence of interpersonal distress, supporting theorists who suggest that deficits are not the opposite of strengths (Horowitz, 2004).

Emotion Regulation: Self-Report

Mounting findings suggest that various aspects of emotional functioning are associated with resiliency. For example, a rare prospective assessment of resilience following the September 11th terrorist attacks suggested positive emotions such as gratitude, interest, and love mediated the predictive relationship between precrisis trait resilience and depressive symptoms postcrisis (Fredrickson, Tugade, Waugh, & Larkin, 2003). Further studies suggest that positive emotionality may provide a buffer against the negative impact of traumatic events (Ong, Fuller-Rowell, & Bonanno, 2010). Relatedly, accumulating evidence suggests that cognitive reappraisal strategies are effective means of reducing arousal in response to negative stimuli (Ayduk & Kross, 2010; Kross, Davidson, Weber, & Ochsner, 2009; Ong, Fuller-Rowell, & Bonanno, 2010). Finally, emotional suppression has been linked with increased severity of PTSD symptoms (Boden, Bonn-Miller, Kashdan, Alvarez, & Gross, 2012).

Emotion Regulation Questionnaire

The Emotion Regulation Questionnaire (ERQ; Gross & John, 2003) is a 10-item self-report questionnaire scaled on a 7-point spread. It is designed to assess individual differences in the habitual use of cognitive reappraisal and expressive suppression. Psychometric analyses support the hypothesized two-factor structure: a *reappraisal* factor demonstrating good reliability (alpha = .80) and a suppression factor producing adequate reliability (alpha = .73). Though not widely used in the clinical context, it has demonstrated the ability to identify a group of military veterans who show lower PTSD severity as a result of the increased use of cognitive reappraisal and reduced alexithymia (Boden, Bonn-Miller, Kashdan, Alvarez, & Gross, 2012). Preliminary analyses suggest that this clinical tool may be useful in identifying mechanisms of resilience in a trauma-exposed population and that it accordingly warrants further research.

Coping: Self-Report

Another important feature of resilient adjustment following a traumatic stressor involves individual differences in coping, with some specific forms of coping identified as particularly relevant. Skodol (2010) distinguishes between trait resilience and coping styles, separating from one another by the extent to which they represent stable patterns of functioning across different contexts. For example, personality characteristics are relatively enduring qualities that may influence the extent to which particular coping strategies are available across varying contexts. The following section reviews instruments that are developed to assess two specific coping strategies linked with resilient trajectories: flexible/pragmatic coping and repressive coping.

Perceived Ability to Cope with Trauma Scale

The Perceived Ability to Cope with Trauma Scale (PACT; Bonanno, Pat-Horenczyk, & Noll, 2011) is a theoretically derived two-factor scale that integrates seemingly disparate perspectives on coping with PTEs. Both of these perspectives show strong support for the advantages of deliberate focus on the trauma itself (Foa & Kozak, 1986; Gortner, Rude, & Pennebaker, 2006; Smyth, Pennebaker, & Arigo, 2012) as well as benefits associated with minimizing trauma focus using distraction or avoidance (for reviews, see Bonanno, 2004). These seemingly disparate strategies are integrated through a hypothesized flexibility mechanism which proposes that the ability to flexibly utilize both coping strategies predicts adjustment to PTEs (Bonanno, Pat-Horenczyk, & Noll, 2011).

In order to develop an instrument that might be more practical for use in large samples and the field, Bonanno et al. (2011) developed a measure that explicitly measures beliefs about one's ability to use different types of coping strategies. By not assessing specific coping strategies, this measure avoids confounds introduced by retrospective bias. The scale is scored using a previously utilized algorithm that combines sum and discrepancy scores into a single variable (Thompson & Zanna, 1995). The calculation involves a multistep process by which a coping polarity score (the absolute value of the discrepancy between the standardized scores for each scale) is subtracted from the sum coping ability score (the sum of the standardized scores from each of the two factors). The authors found that the polarity score, which represents the extremes of either coping style relative to the other, was positively correlated with posttraumatic stress severity, suggesting that overreliance on any one strategy may be associated with posttraumatic stress (Bonanno et al., 2011).

Repressive Coping Style

A second type of coping style associated with resilient adjustment is repressive coping. A growing body of literature suggests that individuals who employ coping mechanisms that minimize negative affect by avoiding threatening stimuli while simultaneously experiencing increased physiological arousal experience resilient outcomes (Hock & Krohne, 2004; Tomarken & Davidson, 1994; Weinberger, Schwartz, & Davidson, 1979). Among bereaved men, for example, individuals who reported fewer clinical symptoms associated with the death of a partner and also demonstrated increased heart rate and skin conductance while describing their emotions demonstrated improved adjustment to loss compared to the nonrepressors over time (Bonanno, Keltner, Holen, & Horowitz, 1995). Because repression is a largely automatic process and requires little cognitive resources, one hypothesized mechanism is that repressive copers ease the threatening nature of stimuli by undergoing cognitive reappraisal, involving construing a stimulus in a way that changes its emotional impact (Folkman, Lazarus, Dunkel-Schetter, DeLongis, & Gruen, 1986; Lazarus & Alfert, 1964; Olff, Langeland, & Gersons, 2005).

Repressive coping is measured through use of a self-report questionnaire developed by Weinberger et al. (1979) that combines a scale of manifest anxiety (Taylor Manifest Anxiety Scale; Taylor, 1953) with a measure of defensiveness (the Marlowe–Crowne Social Desirability Scale; Crowne & Marlowe, 1960). The combined final scale consists of 58 items and is scored by comparing respondents' responses across the two scales with a median value. For example, repressors are those whose anxiety score is lower than a median level in a normal population and whose defensiveness score is higher than the median. Repressive coping has been associated with fewer PTSD symptoms among Israeli volunteers who handled bodies injured in a disaster (Solomon, Berger, & Ginzburg, 2007).

Knowledgeable-Informant Ratings

Knowledgeable-informant strategies are commonly employed to overcome the limits associated with self-report and are frequently employed in the clinical setting to assess trauma-related psychiatric symptoms (Litz et al., 2011; Litz, Penk, Gerardi, & Keane, 1992). In other settings, knowledgeable-informant ratings have been completed by friends of the trauma-exposed individual and those ratings have demonstrated high reliability and convergent validity (Bonanno, Rennicke, & Dekel, 2005). For example, among friends and relatives who rated the adjustment of individuals in or near the World Trade Center during the September 11th terrorist attacks, correct matches between friend and relative ratings and clinical assessment was achieved in 8 out of 10 resilient participants (Bonanno, Rennicke, et al., 2005). In another study of bereaved spouses, friends provided higher ratings of adjustment among resilient individuals before and after the loss compared to other bereaved individuals (Bonanno, Moskowitz, Papa, & Folkman, 2005). Taken together, results suggest that resilient individuals tend to maintain a characteristic level of healthy functioning even in the aftermath of loss. The promising reliability and validity of friend ratings suggests that a multimethod battery would benefit from including knowledgeable-informant ratings.

How can knowledgeable-informant ratings be obtained? One approach that has been employed by Bonanno, Rennicke, et al. (2005) is to provide persons who have experienced an acute stressor with stamped and addressed envelopes that include a brief measure of functioning. The participants give these measures to friends or family who know them well, and they are asked to complete and return them. The value of friend/family ratings of functioning is considerable, offering information on whether their perceptions are consistent with those of the client.

Performance-Based and Implicit Assessment of Resilience

Very little research effort has focused on implicit processes in resilience, including assessment measures that employ performance-based techniques. Given the mixed findings and controversy that characterizes performance-based techniques, it is no surprise that this assessment approach has not been explored more broadly in the context of resilience (Lilienfeld, Wood, & Garb, 2000). However, a review of the empirical literature suggests that specific indices of the Rorschach Inkblot Method (RIM) have demonstrated adequate empirical support to warrant reliable and valid assessment (Bornstein, 2007, 2012; Mihura, Meyer, Dumitrascu, & Bombel, 2013). The use of perfomance-based tasks in personality assessment rests on the assumption that ambiguous stimuli activate psycholgical structures that tend to produce specific patterns of thinking, feeling, and behaving. The generation of a meaningful percept from an ambiguous stimulus is a multistep process involving various stages of directed attention and self-monitoring (Bornstein, 2009).

A specific advantage of incorporating implicit and performance-based measures from the multimethod perspective is that a number of studies have demonstrated that these measures introduce incremental validity in the assessment of real-world behaviors, the prediction of which is especially important when assessing resiliency. More specifically, implicit assessment can be better at predicting operant behavior, whereas self-attributed (self-report) measures are typically better at predicting cognitively guided behavior such as choice, attributions, and values (McClelland, 1985). McClelland suggested that implicit motives tend to sustain behavioral trends over time (operant act frequency), whereas self-attributed motives tend to predict reactions to structured situations where cognitively based choices serve as a determinant (respondent behaviors). For example, McClelland, Koestner, and Weinberger (1989) found that college students who described themselves as achievement oriented in a self-report measure performed best on a word recall task in the presence of an external social incentive compared to those low in self-attributed achievement orientation. Second, those inviduals high in performance-based achievement (assessed using the Thematic Aperception Test) perfomed better on puzzles with increasing difficulty, whereas those with lower scores performed no better. Similar effects have been demonstrated with power motivation (McClelland, 1985). Likewise, among inpatient borderline invividuals, dependency as assessed by the Rorschach Oral Dependency Scale (ROD; Masling, Rabie, & Blondheim, 1967) demonstrated superior prediction of help-seeking behaviors compared to predication generated by a measure of self-attributed dependency (Fowler, Brunnschweiler, Swales, & Brock, 2005).

Performance-Based Assessment: The RIM

Although the research on Rorschach-assessed resilient functioning in the aftermath of a PTE has been sparse, initial case studies suggest that further research may be warranted (Odendaal, Brink, & Theron, 2011; Viglione, 1990; Viglione & Kates, 1997). One case study of an 11-year-old child recently experiencing a PTE incorporated a longitudinal design across three assessment periods: 7 months after the initial assessment and then again at a 4-year follow up (Viglione, 1990). Clinical and behavioral observations confirmed that the child was not presenting with clinical impairment, though his initial Rorschach battery contained several indicators of pathology. These initial indicators were reduced by the next administration and at a four-year follow up declined further. Results are consistent with resilience hypotheses suggesting that resilient individuals may experience internal distress associated with exposure to a PTE, but they are able to maintain functioning. Viglione (1990) cautioned that contradictory and confusing data reflected in a Rorschach protocol administered after exposure to a trauma may lead clinicians to overdiagnose psychopathology among individuals who have recently experienced a PTE. Furthermore, complexity in a Rorschach record to include responses to the trauma (e.g., morbid responses, high trauma index) may function as indicators of resilience when assessed postexposure because openness to experience and the ability to tolerate some internal disorganization may be features of resilient mechanisms.

Further studies have examined the use of the Rorschach to detect resilience among military veterans. Among combat-exposed individuals without PTSD symptoms and a comparison group of combat-exposed veterans with PTSD, the non-PTSD group reported less traumatic content responses to the Rorschach, in addition to decelerated heart rate when producing combat-related content responses (Goldfinger, Amdur, & Liberzon, 1998). Interestingly, when combat controls were producing diffuse shading (Y) responses (associated with stress-related feelings; Weiner, 2003) or combat-related content, they displayed a drop in heart rate. Taken in consideration with previous findings demonstrating heart rate deceleration during tasks of sustained attention, the authors suggested that combat controls who demonstrate resistance to PTSD may have the ability to evoke a state of sustained attention during anxiety-provoking tasks (Goldfinger et al., 1998).

Implicit Assessment: The Implicit Associations Test

Social cognitive perspectives have accrued ample evidence to suggest that social behavior operates under implicit or unconscious influences that can be reliably assessed (Greenwald & Banaji, 1995; Kihlstrom, 1994). The Implicit Association Test (IAT; Greenwald, McGhee, & Schwartz, 1998) is widely used and is based on the underlying assumption that when two concepts are strongly associated, processing time associated with a sorting task is reduced, resulting in faster reaction times (Greenwald et al., 2002). The IAT has demonstrated the ability to predict stereotype influences on performance such as voting behavior (Greenwald, Smith, Sriram, Bar-Anan, & Nosek, 2009), condom use (Czopp, Monteith, Zimmerman, & Lynam, 2004), and performance anxiety (Egloff & Schmukle, 2002) among others (see Greenwald et al., 2009, for a review). A meta-analysis of predictive validity of the IAT concluded that the IAT demonstrated average ($r = .27$) prediction of behavioral, judgment, and physiological measures. Parallel self-report measures also demonstrated predictive validity ($r = .36$), but with more variability. However, in circumstances of social sensitivity or where impression management is important, IAT exceeded self-report measures in predictive validity (Greenwald et al., 2009).

Some studies have employed the IAT to assess resilience (Ihaya, Yamada, Kawabe, & Nakamura, 2010; Xi, Zuo, & Sang, 2011). In one study conducted on 24 Japanese undergraduate and graduate students, researchers measured the reaction time of attitudes toward targets that represented different types of social support (Ihaya et al., 2010). The study hypothesized that resilience represented both recognition and utilization of social resources (Ihaya & Nakamura, 2008). Results suggested significant group differences in IAT performance between high- and low-resilient groups across recognition conditions (family, friend, or companion). Specifically, participants who explicitly answered that they did not consider companions as sources of support (e.g., low resilient in this study) associated those same targets with calm attitudes in the IAT. Results are difficult to interpret given the operationalization of resilience as an ability to rely on others for social support, but nonetheless provide preliminary evidence suggesting individual differences in attitudes toward social support among resilient versus nonresilient individuals.

A second study compared observed, self-assessed, and implicit competence among 523 children between grades 3 and 8 (Xi et al., 2011). The study identified resilient children based on psychosocial functioning in the context of reported stress and adversity. Resilient children demonstrated significantly shorter reaction times to competence terms (e.g., independence) in a self-congruent condition compared to nonresilient children.

Results suggest that individuals who demonstrate resilience in stressful and adverse conditions are not falsely describing themselves as overconfident or avoiding negative symptoms, but rather are drawing upon stable resources of competence and efficacy in order to demonstrate resilient outcomes (Xi et al., 2011).

Psychophysiological Assessment

Given the mounting evidence suggesting unique patterns of physiological arousal between PTSD and trauma-exposed individuals, it appears that more widespread use of these instruments could increase accurate differentiation of trauma-exposed individuals (Goldfinger et al., 1998). However, psychophysiological markers of PTSD and asymptomatic trauma are not widely used in clinical assessment. Although limitations in the clinical setting typically restrict the extent to which these measures can be used, some evidence suggests that psychophysiological measures can offer incremental validity to predicting outcome after a PTE.

One group-design study compared psychophysiological markers among veterans diagnosed with PTSD, psychiatric inpatients with non-PTSD disorders, and combat-exposed veterans with no clinical symptoms (Malloy, Fairbank, & Keane, 1983). Using behavioral, psychophysiological, and self-report measures of PTSD results demonstrated that psychophysiological markers of heart rate arousal and skin conductance accurately discriminated between the three study groups. Behavioral measures of seconds taken to terminate viewing of combat videotapes revealed that the PTSD group terminated the tape in 8 of 10 cases, compared to no terminations among the asymptomatic or psychiatric comparison groups. Additionally, the combat videotape elicited significantly higher heart rates among PTSD veterans than among the other two study groups. Finally, the PTSD group also reported increased fear compared to the two other study groups. Discriminant analyses resulted in 100% accurate classification of the PTSD individuals when psychophysiological, self-report, and behavioral indicators were used in concert. However, the authors did not evaluate the incremental validity of each assessment approach to distinguishing groups. Therefore, no interpretations can be made as to the relative benefit of one assessment approach over the other.

Integrating Multimethod Resilience Data

Integration of data from multiple modalities is the defining feature of multimethod assessment and requires that information must be combined in a meaningful way (Blais & Baity, 2008; Campbell & Fiske, 1959). In the specific case of resilience, assessment data obtained from self-report, knowledgeable informants, and performance-based measures provide incremental data about symptomatic functioning, adaptive functioning, and contributing factors that accurately identify the resilient trajectory only when considered together (see Table 9.1). For example, high self-report resiliency combined with high levels of semistructured clinical interview-assessed PTSD symptomatology would not meet the definitional criteria for an individual displaying a resilient trajectory.

The different modalities outlined in this chapter complement each other in the accurate identification of resilient individuals. For example, self-report and knowledgeable-informant data, when used in combination, are better than either used in isolation because together they provide converging lines of evidence for resilience defined by observable functioning (Bonanno, 2004) and self-attributed ability to cope with adversity (Luthar et al., 2000). Similarly, the combination of self-report and performance-based data is superior to either method used in isolation (Blais & Baity, 2008). For example, when performance data capturing the ability to perceive support (Ihaya et al., 2010) is combined with self-report data that appraises the ability to effectively recruit that support (e.g., Hatcher & Rogers, 2009), assessments more accurately represent resilience functioning.

Challenges Facing Multimethod Assessment

We have reviewed the advantages of a multimethod approach to the assessment of resilience, addressing the incremental validity that self-report, observer, and performance-based measures provide in accurately capturing the resilient trajectory. We have argued that such an approach advances both clinical and theoretical conceptualizations of functioning after extremely aversive events. However, the widespread use of multimethod assessment faces substantial hurdles that must be faced if this approach is to gain currency. Specific obstacles include resource burden, potential lack of compensation, training requirements, and assessee (those individuals going through the assessmenet process) fatigue.

First, although psychological interventions that treat mental illness have seen remarkable advances in the past decade, the existing systems that deliver care are overburdened and reach only a relative minority of those suffering (Kazdin & Blase, 2011). Those resource limitations include a lack of access to full assessment, with few clinics equipped to provide the financial and clinical resources necessary to conduct a multimethod battery. However, the advances being made in other clinical populations suggest that a resolution to this dilemma lies in the near future. For example, Widiger and Samuel (2005) provide a foundation for developing evidence-based guidelines for assessing personality disorders that may have potential applicability in assessing resilience.

Second, managed care has resulted in increased restrictions of reimbursable mental health services. Personality assessment is among the most affected service, with requirements for a shift from lengthy measures to symptom-focused brief instruments (Piotrowski, 1999). However, research is reversing this trend through empirical validation, as in the case of studies demonstrating the utility of personality assessment in developing empirically guided treatment planning and intervention (Ben-Porath, 1997). As a result of such studies, fair compensation for assessment has seen some advances. Furthermore, gains in this area are seen as a result of the mental health parity law and ongoing advocacy.

Third, adequate training for graduate students in multimethod assessment is essential. However, surveys have found that while graduate programs continue to emphasize training in psychological assessment, some declines in these programs have been noted. This may leave students inadequately prepared to meet expectations while on internship (Belter & Piotrowski, 2001). To address this emerging gap in assessment training, Krishnamurthy et al. (2004) outlined a number of recommendations that would improve the preparation of graduate students to conduct psychological assessment, including multimethod assessment. If applied to multimethod assessment, execution of these recommendations could strengthen the skills of the next generation of personality assessors.

Finally, assessee fatigue is a fourth issue that multimethod assessment approaches must address if continued advances are to be made. In this domain as well, gains in related assessment techniques suggest possible solutions for multimethod assessment. For example, techniques employed in therapeutic assessment (Finn, 2007) that emphasize the assessor–client relationship by encouraging active client participation in all phases of assessment, including determination of goals, interpretation of test results, and communicating test results alter the traditional paradigm whereby individuals are passive recipients of multiple batteries over which they have relatively little ownership. Re-envisioning the role of assessee in the multimethod process holds promise for reducing the untoward consequences of lengthy batteries, such as assessee fatigue.

REFERENCES

Al-Naser, F., & Sandman, M. (2000). Evaluating resiliency patterns using the ER-89: A case study from Kuwait. *Social Behavior and Personality, 28*, 505–514.

Alessandri, G., Vecchione, M., Caprara, G., & Letzring, T. D. (2012). The Ego Resiliency Scale revised: A crosscultural study in Italy, Spain, and the United States. *European Journal of Psychological Assessment, 28*, 139–146.

American Psychiatric Association. (2000). *Diagnostic and statistical manual of mental disorders* (4th ed., text rev.). Washington, DC: Author.

Ayduk, Ö., & Kross, E. (2010). Analyzing negative experiences without ruminating: The role of self-distancing in enabling adaptive self-reflection. *Social and Personality Psychology Compass, 4*, 841–854.

Barlow, D. H., & Wolfe, B. E. (1981). Behavioral approaches to anxiety disorders: A report on the NIMH-SUNY, Albany, Research Conference. *Journal of Consulting and Clinical Psychology, 49,* 448–454.

Barron, F. (1953). An ego-strength scale which predicts response to psychotherapy. *Journal of Consulting Psychology, 17,* 327–333.

Beck, A. T. (1961). *Beck Depression Inventory.* Philadelphia: Center for Cognitive Therapy.

Beck, A. T., Steer, R. A., & Carbin, M. G. (1998). Psychometric properties of the Beck Depression Inventory: Twenty-five years of evaluation. *Clinical Psychology Review, 8,* 77–100.

Belter, R. W., & Piotrowski, C. (2001). Current status of doctoral-level training in psychological testing. *Journal of Clinical Psychology, 57,* 717–726.

Ben-Porath, Y. S. (1997). Use of personality assessment instruments in empirically guided treatment planning. *Psychological Assessment, 9,* 361–367.

Berzon, R. A., Donnelly, M. A., Simpson, R. L., Simeon, G. P., & Tilson, H. H. (1995). Bibliography: Quality of life bibliography and indexes: 1994 update. *Quality of Life Research, 4,* 547–569.

Blais, M. A., & Baity, M. R. (2008). The projective assessment of personality structure and pathology. In G. J. Boyle & G. Matthews (Eds.), *The Sage handbook of personality theory and testing* (Vol. 2: Personality Measurement and Testing, pp. 556–586). Thousand Oaks, CA: Sage.

Blais, M. A., Hilsenroth, M. J., Castlebury, F., Fowler, J. C., & Baity, M. R. (2001). Predicting DMS-IV cluster B personality disorder criteria from MMPI-2 and Rorschach data: A test of incremental validity. *Journal of Personality Assessment, 76,* 150–168.

Blake, D. D., Weathers, F. W., Nagy, L. M., Kaloupek, D. G., Gusman, F. D., Charney, D. S., et al. (1995). The development of a clinician-administered PTSD scale. *Journal of Traumatic Stress, 8,* 75–90.

Blanchard, E. B., Jones-Alexander, J., Buckley, T. C., & Forneris, C. A. (1996). Psychometric properties of the PTSD checklist (PCL). *Behaviour Research and Therapy, 34,* 669–673.

Block, J., & Kremen, A. M. (1996). IQ and ego-resiliency: Conceptual and empirical connections and separateness. *Journal of Personality and Social Psychology, 70,* 349–361.

Boden, M. T., Bonn-Miller, M. O., Kashdan, T. B., Alvarez, J., & Gross, J. J. (2012). The interactive effects of emotional clarity and cognitive reappraisal in posttraumatic stress disorder. *Journal of Anxiety Disorders, 26,* 233–238.

Bonanno, G. A. (2004). Loss, trauma, and human resilience: Have we underestimated the human capacity to thrive after extremely aversive events? *American Psychologist, 59,* 20–28.

Bonanno, G. A. (2012). Uses and abuses of the resilience construct: Loss, trauma, and health-related adversities. *Social Science and Medicine, 74,* 753–756.

Bonanno, G. A., Brewin, C. R., Kaniasty, K., & Greca, A. M. L. (2010). Weighing the costs of disaster: Consequences, risks, and resilience in individuals, families, and communities. *Psychological Science in the Public Interest, 11,* 1–49.

Bonanno, G. A., Galea, S., Bucciarelli, A., & Vlahov, D. (2007). What predicts psychological resilience after disaster?: The role of demographics, resources, and life stress. *Journal of Consulting and Clinical Psychology, 75,* 671–682.

Bonanno, G. A., Ho, S. M. Y., Chan, J. C. K., Kwong, R. S. Y., Cheung, C. K. Y., Wong, C. P. Y., et al. (2008). Psychological resilience and dysfunction among hospitalized survivors of the SARS epidemic in Hong Kong: A latent class approach. *Health Psychology, 27,* 659–667.

Bonanno, G. A., Keltner, D., Holen, A., & Horowitz, M. J. (1995). When avoiding unpleasant emotions might not be such a bad thing: Verbal autonomic response dissociation and midlife conjugal bereavement. *Journal of Personality and Social Psychology, 69,* 975–989.

Bonanno, G. A., Kennedy, P., Galatzer-Levy, I. R., Lude, P., & Elfström, M. L. (2012). Trajectories of resilience, depression, and anxiety following spinal cord injury. *Rehabilitation Psychology, 57,* 236–247.

Bonanno, G, A., Mancini, A. D., Horton, J. L., Powell, T. M., Leardmann, C. A., Boyko, E. J., et al. (2012). Trajectories of trauma symptoms and resilience in deployed U.S. military service members: Prospective cohort study. *British Journal of Psychiatry: Journal of Mental Science, 200,* 317–323.

Bonanno, G. A., Moskowitz, J. T., Papa, A., & Folkman, S. (2005). Resilience to loss in bereaved spouses, bereaved parents, and bereaved gay men. *Journal of Personality and Social Psychology, 88,* 827–843.

Bonanno, G. A., Papa, A., Lalande, K., Westphal, M., & Coifman, K. (2004). The importance of being flexible: The ability to both enhance and suppress emotional expression predicts long-term adjustment. *Psychological Science, 15,* 482–487.

Bonanno, G. A., Pat-Horenczyk, R., & Noll, J. (2011). Coping flexibility and trauma: The Perceived Ability to Cope with Trauma (PACT) scale. *Psychological Trauma: Theory, Research, Practice, and Policy, 3,* 117–129.

Bonanno, G. A., Rennicke, C., & Dekel, S. (2005). Self-enhancement among high-exposure survivors of the September 11th terrorist attack: Resilience or social maladjustment? *Journal of Personality and Social Psychology, 88,* 984–998.

Bonanno, G. A., Westphal, M., & Mancini, A. D. (2011). Resilience to loss and potential trauma. *Annual Review of Clinical Psychology, 7,* 511–535.

Bonanno, G. A., Wortman, C. B., Lehman, D. R., Tweed, R. G., Haring, M., Sonnega, J., et al. (2002). Resilience to loss and chronic grief: A prospective study from preloss to 18-months postloss. *Journal of Personality and Social Psychology, 83,* 1150–1164.

Bornstein, R. F. (2007). Might the Rorschach be a projective test after all?: Social projection of an undesired trait alters Rorschach oral dependency scores. *Journal of Personality Assessment, 88,* 354–367.

Bornstein, R. F. (2009). Heisenberg, Kandinsky, and the heteromethod convergence problem: Lessons from within and beyond psychology. *Journal of Personality Assessment, 91,* 1–8.

Bornstein, R. F. (2012). Rorschach score validation as a model for 21st-century personality assessment. *Journal of Personality Assessment, 94,* 26–38.

Campbell, D. T., & Fiske, D. W. (1959). Convergent and discriminant validation by the multitrait-multi-method matrix. *Psychological Bulletin, 56,* 81–105.

Campbell-Sills, L., & Stein, M. B. (2007). Psychometric analysis and refinement of the Connor–Davidson Resilience Scale (CD-RISC): Validation of a 10-item measure of resilience. *Journal of Traumatic Stress, 20,* 1019–1028.

Charuvastra, A., & Cloitre, M. (2008). Social bonds and posttraumatic stress disorder. *Annual Review of Psychology, 59,* 301–328.

Colligan, R. C., & Offord, K. P. (1987). Resiliency reconsidered: Contemporary MMPI normative data for Barron's Ego Strength Scale. *Journal of Clinical Psychology, 43,* 467–472.

Colligan, R. C., Osborne, D., Swenson, W. M., & Offord K. P. (1983). *The MMPI: A contemporary normative study.* New York: Praeger.

Connor, K. M., & Davidson, J. R. T. (2003). Development of a new resilience scale: The Connor–Davidson Resilience Scale (CD-RISC). *Depression and Anxiety, 18,* 76–82.

Consedine, N. S., Magai, C., & Bonanno, G. A. (2002). Moderators of the emotion inhibition–health relationship: A review and research agenda. *Review of General Psychology, 6,* 204–228.

Costa, P. T., & McCrae, R. R. (1992). Normal personality assessment in clinical practice: The NEO Personality Inventory. *Psychological Assessment, 4,* 5–13.

Crowne, D. P., & Marlowe, D. A. (1960). A new scale of social desirability independent of psychopathology. *Journal of Consulting Psychology, 24,* 349–354.

Cumberland-Li, A., Eisenberg, N., & Reiser, M. (2004). Relations of young children's agreeableness and resiliency to effortful control and impulsivity. *Social Development, 13,* 193–212.

Czopp, A. M., Monteith, M. J., Zimmerman, R. S., & Lynam, D. R. (2004). Implicit attitudes as potential protection from risky sex: Predicting condom use with the IAT. *Basic and Applied Social Psychology, 26,* 227–236.

Davey, M., Eaker, D. G. R., & Walters, L. H. (2003). Resilience processes in adolescents: Personality profiles, self-worth, and coping. *Journal of Adolescent Research, 18,* 347–362.

deRoon-Cassini, T. A., Mancini, A. D., Rusch, M. D., & Bonanno, G. A. (2010). Psychopathology and resilience following traumatic injury: A latent growth mixture model analysis. *Rehabilitation Psychology, 55,* 1–11.

Deshields, T., Tibbs, T., Fan, M. Y., & Taylor, M. (2006). Differences in patterns of depression after treatment for breast cancer. *Psycho-Oncology, 15,* 398–406.

Diener, E., Emmons, R. A., Larsen, R. J., & Griffin, S. (1985). The Satisfaction with Life Scale. *Journal of Personality Assessment, 49,* 71–75.

Dienstbier, R. A. (1989). Arousal and physiological toughness: Implications for mental and physical health. *Psychological Review, 96,* 84–100.

Duckworth, A. L., Peterson, C., Matthews, M. D., & Kelly, D. R. (2007). Grit: Perseverance and passion for long-term goals. *Journal of Personality and Social Psychology, 92,* 1087–1101.

Duckworth, A. L., Steen, T. A., & Seligman, M. E. (2005). Positive psychology in clinical practice. *Annual Review of Clinical Psychology, 1,* 629–651.

Egloff, B., & Schmukle, S. C. (2002). Predictive validity of an implicit association test for assessing anxiety. *Journal of Personality and Social Psychology, 83,* 1441–1455.

Finn, S. E. (2007). *In our clients' shoes: Theory and techniques of therapeutic assessment.* Mahwah, NJ: Erlbaum.

Fiori, K. L., & Denckla, C. A. (2012). Social support and mental health in middle-aged men and women: A multidimensional approach. *Journal of Aging and Health, 24,* 407–438.

First, M. B., Spitzer, R. L., Gibbon, M., & Janet, W. B. (2002). *Structured clinical interview for DSM-IV-TR Axis I Disorders.* New York: Biometrics Research, New York State Psychiatric Institute.

Flanagan, J. C. (1978). A research approach to improving our quality of life. *American Psychologist, 33,* 138–147.

Foa, E. B., & Kozak, M. J. (1986). Trauma focus of fear: Exposure to corrective information. *Psychological Bulletin, 99,* 20–35.

Folkman, S. L., Dunkel-Schetter, C., DeLongis, A., & Gruen, R. J. (1986). Dynamics of a stressful encounter: Cognitive appraisal, coping, and encounter outcomes. *Journal of Personality and Social Psychology, 50*, 992–1003.

Folkman, S., Lazarus, R. S., Dunkel-Schetter, C., DeLongis, A., & Gruen, R. J. (1986). Dynamics of a stressful encounter: Cognitive appraisal, coping, and encounter outcomes. *Journal of Personality and Social Psychology, 50*, 992–1003

Fowler, J. C., Brunnschweiler, B., Swales, S., & Brock, J. (2005). Assessment of Rorschach dependency measures in female inpatients diagnosed with borderline personality disorder. *Journal of Personality Assessment, 85*, 146–153.

Fredrickson, B. L., Tugade, M. M., Waugh, C. E., & Larkin, G. R. (2003). What good are positive emotions in crisis?: A prospective study of resilience and emotions following the terrorist attacks on the United States on September 11th, 2001. *Journal of Personality and Social Psychology, 84*, 365–376.

Friborg, O., Hjemdal, O., Rosenvinge, J. H., & Martinussen, M. (2003). A new rating scale for adult resilience: What are the central protective resources behind healthy adjustment? *International Journal of Methods in Psychiatric Research, 12*, 65–76.

Friborg, O., Hjemdal, O., Rosenvinge, J. H., Martinussen, M., Aslaksen, P. M., & Flaten, M. A. (2006). Resilience as a moderator of pain and stress. *Journal of Psychosomatic Research, 61*, 213–219.

Funder, D. C., & Block, J. (1989). The role of ego-control, ego-resiliency, and IQ in delay of gratification in adolescence. *Journal of Personality and Social Psychology, 57*, 1041–1050.

Garmezy, N. (1991). Resilience in children's adaptation to negative life events and stressed environments. *Pediatric Annals, 20*, 459–466.

Goldfinger, D. A., Amdur, R. L., & Liberzon, I. (1998). Psychophysiologic responses to the Rorschach in PTSD patients, noncombat and combat controls. *Depression and Anxiety, 8*, 112–120.

Gortner, E., Rude, S. S., & Pennebaker, J. W. (2006). Benefits of expressive writing in lowering rumination and depressive symptoms. *Behavior Therapy, 37*, 292–303.

Graham, J. R., Ben-Porath, Y. S., & McNulty, J. L. (1997). *MMPI-2 correlates for outpatient mental health settings.* Minneapolis: University of Minnesota Press.

Greenwald, A. G., & Banaji, M. R. (1995). Implicit social cognition: Attitudes, self-esteem, and stereotypes. *Psychological Review, 102*, 4–27.

Greenwald, A. G., Banaji, M. R, Rudman, L. A., Farnham, S. D., Nosek, B. A., & Mellott, D. S. (2002). A unified theory of implicit attitudes, stereotypes, self-esteem, and self-concept. *Psychological Review, 109*, 3–25.

Greenwald, A. G., McGhee, D. E., & Schwartz, J. L. K. (1998). Measuring individual differences in implicit cognition: The implicit association test. *Journal of Personality and Social Psychology, 74*, 1464–1480.

Greenwald, A. G., Poehlman, T. A., Uhlmann, E. L., & Banaji, M. R. (2009). Understanding and using the Implicit Association Test: III. Meta-analysis of predictive validity. *Journal of Personality and Social Psychology, 97*, 17–41.

Greenwald, A. G., Smith, C. T., Sriram, N., Bar-Anan, Y., & Nosek, B. A. (2009). Implicit race attitudes predicted vote in the 2008 U.S. presidential election. *Analyses of Social Issues and Public Policy, 9*, 241–253.

Grilo, C. M., Masheb, R. M., & Wilson, G. T. (2001). A comparison of different methods for assessing the features of eating disorders in patients with binge eating disorder. *Journal of Consulting and Clinical Psychology, 69*, 317–322.

Gross, J. J., & John, O. P. (2003). Individual differences in two emotion regulation processes: Implications for affect, relationships, and well-being. *Journal of Personality and Social Psychology, 85*, 348–362.

Hatcher, R. L., & Rogers, D. T. (2009). Development and validation of a measure of interpersonal strengths: The Inventory of Interpersonal Strengths. *Psychological Assessment, 21,* 554–569.

Hatcher, R. L., & Rogers, D. T. (2012). The IIS–32: A Brief Inventory of Interpersonal Strengths. *Journal of Personality Assessment, 94,* 638–646.

Hjemdal, O., Friborg, O., Braun, S., Kempenaers, C., Linkowski, P., & Fossion, P. (2011). The Resilience Scale for Adults: Construct validity and measurement in a Belgian sample. *International Journal of Testing, 11,* 53–70.

Hock, M. L., & Krohne, H. W. (2004). Coping with threat and memory for ambiguous information: Testing the repressive discontinuity hypothesis. *Emotion, 4,* 65–86.

Hopwood, C. J., Morey, L. C., Edelen, M. O., Shea, M. T., Grilo, C. M., Sanislow, C. A., et al. (2008). A comparison of interview and self-report methods for the assessment of borderline personality disorder criteria. *Psychological Assessment, 20,* 81–85.

Horowitz, L. M. (2004). *Interpersonal foundations of psychopathology.* Washington, DC: American Psychological Association.

Horowitz, M. J., Bonanno, G. A., & Holen, A. (1993). Pathological grief: Diagnosis and explanation. *Psychosomatic Medicine, 55,* 260–273.

Ihaya, K., & Nakamura, T. (2008). Four scales measuring four aspects of resilience: Understanding and utilization of intra- and inter-personal resources. *The Japanese Journal of Personality, 17,* 39–40.

Ihaya, K., Yamada, Y., Kawabe, T., & Nakamura, T. (2010). Implicit processing of environmental resources in psychological resilience *Psychologica, 53,* 102–113.

Joseph, S., Maltby, J., Wood, A. M., Stockton, H., Hunt, N., & Regel, S. (2011). The Psychological Well-Being–Post-Traumatic Changes Questionnaire (PWB-PTCQ): Reliability and validity. *Psychological Trauma: Theory, Research, Practice, and Policy.* 4, 420–428.

Jowkar, B., Friborg, O., & Hjemdal, O. (2010). Cross-cultural validation of the Resilience Scale for Adults (RSA) in Iran. *Scandinavian Journal of Psychology, 51,* 418–425.

Kazdin, A. E., & Blase, S. L. (2011). Rebooting psychotherapy research and practice to reduce the burden of mental illness. *Perspectives on Psychological Science, 6,* 21–37.

Keane, T. M., Malloy, P. F., & Fairbank, J. A. (1984). Empirical development of an MMPI subscale for the assessment of combat-related posttraumatic stress disorder. *Journal of Consulting and Clinical Psychology, 52,* 888–891.

Kessler, R. C., Sonnega, A., Bromet, E., Hughes, M., & Nelson, C. B. (1995). Posttraumatic stress disorder in the National Comorbidity Survey. *Archives of General Psychiatry, 52,* 1048–1060.

Kihlstrom, J. F. (1994). The cognitive unconscious. *Science, 237,* 1445–1452.

Klohnen, E. C. (1996). Conceptual analysis and measurement of the construct of ego-resiliency. *Journal of Personality and Social Psychology, 70,* 1067–1079.

Klopfer, B., Kirkner, F. J., Wishman, W., & Baker, G. (1951). Rorschach Prognostic Rating Scale. *Journal of Personality Assessment, 15,* 425–428.

Kobasa, S. C. (1979). Stressful life events, personality, and health: An inquiry into hardiness. *Journal of Personality and Social Psychology, 37,* 1–11.

Krishnamurthy, R., Vandecreek, L., Kaslow, N. J., Tazeau, Y. N., Miville, M. L., Kerns, R., et al. (2004). Achieving competency in psychological assessment: Directions for education and training. *Journal of Clinical Psychology, 60,* 725–739.

Kross, E., Davidson, M., Weber, J., & Ochsner, K. (2009). Coping with emotions past:

The neural bases of regulating affect associated with negative autobiographical memories. *Biological Psychiatry, 65*, 361–366.

Lam, W. W. T., Bonanno, G. A., Mancini, A. D., Ho, S., Chan, M., Hung, W. K., et al. (2010). Trajectories of psychological distress among Chinese women diagnosed with breast cancer. *Psycho-Oncology, 19*, 1044-1051.

Lazarus, R. S., & Alfert, E. (1964). Short-circuiting of threat by experimentally altering cognitive appraisal. *Journal of Abnormal and Social Psychology, 69*, 195–205.

Leary, T. (1957). *Interpersonal diagnosis of personality.* New York: Ronald Press.

Letzring, T. D., Block, J., & Funder, D. C. (2005). Ego-control and ego-resiliency: Generalization of self-report scales based on personality descriptions from acquaintances, clinicians, and the self. *Journal of Research in Personality, 39*, 395–422.

Lilienfeld, S. O., Wood, J. M., & Garb, H. N. (2000). The scientific status of projective techniques. *Psychological Science in the Public Interest, 1*, 27–66.

Litz, B. T., Gray, M. J., Bryant, R. A., & Adler, A. B. (2002). Early intervention for trauma: Current status and future directions. *Clinical Psychology Science and Practice, 9*, 112–134.

Litz, B. T., & Maguen, S. (2010). Early intervention for trauma. In M. J. Friedman, T. M. Keane, & P. A. Resick (Eds.), *Handbook of PTSD science and practice* (pp. 322–346). New York: Guilford Press.

Litz, B. T., Miller, M. W., Ruef, A. M., & McTeague, L. M. (2011). Exposure to trauma in adults. In M. M. Anthony & D. H. Barlow (Eds.), *Handbook of assessment and treatment planning for psychological disorders* (2nd ed., pp. 215–258). New York: Guilford Press.

Litz, B. T., Penk, W. E., Gerardi, R., & Keane, T. M. (1992). Behavioral assessment of PTSD. In P. Saigh (Ed.), *Post-traumatic stress disorder: A behavioral approach to assessment and treatment* (pp. 50–84). New York: Pergamon Press.

Lucas, R. E., & Baird, B. M. (2006). Global self-assessment. In M. Eid & E. Diener (Eds.), *Multi-method measurement in psychology* (pp. 29–42). Washington, DC: American Psychological Association.

Luthar, S. S. (2006). Resilience in development: A synthesis of research across five decades. In D. Cicchetti & D. J. Cohen (Eds.), *Developmental psychopathology, Vol 3: Risk, disorder, and adaptation* (2nd ed., pp. 739–795). Hoboken, NJ: Wiley.

Luthar, S. S., Cicchetti, D., & Becker, B. (2000). The construct of resilience: A critical evaluation and guidelines for future work. *Child Development, 71*, 543–562.

Luthar, S. S., & Cushing, G. (2002). Measurement issues in the empirical study of resilience. In M. D. Glantz & J. L. Johnson (Eds.), *Resilience and development* (pp. 129–160). New York: Springer.

Luthar, S. S., & Zelazo, L. B. (2003). Research on resilience: An integrative review. In S. S. Luthar (Ed.), *Resilience and vulnerability: Adaptation in the context of childhood adversities* (pp. 510–549). New York: Cambridge University Press.

Lyons, J. A. (1991). Strategies for assessing the potential for positive adjustment following trauma. *Journal of Traumatic Stress, 4*, 93–111.

Lyons, J. A., & Wheeler-Cox, T. (1999). MMPI, MMPI-2 and PTSD: Overview of scores, scales, and profiles. *Journal of Traumatic Stress, 12*, 175–183.

Malloy, P. F., Fairbank, J. A., & Keane, T. M. (1983). Validation of a multi-method assessment of posttraumatic stress disorders in Vietnam veterans. *Journal of Consulting and Clinical Psychology, 51*, 488–494.

Mancini, A. D., & Bonanno, G. A. (2006). Resilience in the face of potential trauma: Clinical practices and illustrations. *Journal of Clinical Psychology, 62*, 971–985.

Mancini, A. D., & Bonanno, G. A. (2009). Predictors and parameters of resilience to loss: Toward an individual differences model. *Journal of Personality, 77,* 1805–1832.

Mancini, A. D., & Bonanno, G. A. (2010). Resilience to potential trauma: Toward a lifespan approach. In J. W. Reich, A. J. Zautra, & J. S. Hall (Eds.), *Handbook of adult resilience.* (pp. 258–280). New York: Guilford Press.

Mancini, A. D., Bonanno, G. A., & Clark, A. (2011). Stepping off the hedonic treadmill: Individual differences in response to major life events *Journal of Individual Differences, 32,* 144–1582.

Martin, J. H. (2003). *Neurtoanatomy text and atlas* (3rd ed.). New York: McGraw-Hill.

Masling, J., Rabie, L., & Blondheim, S. H. (1967). Obesity, level of aspiration, and Rorschach and TAT measures of oral dependence. *Journal of Consulting and Clinical Psychology,* 31, 233–239.

Masten, A. S. (2001). Ordinary magic: Resilience processes in development. *American Psychologist, 56,* 227–238.

McClelland, D. C. (1985). How motives, skills and values determine what people do. *American Psychologist, 40,* 812–825.

McClelland, D. C., Koestner, R., & Weinberger, J. (1989). How do self-attributed and implicit motives differ? *Psychological Review, 96,* 690–702.

McDonald, S. D., & Calhoun, P. S. (2010). The diagnostic accuracy of the PTSD checklist: A critical review. *Clinical Psychology Review, 30,* 976–987.

Meyer, G. J. (2000). Incremental validity of the Rorschach Prognostic Rating Scale over the MMPI ego strength scale and IQ. *Journal of Personality Assessment, 74,* 356–370.

Middleton, W., Moylan, A., Raphael, B., Burnett, P., & Martinek, N. (1993). An international perspective on bereavement related concepts. *Australian and New Zealand Journal of Psychiatry, 27,* 457–463.

Mihura, J. L., Meyer, G. J., Dumitrascu, N., & Bombel, G. (2013). The validity of individual Rorschach variables: Systematic reviews and meta-analyses of the comprehensive system. *Psychological Bulletin, 139,* 548–605.

Morey, L. C. (2007). *The Personality Assessment Inventory professional manual.* Lutz, FL: Psychological Assessment Resources.

Morey, L. C., Lowmaster, S. E., Coldren, R. L., Kelly, M. P., Parish, R. V., & Russell, M. L. (2011). Personality Assessment Inventory profiles of deployed combat troops: An empirical investigation of normative performance. *Psychologial Assessment, 23,* 456–462.

Odendaal, I. E., Brink, M., & Theron, L. C. (2011). Rethinking Rorschach interpretation: An exploration of resilient black South African adolescents' personal constructions. *South African Journal of Psychology, 41,* 528–539.

Olff, M., Langeland, W., & Gersons, B. P. R. (2005). Effects of appraisal and coping on the neuroendocrine response to extreme stress. *Neuroscience and Biobehavioral Reviews, 29,* 457–467.

Ong, A. D., Fuller-Rowell, T. E., & Bonanno, G. A. (2010). Prospective predictors of positive emotions following spousal loss. *Psychology and Aging, 25,* 653–660.

Pietrzak, R. H., Russo, A. R., Ling, Q., & Southwick, S. M. (2011). Suicidal ideation in treatment-seeking Veterans of Operations Enduring Freedom and Iraqi Freedom: The role of coping strategies, resilience, and social support. *Journal of Psychiatric Research, 45,* 720–726.

Piotrowski, C. (1999). Assessment practices in the era of managed care: Current status and future directions. *Journal of Clinical Psychology, 55,* 787–796.

Prigerson, H. G., Shear, M. K., Jacobs, S. C., Reynolds, C. F., Maciejewski, P. K.,

Davidson, et al. (1999). Consensus criteria for traumatic grief. A preliminary empirical test. *British Journal of Psychiatry, 174*, 67–73.

Riolli, L., Savicki, V., & Cepani, A. (2002). Resilience in the face of catastrophe: Optimism, personality and coping in the Kosovo crisis. *Journal of Applied Social Psychology, 32*, 1604–1627.

Rutter, M. (1985). Resilience in the face of adversity: Protective factors and resistance to psychiatric disorders. *British Journal of Psychiatry, 147*, 598–611.

Ryff, C. D., & Singer, B. (1996). Psychological well-being: Meaning, measurement, and implications for psychotherapy research. *Psychotherapy and Psychosomatics, 65*, 14–23.

Schuldberg, D. (1992). Ego strength revised: A comparison of the MMPI-2 and the MMPI-1 versions of the Baron Ego Strength scale. *Journal of Clinical Psychology, 48*, 500–505.

Skodol, A. E. (2010). The resilient personality. In J. W. Reich, A. J. Zautra, & J. S. Hall (Eds.), *Handbook of adult resilience* (pp. 112–125). New York: Guilford Press.

Smyth, J. M., Pennebaker, J. W., & Arigo, D. (2012). What are the health effects of disclosure? *Handbook of health psychology* (2nd ed., pp. 175–191). New York: Psychology Press.

Solomon, Z., Berger, R., & Ginzburg, K. (2007). Resilience of Israeli body handlers: Implications of repressive coping style. *Traumatology, 13*, 64–74.

Spitzer, R. L., Kroenke, K., & Williams, J. W. (1999). Validation and utility of a self-report version of PRIME-MD: The PHQ primary care study. *Journal of the American Medical Association, 282*, 1737–1744.

Taylor, J. A. (1953). A personality scale of manifest anxiety. *Journal of Abnormal Psychology, 48*, 285–290.

Tedeschi, R. G., & Calhoun, L. G. (2004). Posttraumatic growth: Conceptual foundations and empirical evidence. *Psychological Inquiry, 15*, 1–18.

Thomas, K. M., Hopwood, C. J., Orlando, M. J., Weathers, F. W., & McDevitt-Murphy, M. E. (2012). Detecting feigned PTSD using the Personality Assessment Inventory. *Psychological Injury and Law, 5*, 192–201.

Thompson, M. M., & Zanna, M. P. (1995). The conflicted individual: Personality-based and domain-specific antecedents of ambivalent social attitudes. *Journal of Personality, 63*, 259–288.

Tomarken, A. J., & Davidson, R. J. (1994). Frontal brain activation in repressors and nonrepressors. *Journal of Abnormal Psychology, 10*, 339–349.

Torgersen, S., & Vollrath, M. (2006). Personality types, personality traits, and risky health behavior. In M. Vollrath (Ed.), *Handbook of personality and health* (pp. 215–233). Chichester, UK: Wiley.

Vaishnavi, S., Connor, K., & Davidson, J. R. (2007). An abbreviated version of the Connor–Davidson Resilience Scale (CD-RISC), the CD-RISC2: Psychometric properties and applications in psychopharmacological trials. *Psychiatry Research, 152*, 293–297.

Viglione, D. J. (1990). Severe disturbance or trauma-induced adaptive reaction: A Rorschach child case study. *Journal of Personality Assessment, 55*, 280.

Viglione, D. J., & Kates, J. (1997). A Rorschach child single-subject study in divorce: A question of psychological resiliency. In J. R. Meloy, M. W. Acklin, C. B. Gacono, J. F. Murray, & C. A. Peterson (Eds.), *Contemporary Rorschach interpretation*. Mahwah, NJ: Erlbaum.

Waaktaar, T., & Torgersen, S. (2010). How resilient are resilience scales?: The Big Five scales outperform resilience scales in predicting adjustment in adolescents. *Scandinavian Journal of Psychology, 51*, 157–163.

Waaktaar, T., & Torgersen, S. (2012). Genetic and environmental causes of variation in trait resilience in young people. *Behavior Genetics, 42,* 366–377.

Wagnild, G. M., & Young, H. M. (1993). Development and psychometric evaluation of the Resilience Scale. *Journal of Nursing Measurement, 1,* 165–178.

Waugh, C. E., Wager, T. D., Fredrickson, B. L., Noll, D. C., & Taylor, S. F. (2008). The neural correlates of trait resilience when anticipating and recovering from threat. *Social Cognitive and Affective Neuroscience, 3,* 322–332.

Weathers, F. W., Keane, T. M., & Davidson, J. R. (2001). Clinician-administered PTSD scale: A review of the first ten years of research. *Depression and Anxiety, 13,* 132–156.

Weinberger, D. A., Schwartz, G. E., & Davidson, R. J. (1979). Low-anxious, high-anxious, and repressive coping styles: Psychometric patterns and behavioral and physiological responses to stress. *Journal of Abnormal Psychology, 88,* 369–380.

Weiner, I. B. (1994). The Rorschach Inkblot Method (RIM) is not a test: Implications for theory and practice. *Journal of Personality Assessment, 62,* 498–504.

Weiner, I. B. (2003). *Principles of Rorschach interpretation* (2nd ed.). New York: Routledge.

Widiger, T. A., & Samuel, D. B. (2005). Evidence-based assessment of personality disorders. *Psychologial Assessment, 17,* 278–287.

Williams, P. G., Rau, H. K., Cribbet, M. R., & Gunn, H. E. (2009). Openness to experience and stress regulation. *Journal of Research in Personality, 43,* 777–784.

Xi, J., Zuo, Z., & Sang, B. (2011). Perceived social competence of resilient children. *Acta Psychologica Sinica, 43,* 1026–1037.

PART III

Clinical Management

CHAPTER 10

Multimethod Assessment and Treatment Planning

Joni L. Mihura and Robert A. Graceffo

The goal of this chapter is to illuminate the relevance of incorporating different methods of assessment into treatment planning. To date, this is a relatively novel endeavor, which may be somewhat surprising given the intuitive link between assessment and treatment. Thus, the present chapter is unique in its attempt to "make the implicit, explicit" regarding the relationship that multimethod assessment has with treatment planning. The basic tenet of this chapter is that different assessment methods tap different aspects of personality and have implications for a person's experiences and functioning, which, in turn, inform case conceptualization and treatment planning. Our transtheoretical approach should make the chapter relevant to a wide range of practitioners and researchers in the field.

The Status of Methods in the Psychological Assessment Literature

In the psychological assessment literature, textbooks vary in how they address the role of method in understanding a person. Basic psychological assessment textbooks often organize the material by test. These tests may not be different—or only minimally different—in their method of assessment. For example, many tests use a self-report or introspective method of assessment (e.g., the Minnesota Multiphasic Personality Inventory, Second Edition [MMPI-2], the Millon Clinical Multiaxial Inventory [MCMI], and the Personality Assessment Inventory [PAI]), yet each test is described in a separate chapter. On the other hand, tests such as the Wechsler Adult Intelligence Scale (WAIS) or the Rorschach, each containing multiple methods of assessment, are typically described as a single entity. Different methods within tests (e.g., rationally and empirically derived scales on the MMPI-2, verbal and performance subtests on the WAIS, and content and structural methods on the Rorschach) might be compared within the test, but the same methods used by different tests (e.g., self-reported depression as measured by the MMPI-2, PAI, and Beck Depression Inventory [BDI]) are not summarized together. When assessment textbook sections are organized per test instead of per method, it can appear that *test* is equivalent to *method*. Obviously, this is not the case.

The clinical implications of diverse psychological assessment methods are typically addressed in the advanced professional literature, targeting audiences who are already familiar with basic psychometrics and the common psychological tests. This advanced professional literature focuses on the applied level—such as conceptualization, report-writing, and treatment implications (Blais & Smith, 2008; Finn, 1996; Ganellen, 1996; Wiggins, 2003). Antithetical to a multimethod approach to psychological assessment is the currently popular atheoretical approach to understanding (or categorizing) people. Here, structured interviews are used to make *Diagnostic and Statistical Manual of Mental Disorders* (DSM) diagnoses in order to assign the client to the appropriate DSM-focused, manualized treatment (Chambless & Ollendick, 2001). The goal of this approach is not to understand the person through the ways the symptoms and behaviors fit together and interact. Instead, structured interviews assess constructs in a molecular, list-like fashion (i.e., the individual DSM criteria) that relies strongly (and often solely) on self-report.

With regard to the relationship of assessment methods to treatment planning, an unrealistic divide has emerged between psychological testing and psychotherapy in the professional literature. Scant literature addresses the role of assessment method in treatment planning. This is unfortunate because when clinicians (of any orientation) begin to consider all available information about a client, including its source or method, it allows them to implement their set of skills more effectively. For example, if a client tells us he is "depressed," his girlfriend tells us that he is usually agitated (other-report), his demeanor in session suggests that he is anxious (observation), and his records indicate he has been diagnosed with bipolar disorder in the past (record review), then we may think differently about him than if we knew only one or two of these things. Regardless of theoretical orientation, using information from all sources helps us to see the problem more accurately for what it is and utilize appropriate treatment methods. Therefore, broadly speaking, there is a need for the professional literature to target the importance of method in treatment planning, regardless of therapy approach. Specific to this chapter, the scarcity of this literature means that we must lay a good deal of groundwork about methods in themselves in order to discuss the broader meaning of assessment methods in relation to treatment planning.

What Are Existing Psychological Assessment Methods?

It is difficult to precisely catalogue the psychological assessment methods, because in the psychological assessment world the term *method* has not been clearly defined. A few psychologists have offered ways of categorizing assessment methods (Bornstein, 2007; Campbell, 1950, 1957; Lilienfeld, Wood, & Garb, 2000; McClelland, Koestner, & Weinberger, 1989; McGrath, 2008; Meyer & Kurtz, 2006), but no universally accepted approach exists. Instead, psychologists have paid more attention to fine-tuning the trait aspect of psychological constructs rather than their associated method. Often, the reified content of the psychological trait (e.g., depression, social support, agreeableness) is viewed as the kernel of truth, while its associated method is immaterial. But this is a rather flat understanding of a person. It is essentially devoid of context. Is it the way he sees himself? Is it how he verbally describes himself? Is it behaviorally how he tries to present himself? Is it how others see him? All of these aspects contribute to an understanding of a person, as explicated by the interpersonal theorist Timothy Leary (1957), who described different interpersonal levels of personality.

Until a comprehensive and coherent model of assessment methods is developed, as a general guideline we recommend that researchers and practitioners map the assessment method's response process (e.g., reporting morbid images to inkblots) onto the psychological characteristic of interest (e.g., having morbid images on one's mind). Based on surveys (e.g., Archer, Buffington-Vollum, Stredny, & Handel, 2006; Archer & Newsom, 2000; Camara, Nathan, & Puente, 2000; Norcross & Karpiak, 2012), we know that the most popular assessment method is self-report, which includes clinical interview and self-report instruments such as the PAI and BDI. In the child and adolescent literature, informant ratings (e.g., teacher, parent) are a regularly used assessment method. Other popular external assessment methods are behavioral observations, intelligence tests, neuroimaging, and the Rorschach. Other method characteristics are the source of the information (e.g., self, spouse, teacher, parent) for self- and informant ratings and the situation from which it was obtained (e.g., work, home, play, hospital).

Statistical Relationship between Methods and Their Incremental Information

Broadly speaking, there are two different types of research in psychological assessment. One type is test-focused, wherein the focus is the psychometrics of the test. The other is criterion-focused, wherein the test is used to study a psychological condition or characteristic. To date, most clinical assessment research has not focused on how the tests' methods relate to different aspects of personality. Instead, different methods of assessment are often discussed in regard to whether they assess what is "real" or "true" about a person versus understanding the different types of information they provide. Especially when discussing the "projective" method, the tests are often pitted against each other instead of considering how the different methods target different aspects of personality (e.g., Lilienfeld et al., 2000). Therefore, we have some idea of the degree to which comparable scales on major tests relate to each other, but less about what this means for personality.

What follows is a brief summary of meta-analytic findings that address assessment methods used in clinical psychology, experimental psychology (social, personality), and organizational management (personnel selection). As effect size benchmarks, the reader can refer to Cohen's (1988) r's of small (.10), medium (.30), and large (.50) or Hemphill's (2003) report of the middle third of validity effect sizes (based on Meyer et al., 2001) in the psychological assessment research literature ($r = .21$ to .33).

Statistical Relationship

Experimental and clinical research often finds small associations between introspected (self-reported) characteristics and behavior or, put more simply, between what people say about themselves and what they do (e.g., Nisbett & Wilson, 1977; Wilson & Dunn, 2004). Several meta-analytic findings illustrate this phenomenon. For example, self-reported achievement motivation has been shown to have a meager relationship ($r = .15$, $k = 104$) with spontaneous achievement behaviors, such as job performance (Meyer et al., 2001, based on Spangler, 1992). Associations between self-reported and behaviorally assessed impulsivity ($r = .10$, $k = 608$; Cyders & Coskunpinar, 2011) and memory ($r = .15$, $k = 673$; Beaudoin & Desrichard, 2011) are small. The relationship (r's) between self-reported characteristics and parallel characteristics on the Rorschach and storytelling narratives (like the Thematic Apperception Test [TAT]) are .08 ($k = 386$) and .09 ($k = 36$), respectively (Meyer et al., 2001, based on Spangler, 1992; Mihura, Meyer, Dumitrascu, & Bombel, 2013). Interestingly, in these same meta-analyses, the Rorschach and the storytelling narratives' associations with externally assessed characteristics and behaviors were significantly higher than with self-reported characteristics (respectively, r's = .27 & .22, k's = 770 & 82). Lastly, in examining this phenomenon (i.e., what people say versus what they do) in the domain of intelligence, Freund and Kasten (2012) found that self-reported and performance-based intelligence maintain only a moderate relationship ($r = .33$, $k = 154$).

Turning from behavior to informant reports, Klonsky, Oltmanns, and Turkheimer (2002) found a medium association between self and informant ratings of personality disorders when assessed dimensionally (r = .36, k = 11) and a small association when assessed categorically (r = .14, k = 6). In the child and adolescent assessment literature, the range of effect size relationships (r's) between different reporting sources (e.g., child/adolescent, parents, teachers, clinicians, peers) are consistently around .20 to .35 (Achenbach, McConaughy, & Howell, 1987; Meyer, 2002).

Regarding performance personality tests, it is tempting to consider all of the methods that fall into the traditional "projective" category as a unitary method. However, experts have neither historically nor contemporarily considered this to be the case (e.g., Bornstein, 2007; Campbell, 1957; Lilienfeld et al., 2000). As we discuss in subsequent sections, performance-based personality tests use a variety of different methods. To date, no meta-analyses address this topic per se, but the literature supports a more nuanced understanding of implicit methods. For example, a recent meta-analysis found that the Rorschach's Mutuality of Autonomy Scale (Graceffo, Mihura, & Meyer, in press) had a much lower association with the TAT (r = .10, k = 51) than with other criterion variables, such as clinician ratings (r = .25, k = 63) and diagnosis (r = .24, k = 15).

In general, across methods it is logical to expect that the higher the degree of test method overlap on comparable scales, the higher the statistical association should be and vice versa. This is consistent with the argument presented over 50 years ago by Campbell and Fiske (1959) in their description of the multitrait–multimethod matrix (MTMM), in which they describe validity as the agreement between two maximally different methods to assess the same trait. The more similar the method, the more the association represents reliability instead of validity.

In clinical psychology, there has not been a concerted effort to investigate this proposition. However, as an example, Rogers, Salekin, and Sewell (1999) published a meta-analysis of the MCMI in which they equated *test* with *method*. When Mihura et al. (2013) organized Rogers and colleagues' results by method of assessment, the average effect size association (r) between MCMI scales and parallel self-report measures was .57 (k = 118), .36 (k = 105) for semistructured interviews, and was .12 (k = 35) for clinicians' ratings. As a second example, in a comparative meta-analysis of MMPI and Rorschach validity, Hiller, Rosenthal, Bornstein, Berry, and Brunell-Neuleib (1999) found that the MMPI had a significantly stronger association than the Rorschach for studies using diagnosis and other self-report methods as criteria, whereas the Rorschach had larger associations than the MMPI for studies using objective information as criteria (objective meaning real-world events; e.g., number of hospitalizations). These findings are consistent with the idea that the higher the degree of method overlap on comparable scales, the higher the statistical association should be and vice versa.

Mihura et al. (2013) also found that the Rorschach had a moderate association to other external measures of assessment (r = .27, k = 770) but a small association to the MMPI ($r = .07$, $k = 212$). As the authors note, these findings also suggest that to the extent that the MMPI contains valid scales, the Rorschach should logically show incremental validity over the MMPI when jointly predicting a relevant criterion variable.This logic of incremental validity should apply across all valid methods of assessment, a topic to which we now turn.

Incremental Validity

Incremental validity research in psychological assessment targets the question of whether including additional measures can improve our ability to predict a criterion, such as diagnosis or treatment outcome (Hunsley & Meyer, 2003). Sometimes incremental validity studies focus on the *trait* or *symptom* and ignore the implication of using overlapping methods when assessing predictor and criterion variables. For example, if a study investigates the Rorschach's ability to incrementally provide information about diagnosis in addition to a self-report instrument and the diagnosis is obtained from a fully structured interview, then based on method alone (i.e., self-reported information), one would expect the self-report instrument to *statistically* increment over the Rorschach scale in predicting the fully structured interview diagnosis. However, as far as *understanding the person*, incremental information is more minimal. Much of what was gained from the self-report scale had already been gained from the fully structured interview because these methods afford a similar way of knowing the client (i.e., through self-attributed information). Despite statistical evidence of incremental information, clinically, this information has little additive value.

Keeping these issues in mind, a large number of published studies directly or indirectly address the incremental validity of different clinical assessment methods. There are several reviews of these studies (Garb, 1984, 2003; Johnston & Murray, 2003; Lilienfeld et al., 2000; Viglione & Hilsenroth, 2001; Viglione & Meyer, 2008), but none are meta-analytic. A comprehensive summary of these findings is beyond the scope of the present chapter, but just in the past few decades many studies have focused specifically on the incremental validity of different assessment *methods*. For example, studies have shown that Rorschach variables provide incremental validity over self-report measures in predicting suicidal behaviors (Blasczyk-Schiep, Kazén, Kuhl, & Grygielski, 2011; Fowler, Hilsenroth, & Piers, 2001), psychotic diagnoses (Dao, Prevatt, & Home, 2008; Meyer, 2000a; Ritsher, 2004), and treatment outcome (Meyer, 2000b; Perry & Viglione, 1991; Stokes, Pogge, Grosso, & Zaccario, 2001).

In both clinical and nonclinical outlets (e.g., social and personality psychology; personnel selection), a significant amount of research examines the ability of observer judgments to augment what is learned through self-report. In general, the findings suggest that personality characteristics that exist internally and have low observability, such as anxious and depressive thoughts and feelings, are best assessed by self-report methods. However, observer judgments improve upon the self-report method when externally expressed constructs are targeted, such as job performance, intelligence, achievement, and interpersonal functioning (e.g., Connelly & Ones, 2010; Kurtz, Puher, & Cross, 2012; Leising, Krause, Köhler, Hinsen, & Clifton, 2011; Miller, Pilkonis, & Clifton, 2005; Oh, Wang, & Mount, 2011; Vazire, 2010).

Conclusions

While comprehensive mega-analyses evaluating Campbell and Fiske's (1959) MTMM postulates are yet to be published, existing assessment meta-analyses are consistent with the idea that reliability and validity exist along a continuum with method as the moderator. On average, one should expect moderate associations (*r*'s from .21 to .33) across different assessment methods that target similar traits (Hemphill, 2003, based on Meyer et al., 2001). Methods that share the same or very similar methods should show very high associations with each other (along the magnitude found in alternate forms reliability), while more highly disparate methods will show small associations with each other (e.g., Hiller et al., 1999; Meyer, 2002; Mihura et al., 2013; Rogers et al., 1999). Based on empirical findings like these, experts in a variety of areas (e.g., clinical [adult and child], experimental, and organizational management) have argued for a multimethod approach to assessment practice and provided some initial suggestions for integrating methods (e.g., Achenbach, Krukowski, Dumenci, & Ivanova, 2005; Bing, LeBreton, Davison, Migetz, & James, 2007; Chang, Connelly, & Geeza, 2012; Erdberg, 2008; Kraemer et al., 2003; Meyer, 2002). This work is in its early stages and would benefit from interdisciplinary collaboration. But the evidence suggests that clinicians should highlight the unique method of assessment when integrating and applying assessment data to understanding their clients.

Two Major Method Distinctions: Introspectively versus Externally Assessed

The following sections are organized by method of measurement—in particular, whether the information was obtained through introspection (the person's own self-reported evaluation) or external assessment (a source outside of the person), which is a distinguishing property of all psychological information. The historic *objective* and *projective* classes of personality measures, now often referred to as *self-report* and *performance-based* (Meyer & Kurtz, 2006), are subsumed within these categories. Introspective methods include self-report inventories and verbally reported information in a clinical interview. External methods include, but are not limited to, informant ratings, intelligence tests, the Rorschach, the TAT, the Implicit Association Test (IAT; neuroimaging, and institutional records. Clinical interviews typically contain both introspective and external means of attaining client information; therefore, they are discussed in both sections. For each method, we discuss implications for understanding personality and treatment planning.

Introspectively Assessed

Introspective or self-report methods are language-based methods of measurement that acquire information through individuals' verbal descriptions of themselves. Broadly speaking, there are two types of self-report or introspective methods: the clinical interview and the self-report inventory. The clinical interview itself can be conceived as existing along an introspectively-externally assessed continuum defined by the degree of structure imposed on the task. Moving in the direction of increasing structure, this continuum consists of unstructured, semistructured, and fully structured interviews. As the structure in a clinical interview increases, the more the interview can be thought of as a purely introspective method. This means that despite looking different in form, fully structured interviews and self-report inventories share considerable method overlap. Fully structured interviews can be considered more similar to an audio-version of a self-report inventory than to an unstructured interview. Moving toward the externally assessed end of the continuum, the more an interview is unstructured, the more external methods of assessment are introduced, such as clinical judgment and behavioral observations.

In the realm of client self-reported information, there are different types of data that a client might report (e.g., Campbell, 1957; Mayer, 2004, 2005) and not all qualify as introspection. For our purposes, the most relevant type of self-reported data is derived from inferentially abstracting information about one's experiences and behaviors and determining what they mean about one's personality. For example, a client might be asked to report how "modest" he or she is compared to others. This involves evoking one's personal idea of *modesty* (an abstract concept), applying it to oneself and others, and, finally, making comparisons. In contrast, a second type of client-reported data involves concrete, historical information or what Mayer (2004) refers to as "life-space" data (e.g., personal accounts of the number of siblings one has, where one lives, or the type of job one holds). Somewhere between the very concrete and the very abstract is a third type of client-reported data that targets the frequency of certain behaviors, which Mayer calls "act-frequency" data. The events of interest can vary in regard to their abstractness (e.g., how often you attend church services vs. how often you verbally attack someone). Mayer *only* considers assessment methods that produce abstracted information about personality characteristics to be a *self*-report method (a report about the "self"), a convention that we follow here.[1]

With regard to retrospectively reported information, the clinician should be aware that there is a large body of evidence showing low correspondence between recall of past experiences (the retrospective method) and records of that past experience—whether the person's own report at the time; a parent or significant other's report; or medical, legal, and other records (e.g., Hardt & Rutter, 2004; Henry, Moffitt, Caspi, Langley, & Silva, 1994; Widom & Morris, 1997; Widom & Shepard, 1996). For example, Henry et al. (1994) investigated the association between data collected at childhood and recall at age 18. The association between self-reported depression/anxiousness and hyperactivity as a child and the recall of these symptoms at age 18 was only $r = .06$ and $.05$, respectively. The association between the person's recollections and their mother's report of these symptoms when they were a child was only $r = .11$ and $.08$, respectively. Typically, the false-positive error for retrospective recall is smaller than the false-negative rate of error. That is, people are much less likely to report (or recall) an event that happened than they are to not report (or not recall) the event. The clinician should be familiar with the basic findings of this research and the implications of the different kinds of client-reported information

Formal self-report inventories share significant method overlap with fully structured clinical interviews. Key method differences are: (1) in a clinical interview the respondent shares information with a person instead of a self-report inventory (although the respondent is usually aware that the interviewer will know their responses); one implication is that interpersonal dynamics (including personal diversity) might be less likely to affect the self-report inventory method; (2) in contrast to an interview, most broadband self-report inventories include validity scales; and (3) self-report inventories determine the clinical significance of the responses by statistical comparison to norms instead of clinical judgment. There are additional differences, but the take-home message here is that the assessor should be cognizant of the multifaceted nature of the self-report method and its related implications for case conceptualization and related treatment planning.

Popular broadband self-report inventories that contain validity scales are the PAI, MMPI-2, and MCMI-III; popular symptom-focused inventories without validity scales (often used to track treatment progress) are the BDI-II and Beck Anxiety Inventory (BAI) (Archer et al., 2006; Archer & Newsom, 2000; Camara et al., 2000). Across these self-report inventories, a major method distinction is between direct and indirect methods

---

[1]However, in contrast to Mayer, we follow the broader convention in the field that links the self-report method to verbally reported information, whereas Mayer considers self-report to refer to data that has implications about personality that includes both introspective and external methods of assessment.

of assessment. Common indirect self-report items are those used to detect response bias, such as the MMPI validity scales or the Balanced Inventory of Desirable Responding (Paulhus, 2002). Regarding items that indirectly assess psychopathology, the MMPI-2 subtle items qualify. For example, answering false to the item "I like to flirt" is more common when someone is depressed, although it is not immediately obvious that the item would be scored for depression. The subtle items exist on the MMPI-2 clinical scales due to the empirical method of scale construction, not because they were chosen on a rational or theoretical basis. Although such psychopathology items without obvious intent to the respondent have been appealing to clinicians, they have not acquired strong validity support in the research literature (Hollrah, Schlottmann, Scott, & Brunetti, 1995) in contrast to symptom-focused validity scales (Hawes, & Boccaccini, 2009; Nelson, Hoelzle, Sweet, Arbisi, & Demakis, 2010).

General Implications for Understanding Personality

Most psychological assessment writings have focused less on self-report as a method and more on evaluating if it assesses the "truth" with a capital "T," if not for obstacles like impression management and faulty memory (Paulhus & Vazire, 2007; Stone et al., 2000). While it is true that a person can consciously skew how he or she responds to self-report measures (e.g., Hawes & Boccaccini, 2009; Nelson et al., 2010) and a faulty memory can compromise one's ability to recall past events or consolidate information about oneself (Stone et al., 2000), when assessing psychological constructs we emphasize the fact that these constructs by definition are "constructed by the mind." No constructs exist in concrete form for us to "accurately assess." Clients' verbal descriptions of themselves are but one part of understanding them. From this perspective, self-reported information does not reflect an objective thing called *actual* personality; rather, it is *itself* a component of personality. Through self-report, people can show how they see themselves or how they want to be seen, which allows a glimpse into the way their minds have constructed certain concepts (e.g., is "aggression" associated with prideful strength, juvenile immaturity, immorality, or something else?). Toward that goal, a better memory and the absence of a motivating context to dissimulate might provide a clearer glimpse. However, knowing how people present themselves through self-report is indispensable and sheds light on subjective personal meaning. Thus, the question we ask about self-report is this: What does it mean that this person is presenting him- or herself in this particular light, regardless of its "truth" or "falsehood"?

One's conscious self-definition plays a specific role in behavior. For example, research in social cognition has shown that people generally strive for consistency in their behavior (Gawronski, & Strack, 2012) and, therefore, maintain biases such that they differentially attend to certain types of information. Specifically, we tend to focus on and accept behavior that upholds our conscious conception of ourselves and ignore, dismiss, or reject (e.g., rationalize or explain away) that which opposes it. Regardless of the "truth" of the matter, it is important to know a person's conscious self-understanding because it can help us understand the self-view that the person wishes to maintain as well as help to explain how the person interprets reactions from other people.

As noted earlier, introspection or self-report methods are better for assessing internal experiential states like anxiety, while external methods are better at assessing functioning and predicting spontaneous behavior (e.g., Chang, Connelly, & Geeza, 2012; Helzer & Dunning, 2012; McClelland et al., 1989; Mihura et al., 2013; Miller et al., 2004; Schneider & Schimmack, 2009; Vazire, 2010). However, theoretically, if someone were motivated and able to assess and verbalize his or her inner states, he or she could share this information with others, and correspondence of self- and informant-ratings should increase. In support of this idea, Human and Biesanz (2011) found that well-adjusted persons were more likely to share low observability information with new acquaintances, which then allowed the acquaintance to make judgments that were more in line with the person's conscious sense of self (i.e., self- and informant ratings were more closely aligned).

Treatment Implications

As discussed, self-report is an indispensable method for a variety of purposes when assessing personality, which also have implications for treatment. First, self-reported information is an aspect of personality in itself and is not simply a method to obtain "accurate" information. Knowing how a client construes himself and his world helps us understand subjective personal meaning for him. Second, knowing a client's conscious understanding of his personality and related behaviors helps us predict in what domains he might strive for consistency. This striving for consistency can help clients experience a more stable sense of self as well as other benefits. However, these benefits can come at a cost of failing to adjust one's behaviors or perceptions with relevant feedback. It can seem counterintuitive to clients and therapists alike when clients continue to maintain patterns of behaviors that they truly wish to change. Therefore, it is important for clients and therapists to be aware of this human tendency.

Third, knowing how a client attempts to portray herself to others through self-report can help us understand how she expects others to react to her. For example, if a client reports that she is submissive and she truly feels that way, it can be confusing to her when others react to her in a challenging or an aggressive way. Her reaction might be, "I am so shy and unassertive, why would they react to me that way!?" It can also be confusing to the therapist if he or she has also come to view the client as submissive due to their self-report, but then begin to hear client narratives that include challenging, dominating, or defensive reactions from other people. If the therapist can help the client see how his or her dominant or competitive behaviors are evoking these responses from others, it can make the situation less confusing and the client can now choose how to respond, based on that new information. Finally, whether the information goes to a person or to a test, the self-report method can supply information that only the client can know, such as subjective experiences that include negative feelings such as emotional pain or positive feelings such as a sense of awe.

In general, the introspective method is integral to the working alliance, constituting an important common factor across psychotherapies and presenting problems (Flückiger, Del Re, Wampold, Symonds, & Horvath, 2012). For example, the therapist needs to be aware of the client's subjective experience and goals for therapy, whether or not the therapist agrees with the client's self-assessment. Additionally, sharing private, introspected information with the therapist allows the client to achieve a sense of connection and trust that sets the stage for treatment.

At the same time, simply receiving introspective information from a client is not the equivalent of understanding the whole person. To develop real understanding and empathy, the therapist needs to appreciate the underlying dynamics motivating this self-report, as opposed to just the content of it. For example, not all clients stating, "I am unfriendly," have the same motivation or goals in reporting this information. One client might believe the statement and feel comfortable saying so; another client might believe it but wish the therapist would disagree (e.g., a pull for a corrective experience); and still another might not believe it but wish the therapist would agree (e.g., so that he or she can justify subsequently attacking the therapist or portraying himself or herself as wounded).

It is also important to be aware that a client's culture shapes his or her self-construal (Markus & Kitayama, 1991), which impacts self-attributions. This means, for example, that we might expect differential endorsements of "individuality" from a client born in the United States as compared to an Asian American client as a function of cultural differences in the salience of this construct. In addition, the value placed on self-disclosure within a particular culture, community, or family unit is brought to bear on the self-report method, as clients may feel more or less comfortable sharing sensitive information about their lives (see Sue & Sue, 2012, for a discussion of culture and disclosure). Despite all possible motivations for self-report, given that people are better understood in first impressions when they share their less observable traits (Human & Biesanz, 2011), the importance of making a connection with clients and helping them feel safe enough to divulge this material cannot be overstated.

Although our goal is not to compare therapy orientations, it can be illuminating to compare how the introspective method might be conceptualized and applied to a case in different therapy approaches. In cognitive therapy (CT), although self-reported information is the subject matter of treatment, CT is not fully premised on the idea that people know all there is to know of themselves. Clients may not be so aware of their automatic thoughts and must be helped to see them. However, CT does not focus on the possible meaning of this material that exists outside of awareness. In CT, the "stuff" that is missed by a client's self-report is akin to human error. In psychodynamic therapy (PDT), *all* of this information is crucial to understanding the whole person. For example, self-report can reveal the information that people are motivated to keep in consciousness or can show how they wish to appear to others, thereby providing initial clues as to what must be guarded from conscious awareness by defense mechanisms. As therapy develops and the working alliance is established, the therapist can help the client discover their implicit characteristics. In CT, this type of disparity might not be explored because it is viewed as less fundamental to treatment. Thus, self-reported information is important in both CT and PDT, but its implications differ.

Externally Assessed

Many assessment methods use external means of gathering information about clients and their life situations. The great majority of these rely on the judgment of other people. Examples of external methods that utilize the judgment of clinicians include the coding of narrative themes in therapy, clinician rating scales, performance tests such as the WAIS and Rorschach, and the evaluations and notes found in psychiatric records. Examples of external methods that do not utilize clinicians include informant reports provided by parents, teachers, and significant others, as well as medical, legal, and academic records.

The Clinical Interview and Informant Ratings

As in the introspection section, we begin with the clinical interview, but this time we focus on its external methods of assessment. As previously noted, the less structure in an interview, the more external assessment methods are likely to be introduced, such as unstructured behavioral observations and the clinical judgment that directs the interview. Furthermore, psychiatric diagnoses themselves vary in the extent to which their respective sets of symptoms are, by nature, amenable to particular methods. For example, the essence of psychotic diagnoses involves a lack of insight—a judgment that is made by the clinician, not the client. Delusions are fixed, false beliefs, and the clinician must determine their veracity. Hallucinations are experiences created solely by the mind and do not exist in reality. The presence of disorganized speech is another diagnostic judgment made by the clinician. The presence or absence of symptoms in other psychiatric diagnoses, particularly those related to depression and anxiety, rely less on the clinician's judgment and more on the client's own internal experiences, typically accessed by self-report. The variability in assessment method across these psychiatric diagnoses might help explain why external methods like the Rorschach provide incremental prediction over self-report measures for detecting psychosis (Dao et al., 2008; Meyer, 2000a; Ritsher, 2004) and why self-report measures often have a stronger ability than Rorschach measures to detect depressive diagnoses (e.g., Gross, Keyes, & Greene, 2000; Mihura et al., 2013).

Informant reports are much more common in assessments with children than with adults. Meta-analyses of cross-informant agreement for child and adolescent assessments (child/adolescent, parents, teachers, clinicians, peers) reveal validity effect sizes (r's) around .20 to .35. Therefore, many professionals have called for the use of multiple informants in the assessment of children and adolescents (Achenbach et al., 1987; Kraemer et al., 2003; Meyer, 2002). For adult assessments, there are several settings in which informant reports can be helpful, such as forensic and neuropsychological settings. Consistent with this idea, a meta-analysis by Jorm (1997) found that informant ratings performed as well as brief cognitive tests in screening for dementia. Additionally, available studies show that forensic patients report significantly less personality pathology than informants and that the concordance between these ratings is low; in fact, self- and informant ratings were *negatively* related for paranoid personality disorder (Allard & Grann, 2000; Keulen-de-Vos et al., 2011). As previously noted, external evaluations made by others are better than one's own self-report at predicting levels of functioning in a variety of domains—intellectual, interpersonal (social and romantic), occupational, and personality and behavioral impairment more generally—while self-report methods are better for assessing internal experiential states (e.g., Connelly & Ones, 2010; Helzer & Dunning, 2012; Kurtz et al., 2012; Lawton, Shields, & Oltmanns, 2011; Leising et al., 2011; Miller et al., 2004, 2005; Oh et al., 2011; Vazire, 2010).

TREATMENT IMPLICATIONS

These findings have many implications, but a significant one is the importance of understanding the nature of the psychological characteristics that benefit or even require the judgment of a person other than the client. In general, when making diagnoses or conceptualizing a person, clinicians can rely more on the client's self-report when assessing distress but should include their own (and other informants') judgment when assessing dysfunction. For the broad higher-order classifications of psychopathology (Wright et al., 2013), external methods of assessment seem to be more crucial for externalizing and psychotic characteristics than for internalizing symptoms.

As previously discussed, informant reports (and external methods of assessment more generally) may be more important in specific settings, such as forensic and neuropsychological. But in general, the relative congruence of clients' self-report and judgments about them made by others has many treatment implications. Are clients able to understand how others perceive them and why? The ability to do so requires some degree of mentalization and theory of mind. Problems in understanding how others perceive them has negative implications for a client's satisfaction and functioning in interpersonal relationships, which can extend to the therapy relationship. Furthermore, the more such discrepancies affect the goals of therapy—for example, when presenting problems include the client's intimate, social, or work relationships—the more the therapy should focus on helping clients understand how they are experienced by others and why, as well as the implications for their life and their treatment goals.

Practically, clinicians rarely obtain information from informants for their adult clients in general outpatient settings (and it is not always advisable). We have argued that informant reports could be particularly beneficial for certain conditions and settings—largely, externalizing, personality disordered, cognitive impairment, and psychotic conditions and forensic and neuropsychological settings. However, the typical clinician is usually his or her only informant. Therefore, at the very least, clinicians should use the research on self- and informant-report congruence to enhance their empathy for their clients' experiences and perspectives. For instance, it is not noteworthy when other people, including the therapist, have a different perspective on a client's personality and behaviors; it is practically expected. At the same time, this is valuable information when it occurs. In session, the therapist should actively look for discrepancies in self-reported and externally assessed information about their clients. In the clinical interview, this can include noticing when clients' self-report does not match their behavior or the affect that accompanies it or when clients' self-reported experiences seem at odds with a more universal experience of people in a similar situation (e.g., reporting no reaction to the death of a loved one or bullying experiences as a child).

Finally, at times, therapists may experience unusual thoughts and feelings when with a client. This experience with clients can be disorienting, but it can also provide information to further help the therapist understand how others might feel in their client's presence and react. Historically, the psychoanalytic literature has provided the most information on what can be learned in the session about a client's intrapsychic and interpersonal dynamics (Eagle, 2000; Gabbard, 1995). But this knowledge and the related research should extend beyond the brand name of therapy. All in all, when making judgments such as these, the clinician should be familiar with the literature on the biases that people commit when making judgments (e.g., Garb, 1998). With regard to therapist errors in particular, a study by Hamilton and Kivlighan (2009) found that therapists were prone to project their own interpersonal dynamics onto their clients. Therapists who engaged in their own personal therapy were less likely to project their own dynamics onto their clients, an important finding that should be replicated. We emphasize learning a standardized approach to conceptualizing clients' interpersonal dynamics, which leads us to our next section.

Narrative Approaches

There are several narrative approaches in assessment but basically two main methods. The first consists of imaginary narratives ascribed to picture stimuli (e.g., TAT cards or the newer Adult Attachment Projective Picture System [AAP]; George & West, 2012), and the second entails real-life narratives, such as the core conflictual relationship theme method (CCRT; Luborsky, Popp, Luborsky, & Mark, 1994) or McAdams's (2012) life narrative stories. Social cognition research suggests that one's narratives denote a unique aspect of self, in particular the mental representation of self across time, which is different from conceptual self-knowledge (Prebble, Addis, & Tippett, 2013). Therefore, narrative approaches tap a unique aspect of personality distinct from self-report instruments. Abstracted and summarized narratives also impart meaning to one's life.

TREATMENT IMPLICATIONS

Relationship narratives are particularly relevant when interpersonal relationships constitute a client's key focus in therapy. But narrative methods in general are applicable across virtually every therapy orientation. For example, even if a cognitive-behavioral therapy (CBT) focus is on the more concrete amelioration of symptoms such as panic attacks or compulsions, if the client thereby obtains significant improvement on long-standing symptoms, it stands to reason that building this new sense of self into their narrative should help them maintain these changes. Regardless, narrative approaches constitute a unique method with unique implications for treatment.

Performance Tests

Performance tests ask the person to "do" something in order to provide information, in contrast to self-report methods that rely on verbal self-descriptions. Examples of cognitive performance tests include intelligence and achievement tests. Many contemporary psychologists consider projective measures to fall within the domain of performance-based personality tests (e.g., McGrath, 2008; Meyer & Kurtz, 2006).

Within the performance method domain, intelligence tests differ from personality tests in that they use objective criteria. Intelligence tests ask people to perform so that their *abilities* can be tested. There are right and wrong answers, in contrast to a person's performance on personality tests such as the Rorschach and storytelling tests. Campbell (1957) referred to this method distinction as *objective*—where the client's task is to provide the correct answers—versus *voluntary*—where the client's task is to provide his or her own personal interpretation of the stimulus. Bornstein (2007) refers to this latter process as "stimulus attribution" for tests like the Rorschach or TAT. For example, if a client reports seeing many morbid percepts on the Rorschach, this finding would be considered only in terms of its psychological implications, not in terms of its accuracy (e.g., as in the WAIS).

INTELLIGENCE

Generally speaking, there is no obligation to consider intelligence as something separate from personality. Historically, intelligence tests were frequently included in psychological testing batteries to provide an understanding of the whole person (Rapaport, Gill, & Schafer, 1945/1946). Now, especially as assessment batteries use briefer instruments due to time and money considerations (Piotrowski, Belter, & Keller, 1998), performance tests in general (both intelligence and personality tests) are much less likely to be included in a testing battery. Nevertheless, many prominent assessment psychologists have viewed intelligence as a component of personality and have included its construct in personality self-report inventories (e.g., Cattell, 1973; Wechsler, 1950; see also Austin et al., 2011). More contemporaneously, *Intellect*, the fifth factor of the Big Five model of personality (Goldberg, 1992) is largely grounded in the perception of a person's intellectual abilities and interests.

Intelligence tests measure various mental operations, each of which requires its own method of external assessment. Therefore, an intelligence test itself is a multimethod assessment measure. For example, "verbal intelligence" and "nonverbal intelligence" are distinct facets of the (traditional) intelligence construct. In reasoning through a problem verbally, different cognitive functions are used than when reasoning through a problem perceptually. Therefore, intelligence tests must require examinees to perform tasks that tap both verbal (e.g., WAIS-IV–Vocabulary) and nonverbal (e.g., WAIS-IV–Matrix Reasoning) functioning.

There are also other intelligence-related constructs that have a more obvious conceptual overlap with personality constructs—*emotional intelligence* (Mayer, Roberts, & Barsade, 2008) and, a newer construct, *personal intelligence* (Mayer, Panter, & Caruso, 2012). Emotional intelligence is the ability to perceive, understand, and manage one's own and others' emotions and feelings. Personal intelligence is the ability to reason about personality and personality-related information. Emotional intelligence can be estimated by self-report measures, but self-report and performance measures of emotional intelligence show a minimal relationship ($r = .12$, $k = 14$) to each other (Joseph & Newman, 2010). As abilities, emotional and personal intelligence are best assessed by performance measures that have right and wrong answers.

Finally, *psychological mindedness* is the ability to identify dynamic or intrapsychic components and relate them to a person's difficulties (McCallum & Piper, 1990). Although not part of the construct's label, psychological mindedness is effectively a form of *intelligence* or type of *ability* that could just as well be called something like "psychodynamic intelligence." It is the ability to think about oneself and others as having wishes, needs, fears, intentions, conflicts, and defenses.

Treatment Implications. Cognitive abilities are important for clients to succeed in various kinds of psychological treatment. The importance of a client's intelligence varies in relation to the complexity of the therapy requirements, ranging from complex tasks such as psychoanalysis or coordinating multiple psychiatric medications with varying schedules that each have different precautions, interactions, and side effects, to treatments that are not dependent on cognitive abilities such as behavioral modification therapy for clients with developmental disorders (e.g., Gale, Batty, Tynelius, Deary, & Rasmussen, 2010; Green, Kern, Braff, & Mintz, 2000; McCallum, Piper, Ogrodniczuk, & Joyce, 2003; Stilley, Bender, Dunbar-Jacob, Sereika, & Ryan, 2010; Valbak, 2004). Interestingly and perhaps not surprisingly, research has shown that the emotional intelligence of *therapists* predicts positive treatment outcome for their clients (Kaplowitz, Safran, & Muran, 2011; Rieck & Callahan, 2013). This finding argues for the use of psychological assessment in the selection and training of psychotherapists. The broader emerging research in the field indicates that the therapist should be included in the formula when planning treatment and evaluating its effects (Del Re, Flückiger, Horvath, Symonds, & Wampold, 2012).

INKBLOT TESTS

As previously noted, the Rorschach has traditionally been classified as a projective method, but contemporary psychologists use terms such as *performance-based* or *stimulus-attribution* (Bornstein, 2007; Meyer & Kurtz, 2006). Even further extending this contemporary view of Rorschach, we propose that—like intelligence tests—the Rorschach actually uses *more than one* method, each with different implications. For example, some of the methods with the most empirical support (Mihura et al., 2013) that are also preferred by clinicians (Meyer, Hsiao, Viglione, Mihura, & Abraham, 2013) include those that assess mental complexity, the psychotic indicators of distorted perceptions and thought disturbance (or coherence and clarity of communication), and implicit mental representations. Each of these Rorschach methods is discussed separately in the next section.

Treatment Implications. The interpretations of Rorschach variables that assess mental complexity share many similarities with the interpretations of intelligence test variables. There are various types of Rorschach complexity variables (e.g., *Synthesis, Blends, Form%*), but the production of these responses in general suggests higher-order cognitive processes (i.e., seeing the relationship between things, attending to nuances, articulating more complex ideas). The Rorschach complexity variables are positively related to externally assessed measures of intelligence and cognitive ability, such as IQ and education level, and negatively related to indicators of cognitive deficits, like Alzheimer's and closed head injury (Meyer, Viglione, Mihura, Erard, & Erdberg, 2011; Mihura et al., 2013). Research indicates that Rorschach complexity variables serve as positive indicators of a client's ability to engage in psychotherapy and to benefit from it (Alpher, Perfetto, Henry, & Strupp, 1990; Gerstle, Geary, Himelstein, & Reller-Geary, 1988; LaBarbera & Cornsweet, 1985; Nygren, 2004).

The Rorschach measures of distorted perception—or reality-testing problems—use a method that includes the response's perceptual fit to the blot (e.g., "a bat") as well as how common and easy it is for other people to see it at that blot location (Meyer et al., 2011). Therefore, these scores indicate the degree to which the client sees things the same way as other people do (FQo%) – or that others can easily see with just a little effort (FQu%). If a client has problems with reality testing, it can result in understanding a situation very differently than others, including the therapist. Clients will vary in regard to how much they are willing and able to explore the impact and meaning of their distorted perceptions. But with some reflection, many clients can relate to this finding and give examples of it in their everyday lives—typically in interpersonal relationships in which they do not see eye to eye with others. However, the more extreme and rigid the misperceptions, the more difficult it can be for clients to progress in any type of therapy that requires taking perspective on their experiences.

Thought disturbance on the Rorschach is indicated by problems in the coherence and clarity of a client's communication while responding to the inkblots (*Cognitive Scores*)—more specifically, by verbiage and/or perceptual images that are unrealistic, confused, or put together in a way that doesn't make sense. Reviewing these responses can serve as a bridge to talk about parallel experiences in everyday life and to explore this phenomenon when it occurs in therapy. Clients who show psychotic levels of thought disturbance on the Rorschach might also be good candidates for antipsychotic medication, although use of the Rorschach to predict medication response has not yet been thoroughly researched.

Finally, Rorschach variables assess clients' implicit mental representations by the thematic content of their responses, such as when damaged objects are seen (*Morbid*) or when people are seen as overpowering or destructive (*Mutuality of Autonomy Pathology*). The interpretation of these responses relies heavily on the method with which they were assessed. That is, these responses imply that clients have these images on their mind, but they do not indicate the client's attitudes toward the images or their related behavior. If a client sees many damaged objects, it might indicate that the client is afraid of being damaged, enjoys damaging others, or wishes to crusade against war or abuse. Various contemporary psychotherapies focus largely on a client's cognitions, including both psychodynamic and cognitive therapies. However, in general, imagery has central importance in people's day-to-day lives. And with clients there are many situations in which imagery is a key focus of therapy (e.g., flashbacks, nightmares, dreams, fantasies, obsessions). Therefore, the information gained by this Rorschach method can be especially and incrementally helpful for many clients. The two cases presented at the end of this chapter provide some examples.

Other Assessment Methods

We have covered many assessment methods, but multiple other methods exist. Another popular method of assessment involves the use of biomarkers, which are biochemical, genetic, or molecular indicators (e.g., using neuroimaging, neurophysiological, or neuropsychological assessment) of a particular biological condition or process. Currently popular and fruitful areas for the use of biomarkers are in assessment and treatment planning for dementia, schizophrenia, and depression—for example, screening individuals at risk for psychosis (Carter et al., 2011; Klöppel et al., 2012; Luck et al., 2011). While neuroimaging and neurophysiological methods are popular, neurocognitive pattern recognition using traditional neuropsychological assessment measures also holds promise (Koutsouleris et al., 2012).

Harnessing the power of our digital age, we could also employ other assessment methods such as IATs (Greenwald, McGhee, & Schwartz, 1998), electronic diaries (Piasecki, Hufford, Solhan, & Trull, 2007), and virtual reality environments (Schönbrodt & Asendorpf, 2011, 2012). For example, Schönbrodt and Asendorpf (2011, 2012) describe and test an interactive, virtual social environment that can be used to assess a client's attachment dynamics. Clients can interact in a dynamic virtual relationship environment to learn how they react and what they experience when behaving spontaneously and when attempting to change a problematic behavior pattern. In addition to programming common relationship scenarios so that norms can be collected, one could program more personal scenarios that target the client's idiosyncratic relationship patterns. A significant benefit of using a virtual reality method is that it allows therapists to understand the person in different situations. Such a benefit is not afforded to us in traditional clinical settings but is an important component of personality (Mischel, 1973; Mischel & Shoda, 1995). Finally, of course, beyond the realm of the assessment methods used in psychology and psychiatry, we can learn about people from their academic, medical, and legal records.

Practical Challenges to the Multimethod Approach to Treatment Planning

Despite the benefits that multimethod assessment can bring to a clinical case, there are real-world impediments to applying this model as freely as one may deem necessary. First are the practical challenges to the individual clinician on the front lines. An obvious practical concern is financial (Yates & Taub, 2003), including the limitations of third-party reimbursements when adding psychological assessment procedures (Piotrowski et al., 1998). Clinicians must make tough choices in prioritizing which instruments to use with each individual client. Another financial concern is the cost of purchasing testing supplies. To conduct client-focused, multimethod assessments, one must have a wide range of assessment tools on hand. This is further exacerbated due to the need to update tests, which requires clinicians to make continued additional expenditures. Clinicians are also challenged by the burden of having to learn so many different testing procedures, which includes learning the psychometrics and administration, scoring, and interpretation—as well as keeping up with the empirical literature on each test. Hopefully, the emphasis on dissemination of information in the health field will eventually result in a more efficient way for clinicians to do so.

Changing professional ideologies are seen in the training emphases of clinical psychology training programs, where those with a practice focus (e.g., practitioner-scientist or practitioner-scholar) place more emphasis on personality assessment than do other programs (e.g., clinical scientist or scientist-practitioner) (Mihura, Graceffo, & Smith, 2014). Surveys show that doctoral programs have reduced the role of these tests due to changes in their faculty and theoretical orientation (Belter & Piotrowski, 2001). In this regard, the debate between medical-model and person-centered models of clinical treatment shows itself in assessment training decisions to the extent that these ideologies differentially weight the importance of idiographic information (see Westen, Novotny, & Thompson-Brenner, 2004, for a review of this debate).

One practical consequence of the decline in personality assessment training in the programs that produce the most research is the concomitant decline in personality assessment research. Without continued research, psychological assessment cannot exist. The benefits of psychological assessment in terms of treatment planning are already challenging to research. This challenge is paralleled by the economic costs to continue developing evidence-based assessment procedures that target a variety of problems using multiple methods. One solution would be for the field in general to focus more on the response process for each assessment method instead of the name of the test or scale (see also Borsboom, Mellenbergh, & van Heerden, 2004). This would be similar to the approach in psychotherapy research to move beyond the brand names of the different therapies (e.g., CBT, psychodynamic, interpersonal) and focus on what actually happens in the therapy (e.g., Ablon, Levy, & Katzenstein, 2006; Thoma & Cecero, 2009). In this way, the basic processes that are common across different psychological methods and tests could be studied and the findings generalized, instead of concretely focusing on their brand-name packaging.

Guidelines to Using a Multimethod Approach in Treatment Planning

The current state of clinical practice and the economy does not allow every person who presents for treatment to receive an extensive multimethod psychological assessment. Nevertheless, we maintain that clinicians must still use a multimethod assessment framework with every client when conceptualizing the case, communicating with the client, and formulating treatment goals. Clinicians must remember the source of their information. For example, if a client states that his wife was sullen and angry at him last weekend, the clinician would not communicate in an assessment report that his client's wife behaved in a sullen and angry manner because the information was based on self-report, not observation. Or if a clinician observes her client's eyes well up with tears, she cannot assume that her client *feels* sad. Much of this surely seems obvious or intuitive, but sometimes clinicians endow psychological tests or interviews with a magical quality that reifies the construct into a thing-in-itself.

So how do clinicians decide to include methods of assessment beyond the clinical interview? Psychologists have recommended conducting a more extensive multimethod assessment when clients (1) have complex problems, (2) have encountered difficulties making progress in therapy, and (3) are motivated to understand themselves better (Finn, 2007; Fischer, 1994; Haynes, Leisen, & Blaine, 1997; Meyer et al., 2001). In addition, we propose including other methods of assessment when the client's self-reported information is at odds with the therapist's behavioral observations or when the client's descriptions of their experiences outside of therapy do not seem plausible as a way to understand the presenting problem. A body of personality research exists that is consistent with these recommendations. Specifically, the research shows that self-reported information may be less than adequate for clients who (a) present with personality dysfunction and (b) have difficulty making sense of and conveying their inner experiences (e.g., Berant, Newborn, & Orgler, 2008; Human & Biesanz, 2011; Lawton et al., 2011; Meyer, Riethmiller, Brooks, Benoit, & Handler, 2000).

What additional methods and tests should one include? For cognitive assessments, there is typically a focused target of the assessment (e.g., memory, attention, and concentration) and the related options for tests are fairly circumscribed. For personality assessments, there are many more options when choosing the methods and related tests. For complex cases, we recommend a broadband approach with a wide range of constructs obtained by many different methods and tests that include validity scales. Our chapter provides many potential assessment methods. We recommend including at least one self-report and one performance test (Mihura, 2012; Weiner, 2005). The clinician should certainly include methods that target the most important issues for the client. For example, inner experiences and act frequency data can be assessed by self-report (either in the interview, by questionnaire, or by keeping a diary account); thought disorder can be assessed by evaluating the clarity and coherence of the client's speech in the interview and to the Rorschach test; relational problems can be assessed by the CCRT and by a storytelling task that focuses on interpersonal themes, such as the TAT or AAP; and attention and concentration can be assessed by performance-based cognitive assessment methods.

Before conducting the assessment, it is important to formulate hypotheses that take into account the assessment context and related methods. When doing so, the clinician should attempt to predict the client's test results, emphasizing the method by which the results will be obtained. For example, the clinician might predict that the client's PAI aggression scores might be below average given his or her self-report in the interview of being a peaceful person. But given the client's frequent topics of aggressive events in the news and in their childhood, the clinician might predict a higher than average number of aggressive images on the Rorschach. This practice will help the clinician start conceptualizing the client in a rich, three-dimensional manner. Working through the hypotheses in this way can also alert the clinician to which areas may or may not need additional assessment tools. When the test results are obtained, you will learn where you were "wrong," which will teach you more about your client.

After conducting the assessment, the findings should be integrated based on both method and content. For example, when conducting assessments of attention-deficit/hyperactivity disorder, the information should be broadly organized by self-report (interview and questionnaire), informant-report, and performance methods. Clinicians can also refer to the guidelines on integrating MMPI-2 and Rorschach data provided by Ganellen (1996) and Finn (1996). Whether or not these two specific tests are used, these sources provide a framework for how to integrate data derived from introspective and external methods of assessment, including how to make sense of divergent and convergent findings across methods. For instance, Ganellen instructs clinicians to consider whether divergent findings on two similarly named scales on the MMPI-2 and Rorschach might be due to (1) slightly different content domain, (2) varying psychometric properties, (3) a psychological conflict, (4) different levels of awareness, or (5) the client consciously skewing their results. When the methods agree, Ganellen suggests that the clinician can be more confident in his or her findings, and Finn notes that it is easier to give feedback. We emphasize that clinicians continue to respect the context of the assessment method when discussing assessment findings with their clients. Focus on what the different methods might mean for the client. The descriptive terms should not be divorced from their method (Kagan, 1988).

Throughout the therapy process, it is important to keep in mind the wealth of information that the clients provide you through their multi-method assessment. To assist this process, clinicians should periodically refresh themselves with their clients' assessment data. Especially when clients are starting to understand something that they expressed in their assessment via a method other than their self-report, it is an excellent opportunity to weave this material into the therapy. For example, if a client describes images that are on his or her mind and also described similar images on the Rorschach, the therapist would mentally recall this link. We provide examples of this procedure in the brief case examples that follow.

Clinical Applications: Two Related Case Examples

To illustrate the importance of the assessment method for case conceptualization and intervention, we have chosen two actual clients with low Aggression scores on the PAI but who report many aggressive images on the Rorschach. Here, the two methods appear to be in conflict regarding the degree of the client's aggressivity. But when trying to understand the meaning of these findings for each client, we do not limit our options to deciding which finding is "right." Instead, we consider the method of assessment as vital to understanding these assessment results. In doing so, we focus on the response process and its potential interplay with client characteristics (e.g., gender, education, cultural background), presenting problem (e.g., depression, nightmares, trauma), and reason for the assessment (e.g., clinical, forensic). For the PAI Aggression Scale, the client is responding to verbal statements (e.g., "People are afraid of my temper." "I always avoid arguments if I can.") that he or she must verbally comprehend, evaluate self and others based on that understanding, and decide how the statement applies to himself or herself on a four-point scale of false to very true. Given the high face validity of these aggression items, clients can also determine how they wish to portray themselves. On the Rorschach, clients report the images that the inkblots look like to them. This can reflect the degree to which aggressive images are on their mind. However, as previously noted, it is not clear if the client identifies with these images, are afraid of these images, or what their attitude is toward them. Now we turn to describing our two clients and discussing how the assessment method affects the understanding of their case and related interventions.

Case 1

Our first client, an adult male, presents for therapy as very meek and mild-mannered. He reports that he has been depressed for months. His depression started shortly after his wife was assaulted and robbed by two men while he stood by watching helplessly. In addition to the depression, he is experiencing nightmares that are disrupting his sleep. The nightmares terrify him. A thematic analysis of the nightmares indicates that they revolve around the client violently attacking a varying number of men who appear unexpectedly and threaten to hurt a woman he cares about. After the nightmares, he always gets out of bed to make sure the doors are locked. In discussing this material along with his test results, you mention his low PAI Aggression score and wonder what this means to him. You learn that he prides himself in being very calm and level headed. When growing up, he described his mother as emotionally unstable and volatile. He judges her for this and does not "want to be like her." Even though it seems obvious to reason that the anger he felt and did not express during the assault on his wife is now being repetitively played out in the nightmares, the client does not want to explore this possibility and asserts that he really just does not feel angry. He is a calm person. He cannot understand how he could be having these dreams in which he feels rage and commits violent acts.

To address the nightmares, the therapist teaches him the imagery rehearsal technique (IRT; Krakow, Kellner, Pathak, & Lambert, 1995), a technique that can be learned in one session. In IRT the client "rescripts" his nightmares in any manner he finds desirable and mentally rehearses the new story and related images on a daily basis. For the present client, the therapist also hopes that this intervention will help process the trauma on which his nightmares are presumably based. In a very short time, this intervention is completely effective for his nightmares and his depression lessens but does not completely remit. His sense of himself as a failure in being a protective male figure is still causing some depression, which is largely based on shame and is resulting in impotence. The therapy then turns to address this conflict for him.

Case 2

The second client, another adult male, presents as depressed and anxious. He is submissive and placating, and appears somewhat furtive and wound up. A main presenting problem is his reported experience of having no thoughts or images on his mind, which makes him think he has lost these faculties. He is very worried. He meets the criteria for major depression. As therapy commences, the therapist instructs him to engage in behavioral activation to address the depression. As one of his goals, the client schedules workout sessions at a fitness center. At his next session, the client anxiously reports that when he was on the treadmill, images of murdering his brother came to mind. This frightened him and he stopped going to the gym. He became despondent. He is afraid of himself and his aggression. The client has good psychological mindedness and a motivation to understand. Therefore, in the session, you remind him of the aggressive images that he reported on the Rorschach—which involved initially pointing a gun at someone and then the image changed to the gun passively hanging in the air and then to it pointing at the person's own neck. You note the similarity in the process of aggression aimed at someone else that he eventually turns toward himself. You also recall his PAI results in which he reported very few aggressive feelings, thoughts, or actions.

As the client has now started to trust you more, he reveals that he does have these aggressive thoughts and feelings, but he was afraid you would be scared of him if you knew. He also associates to a time in junior high when his older brother and his friends started taunting him. At one point, he experienced so much rage that he thought he was going to lose control, so he went home to his room until he could make the scary feeling go away. The aggressive image on the Rorschach and its theme are explored in therapy as a way of understanding this process. The client finds this very helpful and appreciates you remembering his Rorschach response. You learn that the client also has other ego-dystonic images and urges that come to mind, and he meets the criteria for obsessive–compulsive disorder (OCD). The therapy then has a two-pronged approach: to process the strong feelings of rage toward his brother and to use a mindfulness approach to address his obsessions. This approach helps not only his OCD symptoms but his "blank mind" as he becomes able to experience in the moment.

Conclusions

Our case examples illustrate the importance of understanding the construct—in this instance, aggression—in the context of the method by which it is assessed and tailoring the interpretation to the individual case. In general, the assessment situation and the resulting data should be viewed as a microcosm of the client's life. The meaning that we make out of our lives is based on many types of information, including a linguistic understanding of ourselves and others, behavioral observations of ourselves and others, mental images and representations, others' reactions to us, and our performance on various tasks. Each of these types of information has its place in a psychological assessment. Clinicians and researchers should pay special attention to the method by which we understand ourselves and our clients. As stated at the beginning of this chapter, different assessment methods tap different aspects of personality and have implications for a person's experiences and functioning, which, in turn, should inform case conceptualization and treatment planning.

ACKNOWLEDGMENT

The original version of this chapter was presented at the annual meeting of the Society for Personality Assessment, San Diego, California, March 22, 2013.

REFERENCES

Ablon, J. S., Levy, R. A., & Katzenstein, T. (2006). Beyond brand names of psychotherapy: Identifying empirically supported change processes. *Psychotherapy: Theory, Research, Practice, and Training, 43,* 216–231.

Achenbach, T. M., Krukowski, R. A., Dumenci, L., & Ivanova, M. Y. (2005). Assessment of adult psychopathology: Meta-analyses and implications of cross-informant correlations. *Psychological Bulletin, 131,* 361–382.

Achenbach, T. M., McConaughy, S. H., & Howell, C. T. (1987). Child/adolescent behavioral and emotional problems: Implications of cross-informant correlations for situational specificity. *Psychological Bulletin, 101,* 213–232.

Allard, K., & Grann, M. (2000). Personality disorders and patient–informant concordance on DIP-Q self-report in a forensic psychiatric inpatient setting. *Nordic Journal of Psychiatry, 54,* 195–200.

Alpher, V. S., Perfetto, G. A., Henry, H. P., & Strupp, H. H. (1990). The relationship between the Rorschach and assessment of the capacity to engage in short-term dynamic psychotherapy. *Psychotherapy: Theory, Research, Practice, Training, 27,* 224–229.

Archer, R. P., Buffington-Vollum, J. K., Stredny, R. V., & Handel, R. W. (2006). A survey of psychological test use patterns among forensic psychologists. *Journal of Personality Assessment, 87,* 84–94.

Archer, R. P., & Newsom, C. R. (2000). Psychological test usage with adolescent clients: Survey update. *Assessment, 7,* 227–235.

Austin, E. J., Boyle, G. J., Groth-Marnat, G., Matthews, G., Saklofske, D. H., Schwean, V. L., et al. (2011). Integrating intelligence and personality. In T. M. Harwood, L. E. Beutler, & G. Groth-Marnat (Eds.), *Integrative assessment of adult personality* (pp. 110–151). New York: Guilford Press.

Beaudoin, M., & Desrichard, O. (2011). Are memory self-efficacy and memory performance related?: A meta-analysis. *Psychological Bulletin, 137,* 211–241.

Belter, R. W., & Piotrowski, C. (2001). Current status of doctoral-level training in psychological testing. *Journal of Clinical Psychology, 57,* 717–726.

Berant, E., Newborn, M., & Orgler, S. (2008). Convergence of self-report scales and Rorschach indexes of psychological distress: The moderating role of self-disclosure. *Journal of Personality Assessment, 90,* 36–43.

Bing, M. N., LeBreton, J. M., Davison, H. K., Migetz, D. Z., & James, L. R. (2007). Integrating implicit and explicit social cognitions for enhanced personality assessment: A general framework for choosing measurement and statistical methods. *Organizational Research Methods, 10,* 346–389.

Blais, M. A., & Smith, S. R. (2008). Improving the integrative process: Data organizing and report writing. In R. P. Archer & S. R. Smith (Eds.), *Personality assessment* (pp. 405–440). New York: Routledge.

Blasczyk-Schiep, S., Kazén, M., Kuhl, J., & Grygielski, M. (2011). Appraisal of suicide risk among adolescents and young adults through the Rorschach test. *Journal of Personality Assessment, 93,* 518–526.

Bornstein, R. F. (2007). Toward a process-based framework for classifying personality tests: Comment on Meyer and Kurtz (2006). *Journal of Personality Assessment, 89,* 202–207.

Borsboom, D., Mellenbergh, G. J., & van Heerden, J. (2004). The concept of validity. *Psychological Review, 111,* 1061–1071.

Camara, W. J., Nathan, J. S., & Puente, A. E. (2000). Psychological test usage: Implications in professional psychology. *Professional Psychology: Research and Practice, 31,* 141–154.

Campbell, D. T. (1950). The indirect assessment of social attitudes. *Psychological Bulletin, 47,* 15–38.

Campbell, D. T. (1957). A typology of tests, projective and otherwise. *Journal of Consulting Psychology, 21,* 207–210.

Campbell, D. T., & Fiske, D. W. (1959). Convergent and discriminant validation by the multitrait-multimethod matrix. *Psychological Bulletin, 56,* 81–105.

Carter, C. S., Barch, D. M., Bullmore, E., Breiling, J., Buchanan, R. W., Butler, P., et al. (2011). Cognitive neuroscience treatment research to improve cognition in schizophrenia II: Developing imaging biomarkers to enhance treatment development for schizophrenia and related disorders. *Biological Psychiatry, 70,* 7–12.

Cattell, R. B. (1973). *Personality and mood by questionnaire.* San Francisco: Jossey-Bass.

Chambless, D. L., & Ollendick, T. H. (2001). Empirically supported psychological interventions: Controversies and evidence. *Annual Review of Psychology, 52,* 685–716.

Chang, L., Connelly, B. S., & Geeza, A. A. (2012). Separating method factors and higher order traits of the Big Five: A meta-analytic multitrait–multimethod approach. *Journal of Personality and Social Psychology, 102,* 408–426

Cohen, J. (1988). *Statistical power analysis for the behavioral sciences* (2nd ed.). Hillsdale, NJ: Erlbaum.

Connelly, B. S., & Ones, D. S. (2010). Another perspective on personality: Meta-analytic integration of observers' accuracy and predictive validity. *Psychological Bulletin, 136,* 1092–1122.

Cyders, M. A., & Coskunpinar, A. (2011). Measurement of constructs using self-report and behavioral lab tasks: Is there overlap in nomothetic span and construct representation for impulsivity? *Clinical Psychology Review, 31,* 965–982.

Dao, T. K., Prevatt, F., & Horne, H. L. (2008). Differentiating psychotic patients from nonpsychotic patients with the MMPI-2 and Rorschach. *Journal of Personality Assessment, 90,* 93–101.

Del Re, A. C., Flückiger, C., Horvath, A. O., Symonds, D., & Wampold, B. E. (2012). Therapist effects in the therapeutic alliance–outcome relationship: A restricted-maximum likelihood meta-analysis. *Clinical Psychology Review, 32,* 642–649.

Eagle, M. N. (2000). A critical evaluation of current conceptions of transference and countertransference. *Psychoanalytic Psychology, 17,* 4–37.

Erdberg, P. S. (2008). Multimethod assessment as a forensic standard. In C. B. Gacono, F. Evans, N. Kaser-Boyd, & L. A. Gacono (Eds.), *The handbook of forensic Rorschach assessment* (pp. 561–566). New York: Routledge.

Finn, S. E. (1996). Assessment feedback integrating MMPI-2 and Rorschach findings. *Journal of Personality Assessment, 67,* 543–557.

Finn, S. E. (2007). *In our clients' shoes: Theory and techniques of therapeutic assessment.* Mahwah, NJ: Erlbaum.

Fischer, C. T. (1994). *Individualizing psychological assessment: A collaborative and therapeutic approach.* Mahwah, NJ: Erlbaum.

Flückiger, C., Del Re, A. C., Wampold, B. E., Symonds, D., & Horvath, A. O. (2012). How central is the alliance in psychotherapy?: A multilevel longitudinal meta-analysis. *Journal of Counseling Psychology, 59,* 10–17.

Fowler, J. C., Hilsenroth, M. J., & Piers. C. (2001). An empirical study of seriously disturbed suicidal patients. *Journal of the American Psychoanalytic Association, 49,* 161–186.

Freund, P. A., & Kasten, N. (2012). How smart do you think you are?: A meta-analysis on the validity of self-estimates of cognitive ability. *Psychological Bulletin, 138,* 296–321.

Gabbard, G. O. (1995). Countertransference: The emerging common ground. *International Journal of Psychoanalysis, 76,* 475–485.

Gale, C. R., Batty, G. D., Tynelius, P., Deary, I. J., & Rasmussen, F. (2010). Intelligence in early adulthood and subsequent hospitalization for mental disorders. *Epidemiology, 21,* 70–77.

Ganellen, R. J. (1996). *Integrating the Rorschach and the MMPI-2 in personality assessment.* Hillsdale, NJ: Erlbaum.

Garb, H. N. (1984). The incremental validity of information used in personality assessment. *Clinical Psychology Review, 4,* 641–655.

Garb, H. N. (1998). *Studying the clinician: Judgment research and psychological assessment.* Washington, DC: American Psychological Association.

Garb, H. N. (2003). Incremental validity and the assessment of psychopathology in adults. *Psychological Assessment, 15,* 508–520.

Gawronski, B., & Strack, F. (Eds.). (2012). *Cognitive consistency: A fundamental principle in social cognition.* New York: Guilford Press.

George, C., & West, M. L. (2012). *The Adult Attachment Projective Picture System: Attachment theory and assessment in adults.* New York: Guilford Press.

Gerstle, R. M., Geary, D. C., Himelstein, P., & Reller-Geary, L. (1988). Rorschach predictors of therapeutic outcome for inpatient treatment of children: A proactive study. *Journal of Clinical Psychology, 44,* 277–280.

Goldberg, L. R. (1992). The development of markers for the Big-Five factor structure. *Psychological Assessment, 4,* 26–42.

Graceffo, R. A., Mihura, J. L., & Meyer, G. J. (in press). A meta-analysis of an implicit measure of personality functioning: The Mutuality of Autonomy Scale. *Journal of Personality Assessment.*

Green, M. F., Kern, R. S., Braff, D. L., & Mintz, J. (2000). Neurocognitive deficits and functional outcome in schizophrenia: Are we measuring the "right stuff"? *Schizophrenia Bulletin, 26,* 119–136.

Greenwald, A. G., McGhee, D. E., & Schwartz, J. L. K. (1998). Measuring individual differences in implicit cognition: The Implicit Association Test. *Journal of Personality and Social Psychology, 74,* 1464–1480.

Gross, K., Keyes, M. D., & Greene, R. L. (2000). Assessing depression with the MMPI and MMPI–2. *Journal of Personality Assessment, 75,* 464–477.

Hamilton, J., & Kivlighan, D. M. (2009). Therapists' projection: The effects of therapists' relationship themes on their formulation of clients' relationship episodes. *Psychotherapy Research, 19,* 312–322.

Hardt, J., & Rutter, H. (2004). Validity of adult retrospective reports of adverse childhood experiences: Review of the evidence. *Journal of Child Psychology and Psychiatry, 45,* 260–273.

Hawes, S. W., & Boccaccini, M. T. (2009). Detection of overreporting of psychopathology on the Personality Assessment Inventory: A meta-analytic review. *Psychological Assessment, 21,* 112–124.

Haynes, S. N., Leisen, M. B., & Blaine, D. (1997). The design of individualized behavioral treatment programs using functional analytic clinical case models. *Psychological Assessment, 9,* 334–348.

Helzer, E. G., & Dunning, D. (2012). Why and when peer prediction is superior to self-prediction: The weight given to future aspiration versus past achievement. *Journal of Personality and Social Psychology, 103,* 38–53.

Hemphill, J. F. (2003). Interpreting the magnitudes of correlation coefficients. *American Psychologist, 58,* 78–79.

Henry, B., Moffitt, T. E., Caspi, A., Langley, J., & Silva, P. A. (1994). On the "remembrance of things past": A longitudinal evaluation of the retrospective method. *Psychological Assessment, 6,* 92–101.

Hiller, J. B., Rosenthal, R., Bornstein, R. F., Berry, D. T. R., & Brunell-Neuleib, S. (1999). A comparative meta-analysis of Rorschach and MMPI validity. *Psychological Assessment, 11,* 278–296.

Hollrah, J. L., Schlottmann, R. S., Scott, A. B., & Brunetti, D. G. (1995). Validity of the MMPI subtle items. *Journal of Personality Assessment, 65,* 278–299.

Human, L. J., & Biesanz, J. C. (2011). Target adjustment and self-other agreement: Utilizing trait observability to disentangle judgeability and self-knowledge. *Journal of Personality and Social Psychology, 101,* 202–216.

Hunsley, J., & Meyer, G. J. (2003). The incremental validity of psychological testing and assessment: Conceptual, methodological, and statistical issues. *Psychological Assessment, 15,* 446–455.

Johnston, C., & Murray, C. (2003). Incremental validity in the psychological assessment of children and adolescents. *Psychological Assessment, 15,* 446–455.

Jorm, A. F. (1997). Methods of screening for dementia: A meta-analysis of studies comparing an informant questionnaire with a brief cognitive test. *Alzheimer Disease and Associated Disorders, 11,* 158–162.

Joseph, D. L., & Newman, D. A. (2010). Emotional intelligence: An integrative meta-analysis and cascading model. *Journal of Applied Psychology, 95,* 54–78.

Kagan, J. (1988). The meanings of personality predicates. *American Psychologist, 43,* 614–620.

Kaplowitz, M. J., Safran, J. D., & Muran,, C. J. (2011). Impact of therapist emotional intelligence on psychotherapy. *Journal of Nervous and Mental Disease, 199,* 74–84.

Keulen-de-Vos, M., Bernstein, D. P., Clark, L. A., Arntz, A., Lucker, T. P. C., & de Spa, E. (2011). Patient versus informant reports of personality disorders in forensic patients. *Journal of Forensic Psychiatry and Psychology, 22,* 52–71.

Klonsky, E. D., Oltmanns, T. F., & Turkheimer, E. (2002). Informant-reports of personality disorder: Relation to self-reports and future research directions. *Clinical Psychology: Science and Practice, 9,* 300–311.

Klöppel, S., Abdulkadir, A., Jack, C. R., Koutsouleris, N., Mourão-Miranda, J., & Vemuri, P. (2012). Diagnostic neuroimaging across diseases. *NeuroImage, 61,* 457–463.

Koutsouleris, N., Davatzikos, C., Bottlender, R., Patschurek-Kliche, K., Scheurecker, J., Petra Decker, P., et al. (2012). Early recognition and disease prediction in the at-risk mental states for psychosis using neurocognitive pattern classification. *Schizophrenia Bulletin, 38,* 1200–1215.

Kraemer, H. C., Measelle, J. R., Ablow, J. C., Essex, M. J., Boyce, W. T., & Kupfer D. J. (2003). A new approach to integrating data from multiple informants in psychiatric assessment and research: Mixing and matching contexts and perspectives. *American Journal of Psychiatry, 160,* 1566–1577.

Krakow, B., Kellner, R., Pathak, D., & Lambert, L. (1995). Imagery rehearsal treatment for chronic nightmares. *Behaviour Research and Therapy, 33,* 837–843.

Kurtz, J. E., Puher, M. A., & Cross, N. A. (2012). Prospective prediction of college adjustment using self- and informant-rated personality traits. *Journal of Personality Assessment, 94,* 630–637.

LaBarbera, J. D., & Cornsweet, C. (1985). Rorschach predictors of therapeutic outcome in a child psychiatric inpatient service. *Journal of Personality Assessment, 49,* 120–124.

Lawton, E. M., Shields, A. J., & Oltmanns, T. F. (2011). Five-factor model personality disorder prototypes in a community sample: Self- and informant-reports predicting interview-based DSM diagnoses. *Personality Disorders: Theory Research and Treatment, 2,* 279–292.

Leary, T. (1957). *Interpersonal diagnosis of personality: A functional theory and methodology for personality evaluation.* New York: Ronald Press.

Leising, D., Krause, S., Köhler, D., Hinsen, K., & Clifton, A. (2011). Assessing interpersonal functioning: Views from within and without. *Journal of Research in Personality, 45,* 631–641.

Lilienfeld, S. O., Wood, J. M., & Garb, H. N. (2000). The scientific status of projective techniques. *Psychological Science in the Public Interest, 1,* 27–66.

Luborsky, L., Popp, C., Luborsky, E., & Mark, D. (1994). The core conflictual relationship theme. *Psychotherapy Research, 4,* 172–183.

Luck, S. J., Mathalon, D. H., O'Donnell, B. F., Hämäläinen, M. S., Spencer, K. M., Javitt, D. C., et al. (2011). A roadmap for the development and validation of event-related potential biomarkers in schizophrenia research. *Biological Psychiatry, 70,* 28–34.

Markus, H. R., & Kitayama, S. (1991). Culture and the self: Implications for cognition, emotion, and motivation. *Psychological Review, 98,* 224–253.

Mayer, J. D. (2004). A classification system for the data of personality psychology and adjoining fields. *Review of General Psychology, 8,* 208–219.

Mayer, J. D. (2005). A tale of two visions: Can a new view of personality help integrate psychology? *American Psychologist, 60,* 294–307.

Mayer, J. D., Panter, A. T., & Caruso, D. R. (2012). Does personal intelligence exist?: Evidence from a new ability-based measure. *Journal of Personality Assessment, 94,* 124–140.

Mayer, J. D., Roberts, R. D., & Barsade, S. G. (2008). Human abilities: Emotional intelligence. *Annual Review of Psychology, 59,* 507–536.

McAdams, D. P. (2012). Exploring psychological themes through life-narrative accounts. In J. A. Holstein & J. F. Gubrium (Eds.), *Varieties of narrative analysis* (pp. 15–32). London: Sage.

McCallum, M., & Piper, W. E. (1990). The Psychological Mindedness Assessment Procedure. *Psychological Assessment, 2,* 412–418.

McCallum, M., Piper, W. E., Ogrodniczuk, J. S., & Joyce, J. S. (2003). Relationships among psychological mindedness, alexithymia and outcome in four forms of short-term psychotherapy. *Psychology and Psychotherapy, 76,* 133–144.

McClelland, D. C., Koestner, R., & Weinberger, J. (1989). How do self-attributed and implicit motives differ? *Psychological Review, 96,* 690–702.

McGrath, R. E. (2008). The Rorschach in the context of performance-based personality assessment. *Journal of Personality Assessment, 90,* 465–475.

Meyer, G. J. (2000a). On the science of Rorschach research. *Journal of Personality Assessment, 75,* 46–81.

Meyer, G. J. (2000b). The incremental validity of the Rorschach Prognostic Rating Scale over the MMPI Ego Strength Scale and IQ. *Journal of Personality Assessment, 74,* 356–370.

Meyer, G. J. (2002). Implications of information-gathering methods for a refined taxonomy of psychopathology. In L. E. Beutler & M. Malik (Eds.), *Rethinking the DSM: Psychological perspectives* (pp. 69–105). Washington, DC: American Psychological Association.

Meyer, G. J., Finn, S. E., Eyde, L. D., Kay, G. G., Moreland, K. L., Dies, R. R., et al. (2001). Psychological testing and psychological assessment: A review of evidence and issues. *American Psychologist, 56,* 128–165.

Meyer, G. J., Hsiao, W., Viglione, D. J., Mihura, J. L., & Abraham, L. M. (2013). Rorschach scores in applied clinical practice: A survey of perceived validity by experienced clinicians. *Journal of Personality Assessment, 95,* 351–365.

Meyer, G. J., & Kurtz, J. E. (2006). Advancing personality assessment terminology: Time to retire "objective" and "projective" as personality test descriptors. *Journal of Personality Assessment, 87,* 223–225.

Meyer, G. J., Riethmiller, R. J., Brooks, R. D., Benoit, W. A., & Handler, L. (2000). A replication of Rorschach and MMPI-2 convergent validity. *Journal of Personality Assessment, 74,* 175–215.

Meyer, G. J., Viglione, D. J., Mihura, J. L., Erard, R. E., & Erdberg, P. (2011). *Rorschach Performance Assessment System: Administration, coding, interpretation, and technical manual.* Toledo, OH: Author.

Mihura, J. L. (2012). The necessity of multiple test methods in conducting assessments: The role of the Rorschach and self-report. *Psychological Injury and Law, 5,* 97–106.

Mihura, J. L., Graceffo, R., & Smith, J. D. (2014). *The current status of psychological assessment training in clinical psychology.* Manuscript in preparation.

Mihura, J. L., Meyer, G. J., Dumitrascu, N., & Bombel, G. (2013). The validity of individual Rorschach variables: Systematic reviews and meta-analyses of the Comprehensive System. *Psychological Bulletin, 139,* 548–605.

Miller, J. D., Pilkonis, P. A., & Clifton, A. (2005). Self- and other-reports of traits from the five-factor model: Relations to personality disorder. *Journal of Personality Disorders, 19,* 400–419.

Miller, J. D., Pilkonis, P. A., & Morse, J. Q. (2004). Five-factor model prototypes for personality disorders: The utility of self-reports and observer ratings. *Assessment, 11,* 127–138.

Mischel, W. (1973). Toward a cognitive social learning reconceptualization of personality. *Psychological Review, 80,* 252–283.

Mischel, W., & Shoda, Y. (1995). A cognitive-affective system theory of personality: Reconceptualizing situations, dispositions, dynamics, and invariance in personality structure. *Psychological Review, 102,* 246–268.

Nelson, N. W., Hoelzle, J. B., Sweet, J. J., Arbisi, P. A., & Demakis, G. J. (2010). Updated meta-analysis of the MMPI-2 symptom validity scale (FBS): Verified utility in forensic practice. *Clinical Neuropsychologist, 24,* 701–724.

Nisbett, R. E., & Wilson, T. D. (1977). Telling more than we can know: Verbal reports on mental processes. *Psychological Review, 8,* 231–259.

Norcross, J. C., & Karpiak, C. P. (2012). Clinical psychologists in the 2010s: 50 years of the APA Division of Clinical Psychology. *Clinical Psychology: Science and Practice, 19,* 1-12.

Nygren, M. (2004). Rorschach Comprehensive System variables in relation to assessing dynamic capacity and ego strength for psychodynamic psychotherapy. *Journal of Personality Assessment, 83,* 277–292.

Oh, I. S., Wang, G., & Mount, M. K. (2011). Validity of observer ratings of the five-factor model of personality traits: A meta-analysis. *Journal of Applied Psychology, 96,* 762–773.

Paulhus, D. L. (2002). Socially desirable responding: The evolution of a construct. In H. Braun, D. Jackson, & D. Wiley (Eds.), *The role of constructs in psychological and educational measurement* (pp. 49–69). Mahwah, NJ: Erlbaum.

Paulhus, D. L., & Vazire, S. (2007). The self-report method. In R. W. Robins, R. C. Fraley, & R. F. Krueger (Eds.), *Handbook of research methods in personality psychology* (pp. 224–239). New York: Guilford Press.

Perry, W., & Viglione, D. J. (1991). The Ego Impairment Index as a predictor of outcome in melancholic depressed patients treated with tricyclic antidepressants. *Journal of Personality Assessment, 56,* 487–501.

Piasecki, T. M., Hufford, M. R., Solhan, M., & Trull, T. J. (2007). Assessing clients in their natural environments with electronic diaries: Rationale, benefits, limitations, and barriers. *Psychological Assessment, 19,* 25–43.

Piotrowski, C., Belter, R. W., & Keller, J. W. (1998). The impact of "managed care" on the practice of psychological testing: Preliminary findings. *Journal of Personality Assessment, 70,* 441–447.

Prebble, S., Addis , D. R., & Tippett, L. J. (2013, October). Autobiographical memory and sense of self. *Psychological Bulletin,139,* 815–840.

Rapaport, D., Gill, M. M., & Schafer, R. (1945/1946). *Diagnostic psychological testing* (2 vols.). Chicago: Year Book.

Rieck, T., & Callahan, J. L. (2013). Emotional intelligence and psychotherapy outcomes in the training clinic. *Training and Education in Professional Psychology, 7,* 42–52.

Ritsher, J. B. (2004). Association of Rorschach and MMPI psychosis indicators and schizophrenia spectrum diagnoses in a Russian clinical sample. *Journal of Personality Assessment, 83,* 46–63.

Rogers, R., Salekin, R. T., & Sewell, K. W. (1999). Validation of the Millon Clinical Multiaxial Inventory for Axis II disorders: Does it meet the *Daubert* standard? *Law and Human Behavior, 23,* 425–443.

Schneider, L., & Schimmack, U. (2009). Self-informant agreement in well-being ratings: A meta-analysis. *Social Indicators Research, 94,* 363–376.

Schönbrodt, F. D., & Asendorpf, J. B. (2011). Virtual social environments as a tool for psychological assessment: Dynamics of interaction with a virtual spouse. *Psychological Assessment, 23,* 7–17.

Schönbrodt, F. D., & Asendorpf, J. B. (2012). Attachment dynamics in a virtual world. *Journal of Personality, 80,* 429–463.

Spangler, W. D. (1992). Validity of questionnaire and TAT measures of need for achievement: Two meta-analyses. *Psychological Bulletin, 112,* 140–154.

Spengler, P. M., White, M. J., Ægisdóttir, S., Maugherman, A. S., Anderson, L. A., Cook, R. S., et al. (2009). The meta-analysis of clinical judgment project: Effects of experience on judgment accuracy. *Counseling Psychologist, 37,* 350–399.

Stilley, C. S., Bender, C. M., Dunbar-Jacob, J., Sereika, S., & Ryan, C. M. (2010). The impact of cognitive function on medication management: Three studies. *Health Psychology, 29,* 50–55.

Stokes, J. M., Pogge, D. L., Grosso, C., & Zaccario, M. (2001). The relationship of the Rorschach schizophrenia index to psychotic features in a child psychiatric sample. *Journal of Personality Assessment, 76,* 209–228.

Stone, A. A., Turkkan, J. S., Bachrach, C. A., Jobe, J. B., Kurtzman, H. S., & Cain, V. S. (Eds.). (2000). *The science of self-report: Implications for research and practice.* Mahwah, NJ: Erlbaum.

Sue, D. W., & Sue, D. (2012). *Counseling the culturally different: Theory and practice* (6th ed.). Hoboken, NJ: Wiley.

Thoma, N. C., & Cecero, J. J. (2009). Is integrative use of techniques in psychotherapy the exception or the rule?: Results of a national survey of doctoral-level practitioners. *Psychotherapy, 46,* 405–417.

Valbak, K. (2004). Suitability for psychoanalytic psychotherapy: A review. *Acta Psychiatrica Scandanavica, 109,* 164–178.

Vazire, S. (2010). Who knows what about a person?: The self–other knowledge asymmetry (SOKA) model. *Journal of Personality and Social Psychology, 98,* 281–300.

Viglione, D. J., & Hilsenroth, M. J. (2001). The Rorschach: Facts, fictions, and future. *Psychological Assessment, 13,* 452–471.

Viglione, D. J., & Meyer, G. J. (2008). An overview of Rorschach psychometrics for forensic practice. In C. B. Gacono & F. B. Evans with N. Kaser-Boyd & L. A. Gacono (Eds.), *Handbook of forensic Rorschach psychology* (pp. 21–53). Mahwah, NJ: Erlbaum.

Wechsler, D. (1950). Cognitive, conative, and non-intellective intelligence. *American Psychologist, 5,* 78–83.

Weiner, I. B. (2005). Integrative personality assessment with self-report and performance-based measures. In S. Strack (Ed.), *Handbook of personology and psychopathology* (pp. 317–331). Hoboken, NJ: Wiley.

Westen, D., Novotny, C. M., & Thompson-Brenner, H. (2004). The empirical status of empirically supported psychotherapies: Assumptions, findings, and reporting in controlled clinical trials. *Psychological Bulletin, 130,* 631–663.

Widom, C. S., & Morris, S. (1997). Accuracy of adult recollections of childhood victimization: Part 2. Childhood sexual abuse. *Psychological Assessment, 9,* 34–46.

Widom, C. S., & Shepard, R. L. (1996). Accuracy of adult recollections of childhood victimization: Part 1. Childhood physical abuse. *Psychological Assessment, 8,* 412–421.

Wiggins, J. S. (2003). *Paradigms of personality assessment.* New York: Guilford Press.

Wilson, T. D., & Dunn, E. W. (2004). Self-knowledge: Its limits, value, and potential for improvement. *Annual Review of Psychology, 55,* 493–518.

Wright, A. G. C., Krueger, R. F., Hobbs, M. J., Markon, K. E., Eaton, N. R., & Slade, T. (2013). The structure of psychopathology: Toward an expanded quantitative empirical model. *Journal of Abnormal Psychology, 122,* 281–294.

Yates, B. T., & Taub, J. (2003). Assessing costs, benefits, cost-effectiveness, and cost-benefit of psychological assessment: We should, we can, and here's how. *Psychological Assessment, 15,* 478–495.

CHAPTER 11

Psychotherapy Progress and Process Assessment

Antonio Pascual-Leone, Terence Singh, Shawn Harrington, and Nikita Yeryomenko

Why Assess Psychotherapy Progress and Process?

Progress and process assessment in psychotherapy is the project of collecting and examining data to inform ongoing treatment. On one hand, the assessment of psychotherapy *progress* involves the ongoing periodic collection of data to track short-term outcomes (e.g., a client's level of depressive symptomology following every few sessions). This evaluation can be differentiated from final outcome assessment, which typically employs a pre–post measurement design and focuses on questions of treatment efficacy (e.g., "Did the client improve?") and/or program evaluation (e.g., "Was the treatment effective?"). On the other hand, the assessment of psychotherapy *process* does not concern itself with outcome per se, but rather with moment-by-moment events within a given session—key events, that are thought to predict outcome based on either research or theory. Psychotherapy process variables are typically either (1) assessments of a client's (or therapist's) internal experience, such as an emotional state, or (2) observations of moment-by-moment events, such as a therapist's focus on client cognition.

These approaches to psychotherapy assessment explicitly involve the systematic measurement and communication of evolving change mechanisms and client progress. Yet despite their apparent clinical utility, the majority of the progress and process assessment discourse to date has been confined to research programs and our theoretical understanding of psychotherapy change. As such, there has been little discussion of the benefits of and challenges to the incorporation of these techniques from a clinical perspective (Kazdin, 2008). Perhaps as a result, while standardized progress and process assessments have become an essential component of psychotherapy research, the proportion of clinicians who report using such measures in their independent practice remains low (Phelps, Eisman, & Kohout, 1998). Among clinicians who report regularly using treatment progress and process measures, idiosyncratic "measurement chaos" appears to be the norm (Hatfield & Ogles, 2004, p. 489). A wide diversity of measures not common to the research literature are regularly reported as in use, often alongside unstandardized ratings of individualized behavioral targets (Hatfield & Ogles, 2004).

Given that the benefits of adopting particular techniques in clinical practice have not been detailed, it should not come as a surprise that such ongoing assessment is not yet considered a standard of best practice. The most obvious consequence of this disconnect between research and practice is that well-intentioned clinicians, who make idiosyncratic use of such measures, may be arriving at treatment decisions in part on the basis of unreliable information or poorly chosen measures. The decision making regarding ongoing treatment would benefit from a range of reliable and valid outcome measures. This chapter will detail a number of psychometrically sound progress and process measures and provide examples of their appropriate clinical use. However, practicing clinicians who use progress and process assessment are clearly in the minority. Thus, for a much larger proportion of clinicians, a discussion of the issues, purposes, and rationale for doing treatment process assessment is of great value. The following discussion will provide an overview of this rationale for, and clinical utility of, integrating progress and process assessment into treatment. Specifically, we offer recommendations on empirically supported measures and examples of how to integrate such measures into clinical practice.

Integrating Assessment into Psychotherapy: Change from a Clinician's Perspective

As is routinely noted, one of the most challenging issues facing psychologists has been the "gap" between researchers and practitioners, or the failure to see research findings translated into clinicians' regular practice (Teachman et al., 2012). What is not routinely mentioned regarding this ongoing discrepancy is that psychotherapy research has often failed to confirm the importance of treatment factors that are of self-evident importance to practitioners. On a macro level, the so-called dodo bird verdict, which suggests that all psychotherapies are broadly equivalent in terms of efficacy, is not readily accepted within the clinical community (Budd & Hughes, 2009). On a micro level, large swaths of a therapist's contributions to sessions, including therapist interpretations, self-disclosures, and focus on self-image, have failed to demonstrate consistent statistical associations to good therapy outcome (Stiles, Honos-Webb, & Surko, 1998). Similar nonfindings have been observed for a variety of therapist characteristics, including theoretical orientation, years of experience, and level of training, as well as a number of client characteristics, including gender, ethnicity, and age (Bergin & Garfield, 1994). Even so, this lack of findings is all too often at odds with what therapists find as relevant in session.

Two key arguments have been proposed regarding this divergence between research findings and clinical judgment. The first argument, *the responsiveness critique*, highlights the recursive nature of psychotherapy change and the challenges that the process of psychotherapy poses to traditional assessment techniques. If the therapist is appropriately responsive, he or she will match interventions to the needs of a given client. Thus, as Stiles (1996) succinctly points out, "more of a good thing" is only better if the client is not already getting enough. For example, when a client presents with high anxiety, an intensive intervention may be needed to produce a measurable gain. However, when the same intensive intervention is offered to a client with low anxiety, it may be no more effective than a less involved (yet adequate) approach. Were the effects to be averaged, as they often are in research, the net effect is that a more intensive intervention is only loosely statistically associated with a better outcome, if at all. The recognition that psychotherapy unfolds in a way that is influenced by its emerging context helps to demonstrate the importance of client and therapist characteristics, as well as process components (such as therapist interventions) despite the lack of linear relationships to final treatment outcome. The second argument concerns the clinical advantages of *conceptualizing treatment "outcome" on a variety of levels* and the advantages such a marker-based approach to process assessment lends to clinicians in terms of both appraising a client's progress and informing the ongoing clinical case formulation.

Psychotherapy Change Is Not Linear!

In a series of incisive articles, Stiles and colleagues (e.g., Stiles, 1996, 2009; Stiles et al., 1998) have convincingly argued that the interaction between therapist and client in psychotherapy is systematically responsive. *Responsiveness* here refers to the dynamic nature of human interaction and the ways in which both client and therapist are influenced by constantly emerging perceptions of each other's behavior. In psychotherapy, content and process co-emerge as treatment moves forward, and despite the efforts of manualization (or randomized clinical trials), good psychotherapy cannot be planned completely in advance. Clinical axioms such as, "If a client experiences distress, then encourage the client to identify emotional experiences with specific emotion words," reflects in-session clinician responsiveness. Just as no two conversations are alike, neither do any two clients receive identical treatments. While the averaging of group effects as described in outcome research hopes to wash out these differences, these very differences are of most importance when a clinician is confronted with a client's distress and as they sit across from one another.

It follows that the effects of responsiveness inherent in the psycho-therapeutic process risk not being detected by linear assessments of the relationship between therapy process variables and the outcome of treat-ment. This is particularly true because, unlike casual conversationalists, therapists are focused on producing specific outcomes, such as symptom reduction. That is, they demonstrate *appropriate responsiveness*, or the ability to continually monitor the therapeutic dynamic and select treatment strategies appropriate to both the client's treatment issues and his or her current capacity. Such a process demands attunement to a client's emerging presentation.

Understanding psychotherapy change as both nonlinear and respon-sive highlights the importance of progress and process assessment. For example, suggesting that a particular process variable (e.g., anger) is thera-peutically significant means that treatment outcome is affected by the ther-apist's attention to it. However, as Stiles (1996) notes, it does not necessar-ily follow that clients who receive more attention to this component of their experience will necessarily have better treatment outcomes than those who receive less. Increasing therapeutic attention to a given issue is beneficial only when a client is not receiving enough. If a client is already receiving adequate attention to the issue, then increasing attention is not better. Like-wise, for clients already receiving adequate attention to an issue, a decrease in attention will not result in poorer treatment outcomes than those whose treatment incorporates more. Under the common method of linear assess-ment, there is a high potential for responsiveness in the psychotherapeu-tic process to conceal the contextual relationship between therapy process variables and treatment outcome.

What Counts as an Outcome?

An important implication for clinicians is that when change in psycho-therapy is considered nonlinear, the "when," "how," and "why" of change (Hayes, Laurenceau, Feldman, Strauss, & Cardaciotto, 2007; Pascual-Leone, 2009) cannot be interpreted through the designs of a traditional pre–post treatment study. For the clinician seeking to improve treatment for a given client, a different approach to the assessment of psychotherapy change is called for—one with the potential to reveal predictors, mediators, and moderators of a given case's psychotherapeutic change process.

Greenberg and Pinsof (1986), in their discussion of *big* O's and *little* o's, have provided a useful language for distinguishing between treatment "outcome" at various levels of change. Contrasting between in-session event outcomes (i.e., intermediate outcomes, or small o's) and final treatment outcome (i.e., a big O), the authors advance the notion that conceptualizing treatment outcome in this multilevel manner allows for consideration of final treatment outcome (i.e., good vs. poor therapy; a big O), as well as, on a more detailed level of analysis, session outcomes, or even within-session events (i.e., good vs. poor sessions/events; little *o*'s).

Of course, although final outcomes are the objective, a clinician's actual work happens at the level of single sessions and events (little *o*'s). Thus, the assessment of these intermediate outcomes allows clinicians to consider processing events as within-session outcomes in themselves. For example, when, at the end of a specific cognitive-behavioral intervention, a client is able to shift from all-or-nothing thinking to a more balanced thought, this could be considered as either the outcome of the intervention itself (little *o*), or a productive change process that speaks to progress toward a good final treatment outcome itself (big O), or both. This issue of outcomes assessment may be more apparent in interpersonal or experiential therapy with a difficult client, in which establishing a good relationship is both an intermediate outcome (little *o*) and a prerequisite to larger personality changes (big O). Whatever the treatment context, the multilevel assessment strategy allows clinicians to examine both the immediate impact of their interventions (little *o*) and their impact on good outcome (big O) at the end of treatment.

The Utility of Progress Assessment: Keeping Tabs on Client Change

In its consideration of in-session events as intermediate outcomes, the assessment of psychotherapy progress may be used to serve a variety of immediate clinical roles. The provision of timely feedback to clinicians regarding client progress allows for the type of session-by-session monitoring useful in guiding ongoing treatment. This use of progress assessment represents a clinical extension of quality-assurance action research and can similarly serve to enhance client outcomes. Clinical care models in which clinicians work to either step up or step down treatment intensity following the evaluation of clients' treatment response may find this assessment approach a particularly good fit (Otto, Pollack, & Maki, 2000).

The utility of progress assessment is not limited to the session-by-session evaluation of intermediate outcomes. First, progress assessment does not preclude tracking toward final treatment outcome. Rather, these techniques allow for such assessment to be more routine and detailed: The clinician is able to track a nonlinear pattern of client change from intake to final treatment outcome. Such information may be particularly useful with early treatment responders.

In addition to promoting positive outcomes, progress assessment is also effective in alerting clinicians to opportunities for reducing harm. Cutting-edge research has resulted in several very efficient systems that require less than 10 minutes per session to do so. For example, the collection of presession client data through a computerized self-report measure can be used to systematically provide practitioners with presession "alarm signals" about patients who are beginning to veer away from the normative path of positive outcomes. For such clients, the integration of progress assessment into routine mental health care has been found to reliably improve positive outcomes and reduce negative outcomes (Lambert, 2012).

Moreover, many current techniques allow for such tracking without burdening the clinician with significant additional time or labor investments. For example, Lambert (2012) has reported that clinicians utilizing computerized progress assessment software required only an average of 18 seconds to adequately access and assess presession client data. Progress information thus provides meaningful contributions to clinicians' case formulations and in-session feedback in return for a minimal investment of time and energy.

Finally, Finn and Kamphus (2006) noted that an open dialogue between the clinician and the client about results of a psychological assessment can have a beneficial effect in and of itself. They referred to this as *therapeutic assessment*, and since then it has garnered much empirical support (Hanson & Poston, 2011). Similarly, Hilsenroth (2007) has also observed that engaging clients in psychotherapy assessment is itself an intervention that can change the dynamic of treatment in a positive way. In much the same manner as behavioral monitoring can induce a client to pay more attention to specific aspects of their routine, incorporating the assessment of process variables into treatment may engage both the client and clinician more in gaining ongoing knowledge about treatment issues. Thus, regular presentation of process and progress measures to clients can prime clients to become more reflective or self-monitoring during the course of treatment. Furthermore, some clinicians may be reticent or may harbor concerns that introducing measures into the therapy room will be seen as intrusive or derail the therapeutic alliance (Hatcher, 1999). At the same time, clients who report that collaborative feedback sessions were valuable and impactful also tended to report experiencing more positive therapeutic relationships (Stiles & Snow, 1984). Thus, incorporating assessment feedback into treatment may actually enhance the therapeutic alliance.

The Utility of Assessing In-Session Process: Tracking the Client

The use of moment-by-moment process assessments as part of psychotherapy represents a new frontier for research-informed treatment. The central implication of becoming familiar with process measures as tools for moment-by-moment assessment is that it introduces a new and feasible strategy for honing in on key facets of client experience and behavior. Until recently, being well versed in psychotherapy process measures has been a narrow specialization. However, applying process measures to transcript, audio, or video records of therapy is increasingly being viewed as a fruitful strategy for the continuing education of clinicians (i.e., Hilsenroth, 2007) as well as the monitoring and quality control of treatment.

Being Marker-Driven and Process-Directive

Using process measures as formal indicators for helping therapists to get oriented in session is essentially a "marker-driven" approach to intervention. Although this idea has been most well developed and discussed in emotion-focused therapy, it is compatible with other treatment orientations. Therapists using marker-based interventions conduct a continuous appraisal of different types of emotion states, cognitive strategies, and their associated processing difficulties (Greenberg & Paivio, 1997; Paivio & Pascual-Leone, 2010). Identifying a processing difficulty then serves as an in-session marker for initiating specific therapeutic interventions. This "if–then" approach proposes that, within the broader context of understanding a particular case, "if the client presents marker *X*, then the therapist should do intervention *Y*." Facilitating moments of productive process in this way are themselves considered mini-outcomes (i.e., positive treatment effects). These include accessing adaptive emotions, exploring and changing core dysfunctional beliefs, as well as becoming more mindful of complex difficulties such as transference, self-criticism, or attachment injuries. These processing difficulties cut across, and in terms of intervention are more informative than, global diagnostic categories. For example, as described by Paivio and Pascual-Leone (2010), unresolved attachment injuries and self-critical processes can be at the root of either posttraumatic stress disorder (PTSD) or major depression, but not all clients with PTSD have attachment issues and not all major depressions are generated by self-criticism. However, observing evidence of attachment injuries can (and often should) directly inform moment-by-moment intervention.

Attending to these moment-by-moment processes can result in exceptionally specific use of interventions. In emotion-focused therapy, which uses this approach, therapists are described as making an ongoing "process diagnosis," in which they monitor and attend to the client's unfolding affective state and level of readiness for potential interventions (see Elliott, Watson, Goldman & Greenberg, 2004; Paivio & Pascual-Leone, 2010). Being familiar with "markers" of either productive or problematic client modes of processing can help orient therapists to a client's emerging patterns of change (Pascual-Leone, 2009). Moreover, these markers can help therapists with process-based choices for intervention (e.g., "When the issue arises, would it be more productive to help the client explore the subjective experience of a transgression or the motivation of the perpetrator?"). By tacitly assessing in-session process, therapists increase their awareness of key moments, which leads to more precise interventions.

Tools for Supervision, Training, and Continuing Education

Psychotherapy research has largely focused on developing and testing treatments, with surprisingly little attention given to teaching psychotherapy and examining how to best help professionals develop their skills in the assessment of in-session process (Pascual-Leone & Andreescu, 2013). Despite some advances in training, the pedagogy of psychotherapy has not exploited the dramatic advances made in process research (see Pachankis & Goldfried, 2007). As we will discuss later on, a number of well-known process measures can be used as tools for the clinician's continuing development.

While most process measures were designed in order to explore specific research questions, they also represent a relatively jargon-free operationalization of key constructs and observable in-session events, often offering accessible, intuitive descriptions. This can be an efficient way for clinicians to overcome any limitations in *perceptual acuity* with respect to therapeutic process, a largely unaddressed obstacle when learning to use interventions from new treatment approaches (which often entail different perceptive frameworks). Thus, rather than relying on the slow accumulation of clinical exposure over many years, therapists can directly benefit from the clinical clarity obtained through readily available process research tools.

Progress Assessment: Are We Almost There Yet?

Following the earlier discussion of Greenberg and Pinsof (1986) on big versus little outcomes, *progress assessment* can essentially be thought of as short-term assessments. These periodic assessments, conducted every session or every few sessions at regular intervals, are concerned with ongoing evaluation of the client's progress toward treatment goals. There are three broad categories of progress assessment: (1) therapy satisfaction; (2) symptom change, which is the largest category; and (3) functional assessment from a given theory of change. Therapy satisfaction assessment refers to the client's perceptions of how well therapy is being conducted or progressing. Symptom change assessment is the evaluation of differences in symptoms and functioning from one point in therapy to another. A variety of quantitative, qualitative, structured, semistructured, open-ended, and self-report instruments are available in each category. There are also verbal, paper-and-pencil, and computer methods of administration.

Why Assess Progress?

Assessments of client progress are beneficial to both client and therapist, without much of an added burden to either. First, given what is known about the effect of session outcome on treatment outcome (e.g., Lambert, 2012; Pos, Greenberg, & Warwar, 2009) and the fact that progress assessments enhance treatment (e.g., Shimokawa, Lambert, & Smart, 2010), clients stand to benefit from maximizing their time and money spent on therapy. Second, most progress measures only take between 2 (e.g., the Partners for Change Outcome Management System [PCOMS]; Miller,

Duncan, Sorrell, & Brown; 2005) and 15 minutes (e.g., the Beck Depression Inventory–II [BDI-II]; Beck, Steer, & Brown, 1996) to complete and as such do not require any burdensome time commitment from clients. Neither do they require additional time commitment from therapists, as most modern-day progress measures can be administered online and are scored automatically. Such assessments might even save a therapist time in the long run: A comparative treatment study demonstrated that clients who made the expected gains in therapy and whose therapists also received feedback on their ongoing progress required on average one session less than a control group of clients who similarly made expected gains but whose therapists did not receive feedback on their progress (see Lambert, 2012).

Another benefit of outcome measures is their potential to provide the therapist with the impetus to discuss the client's recent mood, attitudes, or struggles since the last session or progress measurement. Reviewing the client's responses to progress measures before the session allows therapists to be aware of any recent changes. Finally, the therapist's effort in noting client progress and communicating either concerns or client gains has the potential to strengthen the therapeutic alliance, which in turn has a significant impact on therapy outcome (Norcross & Wampold, 2011). Moreover, systematically assessing client progress allows clinicians to more closely monitor and adjust their treatment plans according to the client's needs.

Satisfaction Assessment Tools

Satisfaction assessment tools gauge how content clients are with a therapy session or the degree to which treatment is perceived as helpful. The endorsement of high satisfaction with a given session suggests that client's goals are being met and that therapy is progressing as the client expects. Three differing but widely used client satisfaction assessment tools are the Session Evaluation Questionnaire (SEQ; Stiles, 1980), the Helpful Aspects of Therapy (HAT; Elliott, 1985; Llewelyn, 1988), and the Session Rating Scale (SRS; Miller, Duncan, Sorrell, & Brown, 2005).

The Session Evaluation Questionnaire

The current Form 5 version of the SEQ (Dill-Standiford, Stiles, & Rorer, 1988; Stiles et al., 1994) consists of 21 items rated by clients on a seven-point bipolar scale following a therapy session. This pencil-and-paper questionnaire can be easily adapted to be administered online. Items are divided into two sections: (1) an evaluative section that assesses the value of a session on its depth (i.e., the effectiveness of the session; Stiles, Gordon, & Lani, 2002) and smoothness (i.e., the comfort level experienced in the session; Stiles et al., 2002); and (2) a section that assesses postsession mood on two theoretically established (Larsen & Diener, 1992) dimensions of mood: positivity and arousal.

Scores give mean ratings on each of the four dimensions, where higher scores are indicative of greater depth, smoothness, positivity, and arousal. While the rating of one session is usually not enough, ratings across four to six sessions are considered representative of a client's typical treatment experience (Stiles & Snow, 1984). Internal consistency reliability for the SEQ dimensions is high across a range of settings and conditions (Stiles et al., 2002). Early research has shown mixed findings (e.g., Stiles, Shapiro, & Firth-Cozens, 1990), although a recent study (Pesale, Hilsenroth, & Owen, 2012) on early session progress in psychodynamic therapy has shown a relationship between client progress, as measured by the SEQ, and improved outcome in psychopathology, interpersonal, social, and occupational areas of functioning.

Helpful Aspects of Therapy Questionnaire

The HAT (Elliott, 1985; Llewelyn, 1988) questionnaire is a mixed qualitative–quantitative measure. It asks clients to describe events in the session that were helpful and to indicate how helpful the events were on a four-point scale ranging from 1 = *slightly helpful* to 4 = *extremely helpful*. The next part of the measure asks for a description of any event that was hindering or unimportant, followed by a rating of how hindering it was on a four-point scale from 1 = *extremely hindering* to 4 = *slightly hindering*.

In recent a large-scale study (Castonguay et al., 2010), clients and therapists noted helpful or hindering events following each session using a modified version of the HAT. The results suggested that clients viewed self-awareness, problem clarification, and problem solution as the most helpful events in therapy. Llewelyn's (1988) study found that the most helpful aspects of therapy described by clients were the experience of relief, resolution of a problem, and insight. For a full review of helpful and hindering events for therapists and clients as compared to Llewelyn, see Castonguay and colleagues (2010). Another study (Holowaty & Paivio, 2012) used the HAT to determine the most helpful events in emotion-focused therapy for survivors of child abuse trauma. Exploring child abuse material through an imaginal confrontation, allowing feelings of pain and grieving for the self, and exploring self-conflict via a two-chair dialogue were the most helpful events identified by clients.

The chief utility of this measure in the context of single cases is that it provides therapists with highly personalized and idiosyncratic qualitative feedback about what clients like or dislike about the treatment process and often is suggestive of potential treatment directions. Thus, while research using the HAT has not necessarily been administered in every session, doing so can be palpably useful in clinical practice. Subsequent focus on events the client views as helpful and caution around events the client feels are unhelpful have the added benefit of strengthening the therapeutic alliance (Norcross & Wampold, 2011).

Session Rating Scale

The SRS (part of the PCOMS; Miller et al., 2005) assesses client satisfaction in three therapy domains (Relationship, Goals/Topics, and Approach/Method), in addition to an overall session rating. In each domain, clients are asked to rate the graded extent to which the descriptions were characteristic of their in-session experience (e.g.,"I felt heard, understood and respected"; "We did not work on or talk about what I wanted to work on and talk about"; "The therapist's approach is a good fit for me"). The overall rating includes the stem, "There was something missing in the session today" on one end of a rating scale and "Overall, today's session was right for me" on the other end. The measure is available in online and paper-and-pencil formats and takes less than one minute to complete. It has demonstrated adequate to excellent reliability as well as adequate validity (Campbell & Hemsley, 2009; Duncan et al., 2004).

Measures of Satisfaction: Advantages and Disadvantages

A strength of the SEQ relative to the HAT and the SRS is that it is more comprehensive in its assessment of client satisfaction. Moreover, it is based on theoretically derived domains in comparison to the other two measures and seems to be more quantitatively informative. An advantage of the SRS over the SEQ and the HAT is that it is the most straightforward, user friendly measure of multiple domains and takes the least amount of time to complete. In contrast to the other two measures, the HAT offers an open-ended format for clients to express their satisfaction. Such qualitative information has the potential to inform clinicians of their client's satisfaction in a richer, more descriptive manner.

Symptom Change

Many symptom change measures are classified as "outcome" measures but are used to monitor clients' symptoms throughout the course of therapy either periodically or after every session. For this discussion, such measures can be sorted into two broad classes: (1) the traditional outcome measures originally administered by paper and pencil that most clinicians are familiar with and (2) a number of more contemporary and comprehensive symptom change measures.

Traditional Outcome Measures

A number of commonly known measures are available to track symptom change in clients, many of which were used to establish the validity of more contemporary progress monitoring packages (discussed below). These traditional measures are usually less comprehensive and more specific to target symptom domains. They are also most commonly administered in paper-and-pencil form, and client scores are compared to published cutoffs and clinical norms. Many of the measures will be familiar to clinicians, and for this reason, we only list a selected few: Beck Depression Inventory (BDI-II; Beck, Steer, & Brown, 1996), Beck Anxiety Inventory (BAI; Beck & Steer, 1990), Hamilton Depression Rating Scale (HAM-D; Hamilton, 1960), Hamilton Anxiety Rating Scale (HAM-A; Hamilton, 1959), Center for Epidemiologic Studies Depression Scale—Revised (CES-D-R; Radloff, 1977), and Brief Symptom Inventory (BSI; Derogatis, 1993; a short version of the Symptom Checklist 90–Revised).

With the exception of the BSI, most of the traditional measures are limited to evaluation of either anxiety or depression. Even so, if a clinician is fairly certain that the client is only suffering from anxiety or depression, it is recommended that one of these measures specific to the presenting psychological problems be chosen. An advantage of the HAM-D, HAM-A, and CES-D-R is that they can all be obtained free of charge to clinicians. This also allows clinicians to freely experiment with introducing progress assessment into their routine practice. In deciding to administer more than one of these measures, clinicians should consider their degree of overlap between measures: For example, self-reports of anxiety and depression such as the BDI-II and BAI have a correlation of $r = .66$ (Beck, Steer, Ball, & Ranieri, 1996).

Outcome Questionnaire–45

The Outcome Questionnaire–45 (OQ-45; Lambert et al., 2004) is a 45-item client self-report measure that can be administered prior to therapy sessions via a computer program called the OQ-Analyst (OQ-A; Lambert, 2012). Designed to track adult client progress in therapy, it contains a therapist-friendly interface that alerts them to client improvement or deterioration. The OQ-45 is composed of three subscales assessing three domains: psychological *Symptom Distress* (mostly anxiety and depression), *Interpersonal Relations*, and *Social Role* functioning. Scores are given on each of these subscales as well as an overall score, with higher scores indicating greater disturbance. When administered via the OQ-A, the OQ-45 provides feedback on clients' progress. Progress is considered relative to the clients' previous assessments but also as compared to normative data that has been collected on clients' expected trajectories of change. In this way, the OQ-A uses empirical and rational algorithms to predict which clients are at risk. Thus, by comparing to norms and using a color-coded system, the program gives therapists one of four messages about their clients based on comparisons to a normative sample: (1) the client is in the normal range and termination should be considered; (2) the client is progressing as expected and no changes are required; (3) the client is not progressing as adequately as expected, with recommendation to examine the current treatment and a warning that the client might not gain anything from therapy in its current form; or (4) the client is not progressing as he or she should, with a warning that the client may drop out of treatment and with suggestions for enhancing treatment. The OQ-45 has evidenced strong internal consistency, adequate test–retest reliability, and strong concurrent validity (Lambert et al., 2004). Additionally, research has shown that the measure accurately detects changes in multiple clinical populations but remains stable in a population of untreated individuals (Vermeersch et al., 2004).

Many recent studies have been conducted on the effectiveness of the OQ-45, and the results have been promising. The most recent meta-analytic and mega-analytic review (Shimokawa et al., 2010), has confirmed that clients who were not on track to progress but whose therapists were alerted to this fact fared significantly better than those whose therapists were not given feedback on their progress. Similarly, analyses that look at the OQ-A administration of OQ-45, which includes both feedback and some additional clinical support tools, found similar results. Furthermore, the algorithm used by the OQ-45 was able to identify between 85 and 100% of clients who were at risk for treatment failure *before* they developed negative outcome (Lutz et al., 2006). Furthermore, the OQ-45 was found to be superior to clinical judgments alone in identifying such cases (Spielmans, Masters, & Lambert, 2006). While this tool was developed in the United States, it has also since been introduced in Canada, Europe, and South America, with all studies indicating that using the measure reduces treatment failures.

Clinical Outcomes in Routine Evaluation—Outcome Measure (CORE-OM)

The Clinical Outcomes in Routine Evaluation—Outcome Measure (CORE-OM; Barkham et al., 1998) is a 34-item self-report questionnaire designed to assess treatment outcome but is recommended for use throughout treatment. It is administered by hand or electronically. Clients rate the extent to which they agree with statements in four domains on a five-point scale, from 1 = *not at all* to 5 = *most or all the time*. The CORE-OM measures the domains of (1) subjective well-being; (2) problems/symptoms (mainly depression and anxiety, but also physical problems and trauma); (3) life functioning; and (4) risk to self and others. A total score is also given, with higher scores representing higher levels of distress. Feedback about clients' progress is given to the therapist based on these score. The CORE-OM has evidenced good internal and test–retest reliability as well as good convergent validity (Evans et al., 2002). This tool was standardized in the United Kingdom and has now been adopted on a nationwide basis; it is used in an extensive range of mental health services (Mellor-Clark & Barkham, 2012).

Treatment Outcome Package

The Treatment Outcome Package (TOP; Kraus, Seligman, & Jordan, 2005) consists of 58 questions designed to comprehensively assess psychological functioning. It is administered by computer and processed electronically (or by paper and fax) and assesses 12 domains each on separate scales: depression, panic, psychosis, suicidal ideation, violence, mania, sleep, substance abuse, social conflict, work functioning, sexual functioning, and quality of life (Youn, Kraus, & Castonguay, 2012). Client symptom scores are tracked, and clinicians are informed of the client's progress following each completion. It has demonstrated good test–retest reliability and adequate discriminant and convergent validity (Kraus et al., 2005). The TOP is also able to track reliable change and discriminate between a clinical and nonclinical population.

Measures of Symptom Change: Advantages, Disadvantages, and Suggestions

Compared to traditional and more targeted paper-and-pencil measures, the contemporary and electronically administered progress monitoring packages confer a number of additional advantages. First, they are generally more comprehensive. Second, they are easily administered and tracked by therapists via computer. Third, they automatize the scoring and appraisal of findings by alerting clinicians to the status of a given client's progress. Finally, they offer graphic time-tracking and/or potential recommendations that are easily interpretable.

Each of the three progress monitoring instruments is a strong and convenient measure of symptom change in its own right. As symptom measures, they are atheoretical with respect to treatment orientation and tap into various aspects of the client's experience. All three measures are well supported by research. Compared to the OQ-45, the CORE-OM and the TOP measure symptom change in areas other than anxiety and depression. The TOP is superior in this regard because it assesses many different symptom domains. Although somewhat overlapping with the domains assessed by the CORE-OM and TOP, the OQ-45's emphasis on interpersonal functioning can also be seen as an advantage. Compared to the OQ-45, the CORE-OM and TOP have more items that assess suicidality and violence toward others. A unique feature of the OQ-45 is that its predictive algorithms are designed to identify clients who are at risk for treatment failure, which may be well suited to the needs of the clinician in private practice. In contrast, design of the COPE-OM efficiently allows for multisite comparisons of quality control. Finally, the TOP is a more comprehensive symptom measure, assessing symptoms such as mania, but it has the most items and takes longer to complete. For a more comprehensive overview of these progress monitoring measures and others like it, see Overington and Ionita (2012) or visit *www.mpprg.mcgill.ca/progress%20monitoring.html.*

Functional Change from a Given Theoretical Perspective

Most measures described so far are symptom focused and atheoretical with respect to therapy orientation. However, in reality, many therapists practice, at least to some degree, from a particular approach. Consequently, it is important to be aware of functional changes in the client that might represent progress when viewed from the vantage point of the client's given theoretical orientation. For example, cognitive therapists may find it useful to periodically assess client attitudes. The Dysfunctional Attitude Scale— Short Forms are two nine-item self-reports that have been shown to be a reliable measure of depressive processes as conceptualized by cognitive theory (Beevers, Strong, Myer, Pilkonis, & Miller, 2007).

Similarly, from the perspective of emotion-focused therapy, the extent to which a client has worked through a past interpersonal trauma or grievance (i.e., "unfinished business") represents an important form of progress. The Degree of Resolution Scale (Singh, 1994) consists of 11 items to be completed after key sessions by a client (or in some cases, appraised by a therapist). It assesses the degree to which clients feel troubled by negative feelings and unmet needs, and feel worthwhile in relation to, and accepting of, a specific identified other person. This understanding of progress underpins an important part of case formulation and treatment planning. While the scale is often cited as a research tool, it has also long been used as an index by which clinicians in that approach gauge therapeutic progress. As such, it is reproduced in a number of treatment manuals of emotion-focused therapy (e.g., see Appendix C of Paivio & Pascual-Leone, 2010). By comparison, psychodynamic clinicians see patterns of client transference over the course of therapy as important for client change (e.g., see Gelso, Kivlighan, Wine, Jones, & Friedman, 1997). Such changes will not be captured by atheoretical progress measures but are nonetheless relevant to clinicians, especially when used in evaluating progress and guiding treatment planning from this particular treatment orientation. Although empirically derived measures may be perceived as more accurate than such rational and clinically derived methods, clinical wisdom should not be neglected in assessing client progress.

Concluding Thoughts on Progress Assessment: The Need for a Multimethod Approach

It is also important to be mindful of the distinction between *actual* change and *perceived* change (Kazdin, 1999). Client satisfaction represents perceived change, and perhaps surprisingly, it is not always directly related to actual symptom change (Lunnen & Ogles, 1998). As such, interpreting a client's perspective obviously has its challenges and may contrast with the more objective measure (albeit via self-reports) of symptom change. However, as Kazdin (1999) has observed, emphasis on symptom change, particularly as modeled by rigorous treatment research, often reflects the investigator's perspective. So, reliable as it is, symptom change measures may not always suitably reflect what is actually most important to a given client. Thus, while clinicians would be ill advised to take client satisfaction as a singular measure (despite it being the simplest to begin using), it also seems that getting a sense of the client's perspective is essential, especially for adults in outpatient psychotherapy.

In conclusion, multiple approaches to progress assessment are necessary to appreciate the multifaceted nature of the therapeutic process. Information on targeted symptom change over time, client satisfaction, and measures of client functioning as informed by a given theoretical context, each provide complementary views on progress. When using only one assessment method, clinicians risk missing the forest for the trees, sometimes overlooking clinically relevant variables that are often otherwise within reach. A multimethod assessment provides the clinician with a comprehensive ongoing case conceptualization, helps with treatment planning, and allows a reliable record of change across time, by which clinicians can evaluate their efforts.

Process Assessment: What Is Happening Now?

While progress assessment gages whether a client is "on track" with respect to symptom changes or satisfaction, process is defined by those things that happen moment by moment and are believed (either in theory or given empirical research) as being the "how" and "what" of therapy that predicts progress and outcome. Thus, *process assessments* will usually appraise the client's or therapist's internal experience (e.g., emotional states, interpersonal experiences, transference, insights), or even observations of moment-by-moment events (e.g., observed depth of processing, critical shifts in perspective, or cognitive frames). For example, while the quality of a therapeutic relationship is an integral part of effective treatment (i.e., a process), it is not itself the treatment outcome being sought after. Similarly, when a client gains a new insight, it is a significant in-session event (a process marker, or little o) that mediates but is not to be equated with treatment progress in the sense of behavioral or symptom change (big O). For the purposes of this chapter (and bearing in mind the range of treatment approaches that differentially prize and seek to facilitate distinct in-session processes), we construe two categories of process assessment tools: (1) the therapeutic relationship and (2) a diverse category that we will refer collectively to as in-session client processes, which becomes increasingly critical in the working phase of treatment.

The Therapeutic Relationship

Among known common factors, the therapeutic alliance is the most well-established in-session process that is related to psychotherapy outcomes, with a predictive correlation in the range of .22 to .29 (Horvath, 2005). While there are a number of suitable paper-and-pencil measures, for routine practice settings we recommend the Working Alliance Inventory— Short Revised Version (WAI-SR; Hatcher & Gillaspy, 2006), which is a brief self-report based on Horvath and Greenberg's (1989) original scale. Taking 1 to 2 minutes to complete, WAI-SR is designed to gauge the depth of a therapeutic relationship between client and therapist. The measure consists of 12 Likert scale items, ranging from 1 (*strongly disagree*) to 5 (*strongly agree*), on which clients appraise the collaborative process toward establishing *goals*, the *tasks* to address the problem, and the *bond* in the interpersonal relationship. Reliability coefficients for this measure reach satisfactory levels (between .88 and .92) and construct validity is strong. Therapeutic alliance is often measured pre- or postsession. Often, it is conveniently administered in tandem with progress monitoring measures; however, despite its self-report format, alliance ratings actually describe a variable that is active *during* sessions, making it a process measure (and an intermediate outcome to symptom progress). Assessing for a good relationship early in treatment gives critical and predictive process information, particularly in the first five sessions. While at later stages of treatment, it can still be used to rule out problems since it is often regarded as a sine qua non of good process, one that often mediates other positive process– outcome relationships (see, e.g., mediation models by Pos et al., 2009).

In-Session Client Processes

Why Assess In-Session Process?

It is rare that psychotherapy researchers explicitly recommend re-purposing their process measures either for enriching psychotherapy or for training. Nevertheless, despite the lack of explicit acknowledgment, this often happens in practice, particularly when both research and clinical training are conducted "under the same roof." Hilsenroth (2007) is one of the few researchers who explicitly proposes this kind of transfer: He suggests that the Comparative Psychotherapy Process Scale (CPPS) be used as a training tool to familiarize trainees with discriminating features of cognitive-behavioral versus interpersonal-psychodynamic interventions. But this idea can be further developed: While measures of *therapist* process or intervention (like the CPPS) could help trainees to identify and grasp *what to do* as a therapist, *client* process measures, in contrast, help developing clinicians to *perceive what is happening* in session with the client.

As Pascual-Leone and Andreescu (2013) explain, current approaches to psychotherapy training tend to emphasize intervention skills, while the question of developing a clinician's *perceptual acuity*, or the ability to recognize and orient to key client processes, receives much less attention. They argue that this imbalance may be due to a scarcity of formal strategies, which might otherwise be used to heighten the perceptiveness and sensitivity of clinicians, helping them to recognize and interpret in-session phenomena. Client process measures may turn out to be particularly useful in this regard. One purpose then of formally or informally using process assessment, is for clinicians to hone their ability to see important moment-by-moment therapeutic events during both psychotherapy and diagnostic interviewing.

Using Process Measures

The lion's share of process research measures has emerged from experiential and psychodynamic therapies. For this reason, many of the tools described below are based on constructs from these traditions. Although because they reflect fundamental observations about clients, we believe they can be readily applied to any insight-oriented psychotherapy. Moreover, while all measures have sound psychometrics and are believed to have important relationships to outcome, our aim is only to highlight recommended tools, conveying their basic idea as well as their potential use. Clinicians seeking to improve their assessments of process are advised to examine video or audio recordings of their treatment sessions, while considering the relevant coding criteria for a given measure. Although the coding reliability described by research procedures is uncalled for in this practice, over time, clinicians become sensitized to in-session process markers. This heightens their perceptual acuity and eventually leads to making live in-session observations, or moment-by-moment "process diagnoses."

PROCESS MEASURES OF NARRATIVE AND SPEECH PATTERNS

Developing therapists often do not immediately notice when clients deflect away from evocative ("hot") content; but narrative process measures (Angus, Levitt, & Hartke, 1999) could be used to help sensitize clinicians in attending to their clients' spontaneous shifts in narrative style. First, such research measures can help clinicians to perceive, recognize, and track a client's subtle shifts from external narratives (i.e., plot-and-characters) to more internal narratives (i.e., meaning-and-experiences). Second, this apperceptive framework provides a lens to *help orient clinicians in the moment* as they use interventions to actively facilitate a client's elaboration of more promising process (i.e., internal narratives, hot cognitions).

In a similar example, certain client vocal qualities, such as a highly external, rapid, lecturing voice versus a softer, searching, stop-and-go, and internally focused voice, have also been operationalized and then related to unproductive and productive processes, respectively (Rice & Kerr, 1986). Descriptions of these vocal qualities can provide very intuitive and easy cues to clinicians about a client's internal process and his or her need for moment-by-moment interventions. In the same vein, novice therapists are often anxious about silences during therapy sessions. Familiarizing them with research on the nature of productive versus obstructive client pauses (Levitt, 2001) provides trainees with practical and immediately usable information on what is happening with their clients and how to respond to the pauses in session.

ASSESSING GOOD EXPERIENTIAL PROCESS AND ENGAGEMENT

A client's level of experiencing within psychotherapy refers to the degree to which clients engage and explore their feelings and meaning related to personal distress. The client experiencing scale (Klein, Mathieu-Coughlan, & Kiesler, 1986) is a measure of "depth," whereby certain kinds of processing are considered more engaged and meaningful than others; this seven-point observer rating scale has long been used as a gold standard of good therapeutic process. At the lowest level of experiencing, clients do not speak about their internal experience, including emotions, and instead refer to external events in a removed manner. At the highest level of experiencing, not only are clients engaged with all aspects of their internal experience, but these freshly emerging elements are integrated in an insightful, meaningful manner. Ratings are made passage by passage from written or audio texts, although clinicians who are very familiar with this measure can make rating *in vivo*.

A recent meta-analysis of 11 process–outcome studies and 458 clients (Yeryomenko, 2012) has shown that higher in-session ratings of client's experiencing are predictive of good treatment outcomes in experiential, psychodynamic, and cognitive treatment approaches. Moreover, this predictive effect of the experiencing scale is estimated to be $r = .24$, which is comparable to the predictive strength of the therapeutic alliance (cf. Horvath, 2005). Being competent in the use of this observer rating scale is known (particularly in the experiential tradition) to be helpful in orienting therapists to a client's immediate process and then in deliberately deepening a client's level of meaning exploration in session, whether that be affective or cognitive in nature. However, today clinicians studying emotion-focused therapy are commonly encouraged to practice using the experiencing scale whenever such research training is available. Furthermore, the fact that the rating scale is reprinted in a number of treatment manuals (e.g., Elliott et al., 2004; Paivio & Pascual-Leone, 2010) illustrates its usefulness in assessing process and conducting therapy.

ASSESSING TRANSFERENCE PATTERNS

The core conflictual relationship theme (CCRT; Luborsky, Popp, Luborsky, & Mark, 1994) method was first introduced as a new psychotherapy process research tool for testing and verifying Freud's hypothesis of transference. Since then, it has been increasingly used as a way of palpably introducing clinicians who are learning dynamic therapy to the construct of transference and supporting the development of case formulations. This seamless shift in use of the CCRT process measure (from research to training and practice purposes) is not often acknowledged in treatment manuals or training literature. Nevertheless, becoming proficient in using the CCRT by applying it to transcripts can sensitize clinicians to the *perceptual framework* that is important to a psychodynamic therapy. A perceptual framework of this sort is central to the training and continuing education strategy we are proposing.

APPRAISING IN-SESSION RELATIONAL RUPTURES

Although the general status of the therapeutic relationship may be assessed using client reports as described earlier, research suggests that clients are much less likely to disclose relationship ruptures when they occur (Safran, Samstag, Muran, & Stevens, 2001). However, research criteria used to study in-session relationship ruptures (Safran et al., 2001) have now been assimilated into some of the best practices. Thus, the original research criteria for recognizing and managing interpersonal ruptures have influenced a range of dynamic, experiential, and integrative-cognitive approaches (e.g., Castonguay et al., 2004). Familiarizing clinicians with the original research criteria that have been used for detecting and classifying different types of relationship ruptures between clients and their therapists, as well as the steps in repairing a therapeutic relationship, offers them concrete instruction for *identifying* as well as addressing key relational features.

EVIDENCE FOR THE USE OF PROCESS ASSESSMENT TOOLS

For all the process assessment tools we have discussed, rather than simply learning the evidence related to a given phenomenon, clinicians would do well to engage in a research-like didactic exercise of coding or rating audio or video segments taken from their clinical practice, to provide the kind of perceptual training that is prerequisite to the incisive and timely use of interventions. Although a number of these tools have already been assimilated into treatment approaches or are being used in a relatively undeclared way among process researchers and their students, there is still little empirical research. One study by Pascual-Leone and Andreescu (2013), however, has shown that this approach can be easily integrated into the training of novice clinicians in a modular way over 8 to 10 weeks.

Integrated Application in Practice Settings

A number of practice research networks, many in university-based clinics, are now introducing standardized measures of progress and process used for both research and therapist training (e.g., see Castonguay et al., 2010). Examples of clinical protocols in these settings help illustrate how clinicians may bridge the research–practice gap (Teachman et al., 2012). Recently, we introduced these routine assessments at our university treatment clinic. In one case, the treatment of "Stacey," a 22-year-old female suffering from moderate depression, frequent bouts of alcohol abuse, and some history of self-harm, was clearly facilitated by the use of progress and process assessments. Even prior to the beginning of therapy she expressed strong ambivalence about seeking help, so the risk of dropout was a present issue. However, in keeping with routine progress assessments at our clinic, Stacey was asked to come to therapy sessions 10 minutes early. While in the waiting room, she completed a progress measure (OQ-45) on a netbook computer via the Internet. Instant scoring and feedback was then available for her therapist to view in his office a few minutes prior to seeing her. This tool alerted the clinician to any significant changes in Stacey's situation, including her general functioning, as well as highlighting any critical items she endorsed (e.g., regarding her bouts of heavy drinking, or suicidal ideations). At the end of each session Stacey took another 5 minutes to fill out a qualitative measure of client satisfaction (HAT), and a process measure of the therapeutic alliance (WAI-RS).

When Stacey's progress stagnated after the first few sessions, the OQ-A's algorithm gave a "red flag," indicating that she was not progressing as she should when compared to standard trajectories, and it warned of the risk of client dropout. As a result, the therapist was able to explore this concern with more urgency, while the WAI-RS and HAT provided feedback at the end of each session for monitoring the fragile therapeutic relationship in addition to the client's impressions of the treatment. In her particular case, the measures showed a slow but steady increase in alliance (WAI-RS scores had moved from a 24/60 to 36/60, which was an improvement but was still modest). However, Stacey's feedback on the HAT indicated that she felt that "homework exercises let me feel in control of my problems," and that she yearned to disclose but seemed hesitant (e.g., "unable to talk about what's really bothering me"). This information led the therapist to suggest new tasks for therapy and explicitly discuss the relationship in an inviting manner.

Therapists in our clinic have also trained to be able to make sufficient use of key process measures and are encouraged to use these measures in identifying in-session markers of noteworthy processes when reviewing their session videos prior to supervision. In an effort to help Stacey make sense of her distress, her therapist used moment-by-moment observational process measures (the client experiencing scale and the CCRT) as perceptual guides for becoming oriented to fleeting client processes. The supervisor also used process tools to help highlight key events in therapy (e.g., a period of low experiencing, difficulties with the alliance), along with anchored suggestions for the therapist to address Stacey's treatment needs. With changes to the treatment approach, the alliance rating improved (51/60), and the OQ-A indicated that Stacey was back "on track." The risk of dropout had been averted. These measures essentially provided a set of tools for appraising the vital signs of therapy: information that helps to refine a diagnosis, contribute to treatment planning, monitor risk, and clarify the meaning, context, or motivations underlying real world behavior.

Conclusion

Ongoing assessments of this kind are not yet widely practiced. While the resource burden associated with administering measures (e.g., potential lack of compensation, client fatigue, data storage, and management) may seem like an obvious obstacle to adopting such measures, this is not, in fact, so substantial—as we have seen. Based on informal surveys and our involvement in conference discussions, the most prominent obstacle to introducing progress and process measures into practice may actually be the learning curve. This issue entails the lack of familiarity with new instruments, the need for training, and concern that until it becomes routine, ongoing assessment risks pulling focus away from the actual work to be done in treatment.

Even so, while progress and process assessments do mean making changes to established practices, they offer a number of distinct advantages to clinical work. Unlike the pre–post outcomes used in research and quality control programs, progress monitoring allows regular feedback about clients' satisfaction with therapy and their symptom changes over the course of treatment. In one form or another, use of routine assessments in therapy allows clinicians to become aware of any significant changes (e.g., in symptoms and satisfaction with treatment) that may need to be quickly addressed in a following session.

To date, client process measures have only incipiently and informally been integrated as methods for improving psychotherapy, although along with progress monitoring this is clearly the frontier of psychotherapy assessment. Process assessment tools offer a very unique set of benefits and perhaps are most useful in developing one's incisiveness as a practicing therapist, as well as for the formal purposes of training and supervision. These tools sensitize and orient clinicians to relevant in-session phenomena and can help supervisors suggest specific interventions given the observation of a relevant marker in client process. As in the described clinic example, we recommend that practitioners judiciously select a few measures and keep in mind that the purpose of such assessments is to facilitate therapy. Exploring progress and process assessment tools should be thought of as adjuncts to routine psychotherapy, as they are emerging on the leading edge of the best treatment practices.

REFERENCES

Angus, L., Levitt, H., & Hartke, K. (1999). The narrative processes coding system: Research applications and implications for psychotherapy practice. *Journal of Clinical Psychology, 55*(10), 1255–1270.

Barkham, M., Evans, C., Margison, F., Mcgrath, G., Mellor-Clark, J., Milne, D., et al. (1998). The rationale for developing and implementing core outcome batteries for routine use in service settings and psychotherapy outcome research. *Journal of Mental Health, 7*(1), 35–47.

Beck, A. T., & Steer, R. A. (1990). *Manual for the Beck Anxiety Inventory.* San Antonio, TX: Psychological Corporation

Beck, A. T., Steer, R. A., Ball, R., & Ranieri, W. F. (1996). Comparison of Beck Depression Inventories–IA and –II in psychiatric outpatients. *Journal of Personality Assessment, 67*(3), 588–597.

Beck, A. T., Steer, R. A., & Brown, G. K. (1996). *Manual for the Beck Depression Inventory* (3rd ed.). San Antonio, TX: Psychological Corporation.

Beevers, C. G., Strong, D. R., Myer, B., Pilkonis, P. A., & Miller, I. W. (2007). Efficiently assessing negative cognition in depression: An item response theory analysis of the dysfunctional attitude scale. *Psychological Assessment, 19*, 199–209.

Bergin, A. E., & Garfield, S. L. (1994). *Handbook of psychotherapy and behaviour change* (4th ed). New York: Wiley.

Budd, R., & Hughes, I. (2009). The dodo bird verdict—controversial, inevitable and important: A commentary on 30 years of meta-analyses. *Clinical Psychology and Psychotherapy, 16*, 510–522.

Campbell, A., & Hemsley, S. (2009). Outcome Rating Scale and Session Rating Scale in psychological practice: Clinical utility of ultra-brief measures. *Clinical Psychologist, 13*(1), 1–9.

Castonguay, L. G., Boswell, J. F., Zack, S. E., Baker, S., Boutselis, M. A., Chiswick, N. R., et al. (2010). Helpful and hindering events in psychotherapy: A practice research network study. *Psychotherapy: Theory, Research, Practice, Training, 47*(3), 327–344.

Castonguay, L. G., Schut, J. A., Aikins, E. D., Constantino, J. M., Laurenceau, P. J., Bologh, L., et al. (2004). Integrative cognitive therapy for depression: A preliminary investigation. *Journal of Psychotherapy Integration, 14(1),* 4–20.

Derogatis , L. R. (1993*). Brief Symptom Inventory: Administration, scoring and procedures manual,* (4th ed.) Minneapolis, MN: NCS, Pearson.

Dill-Standiford, T. J., Stiles, W. B., & Rorer, L. G. (1988). Counselor-client agreement on session impact. *Journal of Counseling Psychology, 35*(1), 47–55

Duncan, B. L., Miller, S. D., Reynolds, L., Sparks, J., Claud, D., Brown, J., et al. (2004). The session rating scale: Psychometric properties of a "working" alliance scale. *Journal of Brief Therapy, 3*(1), 3–12.

Elliott, R. (1985). Helpful and nonhelpful events in brief counseling interviews: An empirical taxonomy. *Journal of Counseling Psychology, 32*(3), 307–322.

Elliott, R., Watson, J., Goldman, R. N., & Greenberg, L. S. (2004). *Learning emotion focused therapy: A process experiential approach to change.* Washington, DC: American Psychological Association.

Evans, C., Connell, J., Barkham, M., Margison, F., McGrath, G., Mellor-Clark, J., & Audin, K. (2002). Towards a standardised brief outcome measure: Psychometric properties and utility of the CORE—OM. *British Journal of Psychiatry, 180*(1), 51–60.

Finn, S. E., & Kamphus, J. H. (2006). Therapeutic assessment with the MMPI-2. In J. N. Butcher (Ed.), *MMPI-2: A practitioner's guide* (pp. 165–191). Washington, DC: American Psychological Association.

Gelso, C. J., Kivlighan, D. M., Wine, B., Jones, A., & Friedman, S. C. (1997). Transference, insight, and the course of time-limited therapy. *Journal of Counseling Psychology, 44,* 209–217.

Greenberg, L. S., & Paivio, S. C. (1997). *Working with emotions in psychotherapy.* New York: Guilford Press.

Greenberg, L. S., & Pinsof, W. M. (1986). Process research: Current trends and future perspectives. In L. S. Greenberg & W. M. Pinsof (Eds.), *The psychotherapeutic process: A research handbook* (pp. 3–20). New York: Guilford Press.

Hamilton, M. (1959). The assessment of anxiety states by rating. *British Journal of Medical Psychology, 32,* 50–55.

Hamilton, M. (1960). A rating scale for depression. *Journal of Neurology, Neurosurgery, and Psychiatry, 23,* 56–62.

Hanson, W. E., & Poston, J. M. (2011). Building confidence in psychological assessment as a therapeutic intervention: An empirically based reply to Lilienfeld, Garb, and Wood (2011). *Psychological Assessment, 23*(4), 1056–1062.

Hatcher, R. (1999). Therapists' views of treatment alliance and collaboration in therapy. *Psychotherapy Research, 9,* 405–423.

Hatcher, R. L., & Gillaspy, J. A. (2006). Development and validation of a revised short version of the working alliance inventory. *Psychotherapy Research, 16*(1), 12–25.

Hatfield, D. R., & Ogles, B. M. (2004). The use of outcome measures by psychologists in clinical practice. *Professional Psychology: Research and Practice, 35*(5), 485–591.

Hayes, A. M., Laurenceau, J., Feldman, G., Strauss, J. L., & Cardaciotto, L. (2007). Change is not always linear: The study of nonlinear and discontinuous patterns of change in psychotherapy. *Clinical Psychology Review, 27,* 715–723.

Hilsenroth, M. J. (2007). A programmatic study of short-term psychodynamic psychotherapy: Assessment, process, outcome, and training. *Psychotherapy Research, 17*(1), 31–45.

Holowaty, K. A. M., & Paivio, S. C. (2012). Characteristics of client-identified helpful events in emotion-focused therapy for child abuse trauma. *Psychotherapy Research, 22*(1), 56–66.

Horvath, A. O. (2005). The therapeutic relationship: Research and theory. An introduction to the special issue. *Psychotherapy Research, 15*(1–2), 3–7.

Horvath, A. O., & Greenberg, L. S. (1989). Development and validation of the Working Alliance Inventory. *Journal of Counseling Psychology, 36,* 223–233.

Kazdin, A. E. (1999). The meanings and measurement of Clinical Significance. *Journal of Consulting and Clinical Psychology, 67* (3), 332–339

Kazdin, A. E. (2008). Evidence-based treatment and practice: New opportunities to bridge clinical research and practice, enhance the knowledge base, and improve patient care. *American Psychologist, 63*(3), 146–159.

Klein, M. H., Mathieu-Coughlan, P., & Kiesler, D. J. (1986). The experiencing scales. In L. S. Greenberg & W. M. Pinsof (Eds.), *The psychotherapeutic process: A research handbook* (pp. 21–71). New York: Guilford Press.

Kraus, D. R., Seligman, D. A., & Jordan, J. R. (2005). Validation of a behavioral health treatment outcome and assessment tool designed for naturalistic settings: The treatment outcome package. *Journal of Clinical Psychology, 61*(3), 285–314.

Lambert, M. J. (2012). Helping clinicians to use and learn from research-based systems: The OQ-analyst. *Psychotherapy, 49*(2), 109–114.

Lambert, M. J., Morton, J. J., Hatfield, D., Harmon, C., Hamilton, S., Reid, R. C., et al. (2004). *Administration and scoring manual for the Outcome Questionnaire-45*. Salt Lake City, UT: OQ Measures.

Larsen, R. J., & Diener, E. (1992). Promises and problems with the circumplex model of emotion. In M. S. Clark (Ed.), *Emotion: Review of personality and social psychology,* No. 13 (Vol. IX, pp. 25–59). Thousand Oaks, CA: Sage.

Levitt, H. M. (2001). Sounds of silence in psychotherapy: The categorization of clients' pauses. *Psychotherapy Research, 11,* 295–309.

Llewelyn, S. P. (1988). Psychological therapy as viewed by clients and therapists. *British Journal of Clinical Psychology, 27*(3), 223–237.

Luborsky, L., Popp, C., Luborsky, E., & Mark, D. (1994). The core conflictual relationship theme. *Psychotherapy Research, 4*(3&4), 172–183.

Lunnen, K. M., & Ogles, B. M. (1998). A multiperspective, multivariable evaluation of reliable change. *Journal of Consulting and Clinical Psychology, 66,* 400–410.

Lutz, W., Lambert, M. J., Harmon, S. C., Tschitsaz, A., Schürch, E., & Stulz, N. (2006). The probability of treatment success, failure and duration: What can be learned from empirical data to support decision making in clinical practice? *Clinical Psychology and Psychotherapy, 13,* 223–232.

Mellor-Clark, J., & Barkham, M. (2012). Using the CORE system to support service quality development. In C. Feltham & I. Horton (Eds.), *Handbook of counselling and psychotherapy* (pp. 210–228). London: Sage.

Miller, S. D., Duncan, B. L., Sorrell, R., & Brown, G. S. (2005). The Partners for Change Outcome Management System. *Journal of Clinical Psychology, 61*(2), 199–208.

Norcross, J. C., & Wampold, B. E. (2011). Evidence-based therapy relationships: Research conclusions and clinical practices. *Psychotherapy, 48*(1), 98–102.

Otto, M. W., Pollack, M. H., & Maki, K. M. (2000). Empirically supported treatments for panic disorder: Costs, benefits, and stepped care. *Journal of Consulting and Clinical Psychology, 68,* 556–563.

Overington, L., & Ionita, G. (2012). Progress monitoring measures: A brief guide. *Canadian Psychology/Psychologie Canadienne, 53*(2), 82–92.

Pachankis, J. E., & Goldfried, M. R. (2007). On the next generation of process research. *Clinical Psychology Review, 27,* 760–768.

Paivio, S. C., & Pascual-Leone, A. (2010). *Emotion focused therapy for complex trauma: An integrative approach.* Washington, DC: American Psychological Association.

Pascual-Leone, A. (2009). Dynamic emotional processing in experiential therapy: Two steps forward, one step back. *Journal of Consulting and Clinical Psychology, 77,* 113–126.

Pascual-Leone, A., & Andreescu, C. (2013). Repurposing process measures to train psychotherapists: Training outcomes using a new approach. *Counselling and Psychotherapy Research, 13*(3), 210–219.

Pesale, F. P., Hilsenroth, M. J., & Owen, J. J. (2012). Patient early session experience and treatment outcome. *Psychotherapy Research, 22*(4), 417–425.

Phelps, R., Eisman, E. J., & Kohout, J. (1998). Psychological practice and managed care: Results of the CAPP practitioner survey. *Professional Psychology: Research and Practice, 29,* 31–36.

Pos, A. E., Greenberg, L. S., & Warwar, S. H. (2009). Testing a model of change in the experiential treatment of depression. *Journal of Consulting and Clinical Psychology, 77*(6), 1055–1066.

Radloff, L. S. (1977). The CES-D scale: A self-report depression scale for research in the general population. *Applied Psychological Measurement, 1,* 385–401.

Rice, L. N., & Kerr, G. P. (1986). Measures of client and therapist vocal quality. In L. S. Greenberg & W. M. Pinsoff (Eds.), *The psychotherapeutic process: A research handbook* (pp. 73–105). New York: Guilford Press.

Safran, J. D., Samstag, W. L., Muran, C. J., & Stevens, C. (2001). Repairing alliance ruptures. *Psychotherapy Research, 28*(4), 406–412.

Shimokawa, K., Lambert, M. J., & Smart, D. W. (2010). Enhancing treatment outcome of patients at risk of treatment failure: Meta-analytic and mega-analytic review of a psychotherapy quality assurance system. *Journal of Consulting and Clinical Psychology, 78*(3), 298–311.

Singh, M. (1994). *Validation of a measure of session outcome in the resolution of unfinished business.* Unpublished doctoral dissertation, York University, Toronto, Canada.

Spielmans, G. I., Masters, K. S., & Lambert, M. J. (2006). A comparison of rational versus empirical methods in the prediction of psychotherapy outcome. *Clinical Psychology and Psychotherapy, 13*, 202–214.

Stiles, W. B. (1980). Measurement of the impact of psychotherapy sessions. *Journal of Consulting and Clinical Psychology, 48*(2), 176–185.

Stiles, W. B. (1996). When more of a good thing is better: Reply to Hayes et al. (1996). *Journal of Consulting and Clinical Psychology, 64*, 915–918.

Stiles, W. B. (2009). Responsiveness as an obstacle for psychotherapy outcome research: It's worse than you think. *Clinical Psychology: Science and Practice, 16*(1), 86–91.

Stiles, W. B., Gordon, L. E., & Lani, J. A. (2002). Session evaluation and the Session Evaluation Questionnaire. In G. S. Tryon (Ed.), *Counseling based on process research: Applying what we know* (pp. 325–343). Boston: Allyn & Bacon.

Stiles, W. B., Honos-Webb, L., & Surko, M. (1998). Responsiveness in psychotherapy. *Clinical Psychology: Science and Practice, 5*, 439–458.

Stiles, W. B., Reynolds, S., Hardy, G. E., Rees, A., Barkham, M., & Shapiro, D. A. (1994). Evaluation and description of psychotherapy sessions by clients using the Session Evaluation Questionnaire and the Session Impacts Scale. *Journal of Counseling Psychology, 41*(2), 175–185.

Stiles, W. B., Shapiro, D. A., & Firth-Cozens, J. A. (1990). Correlations of session evaluations with treatment outcome. *British Journal of Clinical Psychology, 29*(1), 13–21.

Stiles, W. B., & Snow, J. S. (1984). Counseling session impact as viewed by novice counselors and their clients. *Journal of Counseling Psychology, 31*, 3–12.

Teachman, B. A., Drabick, D. A., Hershenberg, R., Vivian, D., Wolfe, B. E., & Goldfried, M. R. (2012). Bridging the gap between clinical research and clinical practice: Introduction to the special section. *Psychotherapy, 49*(2), 97–100.

Vermeersch, D. A., Whipple, J. L., Lambert, M. J., Hawkins, E. J., Burchfield, C. M., & Okiishi, J. C. (2004). Outcome Questionnaire: Is it sensitive to changes in counseling center clients? *Journal of Counseling Psychology, 51*(1), 38–49.

Yeryomenko, N. (2012). Does the depth of client experiencing predict good therapy outcomes?: A meta-analysis of treatment outcomes. (Unpublished master's thesis). University of Windsor, Canada.

Youn, S. J., Kraus, D. R., & Castonguay, L. G. (2012). The treatment outcome package: Facilitating practice and clinically relevant research. *Psychotherapy, 49*(2), 115–122.

CHAPTER 12

Multimethod Assessment of Distortion

Integrating Data from Interviews, Collateral Records, and Standardized Assessment Tools

Danielle Burchett and R. Michael Bagby

Psychological assessment is an endeavor that has the potential to provide critical information to the referral source or other users of such service, including clinicians from other professions (e.g., psychiatrists, social workers, nurses), teachers, employers, and those in the legal arena (e.g., lawyers, judges, correctional officers). Yet, a variety of factors may undermine the validity and usefulness of the outcomes of psychological assessments. There are, for example, the inherent psychometric limitations of the instruments used in an assessment battery, and in many assessment contexts, the utility of psychological test results may be compromised by test response bias (e.g., overreporting or underreporting). For instance, scores from scales designed to assess different forms of psychopathology may be artificially elevated or deflated and, therefore, less predictive of the constructs they were meant to measure due to non–content-based or content-based invalid responding (Burchett & Ben-Porath, 2010; Wiggins, Wygant, Hoelzle, & Gervais, 2012). Thus, when conducting personality assessments, it is critical to examine validity scales—indices of response distortion—to determine whether inaccurate symptom reporting influenced the accuracy of the scales of greatest clinical interest: the substantive measures of psychopathology and personality dysfunction.

In addition to providing information about the predictive validity of substantive scale test scores, validity scales can also provide clinically relevant data about the accuracy of examinee self-report. For instance, overreporting in a clinical setting may be indicative of a "cry for help" (Graham,

2006), a stable personality style (Morey, 2007), or intentional distortion for secondary gain (American Psychiatric Association, 2013). Thus, the assessment of response distortion has two main functions: (1) to determine whether substantive test results are valid measures of genuine symptoms, and (2) to provide information about an examinee's presentation that could impact the course of treatment or legal decisions.

In this chapter we first review different types of invalid responding, symptom domains in which they occur, and extant models explaining their etiology. Next, we address strategies and tools used for the detection of misleading responding and then conclude by recommending multimethod assessment of response distortion and providing an illustrative case example.

Types of Response Distortion

Ben-Porath (2003; Table 12.1) discussed the threats to protocol validity in self-report personality assessment, including *non–content-based* and *content-based* invalid responding. Non–content-based invalid responding

TABLE 12.1. Response Styles That May Invalidate Personality and Psychopathology Assessment Results

Non–content-based invalid (NCBI) responding	
Intentional NCBI responding	Unintentional NCBI responding
Intentional nonresponding	Unintentional nonresponding
Intentional random responding	Unintentional random responding
Intentional fixed responding	Unintentional fixed responding
Intentional acquiescence	Unintentional acquiescence
Intentional counteracquiescence	Unintentional counteracquiescence

Content-based invalid responding	
Intentional overreporting	Unintentional overreporting
Feigning (Rogers & Bender, 2003)	Poor insight
Exaggeration	Negative emotionality
Fabrication	
Malingering (American	
Psychiatric Association, 2013)	
Intentional underreporting	Unintentional underreporting
Impression management	Social desirability/self-deception
Minimization	
Denial	
Defensiveness (Rogers, 1984)	

Dissimulation (Rogers, 2008a)

Hybrid responding (Rogers, 2008a)

Note. Expanded from Ben-Porath (2003).

occurs when an individual's invalid test responses are unrelated to the item content. *Nonresponding, random responding,* and *fixed responding* also compromise protocol validity. Nonresponding occurs when the examinee does not respond to test items, whereas random responding occurs when an examinee indiscriminately responds to items with varying answers (e.g., a random true–false–false–true–true pattern). Fixed responding involves indiscriminately providing the same response to test items and includes *acquiescence* (e.g., all "true" responding) and *counteracquiescence* (e.g., all "false" responding). These response styles occur on Likert-type scales as well, with examinees randomly responding or choosing responses at the same level without considering item content (Ben-Porath, 2003).

When an examinee pays attention to the content of the items but provides responses that depict a distorted picture of their actual functioning, it is commonly referred to as *content-based invalid responding.* This may be intentional or unintentional and includes *overreporting* and *underreporting* of symptoms.[1] *Overreporting* occurs when an examinee's responses lead them to appear worse off than they actually are. *Feigning* (Rogers & Bender, 2003) is the intentional exaggeration or fabrication of symptoms (making no assumption as to the examinee's motivation). *Malingering* is a subcategory of feigning, which is by definition externally motivated, context-specific intentional overreporting of symptoms (American Psychiatric Association, 2013). Unintentional overreporting may occur due to *poor insight* into one's symptoms or *negative emotionality,* which predisposes individuals to believe they are more impaired than is true for them (Ben-Porath, 2003; Tellegen, 1985).

Underreporting occurs when an individual's response style leads them to appear better off than they actually are. *Impression management* involves the intentional minimization (reporting fewer symptoms than are present and/or minimizing the severity of those that are reported) or *denial* (denying all symptoms) of problems (Ben-Porath, 2003) in an attempt to create a positive image or demonstrate mental health. Rogers (1984) described *defensiveness* as the opposite of malingering: intentional minimization of symptoms. Unintentional underreporting has been labeled *self-deception* and *social desirability* and is believed to be an inadvertent masking of symptoms (Strong, Greene, Hoppe, Johnston, & Olesen, 1999). Intentional impression management is considered to be a setting-specific strategy, whereas self-deception is thought to be a stable personality trait

---

[1] Rogers, Sewell, and Gillard (2010) recommend against the labels "overreporting" and "underreporting" because they are nonspecific. They instead recommend "dissimulation" to describe intentional response distortion and "feigning" to describe intentional symptom exaggeration. We retain the terms *overreporting* and *underreporting* in this chapter precisely because test results cannot speak to intent. We recommend that the evaluator specify intent and symptom type (e.g., cognitive, somatic, psychopathology) when each can be determined, and we caution that intent cannot be determined by the test results but rather by other collateral information.

(Paulhus, 1988). Rogers (2008a) notes that it is possible to observe *hybrid responding*, in which an examinee utilizes more than one response style (e.g., honest responding in most domains but underreporting of substance abuse).

Domains of Response Distortion

Content-based invalid responding may occur in three general symptom domains: reported somatic complaints, cognitive complaints, and psychopathology (e.g., Hoelzle, Nelson, & Arbisi, 2012; Rogers, Sewell, & Gillard, 2010). Although the detection of somatic and cognitive response distortion is important, it is beyond the scope of this book.[2] The third domain in which invalid responding may occur—in the reporting of psychopathology—is the focus of this chapter. For brevity, we did not include a discussion of performance-based personality tools (e.g., Rorschach and Thematic Apperception Test).

Models of Response Distortion

Several models have been proposed to explain the source of invalid responding. These models generally fall into three main categories: those that propose (1) underlying psychopathology (e.g., pathogenic model, Bash & Alpert, 1980; interpersonal management model, Heinze, 1999); (2) psychopathy, antisocial personality, and criminal behavior (e.g., criminological model; American Psychiatric Association, 1980); or (3) cost–benefit analysis of potential risks and gains in conjunction with individual factors (e.g., adaptational model, Rogers & Cavanaugh, 1983; interactional model of applicant faking, Snell, Sydell, & Lueke, 1999; interactionist model of item-level response distortion, Tett et al., 2006) as reasons for response distortion (see Rogers, 1990, 2008a).

Although there has been support for the adaptational model (e.g., Thomas-Peter, Jones, Campbell, & Oliver, 2000), DSM-5 (American Psychiatric Association, 2013) subscribes to the criminological model. It defines malingering as the "intentional production of false or grossly exaggerated physical or psychological symptoms, motivated by external incentives" (p. 726), and ignores underreporting altogether. According to the DSM, any combination of the following should arouse suspicion of malingering: (1) medicolegal context of presentation, (2) marked discrepancy between claimed stress or disability and objective findings, (3) lack

---

[2]The interested reader is referred to several sources that review the assessment methods within these domains (e.g., Boone, 2007; Hall & Poirier, 2001; Larrabee, 2007; Morgan & Sweet, 2009).

of cooperation during the diagnostic evaluation and in complying with the prescribed treatment regimen, or (4) presence of antisocial personality disorder. Research indicates that these markers are sensitive, but not specific, predictors of malingering (e.g., Kucharksi, Duncan, Egan, & Falkenbach, 2006; Vitacco, 2008).

Berry and Nelson (2010) outlined additional concerns with the (then) DSM-IV-TR guidelines. For instance, the DSM does not distinguish between domains of overreporting (somatic, cognitive, psychopathology), each of which should be assessed using different techniques. Additionally, the DSM calls for the examiner to determine *intent* and *motivation*, which cannot be assessed by psychopathology overreporting tests and can only sometimes be determined with self-report or collateral information (Rogers et al., 2010). Further, Berry and Nelson (2010) discuss the difficulty in distinguishing between *externally motivated* malingering and *internally motivated* somatoform disorder.

Berry and Nelson (2010) recommended changes to the DSM Malingering V code. Within the psychopathology domain, they recommended a focus on (1) using well-validated techniques without attempting to infer intent or motivation, (2) considering literature on the utility of various detection strategies, (3) employing multiple detection strategies to increase accuracy and minimize false-positive rates, (4) specifying the domain(s) in which false symptoms were documented, and (5) documenting the evaluator's level of certainty (possible, probable, definite) and the severity (mild, moderate, severe) of overreporting. We echo these suggestions and believe clinicians should utilize a variety of well-validated detection strategies in addition to collateral information and behavioral observations to assess for overreporting *and* underreporting across the three domains.

Strategies for Detecting Response Distortion in Personality Assessment

Because examinees may distort their clinical presentation in a variety of ways, several detection strategies have been developed. It is important to understand differences between these strategies because useful multimethod assessment of response distortion will employ several strategies during any given assessment.

Detecting Overreported Psychopathology

Numerous methods have been used to develop validity scales and stand-alone instruments to detect overreported psychiatric symptoms such as psychosis, depression, or anxiety. *Quasi-rare symptoms* scales are made of items reflecting symptoms rarely endorsed in normative samples. Although such scales differentiate between "normal" individuals and those who report severe problems, it can be unclear whether elevations are due to overreporting or genuine psychopathology. *Rare symptoms* scales address this concern by including items reflecting symptoms rarely endorsed in clinical samples. These types of scales are much less confounded by genuine psychopathology. The *improbable symptoms* approach is similar to the rare symptoms approach, except that items are of preposterous or ridiculous nature. Clearly, individuals endorsing many of these items are inaccurately reporting their symptomatology. However, these items tend to be so improbable that even moderately sophisticated malingerers can detect and avoid endorsing them (Rogers, 2008b).

The *symptom combinations* strategy involves creating items involving two symptoms, which may commonly occur but rarely occur in combination. The *spurious patterns of psychopathology* method is similar, but includes item combinations reported by malingerers but not genuine patients. The *indiscriminant symptom endorsement* approach was created with the assumption that malingerers tend to endorse an overall higher rate of symptoms than do individuals with genuine psychopathology. *Symptom severity* scales measure the severity or number of severe symptoms endorsed. Those who endorse many of these items as severe are likely to be overreporting symptoms. The *obvious symptoms* detection method uses face-valid symptoms either alone or in combination with more subtle symptoms to differentiate between genuine patients and overreporters (who are more likely to endorse many symptoms that are obviously related to psychopathology). The *reported versus observed* method measures differences between self-reported problems and clinical observations, with the assumption that individuals who report multiple problems not seen by clinicians are exaggerating or fabricating symptoms. The *erroneous stereotypes* detection method involves asking about symptoms that individuals often believe are related to true psychopathology, but in fact, are not (Rogers, 2008b).

Detecting Underreported Psychopathology

A number of detection strategies have been created to determine when an examinee is minimizing problems or exaggerating positive qualities (Rogers, 2008b). Some validity scales utilize a *denial of minor flaws/personal faults* strategy to detect underreporting. Individuals who do not admit to such minor flaws are likely intentionally presenting themselves in a favorable light (Graham, 2006). The *spurious patterns of simulated adjustment* strategy identifies scale configurations that occur in defensive patients but that are uncommon in clinical and community samples. The *denial of psychopathology/patient characteristics* method uses items that differentiate between individuals with known psychopathology who score within normal limits (and are thus believed to be underreporting) and normative samples. The goal of this method is to distinguish between those who *are* generally asymptomatic and those who have symptoms but deny them. The *social desirability* method attempts to identify examinees who present with a highly favorable image. Rogers (2008b) also described a *blended affirmation of virtuous behavior and denial of personal faults* method that combines items about virtuous behaviors and personal faults on the same scale.

Use of Multiple Methods to Detect Distortion

Given the complex nature of response distortion, many researchers have advocated for a multifaceted approach to its detection (e.g., Bender & Rogers, 2004; Mihura, 2012; Ray, 2009). Below we discuss the information that can be gained from clinical interviews, behavioral observations, and collateral sources and provide information about several tools used to detect response distortion. These scales and the domains of response distortion they purport to measure are displayed in Table 12.2.

Clinical Interview and Behavioral Observations

Ironically, perhaps the best-known advocate for the utility of standardized assessment methods, Paul Meehl (1996) stated, "if I were asked to diagnose a mental patient and told that I could either have an MMPI profile or conduct a mental status examination, I would prefer the latter." He appreciated the immensely rich information that can be gathered from a discussion with the examinee and from observing their behaviors. In the context of response distortion, it is important to be attuned to patterns of behavior inconsistent with major mental health conditions and observe whether distractibility, personality patterns, or other factors may be contributing to inaccurate test results. Further, when the setting permits, it can be helpful to observe the examinee's behaviors outside of the formal testing session because they may not think to distort their presentation at those times. Observing discrepancies in and out of the testing setting may provide evidence that the examinee's distortion is *intentional*.

Collateral Information

Treatment records and discussions with staff and family members may provide important background information about an examinee's history. Records may document mental status and behaviors around the time of the evaluation and may help inform whether behaviors are inconsistent with self-reported problems during the evaluation. Of note, while family members may provide information about the examinee's mental health history, they may have agendas in support of (or against) their relative or a poor understanding of the examinee's mental health history. Finally,

TABLE 12.2. Domains of Response Distortion Measured by Common Personality and Psychopathology Inventories and Standalone Measures

	Non–content-based invalid responding			Overreporting			Underreporting	
	Nonresponding	Random responding	Fixed responding	Psychopathology	Cognitive complaints	Somatic complaints	Uncommon virtues	Denial of psychopathology
MMPI-2	CNS/(?)	VRIN	TRIN	F, FB, FP	FBS	FBS	L, S	K, S
MMPI-2-RF	CNS/(?)	VRIN-r	TRIN-r	F-r, FP-r	FBS-r, RBS	FBS-r, FS	L-r	K-r
PAI	Missing items	ICN, INF		NIM, MAL, RDF		MPRDF	PIM, DEF, CDF	DEF, CDF
MCMI-III		V		X, Z			X (low), Y	X (low), Y
SNAP		VRIN, II	TRIN, II	DEV, II			DRIN, RV, II	DRIN, II
SNAP-2		VRIN, II	TRIN, II	DEV, BDEV, II			DRIN, RV, II	DRIN, II
NEO-PI-R	Response count; items A, B, and C	Response Count; items A, B, and C	Response count; items A, B, and C	Item A			Item A	Item A
SIRS		INC		RS, SC, IA, BL, SU, SEL, SEV, RO, DA, OS, SO			DS	
SIRS-2		INC		RS, SC, IA, BL, SU, SEL, SEV, RO, DA, OS, RS, Total, MT Index, SS Index	IF		DS	
SIMS				P, Af	N, Am, LI			
M-FAST				RO, ES, RC, UH, USC, NI, S, Total Score				

Note. Refer to the text for full-scale names and descriptions. II is a composite score indicating protocol invalidity and is elevated in part due to several types of response distortion.

understanding contextual information (e.g., whether evaluation results will impact the examinee's freedom), it is possible to identify *potentially* motivating factors.

Embedded Validity Indices on Self-Report Measures

Minnesota Multiphasic Personality Inventory–2[3]

The Minnesota Multiphasic Personality Inventory–2 (MMPI-2; Butcher et al., 1989, 2001) is a 567-item self-report personality and psychopathology inventory. It includes three scales designed to measure non–content-based invalid responding. Cannot Say (CNS/?) is a count of the number of items omitted or marked as *both* true and false. If many items are omitted or double-marked, the validity of the scale scores is called into question because substantive scale scores will be based on incomplete information. Variable Response Inconsistency (VRIN), designed to measure variable responding, consists of item pairs with similar or opposite content. Points are scored when individuals endorse these pairs in an empirically and conceptually inconsistent manner. True Response Inconsistency (TRIN) consists of item pairs opposite in content. Points are scored when individuals answer both items in the same direction. It is designed to measure both acquiescence and counteracquiescence.

The MMPI-2 also includes several overreporting indices. Infrequency (F), developed using the *quasi-rare symptoms* strategy, consists of items rarely endorsed in the MMPI-2 normative sample. Also developed using the *quasi-rare symptoms* approach, Back Infrequency (F_B) supplements F because it consists of infrequently endorsed items found in the latter part of the MMPI-2 booklet. Infrequency Psychopathology (F_P; Arbisi & Ben-Porath, 1995), developed using the *rare symptoms* approach, consists of items infrequently endorsed in both the MMPI-2 normative sample and by psychiatric inpatients. Its design makes it less likely than F to be elevated due to psychopathology, resulting in fewer false-positive results. Symptom Validity (FBS; Lees-Haley, English, & Glenn, 1991) was developed from rational item selection using the *unusual symptom combinations* approach. Originally designed to detect malingered emotional distress in individuals undergoing personal injury litigation, FBS has been shown to be useful in detecting somatic and cognitive overreporting (Ben-Porath, Graham, & Tellegen, 2009).

The MMPI-2 also includes scales intended to detect underreporting. Lie (L) was developed to assess defensiveness (underreporting). Developed using the *denial of minor flaws* method, it includes items that describe desirable but uncommon features. The *denial of psychopathology* method

---

[3]Despite the existence of several additional MMPI-2 validity scales in the literature, for brevity only those included in the standard test protocol are discussed.

was utilized to develop Correction (K), which was designed to distinguish between those who are genuinely asymptomatic and those who have symptoms but deny them. Butcher and Han (1995) used the *blended affirmation of virtuous behavior and denial of personal faults* strategy to develop the Superlative (S) scale, which includes items that differentiated between airline pilot applicants and individuals in the normative sample. Later research indicated that S is an effective indicator of underreporting (Ben-Porath, 2012).

Relatively few studies have examined the utility of MMPI-2 non–content-based invalid responding validity scales. Dragon, Ben-Porath, and Handel (2012) examined the impact of CNS elevations on the MMPI-2/MMPI-2-RF Restructured Clinical (RC) scales. They found the validity of substantive scales to be relatively robust to increasing missingness, but that the missingness tended to deflate scores to the point of changing the interpretation of test protocols. Several studies have demonstrated the sensitivity of VRIN to random responding (e.g., Berry et al., 1992; Gallen & Berry, 1996). Handel, Arnau, Archer, and Dandy (2006) demonstrated that TRIN is sensitive to simulated insertion of true or false item responses. A limitation of the extant literature has been the need to rely upon simulation designs to create missing, random, or fixed responses due to the difficulty in obtaining an external criterion of such response styles.

The MMPI-2 overreporting validity scales have been shown to distinguish between college students asked to respond honestly and those asked to overreport symptoms (Bagby, Buis, & Nicholson, 1995) as well as forensic pretrial defendants and psychiatric inpatients (Nicholson et al., 1997). They also appear to be effective in distinguishing between genuine psychopathology and simulated depression (Bagby, Marshall, & Bacchiochi, 2005) as well as simulated posttraumatic stress disorder (PTSD; e.g., Arbisi, Ben-Porath, & McNulty, 2006; Bury & Bagby, 2002; Elhai, Gold, Sellers, & Dorfman, 2001; Marshall & Bagby, 2006), and they show strong classification accuracy in distinguishing between Structured Interview of Reported Symptoms (SIRS)-classified overreporters and honest responders (Barber-Rioja, Zottoli, Kucharski, & Duncan, 2009). Based on meta-analytic findings, Rogers, Sewell, Martin, and Vitacco (2003) recommended the clinical use of F_P over F or F_B because the former had good classification rates and the latter appeared to be confounded by genuine psychopathology.

The MMPI-2 underreporting validity scales have been shown to distinguish between college student underreporting simulators and standard-instruction controls (e.g., Baer, Wetter, Nichols, Greene, & Berry, 1995; Bagby, Buis, & Nicholson, 1995). Baer and Miller's (2002) meta-analytic review of the MMPI-2 underreporting validity scale literature noted that several scales had moderately effective classification accuracy but were less effective in the presence of validity scale coaching. They recommended future research using known groups, differential prevalence, and nonstudent simulation designs and examining the impact of coaching and the combined use of multiple MMPI-2 standard and supplementary underreporting validity scales.

Minnesota Multiphasic Personality Inventory–2 Restructured Form

The 338-item MMPI-2 Restructured Form (MMPI-2-RF; Ben-Porath & Tellegen, 2008) includes several revised MMPI-2 validity scales (CNS, VRIN-r, TRIN-r, F-r, F_P-r, FBS-r, L-r, K-r). Additionally, Infrequent Somatic Responses (F_S; Wygant, Ben-Porath, & Arbisi, 2004) was designed to identify individuals overreporting somatic complaints using the *rare symptoms* strategy and includes somatic items uncommonly endorsed by medical patients. The Response Bias Scale (RBS; Gervais, Ben-Porath, Wygant, & Green, 2007) was empirically derived by selecting items that differentiated between disability claimants who failed and those who passed symptom validity tests.

Some research has examined the utility of this relatively new instrument in detecting non–content-based and content-based invalid responding. Dragon et al. (2012) found that MMPI-2-RF CNS elevations changed the interpretability of substantive test results. Handel, Ben-Porath, Tellegen, and Archer (2010) examined the effect of increasing levels of simulated random and fixed responding on VRIN-r and TRIN-r scores, finding that the scales were indeed sensitive to simulated non–content-based invalid responding. Ben-Porath (2012) reported that F-r is most sensitive to broad-range overreporting, while F_P-r is especially sensitive to overreported psychopathology. Sellbom and Bagby (2008b) found that L-r and K-r distinguish between patients with schizophrenia who completed the test under standard or underreporting instructions. They found similar support for the scales in distinguishing between students who took the test under standard instructions and (1) college student underreporting simulators as well as (2) child custody litigants. Although the extant literature is promising, more research is needed to examine the incremental utility and validity of the MMPI-2-RF validity scales across settings.

Personality Assessment Inventory

The Personality Assessment Inventory (PAI; Morey, 1991, 2007) is a 344-item personality and psychopathology self-report inventory with eight validity scales and indexes. Similar to the MMPI-2 VRIN scale, Inconsistency (ICN) was designed to detect inconsistent responding using item pairs of similar or opposite content.

Infrequency (INF), designed to detect careless responding, consists of items that are not indicative of psychopathology but are so bizarre as to be rarely endorsed by individuals in normative and clinical samples. Negative Impression (NIM), developed using the *rare symptoms* overreporting detection strategy, consists of items with psychopathology or personal problem content that is unrealistically severe and not specific to any particular kind of psychopathology. The Malingering Index (MAL; Morey, 1993) was created using the *spurious patterns of psychopathology* strategy. Points are scored when an individual profile meets any of eight criteria that are more commonly endorsed by simulated overreporters than by honest responders (Morey, 1996). The Rogers Discriminant Function (RDF; Rogers, Sewell, Morey, & Ustad, 1996) was also developed using the *spurious patterns of psychopathology* strategy and includes indices that best distinguished between simulators instructed to feign specific disorders and those asked to respond honestly. Positive Impression Management (PIM) was developed utilizing the *denial of minor flaws* underreporting detection strategy, and is made of self-favorable items infrequently endorsed in normative and clinical samples. The Cashel Discriminant Function (CDF; Cashel, Rogers, Sewell, & Martin-Cannici, 1995) was developed utilizing an empirical approach that identified six scales (PIM and five substantive scales), which best distinguished between honest responding and simulated underreporting (Morey, 1996). The Defensiveness Index (DEF; Morey, 1993) is made of eight profile criteria, which occur more frequently with underreporting than with honest responding (Morey, 1996). DEF does not adhere to a particular underreporting detection strategy, but resembles the *blended affirmation of virtuous behavior and denial of personal faults* strategy (Sellbom & Bagby, 2008a). Recently, Mogge, Lepage, Bell, and Ragatz (2010) developed the Negative Distortion Scale (NDS) utilizing a *rare symptoms* approach, and Hopwood, Orlando, and Clark (2010) created the Malingered Pain-Related Disability-Discriminant Function (MPRDF) using a *spurious patterns of psychopathology* approach. Although initial results are promising, more research is needed to validate these validity indicators before they can be recommended for routine clinical use.

Sellbom and Bagby (2008a) reviewed the PAI literature on response distortion, noting that there was strong support for INF as an indicator of random responding, but that ICN had weaker classification accuracy results. They stated that INF and ICN were unable to identify partial random responding except at high levels. A new strategy developed by Morey and Hopwood (2004) shows promise in detecting back random responding, but more research is needed to replicate their findings.

Hawes and Boccaccini (2009) conducted a meta-analysis on the use of NIM, MAL, and RDF in the detection of overreported psychopathology, finding that all three differentiated between overreporters and standard-instruction responders with large effects. Further, research has demonstrated mean PAI validity scale score elevations in the overreporting of specific disorders, including psychosis, depression, generalized anxiety disorder, and posttraumatic stress disorder (e.g., Lange, Sullivan, & Scott, 2010; Rogers et al., 1996; Thomas, Hopwood, Orlando, Weathers, & McDevitt-Murphy, 2012). Of note, Sellbom and Bagby (2008a) concluded that high false-positive rates indicate that the PAI may be effective at *screening out* but less effective at *screening in* malingering. Similarly, they concluded that the PAI demonstrates high false-positive rates in the detection of underreporting, but demonstrates promise as a screening tool.

The PAI validity scales were designed using a variety of detection strategies and are some of the most well-researched response distortion tools available. However, findings are mixed regarding the ability of the PAI to detect coached or sophisticated overreporting (Rogers et al., 1996; Thomas et al., 2012; Veltri & Williams, 2013) or underreporting (Baer & Wetter, 1997). Additional research on the impact of coaching and the incremental utility of each scale would be useful in further evaluating the utility of the PAI in multimethod assessment of response distortion (Sellbom & Bagby, 2008a).

Millon Clinical Multiaxial Inventory–III

The Millon Clinical Multiaxial Inventory–III (MCMI-III; Millon, 1994; Millon, Davis, & Millon, 1997), a self-report inventory designed to measure psychopathology and personality dysfunction in clinical settings, includes four validity indices. The Validity Index (Scale V) consists of three very *improbable symptoms* to assess for non–content-based invalid responding. The Disclosure Index (Scale X) was developed using the *indiscriminant symptom endorsement* strategy to detect whether the patient responded in an open and self-revealing or secretive manner. The Desirability Index (Scale Y) was developed using the *denial of minor flaws* strategy to measure "the patient's inclination to appear socially attractive, virtuous, or emotionally well composed" (Millon, 1994) and the Debasement Index (Scale Z) was designed using a simulated *rare symptoms* strategy (see Sellbom & Bagby, 2008a) to detect "an inclination to deprecate or devalue oneself by presenting more troublesome or emotional and personal difficulties than are likely to be uncovered upon objective review" (Millon, 1994).

Despite being developed to measure different aspects of invalid responding, X, Y, and Z appear to be intercorrelated and associated with MMPI-2 F and F_B, suggesting that all three are sensitive to quasi-rare overreported psychopathology (Craig, 1999; Morgan, Schoenberg, Dorr, & Burke, 2002). Scale Y appears to be modestly associated with MMPI-2 underreporting validity scales, indicating that it may be more sensitive to overreporting than to underreporting (Craig, 1999). These results were consistent with simulation studies that found X, Y, and Z to be associated with overreporting *and* underreporting (e.g., Bagby, Gillis, Toner, & Goldberg, 1991; Daubert & Metzler, 2000). Sellbom and Bagby (2008a) reviewed the MCMI-III literature, concluding that the extant literature on Scale Y indicated it was an inadequate measure of underreporting, with problematic classification accuracy results. They also noted that Scale X (intended to measure disclosure) may be a stronger indicator of overreporting than Scale

Z (intended to measure overreporting). They recommended against routine use of these scales because of problematic classification accuracy findings. In addition, they called for more cross-validation research as well as studies utilizing known groups and an examination of the effects of coaching.

Schedule for Nonadaptive and Adaptive Personality–2nd Edition

The Schedule for Nonadaptive and Adaptive Personality (SNAP; Clark, 1993) and its second edition (SNAP-2; Clark, Simms, Wu, & Casillas, in press) are self-report instruments designed to measure traits associated with personality disorders. Similar to the MMPI family, the SNAP instruments include VRIN and TRIN scales to measure variable and fixed non–content-based invalid responding, respectively. Desirable Response Inconsistency (DRIN) was designed to detect whether examinees inconsistently endorse socially desirable items while denying less socially desirable items of similar content. Conceptually similar to the MMPI-2 L Scale, Rare Virtues (RV) was designed using the *denial of personal faults* strategy and consists of rare and highly socially desirable items. Deviance (DEV) utilizes a *quasi-rare symptoms* approach to detect overreported problems. New to the SNAP-2, Back Deviance (BDEV) utilizes a *quasi-rare symptoms* approach to detect overreporting on the latter portion of the instrument.

VRIN, RV, DEV, BDEV, II, and to some degree, DRIN, are sensitive to extreme levels of non–content-based invalid responding. Most of the scales are sensitive to 100% acquiescent and 100% counteracquiescent responding as well as alternating response patterns (Clark et al., in press). Mean DEV and RV scores differ when comparing simulators and controls, with DEV evidencing strong sensitivity and specificity and RV evidencing strong specificity but modest sensitivity. Further, DEV appears to be associated with MMPI-2 F, whereas RV is associated with a variety of underreporting measures. At present, there is little support for the utility of DRIN, and users are urged to look for corroborating evidence of socially desirable responding (Clark et al., in press; Simms & Clark, 2001). Although initial studies show promise, more research is needed to validate the SNAP and SNAP-2 validity indices across settings.

Revised NEO Personality Inventory

The Revised NEO Personality Inventory (NEO PI-R; Costa & McCrae, 1992) is a 240-item measure of five personality domains. The authors included three one-item "Validity Checks" to screen out clearly invalid tests and guidelines for detecting random responding, but intentionally left out more comprehensive validity scales for the detection of underreporting or overreporting. Rather, they cautioned against administration of the self-report form "if the respondent is unlikely to understand the test or is intensely motivated to present a false picture of himself or herself" (Costa & McCrae, 1992). In response to criticism regarding the lack of validity scales (e.g., Ben-Porath & Waller, 1992) and demonstrations that the NEO substantive scales are susceptible to response distortion (e.g., Paulhus, Bruce, & Trapnell, 1995), Schinka, Kinder, and Kremer (1997) developed three NEO PI-R validity scales: Inconsistency (INC; consisting of item pairs of similar content), Positive Presentation Management (PPM; consisting of quasi-rare positive qualities indicative of *social desirability*), and Negative Presentation Management (NPM; consisting of *quasi-rare symptoms* items) from the extant item pool. As these validity scales are neither part of the test report nor endorsed by either Pearson or the authors of the NEO PI-R, we do not review them here.

Standalone Measures for the Detection of Response Distortion

Structured Interview of Reported Symptoms

The Structured Interview of Reported Symptoms (SIRS; Rogers, Bagby, & Dickens, 1992) is a 172-item structured interview designed to detect feigned psychopathology. The SIRS Primary Scales were designed using eight overreporting detection strategies and include: Rare Symptoms (RS), Symptom Combinations (SC), Improbable or Absurd Symptoms (IA), Blatant Symptoms (BL), Subtle Symptoms (SU), Severity of Symptoms (SEV), Selectivity of Symptoms (SEL), and Reported versus Observed Symptoms (RO). The test also includes a number of supplementary scales to provide additional information about the examinee's response style.

Research has demonstrated that SIRS factor scores are associated with MMPI-2 F and F_p scores (McCusker, Moran, Serfass, & Peterson, 2003). As presented in other sections, the SIRS has often been considered the overreporting gold standard, used to classify patients into criterion groups so that the utility of other tests (e.g., SIMS, M-FAST, MMPI-2, PAI) could be evaluated. To date, the most comprehensive analysis of the classification accuracy of the SIRS is a meta-analysis conducted by Green and Rosenfeld (2011), who examined SIRS studies and dissertations published from 1990 to 2009. The studies examined included original SIRS validation studies as well as replication analyses conducted after the test was published in 1992; the later studies demonstrated lower specificity but higher sensitivity values as compared to the original research. Composite effect sizes for the SIRS Total Score and averaged Primary Scales were notably large. The authors concluded that there is significant support for use of the SIRS, but that caution should be used in designating it as the gold standard of malingering detection, as other tools (e.g., MMPI-2) have demonstrated comparable utility and may be better suited for the detection of feigned cognitive deficits.

Structured Interview of Reported Symptoms, 2nd Edition

Four major changes were implemented in the development of the Structured Interview of Reported Symptoms, 2nd edition (SIRS-2; Rogers, Sewell, & Gillard, 2010): adding a classification scale (Rare Symptoms Total designed to differentiate between genuine but atypical and feigned presentations), two indices (Modified Total Index and Supplementary Scale Index), a supplementary scale for cognitive distortion (Improbable Failure), and a Decision Model to assist the clinician in making conclusions.

Since its release in 2010, the SIRS-2 and its manual have come under notable criticism. DeClue (2011) and Rubenzer (2010) noted such concerns as the use of only 36 suspected feigners in the development of the SIRS-2 decision rules, lack of information on the creation of criterion groups, questionable generalizability of the clinical normative sample (with half of patients diagnosed with dissociative identity disorder), and inflated sensitivity estimates due to the large number of indeterminate cases excluded from classification accuracy analyses. Further, DeClue (2011) reported that information comparing the classification accuracy of the SIRS and SIRS-2 on the same data is not available. Green, Rosenfeld, and Belfi (2013) compared SIRS and SIRS-2 scores in a criterion-group study of forensic inpatients and community overreporting simulators. The SIRS-2 tended to categorize more pretrial forensic patients as genuine or indeterminate responders as compared to SIRS-based classifications of the same scores. The SIRS-2 had excellent specificity but poor sensitivity, which was much lower than for the SIRS. They also found the SIRS Total Score was more useful than was the new SIRS-2 MT Index. More research is needed to inform clinicians about the utility this new instrument across a variety of settings.

Structured Inventory of Malingered Symptomatology

The Structured Inventory of Malingered Symptomatology (SIMS; Widows & Smith, 2005) is a 75-item self-administered inventory designed to measure overreported psychopathology and neuropsychological symptoms in clinical and forensic settings. The instrument has five scales designed to screen for various subdomains of overreported psychopathology, including Psychosis (P; bizarre psychotic symptoms not common in actual psychiatric patients), Neurologic Impairment (N; highly atypical or illogical neurological problems), Amnestic Disorders (Am; memory impairment not seen in individuals with actual brain injury), Low Intelligence (LI; simple, general fund of knowledge), and Affective Disorders (Af; atypical presentation of depression and anxiety). These scales were designed using a combination of detection strategies such as *improbable symptoms* and *close approximations to genuine symptoms* (Smith & Burger, 1997). Scores contribute to a Total Score that helps determine whether a more complete assessment of malingering is warranted (Smith, 2008).

The SIMS scales demonstrate expected associations with PAI and SIRS scales (Edens, Poythress, & Watkins-Clay, 2007). Further, SIMS is able to distinguish between simulated psychopathology overreporters and controls (e.g., Clegg, Fremouw, & Mogge, 2009; Edens, Otto, & Dwyer, 1999; Smith & Burger, 1997), as well as overreporting and honest groups as classified by SIRS scores (e.g., Alwes, 2006; Lewis, Simcox, & Berry, 2002) and by clinicians (Heinze & Purisch, 2001). Lewis et al. (2002) found that SIMS sensitivity and NPP were excellent, but specificity and PPP were low, supporting use of the SIMS as a screener that should be followed up with more extensive testing in the event of elevated scores. Presently, the body of literature on the SIMS is quite limited; more research would inform clinicians about its classification accuracy across settings.

Miller Forensic Assessment of Symptoms Test

The Miller Forensic Assessment of Symptoms Test (M-FAST; Miller, 2001) is a 25-item structured interview created to screen for overreported psychopathology in forensic settings. The instrument contains seven validity indices developed using a variety of overreporting strategies. The M-FAST scales include: Reported versus Observed (RO), Extreme Symptomatology (ES), Rare Combinations (RC), Unusual Hallucinations (UH), Unusual Symptom Course (USC), Negative Image (NI), and Suggestibility (S). The M-FAST scales demonstrate expected associations with MMPI-2, PAI, and SIRS scales (Gaines, 2009; Miller, 2001, 2004; Veazey, Hays, Wagner, & Miller, 2005). Several studies have indicated that the M-FAST is able to distinguish between simulated overreported psychopathology and honest responding (e.g., Guy et al., 2006) as well as between SIRS-classified overreporting and honest groups (e.g., Clark, 2006; Guy & Miller, 2004; Miller, 2004). Because the M-FAST is designed as a screener, it is recommended that a more extensive evaluation of overreporting be conducted if elevated scores occur (Miller, 2001). More research is needed on the utility and susceptibility to coaching of the M-FAST scales, especially those that consist of only one item.

Integrating Multiple Tools

Our aim in this chapter is to recommend sound practice in the multimethod assessment of response distortion. Earlier we reviewed extant research on the individual utility of a variety of standardized tools. Although not reviewed in detail, there is also a substantial literature on the incremental validity of multiple scales *within* many tests (e.g., incremental utility of MMPI-2 F_p over F).

Unfortunately, relatively few studies exist to inform clinicians of the incremental utility of multiple tests used together. Based on this limited literature, it appears that the MMPI-2 and PAI validity indices explain more variance in combination than individually when distinguishing between overreporting simulators and psychiatric inpatients (Blanchard, McGrath, Pogge, & Khadivi, 2003) and between SIRS-identified honest and overreported protocols (Boccaccini, Murrie, & Duncan, 2006). The PAI Malingering Index (MAL) also appears to add incrementally to the M-FAST Total Score (Gaines, 2009). The SIRS adds a statistically significant but practically small increment over SIMS and PAI (Edens, Poythress, & Watkins-Clay, 2007) whereas the M-FAST incrementally improves upon the MMPI-2 in detecting overreporting (Clark, 2006).

Although less is known about the incremental utility of these instruments in detecting underreporting, moderate correlations between PAI and MMPI-2 underreporting validity indices (e.g., Weiss, Serafino, & Serafino, 2000) suggest that these inventories may be measuring unique domains of underreporting. More research is needed to understand whether the combined use of tools improves accuracy in the detection of underreporting.

Recommendations for Multimethod Assessment of Response Distortion

Response distortion is a multifaceted phenomenon that is affected by demand characteristics. Thus, examinees may alter their presentation across multiple evaluations. Further, the specific ways in which examinees will distort their responses is varied and can occur in three domains (psychopathology, cognitive, somatic). Because of the complexity of this phenomenon, we have several recommendations for the multimethod assessment of response distortion in personality and psychopathology evaluations.

• Gather background information that can inform you about potential motivating factors that can provide explanatory evidence regarding intentional or unintentional response distortion (e.g., Is there secondary gain potential? Has the examinee consistently presented in a self-deprecating manner with previous treatment providers?). Developing hypotheses about potentially motivating factors can help create pertinent interview questions and learn which domains of response distortion may be in need of greatest attention.

• Consider the evaluation to be an iterative process. Situational factors, referral questions, and initial information may inform the selection of interview questions, screening tools used, and collateral sources contacted. Initial test results may indicate the need for more comprehensive testing. Once sufficient evidence of response distortion is documented (utilizing validated measures with known error rates), further testing may be excessive and unnecessary. It is important to be prepared to alter planned test administration based on early results.

• Assess for reading level (when administering self-report instruments) and non–content-based invalid responding. Use interview responses and behavioral observations to bolster conclusions about the examinee's ability to attend to testing.

• At present, the current literature does little to inform clinicians about which *combination* of tools best detects various forms of response distortion. Thus, it may be best to select a variety of tools that have been individually validated in the examination setting of interest. Further, a combination should be selected so that at least one tool is sensitive to each type of response distortion (e.g., underreporting, general overreporting, and overreporting of specific symptoms). Further, it may be useful to select tools that were developed using a variety of detection strategies, as examinees may distort responses in a variety of ways. Because distortion often occurs across domains, at minimum screen for overreporting of cognitive and somatic complaints and refer for a neuropsychological evaluation if necessary.

• As recommended by Meehl (1955) and Ray (2009), use screening instruments in forensic settings in order to identify which examinees should be more comprehensively assessed. Screener cut scores are often set at low values that minimize false negatives at the cost of increased false positives. Thus, while the use of screeners (e.g., M-FAST, SIMS) may be cost-effective, it is important to further evaluate those who test positive with more comprehensive tests that utilize cut scores with lower levels of false positives.

• Select empirically supported tools. As shown in Table 12.2, validity indices measure different areas of response distortion. However, not all have been equally validated or examined across settings. Carefully select those that have been empirically validated in your setting and be aware of published error rates. Further, be cognizant that the base rate of invalid responding varies across settings; classification accuracy results from studies with unrealistic base rates may not generalize to your setting. If using substantive tools that do not have well-supported validity indices (e.g., Rorschach and BDI), also use well-validated validity indices in conjunction to assess for response bias.

• Be aware of the limitations to the DSM-5 Malingering V code. Although clinicians are tasked with using the problematic DSM-5 guidelines for malingering, it may be useful to conceptualize and assess for malingering using recommendations from Berry and Nelson (2010). Also be aware that it may be very difficult to gather information about motivating factors or intent. Thus, differentiating between malingering and other explanations (e.g., somatoform disorder, factitious disorder) without extensive historical information may present a significant challenge.

• Be mindful of the impact that culture may have on response styles. Research has demonstrated that individuals from different cultures tend to vary in the extremity of their responses, level of acquiescence, and tendency to underreport problems (e.g., Aday, Cliu, & Anderson, 1980; Johnson, Kulesa, Cho, & Shavitt, 2005; Jürges, 2007; Mercado, 2000). It is important to gather information about the individual's cultural background to help determine whether their cultural norms may be impacting their presentation of symptoms.

Case Example

We selected a case demonstrating the importance of seven critical concepts in the assessment of response distortion.

Understand the Referral Question

Mr. Shaw is a 33-year-old male forensic hospital patient referred for an evaluation of competency to stand trial (CST) and malingering.

Thoroughly Review Available Background Information I: Previous Evaluations

Mr. Shaw was accused of committing three serious felonies, which, if he is convicted, could send him to prison for several years. He previously underwent seven competency evaluations and a hospital admission evaluation in the 21 months before his current evaluation. Some of the evaluators noted that Mr. Shaw reported a history of severe mental health symptoms, including believing he could speak with deceased people, appearing anxious, hypervigilant, agitated, paranoid, unable to sit still, and responding to internal stimuli. He also told an evaluator he was experiencing auditory hallucinations, including getting messages from the television to kill himself. Further, two evaluators noted that Mr. Shaw had difficulty recalling detailed information regarding his case and appeared confused. During one evaluation, he reported he could not remember the alleged offenses.

During other evaluations, it was noted that Mr. Shaw reported symptoms that appeared contrived (e.g., holding conversations with deceased people upon request by the examiner, delaying answers to give the impression of slowed cognitive processing). One examiner noted that he appeared conversational with peers but changed his mood to appear depressed and impaired when speaking with clinical staff. He was administered the M-FAST and received an overall score of 15, which was "highly suggestive of malingered psychopathology" (Miller, 2001). He did not demonstrate any genuine cognitive deficits. He provided significant historical information about his childhood, hospitalizations, and history of medication management and offered specific information about discussions with court personnel, including his status as an incompetent patient, options for plea deals, and the roles of court personnel. Mr. Shaw was able to state his current charges and the severity of the charges, and to estimate the amount of incarceration time he could face if found guilty. He correctly identified his plea options, explained their meaning, and defined the court personnel, including their roles. He was able to think abstractly and had good insight, judgment, and impulse control.

In sum, the conclusions of previous evaluations were mixed. On several occasions, evaluators opined that Mr. Shaw's psychiatric and cognitive symptoms made him incompetent to stand trial, and he was subsequently transferred from the jail to a psychiatric hospital for competency restoration. Other evaluators opined that Mr. Shaw was competent to stand trial, and so he was returned to jail. Some evaluators suspected him of malingering. At the time of the current evaluation, he had recently been readmitted to the hospital, and his treatment team suspected he was malingering psychopathology and cognitive problems.

Thoroughly Review Available Background Information II: Other Records

Legal History

Records indicated that Mr. Shaw had an extensive history of juvenile and adult arrests and significant experience navigating the legal system and going to court.

Hospital Records Informing Mr. Shaw's Reported and Observed Cognitive Abilities

Hospital records indicated that Mr. Shaw was elected by his peers to be president of his unit, a coveted position that comes with special privileges and requires the ability to navigate the social milieu. The office is not typically obtained by patients who are especially suspicious of others, acutely psychotic, or severely depressed. Records also noted that Mr. Shaw attended court competency and discharge planning groups with little to no participation but took active part in leisure groups, demonstrating interest and being verbally expressive. It was noted that Mr. Shaw claimed to have memory problems, being unable to recall court procedure information. However, he was able to quickly and easily answer other questions about medication history, age of onset of illness, timeline of major events, and his daily schedule.

Hospital Records Informing Mr. Shaw's Reported and Observed Psychopathology

Mr. Shaw reported to staff that he heard voices, but he was never observed to be preoccupied with internal stimuli. He complained about previously being assigned a Malingering V code, but he also admitted that he had fabricated psychotic symptoms during his first admission to the hospital.

Conduct the Clinical Interview

While the purpose of this evaluation was to understand Mr. Shaw's current competency to stand trial, it was essential to ask about his reported history of cognitive and psychopathology symptoms to understand whether he had genuine problems that interfered with his ability to attend to court proceedings and assist his attorney.

Self-Reported Cognitive Deficits

Mr. Shaw reported a history of concussions as a teenager. When asked whether he experienced memory deficits related to his case, he reported he did not know what a jury was or whether it included more than one person. He said he did not know what made him the defendant but that he had "heard of" a judge. He said his public defender is "someone who tries to convict you" and said he is incompetent "because I forget. I don't know all of the material yet."

Self-Reported Psychiatric Symptoms

Mr. Shaw reported that he began hearing voices around age 8 and hears them daily. He said he was previously diagnosed with bipolar disorder and has a history of suicide attempts. In describing his recent symptoms, Mr. Shaw reported, "I thought the government was after my family. Most of the time, I believe it. I can hear agents' names, and I trip out."

Self-Reported Information Regarding Potential Motivation to Distort

Mr. Shaw said he prefers the hospital to the jail because "It's a less stressful environment . . . than being locked in a cell 24 hours a day." He reported he receives better treatment, proper medical care, and therapy at the hospital. He also talked at length about a hospital peer whom he identified as his girlfriend.

Pay Attention to Behavioral Observations

It can help to examine whether an examinee's behaviors are inconsistent with his or her reported symptoms. Such information can be invaluable in determining whether they are reporting false symptoms. For Mr. Shaw, the following behavioral observations were noted:

Cognitive Abilities

A day after the evaluator held a brief conversation with Mr. Shaw to meet him and schedule a time for testing, Mr. Shaw saw the evaluator on hospital grounds. Without prompting, he said, "Tomorrow at 9:30, right?" indicating recognition of an unfamiliar staff member and recall of the time of the scheduled appointment. Despite answering many questions with "I don't know," Mr. Shaw appeared to be very cognizant of the tests being administered. During administration of the M-FAST, he correctly stated, "I already did this one when I got here," indicating he recalled the front page of the test from an evaluation conducted several months earlier. Mr. Shaw was able to attend to items, follow test instructions independently, and maintain focus on test items for up to 90 minutes at a time. He demonstrated good memory, attention, and concentration. In contrast to interview responses that, on the surface, indicated he had little knowledge of the legal system, Mr. Shaw provided significant detail about previous arrests, the crimes committed that led to them, and the negotiation process he experienced for previous plea deals.

Psychopathology

Mr. Shaw reported hearing voices talking and repeating the evaluator's questions during the current interview. However, at no point did he appear to be distracted by internal stimuli during several hours of the evaluation. Despite reporting highly persecutory delusional content about legal players wishing to unjustly give him the death penalty, steal his money, and kill his family, he slouched in his chair and answered questions with his arms crossed and in a relaxed position. He presented as euthymic throughout the interview with no signs of anxious, depressive, or manic symptomatology.

Decide upon Instruments to Administer

Previous evaluators came to a variety of conclusions about the veracity of Mr. Shaw's symptomatology. The only standardized testing available for review was an M-FAST administered during a hospital intake. While his very high score of 15 provided evidence of overreported psychopathology, the M-FAST is a state-dependent screening instrument and further evaluation was necessary to more comprehensively assess for distortion. Further, despite reported memory difficulties, no previous testing assessed for cognitive response distortion.

To accurately assess barriers to Mr. Shaw's current competence to stand trial, it was necessary to assess whether he was *currently* exaggerating or fabricating cognitive or mental health problems. There was no indication of need to comprehensively assess for overreported somatic symptoms or underreporting. As listed in Table 12.3, several detection methods were chosen within the selected domains because feigners may distort responses using several approaches and different tests are sensitive to different distortion approaches. Of note, test and interview question selection is an

TABLE 12.3. Instruments Administered to Mr. Shaw and His Test Results

Name of instrument	Description of instrument	Mr. Shaw's scores	Basic interpretation of scores
		Cognitive domain	
Rey Fifteen Item Memorization Test (FIT)	Screener measure of suspect effort on cognitive tests	Combined Recognition and Recall Score: 23	There was no evidence of suspect effort.
Test of Memory Malingering (TOMM)	Forced-choice screener of suspect effort on memory and other cognitive tests	Trial 1: 41/50 Trial 2: 40/50 Retention: 27/50	Mr. Shaw's test scores indicate he did not put forth maximum effort and may have attempted to appear as though he had memory deficits that were not true for him.
Validity Indicator Profile (VIP)	Forced-choice measure of effort and intent on cognitive tests	Nonverbal: 88; Compliant Verbal: 67; Compliant	Mr. Shaw had a compliant response style. There was no compelling evidence of suppression, random responding, or pronounced inconsistency.
Inventory of Legal Knowledge (ILK)	Forced- choice measure of response style in defendants undergoing adjudicative competence evaluations	28/61 (45.9%)	Mr. Shaw's score of 28/61 was similar to scores obtained by examinees who respond randomly. It was lower than scores obtained by most examinees with bona fide mental disorders. His score suggests he had little investment in demonstrating his true knowledge or abilities and raises significant concerns about a feigned or irrelevant response style.
		Psychopathology domain	
Miller Forensic Assessment of Symptoms Test (M-FAST)	Screener structured interview designed to quickly screen for psychopathology overreporting	Previous: 15 Current: 8 RO: 1	Mr. Shaw endorsed items on the M-FAST that indicate the possibility of malingered mental illness. An M-FAST score of 8 is highly suggestive of malingered mental

		ES: 2 RC: 3 UH: 2	illness. A M-FAST score of 8 is highly suggestive of malingered psychopathology in clinical samples. The Reported versus Observed (RO) Scale includes items indicating self-reported problems are inconsistent with observed behaviors. The Extreme Symptomatology (ES) Scale includes symptoms that are very extreme and uncommon. The Rare Combinations (RC) Scale includes psychological symptoms that are rarely seen in combination. The Unusual Hallucination (UH) Scale includes symptoms that are extremely rare in genuine psychiatric populations. Based on Mr. Shaw's M-FAST scores, additional tests are recommended in order to evaluate the possibility that he is malingering.
Structured Interview of Reported Symptoms (SIRS)	Comprehensive structured interview designed to assess psychopathology overreporting response styles (and, less comprehensively, defensiveness)	1 Definite (Rare Symptoms) and 3 Probable (Blatant Symptoms, Selectivity of Symptoms, and Severity of Symptoms)	Mr. Shaw had a markedly elevated score on Rare Symptoms, which measures the tendency to endorse very severe symptoms, often with psychotic content. This elevation is characteristic of individuals who are feigning a mental disorder and is rarely seen in clients responding truthfully. He also had moderately elevated scores on Blatant Symptoms (endorsing many symptoms associated with major mental illness), Selectivity of Symptoms (endorsing a wide range of psychiatric symptoms), and Severity of Symptoms (endorsing many symptoms as extreme or unbearable). This combination of elevated scores is characteristic of individuals who are feigning a mental disorder and is rarely seen in clients responding truthfully.

iterative process. Mr. Shaw's behaviors and test results earlier in the assessment process influenced the selection of later questions and tests. Table 12.3 provides Mr. Shaw's scores along with basic interpretive results for each test. We will not devote a great deal of attention to Mr. Shaw's results in the cognitive symptoms domain (which suggested he did not attempt to perform as well as he could). Rather, we will turn our attention to Mr. Shaw's results from the psychopathology domain.

Mr. Shaw was first administered the Miller Forensic Assessment of Symptoms Test (M-FAST). While his current score of 8 was much lower than his previous score of 15, it still suggested overreported psychopathology symptoms. Because the M-FAST was designed as a brief screening tool, Mr. Shaw was also administered the Structured Inventory of Reported Symptoms (SIRS). He scored in the "Definite" range of overreporting on one of the eight primary scales and in the "Probable" range of overreporting on three others. This provides more information about his approach, utilizing a more comprehensive measure of psychopathology response distortion. Although not administered during this evaluation, we might have additionally chosen to administer a self-report multiaxial personality instrument (e.g., MMPI-2-RF, PAI) which would utilize a different approach. We refrained from doing so because we had significant evidence of overreported psychopathology and did not wish to subject the patient to unnecessary testing.

Interpret Multimethod Test Results with Behavioral Observations and Records

Based on the available evidence, we concluded that Mr. Shaw was intentionally fabricating or exaggerating cognitive difficulties and psychopathology in an attempt to remain at the hospital. This conclusion can be broken into three main areas of evidence. Of note, not all three will be clearly determined in every evaluation:

Behavior

Mr. Shaw's performance on measures of distortion of cognitive problems, as well as discrepancies between his behavior during testing and when not formally evaluated, indicate that he was overreporting psychopathology symptoms and putting forth less than maximal effort to perform well on cognitive measures. He previously demonstrated good knowledge of the court process, which was much better than his reported level of knowledge during this evaluation. It is doubtful that he forgot such information considering that his memory was observed to be intact and there were no documented physiological or psychiatric problems that would indicate he had forgotten the legal information he previously knew.

Intent to Distort

According to records, Mr. Shaw admitted to intentionally overreporting psychopathology in the past. His test results indicated that he was likely overreporting psychiatric problems and not performing as well as he could on cognitive measures. However, *Mr. Shaw's response distortion test results did not directly speak to his intent.* We had to infer his intent based on discrepancies between his behavior during and outside of formal evaluation as well as discrepancies in demonstrated cognitive abilities.

Motivation for Behavior

According to records and his self-report during this evaluation, Mr. Shaw reported a desire to remain at the hospital as opposed to jail. This (admittedly rare) admission allowed for direct conclusions about his motivation to distort. Less direct evidence (e.g., knowledge that he enjoyed spending time with his girlfriend) or hypotheses (e.g., his desire to delay the trial to avoid being found guilty) may have been *inferred,* but without more direct evidence, such inferences would not confirm his motivation.

Although it could not be concluded certainly as to whether Mr. Shaw had any bona fide psychiatric symptoms, his presentation suggested that he was grossly overreporting symptoms of mental illness and memory deficits due to external incentives. As such, we opined that he was competent to stand trial. Further, we recommended that his treatment team consider adding a Malingering V code to his diagnosis of record.

Conclusions

As highlighted throughout this chapter and case example, the assessment of response distortion is a multifaceted endeavor that involves consideration of information from a variety of sources. This task is made more complex by imperfect guidelines (e.g., DSM-5), which have been described as incomplete and unattainable (e.g., Berry & Nelson, 2010). Fortunately, several well-validated methods exist to guide clinicians willing to take on this challenge. Careful selection of standardized tools in conjunction with information from interview, behavioral observations, and collateral sources can provide rich and useful information about the presence, severity, and type of response distortion in order to inform clinical and forensic practice.

REFERENCES

Aday, L. A., Cliu, G. Y., & Anderson, R. (1980). Methodological issues in health care surveys of the Spanish-descent population. *American Journal of Public Health,* 70, 367–374.

Alwes, Y. R. (2006). *The utility of the Structured Inventory of Malingered Symptomatology as a screen for the feigning of neurocognitive deficit and psychopathology in a civil forensic sample.* Master's Thesis, University of Kentucky (Paper No. 394).

American Psychiatric Association. (1980). *Diagnostic and statistical manual of mental disorders* (3rd ed.). Washington, DC: Author.

American Psychiatric Association. (2013). *Diagnostic and statistical manual of mental disorders* (5th ed.). Arlington, VA: Author.

Arbisi, P. A., & Ben-Porath, Y. S. (1995). An MMPI-2 infrequent response scale for use with psychopathological populations: The Infrequency–Psychopathology Scale, F(p). *Psychological Assessment, 7,* 424–431.

Arbisi, P. A., Ben-Porath, Y. S., & McNulty, J. (2006). The ability of the MMPI-2 to detect feigned PTSD within the context of compensation seeking. *Psychological Services, 3,* 249–261.

Baer, R. A., & Miller, J. (2002). Underreporting of psychopathology on the MMPI-2: A meta-analytic review. *Psychological Assessment, 14,* 16–26.

Baer, R. A., & Wetter, M. W. (1997). Effects of information about validity scales on underreporting of symptoms on the Personality Assessment Inventory. *Journal of Personality Assessment, 68,* 402–413.

Baer, R. A., Wetter, M. W., Nichols, D. S., Greene, R., & Berry, D. T. R. (1995). Sensitivity of MMPI-2 validity scales to underreporting of symptoms. *Psychological Assessment, 7,* 419–423.

Bagby, R. M., Buis, T., & Nicholson, R. A. (1995). Relative effectiveness of the standard validity scales in detecting fake-bad and fake-good responding: Replication and extension. *Psychological Assessment, 7,* 84–92.

Bagby, R. M., Gillis, J. R., Toner, B. B., & Goldberg, J. (1991). Detecting fake-good and fake-bad responding on the Millon Clinical Multiaxial Inventory–II. *Psychological Assessment, 3,* 496–498.

Bagby, R. M., Marshall, M. B., & Bacchiochi, J. R. (2005). The validity and clinical utility of the MMPI-2 Malingering Depression Scale. *Journal of Personality Assessment, 85,* 304–311.

Barber-Rioja, V., Zottoli, T. M., Kucharski, L. T., & Duncan, S. (2009). The utility of the MMPI-2 Criminal Offender Infrequency (F_C) Scale in the detection of malingering in criminal defendants. *International Journal of Forensic Mental Health, 8,* 16–24.

Bash, I. Y., & Alpert, M. (1980). The determination of malingering. *Annals of the New York Academy of Sciences, 347,* 86–99.

Bender, S. D., & Rogers, R. (2004). Detection of neurocognitive feigning: Development of a multi-strategy assessment. *Archives of Clinical Neuropsychology, 19,* 49–60.

Ben-Porath, Y. S. (2003). Assessing personality and psychopathology with self-report inventories. In I. B. Weiner (Series Ed.) & A. M. Goldstein (Vol. Ed.), *Handbook of psychology: Vol. 11. Forensic psychology* (pp. 485–508). Hoboken, NJ: Wiley.

Ben-Porath, Y. S. (2012). *Interpreting the MMPI-2-RF.* Minneapolis: University of Minnesota Press.

Ben-Porath, Y. S., Graham, J. R., & Tellegen, A. (2009). *The MMPI-2 Symptom Validity (FBS) scale development, research findings, and interpretive recommendations.* Minneapolis: University of Minnesota Press.

Ben-Porath, Y. S., & Tellegen, A. (2008). *MMPI-2-RF manual for administration, scoring, and interpretation.* Minneapolis: University of Minnesota Press.

Ben-Porath, Y. S., & Waller, N. G. (1992). "Normal" personality inventories in clinical assessment: General requirements and the potential for using the NEO Personality Inventory. *Psychological Assessment, 4,* 14–19.

Berry, D. T. R., & Nelson, N. W. (2010). DSM-5 and malingering: A modest proposal. *Psychological Injury and Law, 3,* 295–303.

Berry, D. T. R., Wetter, M. W., Baer, R. A., Larsen, L., Clark, C., & Monroe, K. (1992). MMPI-2 random responding indices: Validation using a self-report methodology. *Psychological Assessment, 4,* 340–345.

Blanchard, D. D., McGrath, R. E., Pogge, D. L., & Khadivi, A. (2003). A comparison of the PAI and MMPI-2 as predictors of faking bad in college students. *Journal of Personality Assessment, 80,* 197–205.

Boccaccini, M. T., Murrie, D. C., & Duncan, S. A. (2006). Screening for malingering in a criminal-forensic sample with the Personality Assessment Inventory. *Psychological Assessment, 18,* 415–423.

Boone, K. B. (Ed.). (2007). *Assessment of feigned cognitive impairment: A neuropsychological perspective.* New York: Guilford Press.

Burchett, D. L., & Ben-Porath, Y. S. (2010). The impact of overreporting on MMPI-2-RF substantive scale score validity. *Assessment, 17,* 497–516.

Bury, A. S., & Bagby, R. M. (2002). The detection of feigned uncoached and coached posttraumatic stress disorder with the MMPI-2 in a sample of workplace accident victims. *Psychological Assessment, 14,* 472–484.

Butcher, J. N., Dahlstrom, W. G., Graham, J. R., Tellegen, A., & Kaemmer, B. (1989). *Manual for the restandardized Minnesota Multiphasic Personality Inventory: MMPI-2.* Minneapolis: University of Minnesota Press.

Butcher, J. N., Graham, J. R., Ben-Porath, Y. S., Tellegen, A., Dahlstrom, W. G., & Kaemmer, B. (2001). *MMPI-2 manual for administration, scoring, and interpretation* (rev. ed.). Minneapolis: University of Minnesota Press.

Butcher, J. N., & Han, K. (1995). Development of an MMPI-2 scale to assess the presentation of self in a superlative manner: The S scale. In J. N. Butcher & C. D. Spielberger (Eds.), *Advances in personality assessment* (Vol. 10, pp. 25–50). Hillsdale, NJ: Erlbaum.

Cashel, M. L., Rogers, R., Sewell, K., & Martin-Cannici, C. (1995). The Personality Assessment Inventory and the detection of defensiveness. *Assessment, 2,* 333–342.

Clark, J. A. (2006). *Validation of the Miller Forensic Assessment of Symptoms Test (M-FAST) in a civil forensic population.* Master's Thesis. Retrieved from University of Kentucky (Paper No. 399).

Clark, L. A. (1993). *Schedule for Nonadaptive and Adaptive Personality: Manual for administration, scoring, and interpretation.* Minneapolis: University of Minnesota Press.

Clark, L. A., Simms, L. J., Wu, K. D., & Casillas, A. (in press). *Schedule for Nonadaptive and Adaptive Personality: Manual for administration, scoring, and interpretation* (2nd ed.). Minneapolis: University of Minnesota Press.

Clegg, C. B., Fremouw, W., & Mogge, N. (2009). Utility of the Structured Inventory of Malingered Symptoms (SIMS) and the Assessment of Depression Inventory (ADI) in screening for malingering among outpatients seeking to claim disability. *Journal of Forensic Psychiatry and Psychology, 20,* 239–254.

Costa, P. T., & McCrae, R. R. (1992). *NEO-PI-R and NEO-FFI: Professional manual.* Odessa, FL: Psychological Assessment Resources.

Craig, R. J. (1999). Essentials of MCMI-III assessment. In S. Strack (Ed.), *Essentials of Millon Inventories Assessment* (pp. 1–51). New York: Wiley.

Daubert, S. D., & Metzler, A. E. (2000). The detection of fake-bad and fake-good responding on the Millon Clinical Multiaxial Inventory–III. *Psychological Assessment, 12*, 418–424.

DeClue, G. (2011). Harry Potter and the Structured Interview of Reported Symptoms? *Open Access Journal of Forensic Psychology, 3*, 1–18.

Dragon, W. R., Ben-Porath, Y. S., & Handel, R. W. (2012). Examining the impact of unscorable item responses on the validity and interpretability of MMPI-2/ MMPI-2-RF Restructured Clinical (RC) scale scores. *Assessment, 19*, 101–113.

Edens, J. F., Otto, R. K., & Dwyer, T. (1999). Utility of the Structured Inventory of Malingered Symptomatology in identifying persons motivated to malinger psychopathology. *Journal of the American Academy of Psychiatry and the Law, 27*, 387–396.

Edens, J. F., Poythress, N. G., & Watkins-Clay, M. M. (2007). Detection of malingering in psychiatric unit and general population prison inmates: A comparison of the PAI, SIMS, and SIRS. *Journal of Personality Assessment, 88*, 33–42.

Edwards, A. L. (1970). *The measurement of personality traits by scales and inventories.* New York: Holt, Rinehart, & Winston.

Elhai, J. D., Gold, S. N., Sellers, A. H., & Dorfman, W. I. (2001). The detection of malingered posttraumatic stress disorder with MMPI-2 fake bad indices. *Assessment, 8*, 221–236.

Gaines, M. V. (2009). *An examination of the combined use of the PAI and the M-FAST in detecting malingering among inmates.* Unpublished doctoral dissertation. Texas Tech University, Lubbock, TX.

Gallen, R. T., & Berry, D. T. R. (1996). Detection of random responding in MMPI-2 protocols. *Assessment, 3*, 171–178.

Gervais, R. O., Ben-Porath, Y. S., Wygant, D. B., & Green, P. (2007). Development and validation of a Response Bias Scale (RBS) for the MMPI-2. *Assessment, 14*, 196–208.

Graham, J. R. (2006). *MMPI-2: Assessing Personality and Psychopathology* (4th ed.). New York: Oxford University Press.

Green, D., & Rosenfeld, B. (2011). Evaluating the gold standard: A review and meta-analysis of the Structured Interview of Reported Symptoms. *Psychological Assessment, 23*, 95–107.

Green, D., Rosenfeld, B., & Belfi, B. (2013). New and improved?: A comparison of the original and revised versions of the Structured Interview of Reported Symptoms. *Assessment, 20*, 210–218.

Guy, L. S., Kwartner, P. P., & Miller, H. A. (2006). Investigating the M-FAST: Psychometric properties and utility to detect diagnostic specific malingering. *Behavioral Sciences and the Law, 24*, 687–702.

Guy, L. S., & Miller, H. A. (2004). Screening for malingered psychopathology in a correctional setting: Utility of the Miller-Forensic Assessment of Symptoms Test (M-FAST). *Criminal Justice and Behavior, 31*, 695–716.

Hall, H. V., & Poirier, J. G. (2001). *Detecting malingering and deception* (2nd ed.). Boca Raton, FL: Taylor & Francis.

Handel, R. W., Arnau, R. C., Archer, R. P., & Dandy, K. L. (2006). An evaluation of the MMPI-2 and MMPI—A True Response Inconsistency (TRIN) scales. *Assessment, 13*, 98–106.

Handel, R. W., Ben-Porath, Y. S., Tellegen, A., & Archer, R. P. (2010). Psychometric functioning of the MMPI-2-RF VRIN-r and TRIN-r scales with varying degrees of randomness, acquiescence, and counter-acquiescence. *Psychological Assessment, 22*, 87–95.

Hawes, S. W., & Boccaccini, M. T. (2009). Detection of overreporting of psychopathology on the Personality Assessment Inventory: A meta-analytic review. *Psychological Assessment, 21,* 112–124.

Heinze, M. C. (1999). "Yet there's method in his madness . . .": Dimensions of deception and dangerousness. *Aggression and Violent Behavior, 4,* 387–412.

Heinze, M. C., & Purisch, A. D. (2001). Beneath the mask: Use of psychological tests to detect and subtype malingering in criminal defendants. *Journal of Forensic Psychology, 1,* 23–52.

Hoelzle, J. B., Nelson, N. W., & Arbisi, P. A. (2012). MMPI-2 and MMPI-2-Restructured Form validity scales: Complimentary approaches to evaluate response validity. *Psychological Injury and Law, 5,* 174–191.

Hopwood, C. J., Orlando, M., & Clark, T. C. (2010). The detection of malingered pain-related disability with the Personality Assessment Inventory. *Rehabilitation Psychology, 55,* 307–310.

Johnson, T., Kulesa, P., Cho, Y. I., & Shavitt, S. (2005). The relation between culture and response styles: Evidence from 19 countries. *Journal of Cross-Cultural Psychology, 36,* 264–277.

Jürges, H. (2007). True health vs response styles: Exploring cross-country differences in self-reported health. *Health Economics, 16,* 163–178.

Kucharski, L. T., Duncan. S., Egan, S. S., & Falkenbach, D. M. (2006). Psychopathy and malingering of psychiatric disorder in criminal defendants. *Behavioral Sciences and the Law, 24,* 633–644.

Lange, R. T., Sullivan, K. A., & Scott, C. (2010). Comparison of MMPI-2 and PAI validity indicators to detect feigned depression and PTSD symptom reporting. *Psychiatry Research, 176,* 229–235.

Larrabee, G. L. (Ed.). (2007). *Assessment of malingered neuropsychological deficits.* New York: Oxford University Press.

Lees-Haley, P. R., English, L. T., & Glenn, W. J. (1991). A fake bad scale on the MMPI-2 for personal-injury claimants. *Psychological Reports, 68,* 203–201.

Lewis, J. L., Simcox, A. M., & Berry, D. T. R. (2002). Screening for feigned psychiatric symptoms in a forensic sample by using the MMPI-2 and the Structured Inventory of Malingered Symptomatology. *Psychological Assessment, 14,* 170–176.

Marshall, M., & Bagby, R. M. (2006). The incremental validity and clinical utility of the MMPI-2 Infrequency Posttraumatic Stress Disorder scale. *Assessment, 13,* 417–429.

McCusker, P. J., Moran, M. J., Serfass, L., & Peterson, K. H. (2003). Comparability of the MMPI-2 F(p) and F scales and the SIRS in clinical use with suspected malingerers. *International Journal of Offender Therapy and Comparative Criminology, 47,* 585–596.

Meehl, P. E. (1955). Antecedent probability and the efficiency of psychometric signs, patterns, or cutting scores. *Psychological Bulletin, 52,* 194–216.

Meehl, P. E. (1996). Preface. In *Clinical versus statistical prediction: A theoretical analysis and a review of the evidence.* Northvale, NJ: Jason Aronson. (Original work published 1954)

Mercado, M. M. (2000). The invisible family: Counseling Asian American substance abusers and their families. *Family Journal: Counseling and Therapy for Couples and Families, 8,* 267–272.

Mihura, J. L. (2012). The necessity of multiple test methods in conducting assessments: The role of the Rorschach and self-report. *Psychological Injury and Law, 5,* 97–106.

Miller, H. A. (2001). *Miller-Forensic Assessment of Symptoms Test (M-FAST): Professional manual.* Odessa, FL: Psychological Assessment Resources.

Miller, H. A. (2004) Examining the use of the M-FAST with criminal defendants incompetent to stand trial. *International Journal of Offender and Comparative Criminology, 48,* 268–280.

Millon, T. (1994). *Millon Clinical Multiaxial Inventory–III manual.* Minneapolis, MN: National Computer Systems.

Millon, T., Davis, R., & Millon, C. (1997). *Millon Clinical Multiaxial Inventory–III manual* (2nd ed.). Minneapolis, MN: National Computer Systems.

Mogge, N. L., Lepage, J. S., Bell, T., & Ragatz, L. (2010). The negative distortion scale: A new PAI validity scale. *Journal of Forensic Psychiatry and Psychology, 21,* 77–90.

Morey, L. C. (1991). *Personality Assessment Inventory professional manual.* Odessa, FL: Psychological Assessment Resources.

Morey, L. C. (1993, August). *Defensiveness and malingering indices for the PAI.* Paper presented at the annual convention of the American Psychological Association, Toronto, Ontario, Canada.

Morey, L. C. (1996). *An interpretive guide to the Personality Assessment Inventory.* Odessa, FL: Personality Assessment Resources.

Morey, L. C. (2007). *Personality Assessment Inventory professional manual,* 2nd ed. Odessa, FL: Psychological Assessment Resources.

Morey, L. C., & Hopwood, C. J. (2004). Efficiency of a strategy for detecting back random responding on the Personality Assessment Inventory. *Psychological Assessment, 16,* 197–200.

Morgan, C. D., Schoenberg, M. R., Dorr, D., & Burke, M. J. (2002). Overreport on the MCMI-III: Concurrent validation with the MMPI-2 using a psychiatric inpatient sample. *Journal of Personality Assessment, 78,* 288–300.

Morgan, J. E., & Sweet, J. J. (Eds.). (2009). *Neuropsychology of malingering casebook.* New York: Psychology Press.

Nicholson, R. A., Mouton, G. J., Bagby, R. M., Buis, T., Peterson, S. A., & Buigas, R. A. (1997). Utility of MMPI-2 indicators of response distortion: Receiver operating characteristic analysis. *Psychological Assessment, 9,* 471–479.

Paulhus, D. L. (1988). *Assessing self-deception and impression management in self-reports: The Balanced Inventory of Desirable Responding.* Unpublished manual, University of British Columbia, Vancouver, Canada.

Paulhus, D. L., Bruce, M. N., & Trapnell, P. D. (1995). Effects of self-presentation strategies on personality profiles and their structure. *Personality and Social Psychology Bulletin, 21,* 100–108.

Ray, C. L. (2009). The importance of using malingering screeners in forensic practice. *Journal of Forensic Psychological Practice, 9,* 138–146.

Rogers, R. (1984). Towards an empirical model of malingering and deception. *Behavioral Sciences and the Law, 2,* 93–112.

Rogers, R. (1990). Models of feigned mental illness. *Professional Psychology: Research and Practice, 21,* 182–188.

Rogers, R. (2008a). An introduction to response styles. In R. Rogers (Ed.), *Clinical assessment of malingering and deception* (3rd ed., pp. 3–13). New York: Guilford Press.

Rogers, R. (2008b). Detection strategies for malingering and defensiveness. In R. Rogers (Ed.), *Clinical assessment of malingering and deception* (3rd ed., pp. 14–38). New York: Guilford Press.

Rogers, R., Bagby, R. M., & Dickens, S. E. (1992). *Structured Interview of Reported Symptoms professional manual.* Odessa, FL: Psychological Assessment Resources.

Rogers, R., & Bender, S. D. (2003). Evaluation of malingering and deception. In I. B. Weiner (Series Ed.) & A. M. Goldstein (Vol. Ed.), *Handbook of psychology: Vol. 11. Forensic psychology* (pp. 109–132). Hoboken, NJ: Wiley.

Rogers, R., & Cavanaugh, J. L. (1983). "Nothing but the truth" . . . A reexamination of malingering. *Journal of Law and Psychiatry, 11,* 443–460.

Rogers, R., Sewell, K. W., & Gillard, N. D. (2010). *Structured Interview of Reported Symptoms* (2nd ed.). Odessa, FL: Psychological Assessment Resources.

Rogers, R., Sewell, K. W., Martin, M. A., & Vitacco, M. J. (2003). Detection of feigned mental disorders: A meta-analysis of the MMPI-2 and malingering. *Assessment, 10,* 160–177.

Rogers, R., Sewell, K. W., Morey, L. C., & Ustad, K. L. (1996). Detection of feigned mental disorders on the Personality Assessment Inventory: A discriminant analysis. *Journal of Personality Assessment, 67,* 629–640.

Rubenzer, S. (2010). Review of the Structured Inventory of Reported Symptoms–2 (SIRS-2). *Open Access Journal of Forensic Psychology, 2,* 273–286.

Schinka, J. A., Kinder, B. N., & Kremer, T. (1997). Research validity scales for the NEO-PI-R: Development and initial validation. *Journal of Personality Assessment, 68,* 127–138.

Sellbom, M., & Bagby, R. M. (2008a). Response styles on multiscale inventories. In R. Rogers (Ed.), *Clinical assessment of malingering and deception* (3rd ed., pp. 182–206). New York: Guilford Press.

Sellbom, M., & Bagby, R. M. (2008b). Validity of the MMPI-2-RF (Restructured Form) L-r and K-r scales in detecting underreporting in clinical and nonclinical samples. *Psychological Assessment, 20,* 370–376.

Simms, L. J., & Clark, L. A. (2001). Detection of deception on the Schedule for Non-adaptive and Adaptive Personality: Validation of the validity scales. *Assessment, 8,* 251–266.

Smith, G. P. (2008). Brief screening measures for the detection of feigned psychopathology. In R. Rogers (Ed.), *Clinical assessment of malingering and deception* (3rd ed., pp. 323–342). New York: Guilford Press.

Smith, G. P., & Burger, G. K. (1997). Detection of malingering: Validation of the Structured Inventory of Malingered Symptomatology (SIMS). *Journal of the American Academy of Psychiatry and the Law, 25,* 183–189.

Snell, A. F., Sydell, E. J., & Lueke, S. B. (1999). Towards a theory of applicant faking: Integrating studies of deception. *Human Resource Management Review, 9,* 219–242.

Strong, D. R., Greene, R. L., Hoppe, C., Johnston, T., & Olesen, N. (1999). Taxometric analysis of impression management and self-deception on the MMPI-2 in child custody litigants. *Journal of Personality Assessment, 73,* 1–18.

Tellegen, A. (1985). Structure of mood and personality and their relevance to assessing anxiety, with an emphasis on self-report. In A. H. Tuma & J. D. Maser (Eds.), *Anxiety and the anxiety disorders* (pp. 681–706). Hillsdale, NJ: Erlbaum.

Tett, R. P., Anderson, M. G., Ho, C.-L., Yang, T. S., Huang, L., & Hanvongse, A. (2006). Seven nested questions about faking in personality tests. In R. L. Griffith & M. H. Peterson (Eds.), *A closer examination of applicant faking behavior.* Greenwich, CT: Information Age.

Thomas, K. M., Hopwood, C. J., Orlando, M. J., Weathers, F. W., & McDevitt-Murphy, M. E. (2012). Detecting feigned PTSD using the Personality Assessment Inventory. *Psychological Injury and Law, 5,* 192–201.

Thomas-Peter, B. A., Jones, J., Campbell, S., & Oliver, C. (2000). Debasement and faking bad on the Millon Clinical Multiaxial Inventory III: An examination of characteristics, circumstances and motives of forensic patients. *Legal and Criminological Psychology, 5,* 71–81.

Veazey, C. H., Hays, J. R., Wagner, A. L., & Miller, H. A. (2005). Validity of the Miller Forensic Assessment of Symptoms Test in psychiatric inpatients. *Psychological Reports, 96,* 771–774.

Veltri, C. O. C., & Williams, J. E. (2013). Does the disorder matter?: Investigating a moderating effect on coached malingering using the MMPI-2 and PAI. *Assessment, 20,* 199–209.

Vitacco, M. J. (2008). Syndromes associated with deception. In R. Rogers (Ed.), *Clinical assessment of malingering and deception* (3rd ed., pp. 39–50). New York: Guilford Press.

Weiss, W. U., Serafino, G., & Serafino, A. (2000). A study of the interrelationships of several validity scales used in police selection. *Journal of Police and Criminal Psychology, 15,* 41–44.

Widows, M., & Smith, G. P. (2005). *Structured Inventory of Malingered Symptomatology (SIMS): Professional manual.* Odessa, FL: Psychological Assessment Resources.

Wiggins, C. W., Wygant, D. B., Hoelzle, J. B., & Gervais, R. O. (2012). The more you say the less it means: Overreporting and attenuated criterion validity in a forensic disability sample. *Psychological Injury and Law, 5,* 162–173.

Wygant, D. B., Ben-Porath, Y. S., & Arbisi, P. A. (2004). *Development and initial validation of a scale to detect infrequent somatic complaints.* Poster presented at the 39th annual symposium on recent developments of the MMPI-2/MMPI-A, Minneapolis, MN.

CHAPTER 13

Multimethod Violence Risk Assessment

Michael L. Stanfill, Suzanne O'Brien, and Donald J. Viglione, Jr.

Weiner and Greene (2008) differentiate between personality testing and personality assessment by asserting that "personality testing refers to the use of psychological tests to identify an individual's personality characteristics, whereas personality assessment involves integrating many kinds of information into a set of personality-based conclusions and recommendations concerning a person who has been evaluated" (p. 19). When referral issues include violence risk assessment, the goal of assessment is not just to give a risk estimate in a vacuum, but to comprehend the person in context, in light of his or her culture, background, and life experiences, in order to better understand in what circumstances a person could harm themselves or others. It goes without saying then that to do a thorough risk assessment, it is essential to integrate information from multiple sources, using a variety of modalities.

Generally speaking, when designing a test battery, one should consider issues of reliability and test validity, as well as determine whether information one gathers from different measures is redundant or helps to complete a multifaceted picture of the person being assessed. When similar modality measures are being used to assess an individual, one can expect some information to be redundant and therefore not add much to the richness of the clinical picture. Using a multimethod approach to assessment, one can collect a rich amount of data from multiple sources to create a more cohesive and potentially accurate picture of the individual, and then provide the clearest estimate of risk to self and others.

Frequently used to estimate risk for violence are some measures that estimate risk of re-offense by looking at empirically supported variables that research has shown are relevant to violence. Often these measures, such as the Static-99, Revised Version (Static-99R; Hanson, Phenix, & Helmus, 2009) or Violence Risk Appraisal Guide (VRAG; Quinsey, Harris, Rice, & Cormier, 2006), utilize regression equations to estimate risk and require little to no clinician judgment. It is of note that the VRAG was originally designed via review of the empirical research literature and then later "weighted" consistent with actuarial measures based on the results of several studies (Quinsey et al., 2006). Other researchers in the area of prediction of violence suggest evaluating risk utilizing a classification tree approach (Steadman et al., 2000). Risk assessments utilizing the regression equation approach have shown moderate utility and as such are widely used (Babchishin, Hanson, & Helmus, 2011). Underlying the use of such a measure is the assumption that the risk factors have the same predictive value for the individuals being assessed, and all people evaluated with such an instrument are rated on the same characteristics in the same way. In contrast, a classification tree approach is rather idiographic in that the underlying assumption is that some risk factors are relevant for some, though not for all individuals.

The research literature has consistently identified certain risk factors that are relevant for violence risk analysis. These typically include psychopathy, anger modulation difficulties, delusions or preoccupation with violent thoughts, hallucinations associated with violence, personality disorders, substance abuse disorders, gender, a history of childhood maltreatment, conditional release failure or revocation, and of course a history of previous violence (e.g., Borum, 1996; Gretton, Hare, & Catchpole, 2004; Vitacco, Erickson, Kurus, & Apple, 2012). Gathering information about these variables from varied sources with an emphasis on reviewing documentation is necessary in order to conduct a thorough analysis of violence.

The Role of History, the Clinical Interview, and Actuarial Measures

In completing a violence or suicide risk assessment, the patient's history and, when available, clinical interview are essential for gathering information required for completing various actuarial prediction indices (Harris & Lurigio, 2007). Each of these pieces plays a critical role in comprehensive multimodal risk assessment. However, because of the overlapping variance between each of these pieces, they are best discussed as a whole to illustrate the interrelationship among a patient's history, clinical interview, and actuarial scores.

History and the Clinical Interview

Prior to the early to mid-1990s, many studies assessed the relationship between various historical variables and risk for current and/or future violent acts (Link, Andrews, & Cullen, 1992; Monahan, 1993; Swanson, Holzer, Ganju, & Jono, 1990). However, there was little consistency between studies regarding the populations, sampling techniques, and variables assessed (Harris & Lurigio, 2007). To address these challenges, a group of researchers from across the United States formed to complete a large multiyear study, which later became known as the MacArthur Violence Risk Assessment Study (Monahan et al., 2001). The researchers studied ten categories of variables to determine which risk factors predicted further violence in a one-year period after the individual was released from some type of public health facility (e.g. jail, psychiatric hospital). While the variables were selected a priori, the majority of assessed categories were historical and/or static.

Of the historical variables they assessed, many demonstrated either a positive or an inverse relationships with the risk for future violence. Historical variables that had a positive relationship with risk for future violence were: previous violence acts; serious and frequent physical abuse as a child; having a father who was violent, a substance abuser, or criminal; living in a disadvantaged neighborhood; and having a history of intense anger that was difficult to control or modulate (Monahan et al., 2001). Other variables offered more mixed results. For example, having a previous diagnosis of schizophrenia or other major mental illness decreased violence risk, while having a personality disorder or adjustment diagnosis increased risk. Similarly, being male increased risk of violence toward family members, but not other people.

Other researchers approached assessment of historical risk factors thorough literature review and clinician consideration. During development of the Historical, Clinical, Risk Management–20 (HCR-20; Webster, Douglas, Eaves, & Hart, 1997), which is described in more detail below, the authors of the measure assessed many historical variables. Ultimately, based on their review of the literature, they concluded that special consideration should be given to: previous violence, young age of first violent incident; relationship instability; employment problems; substance abuse problems; major mental illness; psychopathy; early maladjustment; personality disorder; and prior supervision failure (Webster et al., 1997).

Although many of these variables can be obtained from document review and collateral information, it is also imperative to have a strong clinical interview to further assess the evaluee's current psychological state (Papapietro, 2012). The context of risk assessment for dangerousness and/or self-harm is typically adversarial, and often the stakes are high for the individual being assessed. For example, the risk assessment could make the difference between parole versus civil commitment, or being treated in a locked facility versus an outpatient setting. In other situations, it could impact sentencing in court. Given such a context, evaluees may not want to be completely forthcoming in their disclosures. As such, information gathered during the clinical interview should be taken with this adversarial context in mind in terms of the reliability and validity of the statements made by the individual.

Assessing the roles of psychiatric illness, symptoms, characterological concerns, and current coping capacity is essential in thorough risk evaluation (Papapietro, 2012). While there is mixed evidence about the global impact of having a psychotic disorder on violence, or acting out aggressively (Harris & Lurigio, 2007; Monahan et al., 2001), having current delusions of violence or persecution around violence increases risk (Harris & Lurigio, 2007; Monahan, 1993; Monahan et al., 2001). In a similar vein, certain personality disorders increase one's risk (e.g., antisocial or borderline personality disorder), while others (e.g., obsessive–compulsive personality disorder) actually lower risk (Monahan et al., 2001; Torrey, Stanley, Monahan, & Steadman, 2008). While having historical collateral information may help to confirm one of these diagnoses, a clinical interview is also necessary to help determine the role the disorder is playing in the individual's current functioning. If the evaluee's current coping capacity is well established and robust, this may serve as a protective factor even in the presence of other clinical risk factors.

Clinical interviews are also critical for the completion of other measures commonly used in risk evaluations. For example, although the Psychopathy Checklist (PCL-R; Hare, 2003) can be completed with a document review alone, it is difficult to score several of the variables without a clinical interview (Gretton et al., 2004; Hare, 2003). While some of these variables are concerned with the content of the interview (e.g., frequent lying), the majority of variables scored via the interview are concerned with the context and presentation of the evaluee (e.g., grandiose sense of self). By focusing more on the presentation of the evaluee, rather than on the content of the dialogue, more reliable information can be gathered for some of these variables.

It is well known that clinical judgment in the absence of any assessment tool is considered to be unreliable and inaccurate (Meehl, 1954). This holds true especially in risk assessment where clinical judgment in and of itself is often very poor (Grob, 1995). Quinsey et al. (1998) point to myriad examples in the literature demonstrating that mental health professionals' predictions about treatability and violent reoffending are no more accurate than those of laypersons. One of the major issues surrounding the poor prediction by clinicians has to do with many clinicians' limited understanding of base rates and frequencies of certain behaviors. As noted earlier, this is not to say that the clinical interview does not have its place. Rather, it is imperative that clinicians combine a clinical interview with other measures as demonstrated in Table 13.1.

TABLE 13.1. Factors, Measures, and Scales to Consider in Multimodal Risk Assessment

Historical
- History of violent acting out
- Having a father that was abusive or an substance abuser
- Past problems with anger
- Current or past substance abuse
- Living in a disadvantaged neighborhood
- *Gender*
- *Psychiatric diagnosis*

Clinical
- Openness and willingness to participate
- Confabulation or exaggeration in spite of alternative evidence
- Grandiose or callousness
- Self-report consistent with other forms of information

Actuarial and structured professional judgment tools
- PCL-R
- VRAG
- COVR
- Static-99R
- Structured Risk Assessment: Forensic Version—Light
- START
- HCR-20

Self-report
- MMPI-2
  - Scale 4, 6, 8,9
  - *O-H*
- PAI
  - AGG
  - DOM
  - VPI
  - ANT
  - BOR

Performance
- Rorschach Aggression Indicators
  - *AGC, AGM (AG), AGP*, AG Potential
  - *MOR*
  - MAP
- Rorschach Idiographic Assessment of Aggression
  - Cognitive processing (Complexity, R, F%, Blends, Sy, M, MC, MC-PPD)
  - Thought disorder (EII-3, TP-Comp, WSumCog, SevCog, X–%, WD–%)
  - Distress or despair (m, Y, MOR, YTVC', CritCont%
  - Interpersonal relationship (SR, PHR/GPHR, M-, V-Comp, H, MAP, PER, r)

Note. Items that are *italicized* are those for which there is mixed evidence or support based on specific characteristics or circumstance.

With all of the specific instruments that have been validated to assist with risk assessment, in current practice clinical judgment used by itself is considered an unethical practice. As noted by Cote, Crocker, Nicholls, and Seto (2012), risk assessment measures help to ensure that clinicians use systematic, reliable, and valid approaches in making forensic opinions.

Actuarial Methods

In an effort to improve the efficacy as well as the specificity of predicting the likelihood to re-offend, actuarial measures have become quite popular. By utilizing a wide variety of historical variables, many measures were created to address criticisms of the less formal clinical approach (Harris & Lurigio, 2007; Harris, Phenix, Hanson, & Thornton, 2003; Monahan, 1993; Monahan et al., 2001; Torrey et al., 2008). Many of these measures, such as the VRAG or Static-99R (Harris et al., 2003; Quinsey et al., 2006) rely solely on historical or static variables that have been shown in research to predict violent or sexual violent recidivism moderately well. One answers a series of questions about the patient's history and criminal record, and based on a regression analysis, an overall estimate of recidivism is provided.

While these historically grounded predictions are helpful, it is also important to consider dynamic or psychological characteristics, especially from a protective factor standpoint. Beyond prediction, many of these dynamic variables are relevant in the management, supervision, and treatment, and thus the risk mitigation of offenders. However, many of these variables are quite changeable and can fluctuate greatly over time. Moreover, the importance of each may vary from person to person. For example, an offender who is otherwise coherent and not psychotic can relapse on methamphetamine and become quite psychotic, delusional, and potentially violent.

Some have argued that actuarial risk assessment should be used as a primary form of evaluation. For example, in the tradition of Meehl (1954), Quinsey et al. (1998) advise clinicians to completely replace clinical judgment with actuarial methods, noting that "actuarial methods are too good and clinical judgment too poor to risk contaminating the former with the latter" (p. 171). However these measures are not foolproof by any means and do not offer an absolute guaranteed prediction of future violence. Actuarials demonstrate moderate validity (Yang & Mulvey, 2012), and various risk assessment measures have consistently flattened out when measured with receiver operating curves at an area under the curve (AUC) of .70 to .80 (Buchanan, 2008; Mossman, 2009; Yang & Mulvey, 2012). Yang and Mulvey (2012) attribute this to various factors such as: "(i) there may be a class of objective markers not yet identified . . . ; (ii) the variance may be completely aleatory and there is no identifiable regularity; or (iii) individual differences in conditional response to social situations have not yet been accounted for in a sufficiently precise manner" (p. 199). Additionally, the role of increasing age in diminished acting out is demonstrated with several populations (Helmus, Thornton, Hanson, & Babchishin, 2012). Some of these measures have attempted to correct for this declining aggressiveness with age (Hanson & Morton-Bourgon, 2009; Harris et al., 2003) albeit to moderate success. Moreover, relevant to the arguments about clinical judgment is the fact that the PCL-R itself involves a great deal of clinical judgment.

The base rates of certain behaviors are an additional concern with actuarial measures. In discussing the base rate of violence recidivism, it is important to consider the population that is being studied, as well as the rate of re-offense. The base rate of violence recidivism is typically low, though when it does occur the cost can be high, particularly in terms of community safety or the perception of community safety. The literature on violent recidivism or dangerousness is replete with cautions about the difficulties in prediction that occur when the outcome in question has a very low base rate (Tengström, 2001).

While several violence risk measures are available, the advantage of using one measure over another remains unclear. Yang, Wong, and Coid (2010) conducted a meta-analysis of second- and third-generation risk assessment tools and their components, which included the Psychopathy Checklist—Revised (PCL-R; Hare, 2003) the Offender Group Reconviction Scale-Version 2 (OGRS; Copas & Marshall, 1998), the Violence Risk Assessment Guide (VRAG; Harris et al., 1993), the Risk Matrix 2000 for Violence (RM2000V), the Historical, Clinical, and Risk Management Violence (HCR-20; Webster et al., 1997), Psychopathy Checklist: Screening Version (PCL:SV; Hart, Cox, & Hare, 1995), the Level of Service Inventory—Revised (LSI-R; Andews & Bonta, 1995), General Statistical Information for Recidivism (GSIR; Bonta, Harman, Hann, & Cormier, 1996), the Violence Risk Scale (VRS; Wong & Gordon, 2001, 2006), and the Static-99 (Hanson et al., 2009); with the goal of attempting to determine which tools provide the most accurate prediction of violence. The results of the meta-analysis showed that all of the tools included in their study produced medium effect sizes, though no particular measure stood out from the rest. Overall, the authors concluded "that there is no appreciable or clinically significant difference in the violence-predictive efficacies of the nine tools after accounting for differences in study features or other unexplained random effects with multilevel regression analysis" (p. 759). In essence, these measures were thought to be interchangeable in predicting violence. They did recommend choosing one tool over another depending on relevant clinical, criminal justice, or risk management functions the tools can perform. Thus, if a clinician is interested in the case management process; the LS/CMI or HCR-20 might be more helpful than others. Of course, if one is evaluating risk of sexual re-offense, the Static-99R is often a top choice. Alternatively, if one is interested in possible personality characteristics and in whether therapy could be helpful or contraindicated, the PCL-R might be indicated. Measures like the VRAG or HCR-20 incorporate the PCL-R (Hare, 2003) into the scoring of the measure, so it may be necessary to score the PCL-R independent of completing other risk assessment measures.

Although use of some of the actuarial measures designed to assess risk have benefits, such instruments also have some important limitations. For example, the time period for which these measures predict risk is limited. Also, the relative risk estimates obtained for an individual are heavily reliant on whether the individual being assessed matches the sample on which the risk estimates are based or matches research samples. For example, in attempting to assess risk of re-offense for a female sex offender, one cannot reliably depend on the typical actuarial risk assessment measures because validity evidence for these measures is based solely on male offenders, and there is limited research on differentiating characteristics and risk factors between male and female sex offenders. These measures have also been criticized for relying on a single regression equation (Steadman et al., 2000) that is presumed to be useful across diverse populations. That being said, recent research has noted the limitations of these actuarial measures when used by themselves (Hanson & Morton-Bourgon, 2009; Harris & Lurigio, 2007). The field as a whole has moved toward a more structured professional judgment model (Harris & Lurigio, 2007; Torrey et al., 2008).

Structured Professional Judgment

As an alternative to actuarial prediction, another method that has emerged in recent decades and is routinely in practice is the structured professional judgment model (Douglas, Oglaff, & Hart, 2003). This model can be considered a guided clinical approach that focuses on empirically validated risk factors to violence. One of the more widely known structured professional judgment tools commonly utilized with forensic psychiatric patients in California and Washington is the HCR-20 (Webster et al., 1997). HCR-20 considers historical (or static) variables, clinical items, and risk management items. The tool has 20 items. Unlike the actuarial measures, however, it does not combine different risk factors into a regression equation to predict outcome, nor does it provide a specific probability figure regarding re-offense, but instead rates risk categorically (i.e., low, moderate, high). The final determination of risk level is not necessarily finalized by the number of risk factors present, nor does it need to be influenced by each item or score.

When the HCR-20 was in its infancy, Borum (1996) noted that "the promise of this instrument lies in its foundation on a conceptual model or scheme for assessing dangerousness and risk; its basis in the empirical literature; its operationally defined coding system allowing for increased reliability; and its practical use, as evidenced in its brevity and allowance for time-consuming data collection to be done by trained assistants (H and

R variables through record review)" (p. 950). Like actuarial measures, the HCR-20 is capable of providing a moderate degree of accuracy in predicting violence (Mills, Kroner, & Hemmati, 2007).

One potential limitation of the HCR-20, as discussed by Rufino, Boccaccini, and Guy (2011), is that some items on the Clinical and Risk Management scales are subjectively scored—which might compromise its overall predictive validity. Nonetheless, the authors also cite research demonstrating adequate rater agreement, including that of Douglas and Reeves (2010) who had reviewed rater agreement from available HCR-20 studies and found that the median rater agreement coefficient (intra-class correlation coefficient; ICC) for the Total Score was .85. Not surprisingly, the rater agreement coefficient was higher for the Historical items (.86) than for the other two scales that are more subjective in nature (rater coefficients of .74 and .68 for Clinical scale and Risk Management scale, respectively).

Another advantage of the HCR-20 is that it can help identify specific risk factors relevant to the individual, help the clinician identify potential victim pools, and assist in identifying relevant intervention strategies to manage risk while in treatment (Guy, Packer, & Warnken, 2012). In addition, although the HCR-20 has slightly better predictive validity for evaluating future risk in men than in women, unlike most if not all of the actuarial risk assessment measures published today, the HCR-20 can be used with female offenders (de Vogel & de Ruiter, 2004; Garcia-Mansilla, Rosenfeld, & Cruise, 2011).

The field now recognizes the need to balance risk assessment by including protective factors in risk analysis (Rogers, 2000). In response to this need, the Short-Term Assessment of Risk and Treatability (START; Webster, Martin, Brink, Nicholls, & Middleton, 2004; Webster et al., 2009), a structured professional judgment measure was developed to include static as well as dynamic protective and risk factors that capture both client strengths and vulnerabilities (Desmarais, Nicholls, Wilson, & Brink, 2012) across multiple domains related to risk (e.g., risk to others or self). This measure focuses on psychological functioning, adaptability, social functioning, external resources, and overall engagement. By addressing these various domains, the evaluee can rate increased risk on one domain, but have protective factors in another. For example, while a person may have a major mental illness that increases his or her risk for self-harm, this risk can be mitigated by other internal and external resources, as well as their overall adaptability. Preliminary research on this measure has demonstrated predictive and incremental validity over the HCR-20 and PCL:SV.

Self-Report Personality Instruments

One finding from the MacArthur Violence Risk Assessment Study was that chemical abuse comorbidity with certain mental disorders was a risk factor for future violence (Monahan, 1993). In that study, a diagnosis of schizophrenia was not a risk factor for future violence per se, yet command-type auditory hallucinations, violent thoughts, and nondelusional suspiciousness were all associated with future violence. However, psychologists are often called upon to evaluate mentally ill offenders to provide a violence risk analysis. The evaluator should consider the type of illness likely to increase one's risk for violence (e.g., manic episode with comorbid active substance abuse) versus illnesses that would decrease the risk of violence (e.g., severe depression with psychomotor retardation).

Broadband instruments such as the Minnesota Multiphasic Personality Instrument, Second Edition (MMPI-2; Butcher, Dahlstrom, Graham, Tellegen, & Kaemmer, 1989), and the Personality Assessment Inventory (PAI; Morey, 2007) attempt to assess the frequency, depth, breadth, and severity of psychiatric problems or behaviors. They are a staple in clinical evaluations. Understanding the referral questions and the adversarial context of the evaluation helps inform which measures to choose and those that are most appropriate. Although these instruments are not specifically designed to identify who is at risk to become violent, personality assessment instruments provide important and unique contributions in forensic settings, given that the personality data derived from such instruments can help with developing realistic treatment goals and appropriate interventions, and evaluating treatment progress. This in turn can help with handling case management and monitoring the degree of continued risk to the community (Nieberding, Moore, & Dematatis, 2002).

One advantage of broadband psychological tests is their ability to assess response styles. A large amount of research has been done on response-style strategies for both of these instruments (Meyer et al., 2001). Having the ability to assess how accurate or forthcoming a respondent has been in responding can help determine how psychologically disturbed a respondent may be or whether other factors (e.g., poor concentration, poor comprehension, positive or negative impression management) might also need to be considered.

Although most broadband tests were not developed for the purpose of predicting violent behavior, these psychological tests can contribute to a nomothetic understanding of dangerousness and self-harm, given that they provide information about certain constructs that research has shown to be related to dangerousness and self-harm. One such variable is sustained and persistent major mental illness. Although not all individuals with a major mental illness are violent and not all violent people are mentally ill, some research has shown a link between mental illness and violence (Harris & Lurigio, 2007; Link et al., 1992; Monahan, 1993). Broadband personality assessment measures have the potential to contribute a robust amount of information to the clinical/forensic picture concerning psychopathology.

Research has shown that certain clinical conditions are more closely related to risk for dangerousness and/or self-harm than others. For instance, while data are mixed as to whether individuals who are actively experiencing command auditory hallucinations or delusions are at increased risk for violence, individuals with substance use diagnoses, antisocial personality disorder, poor impulse control, or moderate/high psychopathy are more likely to pose a risk to the safety of others (Monahan et al., 2001; Hare, 2003; Harris & Lurigio, 2007). Alternatively, individuals presenting negative symptoms are less likely to be violent (Shah, 1993; Swanson et al., 2006, as quoted in Conroy & Murrie, 2007). By thoroughly examining the clinical picture that emerges from the profile, one can ascertain whether personality factors are present that increase or decrease an individual's risk for dangerousness or self-harm. In particular, if the person has a history of a major mental disorder, it is important to have a clear understanding of the patient's current mental status, mental illness history, and past violence to determine imminent risk (Conroy & Murrie, 2007).

In addition, broadband measures tap other constructs that are associated with risk of violence, such as aggressive behavior, problems with impulse control, antisocial attitudes, impulsivity/recklessness, delusional thoughts, and hallucinations (Butcher et al., 1989). Although these measures are rather face valid regarding substance abuse, they can identify some characteristics that are common among substance abusers, such as risk-taking, excitement-seeking, and impulsivity (Butcher et al., 1989; Meyer et al., 2001).

Graham (2006) noted that numerous studies have found the MMPI-2 to be one of the most widely accepted psychological tests to use in forensic settings. Indeed, because "MMPI-2-based forensic assessment can shed light on the individual's psychological adjustment as he or she sees it and is willing to share self-observations with others" (Pope, Butcher, & Seelen, 2006, p. 37), it has been widely used in personal injury, workers' compensation, family custody, and criminal responsibility cases. Although it does not address issues of dangerousness directly, the MMPI-2 assesses a wide range of serious psychopathology and personality characteristics in the clinical scales and subscales that can affect treatment and risk management (Nieberding et al., 2002). For example, Megargee, Mercer and Carbonell (1999) found that elevations on the following scales are suggestive of deficient inhibitions or behavioral controls, and accordingly could be associated with aggression: infrequency (F), psychopathic deviate (4), paranoia (6), schizophrenia (8), and hypomania (9). Research regarding the Overcontrolled Hostility scale (O-H) is mixed, and Graham concluded that "there is no evidence to suggest that high scores on the O-H scale in groups other than prisoners are associated with violent acts" (p. 203).

The PAI (Morey, 2007) has become increasingly popular in risk assessment evaluations. In addition to validity scales, clinical scales (and their corresponding subscales), treatment consideration scales, and interpersonal scales; the PAI includes other scales of forensic utility to assess potential malingering, as well as scales to assess risk of both dangerousness and self-harm. For instance, the Suicide Potential Index (SPI) was developed to include common features that have been shown to be associated with suicide. Although there is limited research on this index, evidence suggests that the SPI differentiates groups with and without a history of suicidal ideation, attempts, and history of psychiatric hospitalization (Hopwood, Baker, & Morey, 2008; Sinclair et al., 2012). It also was found to be a strong predictor of suicidal behavior in veterans with a history of head injury (Breshears, Brenner, Harwood, & Gutierrez, 2010).

The PAI includes specific indices that were created to assess violence risk, as well as certain interpersonal scales that have been found useful in assessing the likelihood of future violence. The Violence Potential Index (VPI) is in essence a theoretical index that includes PAI variables tapping constructs that the literature has shown to be associated with violence, such as explosive anger, lack of empathy, impulsivity, substance abuse, and sensation seeking (Edens, Hart, Johnson, Johnson, & Oliver, 2000). Research on the utility of the VPI has been mixed (Hopwood et al., 2008; Boccaccini, Murrie, Hawes, Simpler, & Johnson, 2010; Sinclair et al., 2012). On the positive side, Antisocial Behaviors (ANT) was found to be related strongly to the antisocial personality symptom count on the Structured Clinical Interview of DSM Disorders, Second Edition (SCID-II; Guy, Poythress, Douglas, Skeem, & Edens, 2008), and the ANT scale was deemed the best predictor of institutional misconduct in incarcerated women (Skopp, Edens, & Ruiz, 2007). With a population of combat veterans who were being evaluated for posttraumatic stress disorder (PTSD), however, the Aggression (AGG) composite scale provided incremental validity over the effects of PTSD severity, demographic variables, and scales on the MMPI-2 associated with aggression and externalized anger, whereas the VPI did not provide any additional explanatory power over these other predictors (Crawford, Calhoun, Braxton, & Beckham, 2007).

Other PAI variables, including AGG, Dominance (DOM), and ANT, have been found to improve prediction of violence over the Static-99 with sex offenders (Boccaccini et al., 2010). Indeed, these authors cite Walters's (2006) meta-analysis that demonstrates that "scores from content-relevant self-report measures, such as the PAI, tend to predict violence, misbehavior, and recidivism just as well as scores from clinician-scored measures specifically designed to assess violence or recidivism risk" (p. 142). In addition, since the PAI is not a labor-intensive test, it can be used as a screening tool. When violence indicators are elevated, this may signal the need for a more intensive or focused violence risk assessment (Douglas, Hart, & Kropp, 2001).

Performance-Based Personality Instruments

The Rorschach Inkblot Method, as configured by the Rorschach Performance Assessment System (R-PAS; Meyer, Viglione, Mihura, Erard, & Erdberg, 2011) and the Comprehensive System (CS; Exner, 2003), offers distinct opportunities and information when included in an evaluation of dangerousness. Relative to self-report tests, the Rorschach has proven to be less vulnerable to false self-presentation or impression management (Meloy, 1992; Viglione, 1999). For this reason it has often been used in forensic evaluations (Gacono & Evans, 2008). It is not surprising that forensic research practice information supports the view that forensic applications of the Rorschach have a long history. Nevertheless, questions have arisen about using the Rorschach in court. In approximately 8,000 court cases, half of which were criminal, as far back as 1945, Weiner, Exner, and Sciara (1996) found that the Rorschach was rarely challenged (0.08%) and was almost never ruled inadmissible (0.01%). The "legal weight" of the Rorschach was supported in a related survey where it was frequently important enough to be discussed in the legal rulings (Meloy, Hansen, & Weiner, 1997). More recently, Gacono and Evans (2008) detailed the many applications of the Rorschach to forensic use. In 2012, Erard articulated a rationale for using the R-PAS in court (Erard, 2012).

At least seven meta-analyses support the validity of the Rorschach (Atkinson, Quarrington, Alp, & Cyr, 1986; Bornstein, 1996, 1999; Diener, Hilsenroth, Shaffer, & Sexton, 2011; Hiller, Rosenthal, Bornstein, & Berry, 1999; Mihura, Meyer, Dumitrascu, & Bombel, 2013; Parker, Hanson, & Hunsley, 1988). A key finding of these meta-analyses is that many Rorschach variables are valid and useful when one emphasizes externally assessed characteristics rather than self-report scales as criteria. This fact has led to claims that the Rorschach corresponds to ecologically valid real-world behavioral events and life outcomes better than it does self-attributed or introspective characteristics in the form of self-report scales. Thus, in the evaluation of dangerousness, the Rorschach data are likely consistent with what people do rather than with what people say about themselves. In turn, this conclusion supports the idea of classifying the Rorschach as a performance test of personality, in the same way that the Wechsler is a performance test of intelligence (Meyer & Kurtz; 2006; Meyer & Viglione, 2008; Weiner & Greene, 2008, Viglione & Rivera, 2012). These tests involve the respondent's performing tasks to produce a sample of behavior relevant to personality. Thus, the Rorschach involves the induction, observation, characterization, and quantification of the "personality in action," a performance that is then generalized to real-life behaviors. In addition, the Rorschach allows the observation of interpersonal behavior and attitudes, which might expose callous, insensitive, narcissistic, hostile, paranoid, or uncooperative behaviors presumed to accompany some presentations of dangerousness.

The definitive meta-analysis is the Mihura et al. (2013) tome published in *Psychological Bulletin*. This all-inclusive, ambitious project combines 95 individual meta-analyses of peer-reviewed empirical validity literature on CS variables (Exner, 2003). They found that the mean validity coefficient was $r = .27$ for externally assessed characteristics but only $r = .08$ for self-report scales and fully structured interview criteria. The variables with the strongest support were largely those that assess cognitive characteristics or thought perceptual problems and psychotic disturbance. Consistent with other findings (Meyer et al., 2011; Viglione, 1999), those variables whose response process most closely resembled the assessment targets had the best validity (e.g., inaccurate form [FQ–] and psychosis; broken, damaged, injured, sad response attributions and depression [MOR], synthesis responses [Sy or DQ+ in the CS[1]] and sophisticated thinking). However, many CS variables, including some used in evaluations of dangerousness such as indices of self-centeredness (Egocentricity Index in CS, not included in R-PAS) and impulsivity (Zd in CS, not in R-PAS), found essentially no support in the meta-analysis. In turn, this meta-analysis was used as the chief variable selection tool in decisions of what variables to include in the recently published R-PAS (Meyer et al., 2013).

Of course, any claim of superior measurement of real-life behavior would require that the Rorschach demonstrate incremental validity over self-report criteria. Evidence supporting incremental validity is presented by Mihura et al. (2013) and others (e.g., Blais, Hilsenroth, Castlebury, Fowler, & Baity, 2001; Meyer, 2000; Viglione & Hilsenroth, 2001; Weiner, 2001).

A final caution with the Rorschach is that the CS normative data (Exner et al., 2001) have been demonstrated to pathologize interpretations (Meyer, Erdberg, & Shaffer, 2007; Shaffer, Erdberg, & Haroian, 2007; Viglione & Hilsenroth, 2001; Viglione & Meyer, 2008; Wood, Nezworski, Garb, & Lilienfeld, 2001), especially those of protocols produced by respondents from diverse cultural backgrounds. To minimize these difficulties one should use norms from the large sample of international records (Meyer et al., 2007) for the CS or for the R-PAS norms (Meyer et al., 2011); which are also derived from a subgroup of these same international data.

When applying the Rorschach to the evaluation of dangerousness, two major strategies may be used. One involves the direct observation of aggressive references as indicative of aggressive preoccupation or risk. The second involves a more idiographic or individualized approach. In this approach, one evaluates the recurrence of evidence of psychological processes or features associated with previous violence to derive conclusions regarding mechanisms or paths to future violence.

Rorschach Aggression Indicators

Over the years, many overlapping schemes have emerged for scoring aggressive content and references in Rorschach responses (e.g., Elizur, 1949; Exner, 2003; Gacono & Meloy, 1994; Holt, 1977; Meloy & Gacono, 1992). Currently widely available aggression scores in R-PAS and the CS are Aggressive Movement (AGM, AG in CS), Aggression Content (AGC, not in CS, from Gacono & Meloy, 1994; Meloy & Gacono, 1992), and Mutuality of

---

[1]In this chapter R-PAS variable symbols will be listed first, followed by corresponding Comprehensive System (CS) variables if their names differ. These two versions may be coded or calculated slightly differently.

Autonomy Pathology (MAP, not in CS, from Urist, 1977). Encompassing the most severe scores in Urist's Mutuality of Autonomy, MAP involves a reference to a controlling, malevolent, hostile, or destructive relationship or interaction. Infrequently, a person may spontaneously express interest or even enjoyment in damage or injury in Rorschach imagery that is in a morbid response (MOR), so that these responses can indicate aggressive interests. This aggressive component of some MOR responses is recognized in the overlap between MOR and the Aggression Past response (in neither R-PAS nor CS; however, see Gacono & Meloy, 1994, and Meloy & Gacono, 1992).

The theory behind all these scores associates these aggressive references with aggressive ideation and also, to some degree, with aggressive behavior and motives. These aggressive references are also linked to less troublesome characteristics such as competitiveness, interpersonal dominance, and mastery and self-improvement strivings (a potential discriminant validity problem in Rorschach-based risk assessment). Both psychodynamic and cognitive-behavioral theories suggest that aggressive tendencies are associated with aggressive perceptions, which would lead to aggressive interpretation of Rorschach stimuli. Similarly, according to the response process or behavioral representation approach to the Rorschach as a performance test, aggressive responses mirror behaviors in the real world. That is, aggressive perceptions and preoccupations with aggression in processing information on the Rorschach are likely to be expressed in the real world as aggressive cognitions. Conversely, benevolent or cooperative interactions or descriptions (COP) would be less likely among dangerous individuals.

Theoretical linkages notwithstanding, research on these aggressive Rorschach scores and aggression reveals a small and often nonsignificant association between them and actual aggressive or violent behavior (Kiss, Mihura, & Meyer, 2013; Mihura et al., 2013; Viglione, 1999). In related work, Wood et al. (2010) found support for Aggressive Potential, a low base-rate variable (Gacono & Meloy, 1994; Meloy & Gacono, 1992) that is not included in either R-PAS or the CS. It coded for impending or future aggression (e.g., "a bear about to pounce on some fish"). On the other hand, no support was found for AGM as a correlate of psychopathy. In fact, this meta-analysis also found support for the opposite: COP scores of zero were associated with psychopathy. Nevertheless, the effect sizes would not justify using aggressive Rorschach responses alone as suggesting dangerousness potential without other strong indicators.

Research supports the view that respondents can control the expression of aggressive, sexual, and other crude or alternatively overtly pleasing content on the Rorschach (Exner, 2003; Gacono & Meloy, 1994; Meloy, 1992; Viglione, 1999). This ability to screen out the more blatant, socially undesirable contents and references limits the negative predictive power and specificity of these scores. For example, a recent retest study (Benjestorf, Viglione, Lamb, & Giromini, 2013) demonstrated that violent offenders and nonoffenders, when asked to present themselves as posing no threat of dangerousness in a court role-playing context, suppress about half of the aggressive content largely in the form of the frequent AGC. Also, a semantic, textual analysis found that individuals in the suppressive condition tended to add positive and pleasant elaborations while suppressing negative, problematic, threatening, and anatomical content.

The Benjestorf et al. (2013) and Viglione (1999) studies demonstrated that offenders produce more restricted and simplistic records. Such simplicity may be due to (1) an attempt to limit disclosure in an adversarial context, and/or (2) unsophisticated coping and processing abilities that lead to coercive or aggressive instrumental misbehaviors *in vivo*. Taken together, then, the evidence suggests that high levels of Rorschach aggressive content within simplistic records in dangerousness evaluations may be a specific but not a very sensitive indicator of the potential for behavioral dyscontrol and aggressive acts.

Idiographic Assessment of Dangerousness

As noted earlier, the second approach to evaluating dangerousness incorporates an idiographic or individualized perspective involving consideration of how the specific examinee might become aggressive or violent. Typically, it is applied to someone who has previously shown aggressive tendencies or committed a violent act. In accordance with the axiom that previous violence predicts future violence, in such situations one might look for the recurrence of psychological conditions that existed at the time of a previous violent act as an indicator of emergent aggression. In this approach, the examiner evaluates the recurrence of evidence of psychological processes or features associated with previous violence to draw conclusions about mechanisms or paths to future violence.

Accordingly, one would speculate about poor judgment and impulsivity, simplicity, limited processing ability, rigid black and white thinking, and immaturity among the engagement and cognitive processing variables predictive of violence risk. Such a limitation may be expressed as low Complexity (not in CS), the number of responses (R), Form Percentage (F%, Lambda in CS), multiple determinant responses (Blends), synthesized responses (Sy, DQ+ and Dv/+ in CS), human movement (M), total of human movement and weighted sum of color (MC, EA in CS), and difference between MC and potentially problematic determinants (MC–PPD, D-score in CS); as well as more color-dominant versus form-dominant color responses (i.e., CF + C greater than SumC, FC less than CF + C in CS).

To evaluate the current violent risk of an individual whose violence is defined by psychotic episodes, one would examine the perception and thinking problems domain for psychotic, thought disorder, or judgment disturbance indicators, expressed as high scores on the Ego Impairment Index (EII-3, not in CS); Thought and Perception–Composite (TP-Comp, Perception and Thought Index, CS); Weighted Sum of Cognitive Codes

(WSumCog, WSum6 in CS); Severe Cognitive Codes (SevCog, Lvl 2 in CS); proportion of distorted responses (FQ%, X-% in CS); proportion of distorted whole and common detail responses (WD%, WDA% in CS); and low scores in FQo% and P. Moreover, with such cases one can search the response imagery for references to delusions or preoccupations associated with previous violent psychotic episodes (Link et al., 1992; Monahan et al., 2001). Assume in a hypothetical case that statements regarding delusions about "black sprits hiding in the dark" culminated in a murder. If fearful allusions or references to darkness and obscured images appear in a subsequent Rorschach, one may conclude that these dangerous cognitions are again active, thus indicating tangible risk of violence.

Distress and despair, or "emotional collapse," may provoke aggressive acts for some individuals. Thus, in those with such a history, elevated stress and distress variables (inanimate movement [m], diffuse shading [Y], morbid content [MOR], shading and achromatic color [YTVC', sh in CS], and crude and problematic contents [CritCont%, not in CS]) might stimulate aggression. Alternatively, an extreme elevation on the Suicide Concern Scale [SC-Comp, Suicide Constellation in CS], might suggest danger to the self.

Pathways to violence may also be associated with interpersonal relations and self-concept in the form of extreme dependency; conflicted, disturbed, or paranoid interpersonal relatedness; callous or narcissistic inclinations; skillful exploitation of others; or, conversely, misunderstanding of self and other (Gacono, Gacono, Meloy, & Baity, 2008; Meloy & Gacono, 1992). To some degree all of these are accessible among Rorschach self and other representation variables (Space Reversal, [SR, not in CS], Good to Poor Human Representations [PHR/GPHR, HRV in CS], distorted human movement responses [M-], Vigilance Composite [V-Comp, Hypervigilance Index in CS] whole realistic human content [H], and cooperative movement [COP]), as well as the aggression variables discussed earlier, particularly MAP and Mutuality of Autonomy Health (MAH, not in CS) interpreted in terms of relational themes (Bombel, Mihura, & Meyer, 2009; Graceffo, Mihura, & Meyer, in press). In addition, self-concept and interpersonal imagery is expressed qualitatively in the verbatim test record and interaction with the examiner. Relevant to interpersonal problems and violence is research support (Wood et al., 2010) for elevations with elevated Personal Knowledge Justification responses (PER) and low Texture responses, as well as for reflections (r, Mihura et al., 2013), and narcissistic content in the form of idealization and devaluation (Hilsenroth, Fowler, Padawer, & Handler, 1997).

Conclusion

Prediction of future behavior will always be a difficult task that will be compounded by high-risk situations and the pressure to get the prediction "right" the first time. Additionally, over the past 20 years of research, several different research groups have presented a wide range of constructs, which, when combined in various combinations, increase a person's risk for future violence and aggressiveness (Gacono & Evans, 2008; Hare, 2003; Harris & Lurigio, 2007; Harris et al., 2003; Monahan et al., 2001). Though this process is difficult, evaluators should not shy away from or feel overwhelmed by it.

Through the context of a thorough multimodal psychological assessment, many risk factors that contribute to future risk of dangerousness can be assessed. This is not to say that the evaluator should simply assess all available risk factors and sum the total to create a total risk quotient. Not all risk factors are created equal, with some implying more future risk for dangerousness than others (Monahan et al., 2001). Additionally, several risk constructs have shared variance with one another, and so assessment of each of them would be repetitive and potentially confusing if one measure suggested danger while several others measuring the same construct did not.

The completed multimodal psychological risk assessment should contain information from multiple sources and multiple modalities (Meehl, 1954). Completion of a clinical interview offers information regarding the evaluee's approach to the assessment, glibness, overall engagement, and other interpersonal information related to the interaction with the examiner. Additionally, an interview can be helpful to score specific instruments such as the PCL-R (Hare, 2003). This information can then be combined with scores from actuarials and other risk-focused measures to form a structured professional judgment. While initially designed to assess broader range personality constructs, various self-report (e.g., MMPI-2, PAI) and performance-based personality instruments (e.g., the Rorschach) can offer an additional wealth of information when assessing someone's risk. Not only does this effort include the evaluation of specific aggression-created scale scores (e.g., O-H on the MMPI-2, VPI on the PAI, AGC on the Rorschach), but also personality and psychopathology constructs that can contribute to future violence as well (e.g., AAS/APS on the MMPI-2, TPI on the Rorschach). Consistent with other assessment practice, one should take into consideration contradicting information. The importance of protective factors cannot be understated and is an essential part of risk assessment. By taking this approach, the evaluator will be able to address the referral questions around risk with the best known information.

REFERENCES

Andrews, D. A., & Bonta, J. (1995). *Level of Service Inventory—Revised*. Toronto, ON: Multi-Health Systems.

Atkinson, L., Quarrington, B., Alp, I. E., & Cyr, J. J. (1986). Rorschach validity: An empirical approach to the literature. *Journal of Clinical Psychology, 42*, 360–362.

Babchishin, K. M., Hanson, R. K., & Helmus, L. (2011). *The RRASOR, Static-99R and Static-2002R all add incrementally to the prediction of recidivism among sex offenders* (Corrections Research User Report 2011-01). Ottawa, ON, Canada: Public Safety.

Benjestorf, V., Viglione, D. J., Lamb, J. D., & Giromini, L. (2013). Suppression of aggressive Rorschach responses among violent offenders and non-offenders. *Journal of Interpersonal Violence, 28*(15), 2891–3003.

Blais, M. A., Hilsenroth, M. J., Castlebury, F., Fowler, J. C., & Baity, M. R. (2001). Predicting *DSM-IV* Cluster B personality disorder criteria from MMPI-2 and Rorschach data: A test of incremental validity. *Journal of Personality Assessment, 76,* 150–168.

Boccaccini, M. T., Murrie, D. C., Hawes, S. W., Simpler, A., & Johnson, J. (2010). Predicting recidivism with the Personality Assessment Inventory in a sample of sex offenders screened for civil commitment as sexually violent predators. *Psychological Assessment, 22*(1), 142–148.

Bombel, G., Mihura, J. L., & Meyer, G. J. (2009). An examination of the construct validity of the Rorschach Mutuality of Autonomy (MOA) Scale. *Journal of Personality Assessment, 91,* 227–237.

Bonta, J., Harman, W. G., Hann, R. G., & Cormier, R. B. (1996). The prediction of recidivism among federally sentenced offenders: A re-validation of the SIR scale. *Canadian Journal of Criminology, 38,* 61–79.

Bornstein, R. F. (1996). Construct validity of the Rorschach Oral Dependency scale: 1967–1995. *Psychological Assessment, 8,* 200–205.

Bornstein, R. F. (1999). Criterion validity of objective and projective dependency tests: A meta-analytic assessment of behavioral prediction. *Psychological Assessment, 11,* 48–57.

Borum, R. (1996). Improving the clinical practice of violence risk assessment: Technology, guidelines, and training. *American Psychologist, 51,* 945–956.

Breshears, R. E., Brenner, L. A., Harwood, J. E. F., & Gutierrez, P. (2010). Predicting suicidal behavior in veterans with traumatic brain injury: The utility of the Personality Assessment Inventory. *Journal of Personality Assessment, 92,* 349–355.

Buchanan, A. (2008). Risk of violence by psychiatric patients: Beyond the "actuarial versus clinical" assessment debate. *Psychiatric Services, 59*(2), 184–190.

Butcher, J. N., Dahlstrom, W. G., Graham, J. R., Tellegen, A., & Kaemmer, B. (1989). *MMPI-2: Minnesota Multiphasic Personality Inventory-2: Manual for administration and scoring.* Minneapolis: University of Minnesota Press.

Conroy, M. A., & Murrie, D. C. (2007). *Forensic assessment of violence risk: A guide for risk assessment and risk management.* Hoboken, NJ: Wiley.

Copas, J., & Marshall, P. (1998). The Offender Group Reconviction Scale: The statistical reconviction score for use by probation officers. *Journal of the Royal Statistical Society, 47C,* 159–171.

Cote, G., Crocker, A., Nicholls, T., & Seto, M. (2012). Risk assessment instruments in clinical practice. *Canadian Journal of Psychiatry, 57*(4), 238–244.

Crawford, E. F., Calhoun, P. S., Braxton, L. E., & Beckham, J. C. (2007). Validity of the Personality Assessment Inventory Aggression Scales and Violence Potential Index in veterans with PTSD. *Journal of Personality Assessment, 88* (1), 90–98.

Desmarais, N., Nicholls, T. L., Wilson, C. M., & Brink, J. (2012). Using dynamic risk and protective factors to predict inpatient aggression: Reliability and validity of START assessments. *Psychological Assessment, 24*(3), 685–700.

de Vogel, V., & de Ruiter, C. (2004). Differences between clinicians and researchers in assessing risk of violence in forensic psychiatric patients. *Journal of Forensic Psychiatry and Psychology, Crime and Law, 8*, 93–111.

Diener, M. J., Hilsenroth, M. J., Shaffer, S. A., & Sexton, J. A. (2011). A meta-analysis of the relationship between the Rorschach Ego Impairment Index (EII) and psychiatric severity. *Clinical Psychology and Psychotherapy, 18*, 464–485.

Douglas, K. S., Hart, S. D., & Kropp, P. R. (2001). Validity of the Personality Assessment Inventory for forensic assessments. *International Journal of Offender Therapy and Comparative Criminology, 45*(2), 183–197.

Douglas, K. S., Ogloff, J. R., & Hart, S. D. (2003). Evaluation of a model of violence risk assessment among forensic psychiatric patients. *Psychiatric Services, 54*(10), 1372–1379.

Douglas, K. S., & Reeves, K. (2010). The HCR-20 violence risk assessment scheme: Overview and review of the research. In R. K. Otto & K. S. Douglas (Eds.), *Handbook of violence risk assessment* (pp.147–185). New York: Routledge/Taylor and Francis Group.

Edens, J. F., Hart, S. D., Johnson, D. W., Johnson, J., & Oliver, M. E. (2000). Use of the PAI to assess psychopathy in offender populations. *Psychological Assessment, 12*, 132–139.

Elizur, A. (1949). Content analysis of the Rorschach with regard to anxiety and hostility. *Rorschach Research Exchange and Journal of Projective Techniques, 13*, 247–287.

Erard, R. E. (2012). Expert testimony using the Rorschach Performance Assessment System in psychological injury cases. *Psychological Injury and Law, 5*, 122–134.

Exner, J. E. (2003). *The Rorschach: A comprehensive system*: Vol. 1: Basic foundations (4th ed.). Hoboken, NJ: Wiley.

Exner, J. E., Colligan, S. C., Hillman, L. B., Metts, A. S., Ritzler, B., Rogers, K. T., et al. (2001). *A Rorschach workbook for the Comprehensive System* (5th ed.). Asheville, NC: Rorschach Workshops.

Gacono, C. B., & Evans, F. B. (2008), *Handbook of forensic Rorschach psychology*. Mahwah, NJ: Erlbaum.

Gacono, C. B., Gacono, L. A., Meloy, J. R., & Baity, M. (2008) Appendix A: The Rorschach assessment of aggression: The Rorschach extended aggression scores. In C. B. Gacono & F. B. Evans (Eds.), *Handbook of forensic Rorschach psychology*. Mahwah, NJ: Erlbaum.

Gacono, C. B., & Meloy, J. R. (1994). *The Rorschach assessment of aggressive and psychopathic personalities*. Hillsdale, NJ: Erlbaum.

Garcia-Mansilla, M., Rosenfeld, B., & Cruise, K. R. (2011). Violence risk assessment and women: Predictive accuracy of the HCR-20 in a civil psychiatric sample. *Behavioral Sciences and the Law, 29*, 623–633.

Graceffo, R. A., Mihura, J. L., & Meyer, G. J. (in press). A meta-analysis of an implicit measure of personality functioning: The Mutuality of Autonomy Scale. *Journal of Personality Assessment*.

Graham, J. R. (2006). *MMPI-2: Assessing personality and psychopathology* (4th ed.). New York: Oxford University Press.

Gretton, H. M., Hare, R. D., & Catchpole, R. E. H. (2004). Psychopathy and offending from adolescence to adulthood: A 10-year follow-up. *Journal of Consulting and Clinical Psychology, 72*(4), 636–645.

Grob, G. (1995). *The mad among us: A history of the care of America's mentally ill*. Cambridge, MA: Harvard University Press.

Guy, L., Packer, I. K., & Warnken, W. (2012). Assessing risk of violence using structured professional judgment guidelines. *Journal of Forensic Psychology Practice. 12*, 270–283.

Guy, L. S., Poythress, N. G., Douglas, K. S., Skeem, J. L., & Edens, J. F. (2008). Correspondence between self-report and interview-based assessments of antisocial personality disorder. *Psychological Assessment, 20*, 47–54.

Hanson, R. K., & Morton-Bourgon, K. E. (2009). The accuracy of recidivism risk assessments for sexual offenders: A meta-analysis of 118 prediction studies. *Psychological Assessment, 21*, 1–21.

Hanson, R. K., Phenix, A., & Helmus, L. (2009, October). *Static-99(R) and Static-2002(R): How to interpret and report in light of recent research.* Preconference workshop at the 28th Annual Research and Treatment Conference of ATSA, Dallas, TX.

Hare, R. D. (2003). *Manual for the Revised Psychopathy Checklist* (2nd ed.). Toronto, ON: Multi-Health Systems.

Harris, A., & Lurigio, A. J. (2007). Mental illness and violence: A brief review of research and assessment strategies. *Aggression and Violent Behavior, 12*, 542–551.

Harris, A., Phenix, A., Hanson, R. K., & Thornton, D. (2003). *Static-99 coding rules: Revised—2003.* Ottawa, ON: Corrections Directorate.

Harris, G. T., Rice, M. E., & Quinsey, V. L. (1993). Violent recidivism of mentally disordered offenders: The development of a statistical prediction instrument. *Criminal Justice and Behavior, 20*, 315–335.

Hart, S., Cox, D., & Hare, R. (1995). *The Hare Psychopathy Checklist: Screening version* (PCL:SV). Toronto, ON: Multi-Health Systems.

Hastings, M. E., Krishman, S., Tangney, J. P., & Stuewig, J. (2011). Predictive and incremental validity of the Violence Risk Appraisal Guide scores with male and female jail inmates. *Psychological Assessment, 23*(1), 174–183.

Helmus, L., Thornton, D., Hanson, R. K., & Babchishin, K. M. (2012). Improving the predictive accuracy of Static-99 and Static-2002 with older sex offenders: Revised age weights. *Sexual Abuse: A Journal of Research and Treatment, 24*(1), 64–101.

Hiller, J. B., Rosenthal, R., Bornstein, R. F., & Berry, D. T. (1999). A comparative meta-analysis of Rorschach and MMPI Validity. *Psychological Assessment, 11*, 278–296.

Hilsenroth, M. J., Fowler, J. C., Padawer, J. R., & Handler, L. (1997). Narcissism in the Rorschach revisited: Some reflections on empirical data. *Assessment, 9*, 113–121.

Holt, R. R. (1977). A method for assessing primary process manifestations and their control in Rorschach responses. In M. A. Rickers-Ovsinkina (Ed.), *Rorschach psychology* (pp. 375–420). Huntington, NY: Krieger.

Hopwood, C. J., Baker, K. L., & Morey, L. C. (2008). Extra test validity of selected personality assessment inventory scales and indicators in an inpatient substance abuse setting. *Journal of Personality Assessment, 90*, 574–577.

Kiss, A., Mihura, J., & Meyer, G. J. (2013, March). *An expanded meta-analytic review of the AGC Score and its relationship to real life violence.* Paper presented at the annual meeting of the Society for Personality Assessment, San Diego, CA.

Link, B., Andrews, H., & Cullen, F. (1992). The violent and illegal behavior of mental patients reconsidered. *American Sociological Review* (57), 275–292.

Meehl, P. E. (1954). *Clinical versus statistical prediction: A theoretical analysis and a review of the evidence.* Minneapolis: University of Minnesota Press.

Megargee, E. I., Mercer, S. J., & Carbonell, J. L. (1999). MMPI-2 with male and female state and federal prison inmates. *Psychological Assessment, 11*, 177–185.

Meloy, J. R. (1992). *Violent attachments.* Northvale, NJ: Jason Aronson.

Meloy, J. R., Hansen, T. L., & Weiner, I. B. (1997). Authority of the Rorschach: Legal citations during the past 50 years. *Journal of Personality Assessment, 69*, 53–62.

Meloy, J., & Gacono, C. B. (1992). The aggression response and the Rorschach. *Journal of Clinical Psychology, 48*(1), 104–114.

Meyer, G. J. (2000). On the science of Rorschach research. *Journal of Personality Assessment, 75,* 46–81.

Meyer, G. J. (2004). The reliability and validity of the Rorschach and TAT compared to other psychological and medical procedures: An analysis of systematically gathered evidence. In M. Hilsenroth & D. Segal (Eds.), Personality assessment. Volume 2 in M. Hersen (Ed.-in-Chief), *Comprehensive handbook of psychological assessment* (pp. 315–342). Hoboken, NJ: Wiley.

Meyer, G. J., & Archer, R. P. (2001). The hard science of Rorschach research: What do we know and where do we go? *Psychological Assessment, 13,* 486–502.

Meyer, G. J., Erdberg, P., & Shaffer, T. W. (2007). Toward international normative reference data for the Comprehensive System. *Journal of Personality Assessment, 89*(S1), 201–216.

Meyer, G. J., Finn, S. E., Eyde, L. D., Kay, G. G., Moreland, K. L., Dies, R. R., et al. (2001). Psychological testing and psychological assessment: A review of evidence and issues. *American Psychologist, 56*(2), 128–165.

Meyer, G. J., & Kurtz, J. E. (2006). Guidelines Editorial—Advancing personality assessment terminology: Time to retire "objective" and "projective" as personality test descriptors. *Journal of Personality Assessment, 87,* 1–4.

Meyer, G. J., & Viglione, D. J. (2008). An introduction to Rorschach assessment. In R. P. Archer & S. R. Smith (Eds.), *Personality assessment* (pp. 281–336). New York: Routledge.

Meyer, G. J., Viglione, D. J., Mihura, J. L., Erard, R. E., & Erdberg, P. (2011). *Rorschach Performance Assessment System: Administration, coding, interpretation, and technical manual.* Toledo, OH: Rorschach Performance Assessment System.

Mihura, J. L., Meyer, G. J., Dumitrascu, N., & Bombel, G. (2013). The validity of individual Rorschach variables: Systematic reviews and meta-analyses of the comprehensive system. *Psychological Bulletin, 139, 548–605.*

Mills, J. F., Kroner, D. G., & Hemmati, T. (2007). The validity of violence risk estimates: An issue of item performance. *Psychological Services, 4*(1), 1–12.

Monahan, J. (1993). Mental disorder and violence: Another look. In S. Hodgins (Ed.), *Mental disorder and crime* (pp. 287–302). Newbury Park, CA: Sage.

Monahan, J., Steadman, H., Silver, E., Appebaum, A., Robbins, P., Mulvey, E. P., et al. (2001). *Rethinking risk assessment: The MacArthur study of mental disorder and violence.* New York: Oxford University Press.

Morey, L. C. (2007). *The Personality Assessment Inventory professional manual.* Lutz, FL: Psychological Assessment Resources.

Mossman, D. (2009). The imperfection of protection through detection and intervention. Lessons from three decades of research on the psychiatric assessment of violence risk. *Journal of Legal Medicine, 30*(1), 109–140.

Nieberding, R. J., Moore, J. T., & Dematatis, A. P. (2002). Psychological assessment of forensic psychiatric outpatients. *International Journal of Offender Therapy and Comparative Criminology, 46,* 350–363.

Papapietro, D. J. (2012). The value of the clinical interview. *Journal of the American Academy of Psychiatry and the Law, 40,* 215–220.

Parker, K. C. H., Hanson, R. K., & Hunsley, J. (1988). MMPI, Rorschach and WAIS: A meta analytic comparison of reliability, stability and validity. *Psychological Bulletin, 103,* 367–373.

Pope, K. S., Butcher, J. N., & Seelen, J. (2006). *The MMPI, MMPI-2, and the MMPI-A in Court* (3rd ed.). Washington, DC: American Psychological Association.

Quinsey, V. L., Harris, G. T., Rice, M. E., & Cormier, C. A. (2006). Violence risk appraisal guide. In V. L. Quinsey, G. T. Harris, M. E. Rice, & C. A. Cormier (Eds.), *Violent offenders: Appraising and managing risk* (2nd ed.). Washington, DC: American Psychological Association.

Rogers, R. (2000). The uncritical acceptance of risk assessment in forensic practice. *Law and Human Behavior, 24,* 595–605.

Rufino, K., Boccaccini, M., & Guy, L. (2011). Scoring subjectivity and item performance on measures used to assess violence risk: The PCL-R and HCR-20 as exemplars. *Assessment, 18* (4), 453–463.

Shaffer, T. W., Erdberg, P., & Haroian, J. (2007). Rorschach Comprehensive System data for a sample of 283 adult nonpatients from the United States. *Journal of Personality Assessment, 89*(S1), S159–S165.

Shah, A. K. (1993). An increase in violence among psychiatric inpatients: Real or apparent? *Medicine, Science and the Law, 33*(3), 227–230.

Sinclair, S. J., Bello, I., Nyer, M., Slaven-Mulford, J., Stein, M. B., Renna, M., et al. (2012). The Suicide (SPI) and Violence Potential Indices (VPI) from the Personality Assessment Inventory: A preliminary exploration of validity in an outpatient psychiatric sample. *Journal of Psychopathology and Behavioral Assessment, 34,* 423–431.

Skopp, N. A., Edens, J. F., & Ruiz, M. A. (2007). Risk factors for institutional misconduct among incarcerated women: An examination of the criterion-related validity of the Personality Assessment Inventory. *Journal of Personality Assessment, 88*(1), 106–117.

Steadman, H. J., Silver, E., Monahan, J., Appelbaum, P. S., Clark Robbins, P., Mulvey, E. P., et al. (2000). A classification tree approach to the development of actuarial violence risk assessment tools. *Law and Human Behavior, 24*(1), 83–100.

Swanson, J., Holzer, C., Ganju, V., & Jono, R. (1990). Violence and psychiatric disorder in the community: Evidence from the Epidemiologic Catchment Area surveys. *Hospital and Community Psychiatry, 41,* 761–770.

Swanson, J. W., Swartz, M. S., Van Dorn, R. A., Elbogen, E. B., Wagner, H. R., Rosenheck, R. A., et al. (2006). A national study of violent behavior in persons with schizophrenia. *Archives of General Psychiatry, 63,* 490–499.

Tengström, A. (2001). Long-term predictive validity of historical factors in two risk assessment instruments in a group of violent offenders with schizophrenia. *Nordic Journal of Psychiatry, 55,* 243–249.

Tong, D. (2007). The penile plethysmograph, Abel Assessment for Sexual Interest, and MSI-II: Are they speaking the same language? *American Journal of Family Therapy, 35,* 187–202.

Torrey, E. F., Stanley, J., Monahan, J., & Steadman, H. J. (2008). The MacArthur Violence Risk Assessment Study revisited: Two views ten years after its initial publication. *Psychiatric Services, 59,* 147–152.

Urist, J. (1977). The Rorschach test and the assessment of object relations. *Journal of Personality Assessment, 41,* 3–9.

Viglione, D. J. (1999). A review of recent research addressing the utility of the Rorschach. *Psychological Assessment, 11,* 251–265.

Viglione, D. J., & Hilsenroth, M. J. (2001). The Rorschach: Facts, fictions, and future. *Psychological Assessment, 13,* 452–471.

Viglione, D. J. & Meyer G. J (2008). An overview of Rorschach psychometrics for forensic practice. In C. B. Gacono & F. B. Evans with N. Kaser-Boyd (Eds.), *Handbook of forensic Rorschach psychology* (pp. 22–54). Mahwah, NJ: Erlbaum.

Viglione, D. J., & Rivera, B. (2012). Performance assessment of personality and psychopathology. In I. B. Weiner (Ed.-in-Chief), J. R. Graham, & J. A. Naglieri (Vol. Eds.), *Comprehensive handbook of psychology: Assessment psychology* (2nd ed., Vol. 10, pp. 600–621). Hoboken, NJ: Wiley.

Vitacco, M. J., Erickson, S. K., Kurus, S., & Apple, B. N. (2012). The role of the Violence Risk Appraisal Guide and Historical, Clinical, Risk-20 in the U.S. courts: A case law survey. *Psychology, Public Policy and Law, 18*, 361–391.

Walters, G. D. (2006). Coping with malingering and exaggeration of psychiatric symptomatology in offender populations. *American Journal of Forensic Psychology, 24*(4), 21–40.

Webster, C. D., Douglas, K. S., Eaves, D., & Hart, S. D. (1997). *HCR-20: Assessing the risk for violence (Version 2)*. Vancouver: Mental Health, Law, and Policy Institute, Simon Fraser University.

Webster, C. D., Martin, M. L., Brink, J., Nicholls, T. L., & Desmarais, S. L. (2009). *Manual for the Short-Term Assessment of Risk and Treatability (START)* (Version 1.1). Port Coquitlam, Canada: British Columbia Mental Health & Addiction Services.

Webster, C. D., Martin, M. L., Brink, J., Nicholls, T. L., & Middleton, C. (2004). *Manual for the Short-Term Assessment of Risk and Treatability (START)* (Version 1.0 Consultation Edition). Port Coquitlam, Canada: Forensic Psychiatric Services Commission and St. Joseph's Healthcare.

Weiner, I. B. (1999). What the Rorschach can do for you: Incremental validity in clinical applications. *Assessment, 6*, 327–339.

Weiner, I. B. (2001). Advancing the science of psychological assessment: The Rorschach Inkblot Method as exemplar. *Psychological Assessment, 13*, 327–339.

Weiner, I. B., Exner, J. E., & Sciara, A. (1996). Is the Rorschach welcome in the courtroom? *Journal of Personality Assessment, 67*, 422–424.

Weiner, I., & Greene, R. (2008). *Handbook of personality assessment*. Hoboken, NJ: Wiley.

Wong, S., & Gordon, A. (2001). The Violence Risk Scale. *Bulletin of the International Society for Research on Aggression, 23*, 16–20.

Wong, S. C. P., & Gordon, A. (2006). The validity and reliability of the Violence Risk Scale: A treatment friendly violence risk assessment tool. *Psychology, Public Policy and Law, 12*, 279–309.

Wood, J. M., Lilienfeld, S. O., Nezworski, M. T., Garb, H. N., Allen, K. H., & Wildermuth, J. L. (2010). Validity of Rorschach Inkblot scores for discriminating psychopaths from nonpsychopaths in forensic populations: A meta-analysis. *Psychological Assessment, 22*, 336–349.

Wood, J. M., Nezworski, M. T., Garb, H. N., & Lilienfeld, S. O. (2001). The misperception of psychopathology: Problems with norms of the Comprehensive System for the Rorschach. *Clinical Psychology: Science and Practice, 8*(3), 350–373.

Yang, M., Wong, S. C. P., & Coid, J. (2010). The efficacy of violence prediction: A meta-analytic comparison of nine risk assessment tools. *Psychological Bulletin, 136*(5), 740–767.

Yang, S., & Mulvey, E. P. (2012). Violence risk: Re-defining variables from the first-person perspective. *Aggression and Violent Behavior, 17*(3), 198–207.

CHAPTER 14

Integration and Therapeutic Presentation of Multimethod Assessment Results

An Empirically Supported Framework and Case Example

Justin D. Smith and Stephen E. Finn

Psychological assessment instruments are a means of getting into our client's shoes (Finn, 2007). Each assessment method and each instrument provides a unique lens through which to see and understand different aspects of clients' experiences. Because every assessment tool has its own strengths and weaknesses, multimethod assessment provides a more complete picture of the client. This in turn helps when we discuss the findings of the assessment with the client and with significant people in the client's life. Existing research suggests that clinicians using a single assessment method are likely to develop an incomplete or biased understanding of the client (e.g., Meyer, Riethmiller, Brooks, Benoit, & Handler, 2000). During the feedback process, such limited understanding can lead clients to feel misunderstood, disrespected, and not listened to by the assessor, which decreases the chances that the assessment will produce a therapeutic benefit (Finn & Tonsager, 1997).

In this chapter we present an empirically supported framework for providing feedback to clients from a multimethod assessment. We believe that this method leads to clients' feeling understood and that this in turn maximizes the potential that the assessment will lead to real and important changes in clients' lives. The conceptual foundations of our model are self-verification theory (Swann, Chang-Schneider, & McClarty, 2007) and our understanding of the contributions of different methods of assessment, including the neurobiological, interpersonal, and motivational factors involved during their administration. Our conceptualization and techniques are illustrated in the Therapeutic Assessment (TA; Finn, 2007) of an adult woman in psychotherapy for obsessive–compulsive disorder (OCD) and a severe eating disorder who was still mourning the traumatic loss of her mother from when she was a teenager.

Rationale for Multimethod Assessment

Let us first define what we mean by a multimethod assessment. Among personality assessors, the term multimethod assessment is often used for assessments that include a broadband self-report personality inventory, such as the Minnesota Multiphasic Personality Inventory (MMPI; Butcher, Dahlstrom, Grahm, Tellegen, & Kaemmer, 1989) or the Personality Assessment Inventory (PAI; Morey, 1991), *and* a performance-based instrument, such as the Rorschach (Rorschach, 1921/1942). Other psychologists use the term multimethod assessment more broadly, to include assessments based on formal assessment instruments and a clinical interview, or a clinical interview and direct observation of the client. We believe a clinical interview is a necessary but not sufficient element of a comprehensive multimethod assessment, and later in this chapter we will discuss the usefulness of observational assessment techniques, especially in assessments involving multiple participants (i.e., couples and families). As we will discuss, we believe the term multimethod assessment is most applicable when similar constructs (e.g., depression, self-esteem) are formally measured with different methods that have distinct sources of error (e.g., self-report and observational rating, or self-report and performance-based test).

One challenge of multimethod assessment is a skillful integration of the findings from different methods. Beutler and Berren (1995), Finn (1996), Meyer (1997), and others have focused on different aspects of this issue. Integration is particularly challenging when different modalities produce discrepant findings, and research indicates that this is frequently the case. More than a half a century ago, Campbell and Fiske (1959) presented an empirical approach to understanding the common occurrence of multiple methods resulting in relative independence: the multimethod–multitrait matrix, which assesses convergent and discriminant validity. In research circles, the discordance between different types of tests has commonly been referred to as method bias. Meyer et al. (2001) provided a clear and useful discussion of this issue as it applies to clinical assessment. They highlighted the potential biases of monomethod assessments, argued that the construct validity of nomothetic assessment is enhanced by assessors' using multiple methods and operational definitions (see Cook & Campbell, 1979), and emphasized how the complexity of the constructs psychologists commonly assess in clinical practice contributes to low cross-method correlations. Further, Meyer and colleagues (2001) empirically demonstrated that different methods of assessment provide unique and distinctive data that are not available from other sources.

One of the formative works in this area comes from McClelland, Koestner, and Weinberger's (1989) review of the association between behavior and self-attributed and implicit motives, derived by self-report and stories written to pictures, respectively. They concluded that the paucity of significant correlations was due to differences in the motives of the subjects inherent to the two different methods. That is, self-report is likely based on more cognitively elaborated constructs, whereas implicit measures tap into a more primitive, affectively driven system. In keeping with this conclusion, Meyer and Kurtz (2006) argued that the common taxonomy of personality tests as being "objective" or "projective" was outdated and misleading. Accordingly, they proposed new terms they felt more accurately depict the nature of the assessment stimulus and the way in which the assessor interprets the results. The term *performance-based* assessment is increasingly being used in the field of personality assessment to replace the former *projective* label. "Objective" tests are now given more descriptive labels, such as self- or parent report. Complementary classification systems have also been offered. For example, Bornstein's (2002) process-based framework relies on the attribution processes involved in responding. Self-report measures involve a self-attribution process in which the subject consciously assesses the extent to which an adjective, statement of behavior, or other descriptive stimulus applies to them. Assessment methods requiring the subject to respond to the attributed nature of an external stimulus (e.g., inkblot, picture) are labeled as stimulus–attribution tests, with the assumption that subjects draw from nonconscious cognitive systems in the production of verbal responses. Schultheiss (2007) proposed classifying tests according to a widely used model of human memory systems, drawing a distinction between declarative (consciously accessible memory systems) and nondeclarative methods (i.e., nonconscious memory systems whose operation is reflected in the subject's performance).

More recently, Finn (2012) drew from research in attachment, infant development, and developmental neurobiology research to conceptualize the ways in which different psychological assessment methods activate specific brain functions and how assessment psychologists can be more effective agents of therapeutic change. As summarized by Finn, the research of Schore (2003, 2009), Siegel (2012), Cicchetti (1994), and others indicates that attachment relationships in infancy influence critical areas of brain development that provide the foundation for important functions, such as emotion regulation, empathy, social relatedness, moral development, and behavioral control. Underdevelopment of these functions during childhood is implicated in the development and maintenance of a host of problems later in life (e.g., Cicchetti & Toth, 1998; Shaw, Gilliom, Ingoldsby, & Nagin, 2003).

Schore has amassed an impressive amount of evidence showing that the right hemisphere of the brain is dominant in the processing of attachment arousal and other affective experiences, especially those involving trauma. The right hemisphere has dense reciprocal connections to the limbic and subcortical areas of the brain, which process affect and subtle interpersonal signals at a subconscious level and are not readily accessible through language (Schore, 2009). Further, Schore (2009), Bromberg (2006), and others have explained how the successful psychological treatment of individuals with early attachment trauma requires that the therapist form a secure auxiliary attachment relationship with the client and nonverbally relate "right hemisphere to right hemisphere," to use Schore's terminology. This nonverbal communication serves to regulate the client's negative affect states, enhance positive affect states, and reorganize the way in which the right hemisphere processes affect (Schore, 2003). A recent meta-analysis by Diener, Hilsenroth, and Weinberger (2007) revealed that the relationship between affect focus, defined as the therapist drawing the client's attention to his or her affect state in the moment, was significantly correlated with treatment outcomes ($r = .30$), highlighting the importance of activating right-brain processes in psychological interventions.

The implications of this research are numerous and will be enumerated in later sections of this chapter. Returning to the issue at hand, we note that neurobiological research suggests that different assessment methods tap into different areas of the brain (Finn, 2012). The verbal and non-emotionally arousing administration of common self-report instruments, such as the MMPI or PAI, appears to activate more left-hemisphere cortical functions, while tests such as the Rorschach and the Adult Attachment Projective Picture System (AAP; George & West, 2012) activate more right-hemisphere and subcortical functioning due to their visual, emotionally arousing stimulus properties and the interpersonal demands of their administration (see also Fowler, Hilsenroth, & Handler, 1996; Meyer, 1997). As a result, performance-based tests activate implicit schemas about self and other, which are reflected in interpersonal patterns between assessee and assessor as well as in specific responses to test stimuli. In some individuals, such as those with a dismissing attachment status, these implicit patterns are quite discrepant from consciously accessible perceptions reported on self-report inventories (e.g., Dozier & Lee, 1995). Thus, performance-based tests can provide a window into right-hemisphere disorganization and subcortical dysregulation in clients with insecure attachment and developmental trauma histories that would not be readily available otherwise.

Functional magnetic resonance imaging (fMRI) and electroencephalography (EEG) studies using Rorschach inkblots as stimuli have consistently revealed subcortical activation when certain percepts related to emotional arousal are reported. Asari et al. (2008) found that individuals with lower form-quality scores had larger amygdalas—a sign of more frequent amygdalic activation—suggesting that emotional activation greatly influences the extent to which one distorts reality. In a study involving the receipt of negative feedback, Jimura, Konishi, Asari, and Miyashita (2009) found greater activation of the posterior medial prefrontal cortex, an area implicated in the processing of negative emotions, for those individuals with higher C′ scores on the Rorschach. Last, human movement responses (M) on the Rorschach have long been considered an index of developmentally advanced cognitive cognition, such as the ability to imagine (movement from a static stimulus) and the capacity for empathy (due to the implied ability to identify a human being in an ambiguous inkblot). Research using EEG found significant mu wave suppression when subjects perceived human movement (i.e., reported a percept with an M determinant) (Giromini, Porcelli, Viglione, Parolin, & Pineda, 2010). These studies not only provide evidence for the validity of long-held interpretations of these Rorschach scores, but also demonstrate the activation of brain areas associated with salient functions for psychological health and well being, as well as assessment and psychotherapy.

The assessment of attachment security offers a prime example of where activation of different neuroanatomical structures may account for disagreement between methods. Attachment security can be assessed through self-report measures, which yield an attachment "style," or performance-based measures (such as the AAP or the Adult Attachment Interview), which result in an attachment "classification" or "status." A meta-analytic review of the empirical overlap of self-reported attachment style and AAI security classifications showed a trivial association ($r = .09$) (Roisman et al., 2007). These results indicate that these two methods assess different aspects of attachment security and that self-reported attachment styles are not analogous to the results obtained from the AAP.

Neurobiology research findings are again useful in understanding the brain processes involved in the assessment of attachment classification. Buchheim and colleagues (2006) administered the AAP in an fMRI environment. In one study of 16 nonpatient adult women, 6 were classified with an organized attachment status (secure, dismissing, or preoccupied) and 5 were unresolved or disorganized, which is particularly associated with past trauma and various forms of psychopathology. (The scans of five women were not analyzed due to excessive head movement; Buchheim et al., 2006.) The fMRI results showed increased limbic system activation, centered mainly in the right amygdala and hippocampus, in the women classified as disorganized compared to those who were organized. These two brain regions are associated with fear and autobiographical memory, respectively. Thus, the AAP might have reactivated "unresolved" traumatic or negative autobiographical memories in the women with disorganized attachment classifications. A second fMRI study found differences in the neural responses to the "alone" versus "dyadic" pictures of the AAP between a group of 11 women diagnosed with borderline personality disorder (BPD) and 17 nonpatient women. The BPD group had significantly more activation in the anterior midcingulate cortex in response to the alone pictures and more activation of the right superior temporal sulcus and less activation of the right parahippocampal gyrus compared to nonpatients. These activation patterns indicated greater activation of brain areas associated with pain and fear in the BPD group. Further, the BPD group had more traumatic markers in their verbal responses to the alone pictures, an indication of attachment trauma (George & West, 2012). Advances in neurobiology and brain-imaging technology are helping assessment psychologists better understand the processes that are activated when they use different assessment procedures.

Discordance between methods is not limited to comparisons between self-report and performance-based tests. The literature comparing assessment methods, most commonly self-report compared to observation by the clinician or some other informant, often results in small to medium correlations (e.g., Achenbach, McConaughy, & Howell, 1987). A potent example of the clinical implications of multimethod assessment comes from a study examining clients' reports of suicidality and suicidal ideation during a clinical interview and responses to the MMPI-2 (Glassmire, Stolberg, Greene, & Bongar, 2001). The results showed discordance rates between these methods ranging from 9.6% to 19.1%. Glassmire and colleagues concluded that the six suicidality items on the MMPI-2 contributed valuable information above that obtained through verbal self-report.

After the administration of a well-constructed multimethod assessment, the assessor is left with a wealth of actuarial data derived from various sources and assessment methods alongside clinical intuition, observation, and historical information about the client to provide context and ecological validity to the nomothetic results. The ethical principles of the American Psychological Association (American Psychological Association, American Educational Research Association, & National Council on Measurement in Education, 1999) clearly dictate that assessors provide clients with feedback of the results of assessment. So then, the issue at hand is how to best present findings for the benefit of the client.

An Empirically Supported Framework

The importance of a model grounded in empirically derived theory and techniques is evident in the growing evidence base for the therapeutic effectiveness of psychological assessment in general and collaborative and therapeutic models of assessment specifically. In a meta-analysis of 17 studies made up of 1,496 adult and adolescent participants comparing psychological assessment to a comparison condition, Poston and Hanson (2010) found a significant overall effect (Cohen's $d = 0.423$) favoring the therapeutic effectiveness of psychological assessment. They concluded that personalized, collaborative feedback, highly involving the presentation of test findings, results in clinically meaningful effects. Studies included in this meta-analysis employing the empirically supported framework described in this chapter (e.g., Finn & Tonsager, 1992; Newman & Greenway, 1997) resulted in the largest group differences, particularly in reducing distress and increasing self-esteem.

The guiding framework for assessment feedback described in this chapter builds on the work of Finn and colleagues (e.g., Finn, 1996, 2007; Finn & Tonsager, 1992, 1997), which emphasizes clients' motive for self-verification (e.g., Swann et al., 2007). Self-verification theory posits that human beings are inherently motivated to seek confirmation that their views of themselves and their experiences of the world are accurate, or at the very least, shared by others. When people have experiences in which their self-views and preconceptions are challenged or shattered, a very uncomfortable and disorienting feeling can follow, leading the person to experience the world as not real and to feel that he or she is falling apart. Kohut (1977) termed this experience disintegration anxiety. Clients' intrinsic search for self-verification and the related need to defend against disintegration anxiety guides the process of feedback delivery employed a useful heuristic that Finn has termed "levels of information."

Levels of Information

Finn (1996) postulated that test feedback is more powerful and useful for clients when it is ordered according to clients' existing views of themselves. Schroeder, Hahn, Finn, and Swann (1993) found that undergraduates were more positively impacted by receiving feedback about personality traits when they were presented in this manner. As a result, Finn has recommended that, in most cases, information derived from an assessment be presented to clients in increasing "levels." Level 1 (L1) information is congruent with the client's self-view and is generally readily accepted. Level 2 (L2) feedback is mildly discrepant from the client's self-view and often modifies or amplifies clients' usual ways of thinking about themselves. These findings are typically well received when presented as hypotheses for discussion. Clients rarely reject L2 findings because they are unlikely to be a threat to core beliefs or the client's self-esteem. Finn recommended that the majority of the findings in an assessment feedback session should be L2.

Level 3 (L3) findings are those that are highly discrepant from the client's usual way of thinking. This kind of feedback is typically very anxiety provoking for the client and often mobilizes their characteristic coping mechanisms. Assessors need to monitor how overwhelmed the client is becoming as L2 and then L3 information is presented and decide whether to continue presenting a novel way of viewing and understanding the client's situation. The ordering of feedback from L1 to L2 to L3 is one way of titrating clients' emotional arousal by helping them feel understood and supported by the assessor. Finn (2007) recommends discussing assessment findings with clients by taking "half steps," as opposed to jumping directly to the next level. We discuss some of the inherent challenges and potential pitfalls of presenting L3 feedback later in this chapter.

As will be discussed later, although any test can produce L1, L2, or L3 information, there appears to be a correlation between assessment method and the level of results that are produced, with performance-based methods yielding more L2 and L3 information than do self-report tests and self-report tests providing more L1 information. For this reason, Finn (1996) strongly recommended that assessors use a combination of self-report and performance-based tests in most assessments.

Preparing Clients to Accept Feedback

In TA, Finn and his colleagues also paid special attention to how to help clients accept L2 and L3 information. The process of preparing clients for feedback begins in the initial interview and continues throughout the assessment, using various techniques. A complete discussion of this topic is beyond the scope of this chapter, but we wish to mention three techniques that are particularly useful. First, asking clients to pose specific questions about themselves and their situations that they wish to have addressed by the assessment greatly facilitates feedback. Finn (2007) found that getting questions early on enlists clients' curiosity and lowers defensiveness, and that clients' are more willing to accept L2 and L3 information later in an assessment if it is relevant to their questions. Second, engaging clients in discussing their actual test responses, experiences, and test behaviors (generally after standardized administration is completed) can help them grasp information that would be threatening if presented in isolation in a post-testing feedback session (Fischer, 1985/1994; Smith & George, 2012). Finn (2007) calls this technique the "extended inquiry" when it is done spontaneously and without planning, and "an assessment intervention" when it is carefully planned with the goal of highlighting potential L3 findings. (See Finn, 2003, 2011, and Smith, Finn, Swain, & Handler, 2010, for examples.)

Third, a somewhat unique set of procedures is applicable to assessments of couples and families: observation and video feedback. In the child and family TA model, Finn (2007) and Tharinger et al. (2012) invite parents to observe their child's testing from a corner in the room through either a one-way mirror or a video link. This arrangement allows parents to hear and see the results of the assessment themselves, which is less threatening than direct feedback from the assessor. For example, the parents might see their child as being oppositional and noncompliant because he or she is a "bad" child. After witnessing the child seeing "a sad kitty" on Card 1 of the Rorschach and telling stories to picture stimuli with dysphoric themes, they might come to understand the child's problem behaviors as an indicator of underlying depressive affect.

A specific intervention technique in use in a variety of family-based interventions is called video feedback, which involves the parent(s) viewing a videotaped interaction between themselves and their child(ren) alongside the clinician, with the aim of improving parenting skills and the quality of familial relationships. Tharinger et al. (2012) assert that observational techniques help parents "step back" and examine the child and family interactions with new eyes. Smith, Dishion, Moore, Shaw, and Wilson (2013) examined the incremental effects of adding a video feedback component to the feedback session of a family-based collaborative assessment intervention for early childhood problem behaviors. Video feedback given to caregivers when their children were age 2 reduced those caregivers' negative relational schemas (i.e., attributions about the child) at age 3, which in turn led to less caregiver coercive behaviors assessed at age 5. Video feedback involved parents' viewing segments of previously videotaped family interaction tasks that assessors had selected as examples of desired, positive parenting behaviors. Smith et al. (2013) postulated that observational techniques such as video feedback allow parents to disembed from emotionally laden interactions in which their responses are based on overlearned relational patterns that lead to inaccurate beliefs regarding the intent of the child's behaviors. From a neurobiology perspective, we might postulate that such procedures shift information processing from limbic regions to the prefrontal cortex. Smith and colleagues (2013), Tharinger et al. (2009, 2012), and Holigrocki, Crain, Bohr, Young, and Bensman (2009) all found that when assessors support parents in observing their children during an assessment, parents can shift their understanding of their children's problems and the entire family system can change in positive ways.

Integrating Findings of Multimethod Asssessment

As discussed earlier, we believe that multimethod assessment is clinically useful because it helps assessors compensate for the limitations of different assessment methods and integrate their strengths. One instance where this integrative approach has been well articulated concerns the convergence or divergence of findings from self-report and performance-based personality methods. Earlier we reviewed the primary neurobiological, interpersonal, cognitive, and motivational factors of these two assessment methods. Now let us spell out the implications of these factors for understanding different assessment findings and discussing them with our clients. Finn (1996) proposed a model for integrating findings from the MMPI-2 and Rorschach; however, this model is generally applicable to combinations of other self-report and performance-based personality tests. Four primary patterns (see Figure 14.1) can be obtained from considering the level of distress or disturbance on the two tests. Distress and disturbance can be looked at generally or as it regards specific problem areas (e.g., thought disorder, anger

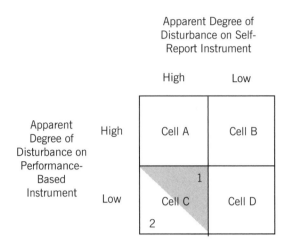

FIGURE 14.1. Configurations of self-report and performance-based assessment findings.

control problems.) The two convergent cells (A and D) represent assessment situations where the results of both tests show either high or low levels of disturbance. These results are relatively easy to interpret and subsequently to discuss with clients. Cell A indicates that clients' problems are clearly evident in their day-to-day functioning, they are aware of these problems, and they are willing and able to report them on a self-report inventory. This is a common pattern among voluntarily referred help-seeking clients. Test results falling in Cell D indicate that clients function well in structured and less structured situations, with and without interpersonal interaction, and are rarely found in clinical settings. In both cases of convergent results, the client is unlikely to be surprised by feedback on the assessment findings.

Two cells, B and C, indicate an apparent disagreement between the two types of tests. Cell B indicates low disturbance on self-report and high disturbance on the performance-based test. This finding suggests that the client has psychopathology that emerges in less structured, interpersonal, emotionally arousing situations. However, the client is believed to function relatively well in structured situations where he or she can enlist intellectual resources to manage emotional arousal. Such clients are often unaware of the full extent of their difficulties and are thus unable to report them directly. Giving feedback to such clients is complex because any discussion of their underlying difficulties may not be self-verifying (i.e., may be L3 information). These clients are also prone to becoming overwhelmed, flooded, confused, or defensive when assessors try to discuss their underlying problems.

Situations where there is high disturbance on self-report instruments and low disturbance on performance-based tests are represented by Cell

C. This is the least common constellation in clinical settings and is more frequently found among clients applying for disability or involved in an assessment for forensic or litigation purposes. Cell C can be further divided to account for the client's level of engagement on the performance-based test. In the case of the Rorschach, for example, the complexity of the protocol is evident in the number of responses (R), the percentage of Pure Form responses, and the amount of color determinants coded. When engagement is adequate on the Rorschach, the distressed and disturbed self-report findings may represent a "cry for help" from the client or the possibility of deliberate malingering—in situations when the assessment context suggests the client may be motivated to present with high psychiatric disturbance. When there is low engagement and complexity in the client's Rorschach responses, the client may have reacted with withdrawal, constriction, or dissociation in response to the highly arousing interpersonal and emotional demands of the performance-based test administration. In such situations it is generally better to believe and affirm the client's distress and disturbance on the self-report test and to hypothesize that others may not always be able to perceive the client's level of distress. The client will feel deeply misunderstood if the assessor mistakenly asserts that symptoms were intentionally overreported on the self-report measure.

Reaching Appropriate Depth Is Necessary for Lasting Change

Lilienfeld, Garb, and Wood (2011) suggested that the therapeutic benefits of assessment feedback evidenced by Poston and Hanson's (2010) meta-analysis could be explained by a phenomenon called the Barnum effect. The Barnum effect refers to a type of subjective validation in which a person finds personal meaning in a statement that likely applies to many people. Such phrases are often called Barnum statements. An example of a Barnum statement would be, "You have a need for people to like and admire you, and yet tend to be critical of yourself." The decade's old assertion that clients' positive reactions to personality test feedback are due to the Barnum effect is not supported by empirical evidence (e.g., Furnham & Schofield, 1987). Recent research on the Barnum effect is scant, likely because it was largely rejected more than a quarter century ago. Studies that have been conducted provide evidence that speaks against the Barnum effect (e.g., Andersen & Nordvik, 2002; Schroeder et al., 1993). The findings of the Schroeder et al. (1993) study indicate that the greatest therapeutic benefits occur when the majority of feedback is L2. Given that L2 feedback is conceptualized as being slightly discrepant from current self-views, which likely raises some anxiety for the client, this finding suggests that therapeutic outcomes of assessment are somewhat contingent upon eliciting moderate emotional arousal during feedback. These results are consistent with the meta-analytic findings of Diener et al. (2007) indicating that better outcomes were related to clients' in-session emotional exposure. In assessment, this occurs when feedback is highly individualized and is presented in accordance with our framework.

Advantages of Multimethod Assessment

In terms of the feedback process specifically, multimethod assessment has some distinct advantages over reliance on a single measure or clinical judgment. One of the challenges of our guiding framework is to determine which levels of information test findings are for each client. Fortunately, the different assessment methods of a multimethod assessment provide a scaffold. The convergence of findings from different methods is a key factor in determining the congruence of a finding with the client's self-view. For example, self-report measures reveal the client's general self-view at the time of testing and their self-representation (how they believe others see them). Thus, the majority of the findings from self-report measures are L1 and L2. Self-report item endorsement can be L2 because of the empirical correlates of response constellations: Although clients endorse certain individual items, they might not fully appreciate their meaning when considered in conjunction with other responses. For example, clients might endorse experiencing fatigue, difficulty sleeping, apathy, and dysphoria on a self-report questionnaire, but they may not have considered that they are depressed. With proper preparation and presentation of the findings, this finding could be easily rejected if the assessor leapt to the conclusion that the finding is L1.

Returning to the model in Figure 14.1, we see that the convergence of test results in Cells A and D suggests that clients are likely to accept the findings of the assessment regardless of the source of the findings (i.e., the instrument). In cases where a discrepancy exists between the findings on multiple methods (Cells B and C), the assessor should begin with an acknowledgment of the self-report findings prior to presenting the results of the performance-based test(s). In the case of Cell B, where there is a suggestion of underlying pathology that the client is unaware of, or at least is reluctant to report, the level of disturbance, the assessor must proceed cautiously and adequately prepare the client. This is illustrated in our case example.

Additionally, the inclusion of performance-based assessment methods affords unique, client-specific material. Finn (1996) suggested presenting assessment findings employing the language, imagery, and metaphors used by the client during clinical interviews and performance-based test responses. For example, we might know from her MMPI-2 that a client is severely depressed, but we may choose to discuss it with her using the language of her first response to Card I of the Rorschach: "The testing suggests that lately you are feeling battered and tired from the 'wars' you have been through, and you're wondering if you're going to be able to keep on going." Using such client-generated languages, images, and metaphors can help clients feel deeply mirrored and understood, and that someone is helping to "hold" or "regulate" difficult emotional sates. This effect can be particularly salient when presenting L3 findings: The client is more likely to accept and integrate L3 findings into their existing self-concepts if they are able to stay interpersonally regulated. The "right-brain to right-brain" communication between the client and assessor serves this function. Metaphor can similarly aid in the client's understanding and acceptance of abstract or complex psychological processes.

Challenges of Multimethod Assessment Feedback

Having made the case for multimethod assessment, it seems important to also acknowledge that it produces a host of challenges for the assessor. This may be one reason why some assessors use only one method, such as an interview or a self-report measure.

Time and Money

First, it must be acknowledged that multimethod assessment, especially when it includes performance-based instruments, takes more time and is therefore more costly than single-method assessment. Luckily, advances such as computer-assisted coding, and a new, leaner system for interpreting the Rorschach—the Rorschach Performance Assessment System (R-PAS; Meyer, Viglione, Mihura, Erard, & Erdberg, 2011)—have increased the efficiency of such methods. Also, the AAP takes much less time than the previous gold-standard measure for determining attachment status, the AAI. Still it is conceivable that in certain settings, where service demands are high and psychologists are in short supply, multimethod assessment will have to be reserved for clients who are particularly difficult or puzzling.

More Skill Is Required in Giving Feedback

Also, because performance-based measures produce more L3 information, it takes a greater level of skill and sensitivity to give feedback to clients about their results. In fact, we believe that assessors who wish to give feedback to clients through multimethod assessment will greatly benefit from training in psychotherapy in addition to training in psychological assessment. And because information from performance-based and implicit methods is more likely to dysregulate clients, assessors need training in techniques that help prepare clients to incorporate L3 information, such as extended inquiries. As mentioned earlier, assessors will need training in how to determine beforehand what is L1, L2, and L3 information and how to present such findings in a feedback session. Last, training in collaborative assessment methods seems crucial. The evidence is now clear that collaborative versus "delivered" (i.e., unilateral) feedback has much more impact on clients (Hanson, Claiborn, & Kerr, 1997). And when assessors help clients tie test findings to events and experiences in their daily lives, test feedback becomes more accessible, memorable, and useful (Fischer, 1985/1994).

Demands on the Assessor

Multimethod assessment is more time consuming than is single-method assessment, and Finn (2007) has asserted that it is more emotionally demanding as well. Assessors find themselves thinking about and feeling more about the clients they assess, and emotionally arousing responses to the EMP, Rorschach, and AAP may be difficult to leave at the office door. Many assessors find it challenging that frequently they cannot tell clients everything they have learned from a multimethod assessment; some L3 information would just be too disruptive for the client at the time of the assessment and needs to be "contained" by the assessor. In such situations, it can be very helpful if one can share such information with a referring professional, if there is one, who can "hold it" until the client is ready to hear it later in psychotherapy. For these reasons, Finn (2007) has suggested that therapeutically oriented multimethod assessment is best practiced in the context of a community of colleagues who share similar goals and training.

Case Example

We illustrate our empirically supported approach to feedback with one of the most common assessment configurations in clinical settings—discordant self-report and performance-based results (Cell B)—and describe how the results of a multimethod assessment clarified the etiology of the client's diagnosis and informed ongoing psychotherapy with the referring psychologist. The first author (JDS) was the assessor in this case, and all first-person pronouns refer to him.

Referral

Karen, a 57-year-old unemployed mother of three young adult daughters, was referred for a psychological assessment in order to help her better understand her diagnosis and clarify the goals and intervention approach of stalled, 2-year-long psychotherapy. Karen was diagnosed with OCD shortly after she began treatment with her current psychologist. Despite what appeared to be an accurate diagnosis, cognitive-behavioral therapy, largely consisting of exposure and cognitive restructuring, had been unable to appreciably reduce Karen's OCD symptoms. Similarly, she was still unable to maintain employment and was forced to rely on disability, alimony, and a dwindling trust fund. In our account, we will focus mainly on the verbal feedback provided to Karen regarding one of her assessment questions: "How did my mother's death affect the development of my OCD?"

Background and Early Memories

Karen was the only child of married parents; her father was a scientist and her mother a high school teacher. Karen's report, and her responses on the Early Memory Procedure (EMP; Bruhn, 1992) painted a picture of her mother as critical and harsh, while her father was detached, analytical, and goal-oriented. Karen recalled that her parents were good functional care-takers but that she never felt emotionally supported. She recalled a number of memories during the EMP consistent with this sentiment. The EMP is a test of early autobiographical memories in which the client is asked to recall the five earliest, specific one-time memories or events and describe these events in as much detail as possible. The EMP can be used as an initial assessment procedure to gather and explore information related to early childhood experiences and family history. One of the most salient memories for Karen was from when she was about 4 years old. The family was eating fish and a small bone became stuck in Karen's throat. She wrote, "My father, the engineer, gets out the needle nosed pliers and a flashlight and tries to get the fishbone out by sticking the pliers down my throat." Karen's parents became annoyed because she kept gagging when the pliers went down her throat, and they eventually had to take her to the emergency room to have it removed. She felt blamed for something she couldn't have avoided. She wrote that she wished her parents had acknowledged her help-lessness and fear rather than blaming her.

On the sixth memory of the EMP, which is a particularly important or vivid memory from any time in the client's life, Karen immediately chose to write about her mother's death. She reported that the images were really fresh in her mind: arriving home from school to find her father on the front porch and knowing that her mother had died (her father was never home after school), running to him and collapsing on the cement as he met her in the driveway, then crying the rest of the night. In discussing this memory with her later, I learned that Karen's mother had been ill with a very pain-ful type of cancer. When morphine failed to ease her pain, she resorted to a drastic measure: surgery to sever her spinal cord below the shoulders, which did not relieve the pain and resulted in her requiring full-time care. During the day a nurse cared for her in their home. When Karen arrived home from school, she took over her mother's care for the 3–4 hours until her father arrived home from work. Karen was just 12 years old. Among other duties, she administered her mother's pain medication, most often morphine, which required very precise measurement: Too little and her mother would be in intense pain; too much and her mother would die.

Karen reported that she never expressed grief following her mother's death because she felt she needed to be strong for her father because he was "falling apart." Her mother's death was never spoken about, and photographs of her were taken down and hidden not long after her passing. Karen's father drank heavily for about 9 months, during which time Karen's issues with perfectionism and body image intensified. When Karen was 11 years old, prior to her mother's being diagnosed, she recalled her mother telling her that she would need to lose weight to be accepted by her peers. She insisted that Karen weigh no more than 95 pounds (Karen was 5′ 2″). As her mother became ill, Karen began restricting and exercising daily. She remembered a time when she was caring for her mother that she went into her room wearing only underwear and a bra. Her mother smiled and remarked that she was beautiful. Karen felt that she had finally achieved the proper weight—she was 90 pounds—and she did whatever was required to maintain that afterward. She struggled with anorexia and binge eating throughout high school, college, and early adulthood, requiring brief hospitalizations more than once during college when her weight became dangerously low. Karen's self-assessment that her mother's death was the catalyst in the development of her OCD appeared plausible.

Summary of Assessment Results

Karen's TA consisted of a multimethod assessment of cognitive functioning, personality characteristics, and attachment status. These areas of functioning were assessed because they mapped onto the full list of Karen's assessment questions. Results of the Wechsler Adult Intelligence Scales, 4th Edition (Wechsler, 2008) indicated a Full-Scale IQ of 115, with a significant discrepancy between her Verbal Comprehension (127) and Perceptual Reasoning (98) indices. Her MMPI-2 profile was valid, but suggested that Karen tended to minimize her distress and socially undesirable problems and tried to present herself as "having it all together" ($L = 52$ [T-score], $F = 44$, $K = 74$, $S = 68$). Consistent with this response set, no Clinical Scales were elevated. Scales 3 ($Hy = 61$) and 7 ($Pt = 62$) were the highest, signifying obsessive–compulsive tendencies, anxiety, phobias, irrational fears, and perfectionism and a tendency to manifest psychological symptoms as physical or health complaints ($HEA = 53$; the highest Content Scales score). Karen's strong dependency needs ($Hy_2 = 63$) and overcontrol of anger ($Hy_5 = 62$, $O\text{-}H = 63$, $AGGR = 38$) are also notable. Among the Supplementary Scales, only the Repression scale ($R = 86$) was clinically elevated; this score suggested that Karen used repression, denial, and rationalization, was overcontrolled, and lacked insight.

The results of the Rorschach, scored using the R-PAS (Meyer et al., 2011), indicated significant psychological impairment. Karen produced a 33-response profile ($R = 124T$; $Pu = 98T$), with evidence of severe perceptual and thinking problems ($EII\text{-}3 = 130T$; $TP\text{-}Comp = 122T$; $WSumCog$

= 129T; *SevCog* = 138T), morbid thoughts, images, and feelings (*MOR* = 123T), a tendency to misperceive the actions and intentions of others (*M*– = 123T), and a preoccupation with the vulnerability of her body or its functions (*An* = 133T). She also scored very high on a measure that is sometimes associated with past trauma (*CritCont%* = 134T).

Karen's AAP was judged to be Unresolved, indicating that she had significant difficulty regulating affect when her attachment system was aroused and a disorganized defensive pattern. People with this result are unable to consistently reorganize after their attachment system is activated and are prone to experiencing unexpected overwhelming and disorienting affect as a result. There was also evidence in the AAP of failed mourning (i.e., the unresolved loss of an attachment figure), which is the prolonged absence of conscious grieving and a detached psychological state involving deactivation defenses (i.e., the avoidance of emotions and a focus on achievement, rules, and doing things the "right" way). This type of Unresolved attachment status has been found to be related to abandonment by an attachment figure that compromises psychological safety. Consistent with empirical research of failed mourning, Karen experienced physical stress reactions, eating problems, and a compulsive need to care for others at the expense of meeting her own needs (see George & West, 2012). When we discussed her AAP stories after the standard administration (i.e., during the extended inquiry), Karen and I were able to connect her current difficulties with her past experiences in a way that validated her experiences and fostered self-compassion. Karen reported that her attempts to control her life had "ballooned" after her mother died, and she agreed that she avoided painful emotions and tried to be entirely self-reliant so that she would not have to risk another devastating loss.

Planning the Feedback

The results of the standardized testing, most notably the discrepancy between self-report and performance-based assessment methods, suggested that it would be very important to order information about Karen's psychological struggles when giving her feedback, in accordance with self-verification theory. We hypothesized that Karen had developed obsessive–compulsive defenses in response to her traumatic attachment experiences and failed mourning, perhaps in combination with a genetic predisposition toward OCD (her father had an OCD diagnosis). Karen's OCD consisted of contamination fears and behavioral and affective avoidance of perceived threats and emotionally arousing situations. Basically, the testing suggested that she avoided emotions because she easily got overwhelmed and dysregulated by strong feelings. When this happened, her obsessive defenses would kick in as a way to manage her emotions ("If I can just control every aspect of my life, I'll be safer"), but these defenses themselves were painful and distressing. The MMPI-2 indicated that her obsessive–compulsive anxiety, perfectionism, and health concerns were congruent with her self-view, while failed mourning and the related need for affection were not well integrated. We now present an abbreviated, annotated transcript of the discussion surrounding Karen's primary question about the effect of her mother's death on the development of her OCD. We note the level of information of each finding as well as how the assessor tired to help Karen feel understood and valued in order to guard against possible disintegration anxiety when presented with feedback that differed from her current self-views.

Multimethod Assessment Feedback Presentation

ASSESSOR: Before I present assessment results related to this question, what is your best guess as to the answer? [This type of inquiry helps the assessor gauge what new information the client has been able to integrate during the assessment and also helps the assessor determine the level of the findings.]

KAREN: I think it had a lot to do with it. I had control issues around food before that, and I always expected myself to be perfect in school, and I mean perfect—it wasn't enough to get an A, I had to get a perfect score. But after my mother died, my OCD took on a life of its own.

ASSESSOR: Karen, the link you are making seems accurate to me based on the assessment and the experiences you shared with me [validating the client's self-view]. Do you have a sense about why the OCD took on a life of its own? [Using client's words helps the client feel understood.]

KAREN: (Laughs). Well, I didn't seem to have much of a choice, did I? My father was falling apart, and I had to keep plugging along for both of us.

ASSESSOR: You were in a really tough situation after your mother passed away. With your father having such a difficult time, someone had to stay strong and make sure the family didn't collapse [L1: Karen feels heard; adding contextual considerations aids in the development of self-compassion.] It seems that you did the best you could at the time to get through a scary situation [introduces the frightening nature of not being cared for by her father following the loss of her primary attachment figure], which was to pull yourself together, focus on school [L1], and try to maintain equilibrium [Karen had used the word *equilibrium* to describe the feeling of being emotionally regulated]. Sometimes the behaviors and thoughts associated with OCD, such as perfectionism in school and focusing on food and your weight, arise out of a need to cope with really intense experiences, emotions, or situations

[L2: introduces OCD as a coping strategy]. Does that seem to fit with your experience?

KAREN: I think so. It was a really terrible time. I didn't know what else to do.

ASSESSOR: It sounds like you were feeling a little helpless and alone [L2: attachment trauma].

KAREN: I was alone. My father was there, but he wasn't himself for a long time after my mother died, especially when he was drinking.

ASSESSOR: I can see why you felt like you had no other options. You did what you had to do to get through [validation]. It's sad that you had to go through that time of your life on your own.

KAREN: (*tearing up*) I just wish someone, anyone, had been there for me to talk with about my mother and how scary it felt to be without her.

ASSESSOR: Absolutely. Losing your mother left you with intense feelings of loss, sadness, and fear about what your life would be like without her. (*Long pause as Karen cries.*) The test results suggest that you still have a lot of intense feelings inside you that threaten your equilibrium if you were to really feel them [L2: affect avoidance; unresolved mourning]. The testing also suggests that the OCD symptoms we have talked so much about are a way to help keep you safe against these painful and frightening feelings that you worry could overwhelm you if you were to let them out of the box [Karen used the metaphor of storing her emotions in a box with a tight-fitting lid during extended inquiry of the EMP]. I see that you don't want to fall apart like your father did when he was grieving [validation]. It takes a lot of energy to keep all these feelings in that little box [understanding].

The assessor went on to connect Karen's OCD behaviors (e.g., avoiding real things that could hurt her, like pesticides and nuclear radiation) to her desire to protect herself from the underlying feelings that were very difficult to manage if she were to let them out all at once and without assistance. This coping mechanism "filled the gap" for the assistance she had longed for from her father but never received. The assessor helped Karen start the process of grieving over this void in her childhood and also the fact that she now found it difficult to see others as sources of emotional support, even her therapist. In this case, the assessor decided that Karen's minimal insight and strong coping mechanisms rendered presentation of L3 information too threatening. The assessor elected to share the L3 finding (Karen's underlying anger toward her parents, which was evident in each of the tests administered) with her therapist to be addressed after Karen was able to manage her grief. Upon seeing the findings of the assessment, the therapist reformulated the treatment goals to reflect a conceptualization of OCD behaviors as affect avoidance, particularly grief and longing for support that threatened her self-reliance and put her at risk for being severely injured again.

Conclusions

The use of an empirically supported guiding framework to multimethod assessment feedback increases the potential of positively affecting the client's life and improving subsequent treatment outcomes. The selection of a multimethod assessment battery consisting of self-report and performance-based tests that tap into complementary neurobiological processes, memory systems, and motivational factors is the key to (1) fully understanding clients' dilemmas of change and (2) determining the level of information of key findings. A core aspect of our framework is the recommendation to first present findings that confirm previously held self-views and then gradually move toward more discrepant findings that require alteration of the client's story. Empirical research shows that assessors should provide mostly L1 and L2 findings, and that L2 findings are necessary to achieve therapeutic outcomes (Schroeder et al., 1993). Last, assessors need to practice the interpersonal behaviors that help regulate clients' negative affect states during assessment feedback. This kind of sensitivity is essential for therapeutic outcomes, as the feedback process is inherently anxiety producing under any circumstance and is even more so when findings diverge from clients' existing self-schemas in the way the case example of Karen illustrates.

ACKNOWLEDGMENTS

Justin D. Smith received support in the preparation of this chapter by research training grant MH20012 from the National Institute of Mental Health, awarded to Elizabeth Stormshak.

REFERENCES

Achenbach, T. M., McConaughy, S. H., & Howell, C. T. (1987). Child/adolescent behavioral and emotional problems: Implications of cross-informant correlations for situational specificity. *Psychological Bulletin, 101*(2), 213–232.

American Psychological Association, Amercian Educational Research Association, & National Council on Measurement in Education. (1999). *Standards for educational and psychological testing.* Washington, DC: American Educational Research Association.

Andersen, P., & Nordvik, H. (2002). Possible Barnum effect in the five factor model: Do respondents accept random NEO Personality Inventory—Revised scores as their actual trait profile? *Psychological Reports, 90*(2), 539–545.

Asari, T., Konishi, S., Jimura, K., Chkazoe, J., Nakamura, N., & Miyashita, Y. (2008). Amygdalar enlargement associated with unique perception. *Cortex, 30*, 1–6.

Beutler, L., & Berren, M. (1995). *Integrative assessment of adult personality.* New York: Guilford Press.

Bornstein, R. F. (2002). A process dissociation approach to objective-projective test score interrelationships. *Journal of Personality Assessment, 78*(1), 47–68.

Bromberg, P. M. (2006). *Awakening the dreamer: Clinical journeys.* New York: Analytic.

Bruhn, A. R. (1992). The Early Memories Procedure: A projective test of autobiographical memory, part 1. *Journal of Personality Assessment, 58*(1), 1–15.

Buchheim, A., Erk, S., George, C., Kächele, H., Ruchsow, M., Spitzer, M., et al. (2006). Measuring attachment representation in an fMRI environment: A pilot study. *Psychopathology, 39*(3), 144–152.

Butcher, J. N., Dahlstrom, W. G., Grahm, J. R., Tellegen, A., & Kaemmer, B. (1989). *The Minnesota Multiphasic Personality Inventory–2 (MMPI-2): Manual for administration and scoring.* Minneapolis: University of Minnesota Press.

Campbell, D. T., & Fiske, D. W. (1959). Convergent and discriminant validation by the multitrait—multimethod matrix. *Psychological Bulletin, 56*, 81–105.

Cicchetti, D. V. (1994). Integrating developmental risk factors: Perspectives from developmental psychopathology. In C. A. Nelson (Ed.), *Minnesota symposium on child psychology: Vol. 27. Threats to optimal development* (pp. 285–325). Mahwah, NJ: Erlbaum.

Cicchetti, D. V., & Toth, S. L. (1998). The development of depression in children and adolescents. *American Psychologist, 53*(2), 221–241.

Cook, T. D., & Campbell, D. T. (Eds.). (1979). *Quasi-experimentation: Design and analysis issues for field settings.* Chicago: Rand-McNally.

Diener, M. J., Hilsenroth, M. J., & Weinberger, J. (2007). Therapist affect focus and patient outcomes in psychodynamic psychotherapy: A meta-analysis. *American Journal of Psychiatry, 164*, 936–941.

Dozier, M., & Lee, S. W. (1995). Discrepancies between self- and other-report of psychiatric symptomatology: Effects of dismissing attachment strategies. *Development and Psychopathology, 7*, 217–226.

Finn, S. E. (1996). Assessment feedback integrating MMPI-2 and Rorschach findings. *Journal of Personality Assessment, 67*(3), 543–557.

Finn, S. E. (2003). Therapeutic assessment of a man with "ADD" [Case Reports]. *Journal of Personality Assessment, 80*(2), 115–129.

Finn, S. E. (2007). *In our client's shoes: Theory and techniques of therapeutic assessment.* Mahwah, NJ: Erlbaum.

Finn, S. E. (2011). Journeys through the valley of death: Multimethod psychological assessment and personality transformation in long-term psychotherapy. *Journal of Personality Assessment, 93*(2), 123–141.

Finn, S. E. (2012). Implications of recent research in neurobiology for psychological assessment. *Journal of Personality Assessment, 94*(5), 440–449.

Finn, S. E., & Tonsager, M. E. (1992). Therapeutic effects of providing MMPI-2 test feedback to college students awaiting therapy. *Psychological Assessment, 4*(3), 278–287.

Finn, S. E., & Tonsager, M. E. (1997). Information-gathering and therapeutic models of assessment: Complementary paradigms. *Psychological Assessment, 9*(4), 374–385.

Fischer, C. T. (1985/1994). *Individualizing psychological assessment.* Mahwah, NJ: Erlbaum.

Fowler, J. C., Hilsenroth, M. J., & Handler, L. (1996). Two methods of early memories data collection: An empirical comparison of the projective yield. *Assessment, 3*(1), 63–71.

Furnham, A., & Schofield, S. (1987). Accepting personality test feedback: A review of the Barnum effect. *Current Psychological Research and Reviews, 6*(2), 162–178.

George, C., & West, M. L. (2012). *The Adult Attachment Projective Picture System: Attachment theory and assessment in adults.* New York: Guilford Press.

Giromini, L., Porcelli, P., Viglione, D. J., Parolin, L., & Pineda, J. A. (2010). The feeling of movement: EEG evidence for mirroring activity during the observations of static, ambiguous stimuli in the Rorschach cards. *Biological Psychology, 85*(2), 233–241.

Glassmire, D. M., Stolberg, R. A., Greene, R. L., & Bongar, B. (2001). The utility of MMPI-2 suicide items for assessing suicidal potential: Development of a suicidal potential scale. *Assessment, 8*(3), 281–290.

Hanson, W. E., Claiborn, C. D., & Kerr, B. (1997). Differential effects of two test-interpretation styles in counseling: A field study. *Journal of Counseling Psychology, 44*, 400–405.

Holigrocki, R., Crain, C., Bohr, Y., Young, K., & Bensman, H. (2009). Interventional use of the Parent–Child Interaction Assessment–II Enactments: Modifying an abused mother's attributions to her son. *Journal of Personality Assessment, 91*(5), 397–408.

Jimura, K., Konishi, S., Asari, T., & Miyashita, Y. (2009). Involvement of the medial prefrontal cortex in emotion during feedback presentation. *NeuroReport, 20*, 886–890.

Kohut, H. (1977). *The restoration of the self.* New York: International Universities Press.

Lilienfeld, S. O., Garb, H. N., & Wood, J. M. (2011). Unresolved questions concerning the effectiveness of psychological assessment as a therapeutic intervention: Comment on Poston and Hanson (2010). *Psychological Assessment, 23*(4), 1047–1055.

McClelland, D. C., Koestner, R., & Weinberger, J. (1989). How do self-attributed and implicit motives differ? *Psychological Review, 96*(4), 690–702.

Meyer, G. J. (1997). On the integration of personality assessment methods: The Rorschach and the MMPI. *Journal of Personality Assessment, 68*(2), 297–330.

Meyer, G. J., Finn, S. E., Eyde, L. D., Kay, G. G., Moreland, K. L., Dies, R. R., et al. (2001). Psychological testing and psychological assessment: A review of evidence and issues. *American Psychologist, 56*(2), 128–165.

Meyer, G. J., & Kurtz, J. E. (2006). Advancing personality assessment terminology: Time to retire "objective" and "projective" as personality test descriptors. *Journal of Personality Assessment, 87*(3), 223–225.

Meyer, G. J., Riethmiller, R. J., Brooks, R. D., Benoit, W. A., & Handler, L. (2000). A replication of Rorschach and MMPI-2 convergent validity. *Journal of Personality Assessment, 74*(2), 175–215.

Meyer, G. J., Viglione, D. J., Mihura, J., Erard, R. E., & Erdberg, P. (2011). *Rorschach Performance Assessment System: Administration, coding, interpretation, and technical manual.* Toledo, OH: Rorschach Assessment System.

Morey, L. C. (1991). *Personality Assessment Inventory professional manual.* Odessa, FL: Psychological Assessment Resources.

Newman, M. L., & Greenway, P. (1997). Therapeutic effects of providing MMPI-2 test feedback to clients at a university counseling service: A collaborative approach. *Psychological Assessment, 9*(2), 122–131.

Poston, J. M., & Hanson, W. E. (2010). Meta-analysis of psychological assessment as a therapeutic intervention. *Psychological Assessment, 22*(2), 203–212.

Roisman, G. I., Holland, A., Fortuna, K., Fraley, R. C., Clausell, E., & Clarke, A. (2007). The Adult Attachment Interview and self-reports of attachment style: An empirical rapprochement. *Journal of Personality and Social Psychology, 92*(4), 678–697.

Rorschach, H. (1921/1942). *Psychodiagnostics* (5th ed.). Berne, Switzerland: Verlag Hans Huber. (Original work published 1921)

Schore, A. N. (2003). *Affect regulation and repair of the self.* New York: Norton.

Schore, A. N. (2009). Right brain affect regulation: An essential mechanism of development, trauma, dissociation, and psychotherapy. In D. Fosha, M. Solomon & D. Siegel (Eds.), *The healing power of emotions: Integrating relationships, body, and mind: A dialogue among scientists and clinicians* (pp. 112–144). New York: Norton.

Schroeder, D. G., Hahn, E. D., Finn, S. E., & Swann, W. B. J. (1993). *Personality feedback has more impact when mildly discrepant from self views.* Paper presented at the fifth annual convention of the American Psychological Society, Chicago, IL.

Schultheiss, O. C. (2007). A memory-systems approach to the classification of personality tests: Comment on Meyer and Kurtz (2006). *Journal of Personality Assessment, 89*(2), 197–201.

Shaw, D. S., Gilliom, M., Ingoldsby, E. M., & Nagin, D. S. (2003). Trajectories leading to school-age conduct problems. *Developmental Psychology, 39*(2), 189–200.

Siegel, D. (2012). *The developing mind: How relationships and the brain interact to shape who we are* (2nd ed.). New York: Guilford Press.

Smith, J. D., Dishion, T. J., Moore, K. J., Shaw, D. S., & Wilson, M. N. (2013). Video feedback in the Family Check-Up: Indirect effects on observed parent–child coercive interactions. *Journal of Clinical Child and Adolescent Psychology, 42*(3), 405–417.

Smith, J. D., Finn, S. E., Swain, N. F., & Handler, L. (2010). Therapeutic assessment in pediatric and primary care psychology: A case presentation of the model's application. *Families, Systems, and Health, 28*(4), 369–386.

Smith, J. D., & George, C. (2012). Therapeutic assessment case study: Treatment of a woman diagnosed with metastatic cancer and attachment trauma. *Journal of Personality Assessment, 94*(4), 331–344.

Swann, Jr., W. B., Chang-Schneider, C., & McClarty, K. (2007). Do people's self-views matter? Self-concept and self-esteem in everyday life. *American Psychologist, 62*(2), 84–94.

Tharinger, D. J., Finn, S. E., Arora, P., Judd-Glossy, L., Ihorn, S. M., & Wan, J. T. (2012). Therapeutic assessment with children: Intervening with parents "behind the mirror." *Journal of Personality Assessment, 94*(2), 111–123.

Tharinger, D. J., Finn, S. E., Gentry, L., Hamilton, A. M., Fowler, J. L., Matson, M., et al. (2009). Therapeutic assessment with children: A pilot study of treatment acceptability and outcome. *Journal of Personality Assessment, 91*(3), 238–244.

Wechsler, D. (2008). *Wechsler Adult Intelligence Scale, 4th edition (WAIS-IV).* New York: Psychological Corporation.

Conclusion

Toward a Framework for Integrating Multimethod Clinical Assessment Data

Christopher J. Hopwood and Robert F. Bornstein

The genesis of this book lies in three facts whose juxtaposition is both ironic and troubling: (1) individual differences in adult personality and psychopathology have been the raw material on which many of the foundational principles and methods of assessment in clinical psychology have been built (Cronbach & Meehl, 1955; Loevinger, 1957); (2) fundamental among these principles—sometimes stated directly, at other times implied—is the value of multimethod assessment (Campbell & Fiske, 1959; Messick, 1995); and (3) clinical assessment of adult personality and psychopathology lags behind neuropsychology, child clinical psychology, and medicine in its use of evidence-based multimethod assessment. By demonstrating the value of multiple assessment methods for adult personality, psychopathology, and treatment, we hope to encourage its use in training, practice, and research.

In this volume we brought together experts with extensive research and clinical experience to describe the potential for multimethod assessment for their particular domains of expertise. We sought to cover the most important domains in adult personality and psychopathology, examine a broad range of traditional and novel assessment methods, and involve individuals with backgrounds in both clinical practice and assessment research, who collectively represent an array of theoretical orientations. In this concluding chapter, we highlight how the contents of the book demonstrate the value of assessment along each of these dimensions, with the hope of contributing to an overarching framework for the application of multimethod assessment in clinical settings. This framework has three steps: (1) determining the major assessment domains relevant to case formulation; (2) linking those domains to empirically validated multimethod assessment procedures; and (3) integrating assessment data using an evidence-based heuristic model that permits rich but efficient formulation and hypothesis testing.

Covering the Major Assessment Domains

In effective assessment, one must balance the ideal (and idealistic) goal of incorporating everything that might be useful with a more realistic focus on what is most important. Assessors who are distractible, use their favored tests regardless of case specifics, or lack an evidence-based heuristic model for organizing test data will not only be inefficient but may also miss some critical aspects of a case formulation. It is predictable based on contemporary reimbursement schedules and training bandwidths that the more common problem is the failure to adequately assess complex patient characteristics that could lend confidence to predictions, recommendations, interventions, and evaluations of progress and change. Mental health professionals routinely shun wide swaths of assessment procedures or psychological domains based on habit, cost, or time—even when research suggests that in the long run such domains and procedures can save time and money. We therefore aimed for broad coverage of assessment constructs and approaches across three domains: Personality and Individual Differences, Psychopathology and Resilience, and Clinical Management.

Thematic across these domains is the interaction between science and practice. One of the underlying goals in the lab, argue Kosloff, Maxfield, and Solomon, is "translating basic experimental findings into practically applicable approaches that foster physical and psychological welfare" (Chapter 4, p. 121). Conversely, they note that one of the underlying goals of practitioners should be to bring lab results from "bench to bedside"— that is, into the consulting room.

We opened with the Personality and Individual Differences section because of our assumption that effective assessment must begin with a sense of who the person being assessed is. This requires understanding the person, not just the person's pathology. In addition to providing a more holistic perspective, personality science has significant untapped potential for improving clinical practice in specific ways. For instance, as Galione and Oltmanns note, "the current direction in the field of personality embraces the variance that multiple measures provide, to the extent that it increases validity" (Chapter 1, p. 22). As this research continues to accumulate, clinical decisions about how to select optimal assessment procedures should become more efficient and evidence based.

One of the most obvious ways in which personality science can have a positive impact on clinical assessment involves the organization of psychopathology. The widely criticized polythetic/categorical model of contemporary psychiatry can be contrasted with the elegant factor models from quantitative psychology that yield largely similar structures in undergraduate self-ratings on dictionary terms and diagnostic data from patients (e.g., Wright et al., 2013). Furthermore, the small collection of higher-order traits identified in these models resemble broad regulatory systems as conceptualized in clinical neuroscience (Patrick & Bernat, 2010). Although the specific structure varies somewhat across methods, in general these domains include biopsychosocial systems involving the experience and regulation of negative emotions (neuroticism, behavioral inhibition, internalizing psychopathology), activation, sensation-seeking, and reward (extraversion, positive temperament, behavioral activation), behavioral regulation and impulse control (constraint/disinhibition, externalizing psychopathology), prosocial behavior (agreeableness/antagonism, personality pathology), and thought quality (openness, intellect, psychoticism) (Harkness, Reynolds, & Lilienfeld, 2014).

The identification of domains that provide a common structure across normal personality, psychiatric symptoms, and neurobehavioral constructs has important implications for the classification of psychopathology (Clark, 2007; Harkness et al., 2014). Specifically, organizing assessment methods around the individual differences identified in this research has the potential to contribute to a more evidence-based model of personality and psychopathology that can solve several problems with the descriptive, symptom-focused approach of the *Diagnostic and Statistical Manual of Mental Disorders* (DSM-5; American Psychiatric Association 2013). One implication is that co-occurrence between disorders such as depression and generalized anxiety can be explained by their being in the same (e.g., neurotic) spectrum of psychopathology (see also Cramer, Waldorp, van der Maas, & Borsboom, 2010). Another implication is that dimensional models help account for diagnostic heterogeneity, which arises in part when diagnostic categories are influenced by multiple underlying domains. For instance, borderline personality disorder is related to both a heightened disposition for negative affect as well as a tendency toward disinhibition (Samuel & Widiger, 2008). It is therefore not surprising that typologies of individuals with that diagnosis tend to include individuals who can be distinguished with these traits (Lenzenweger, Clarkin, Yeomans, Kernberg, & Levy, 2008). Traits that are unrelated to the diagnosis can also be helpful in depicting clinically useful heterogeneity, such as when depressed individuals vary in terms of how dominant or submissive they tend to be with others (e.g., Cain et al., 2012).

The Psychopathology and Resilience section is accordingly organized around evidence-based spectra of psychopathology including internalizing, externalizing, and thought disorder rather than discrete diagnostic categories. Each of the chapters focuses on assessment principles that would generalize to syndromes across and beyond their respective spectra. One domain that is routinely ignored in formal clinical assessment, even though it is a critical element of effective formulation, involves strengths, resources, and other features that speak to the individual's adaptive potential. In order to encourage the multimethod assessment of such features, chapters in this section that focus on problems and symptoms are complemented by a chapter on evidence-based multimethod assessment of resilience. The third section is devoted to issues related to Clinical Management. This section focuses on variables beyond those that are assessed during an intake session for the purpose of diagnosis, including treatment progress, treatment process, risk management, and distortion.

Stable Traits and Dynamic Processes

One of the goals of this book is to encourage the use of measurement methods that more closely approximate the kinds of behaviors that are of clinical interest, at the time scale or level of resolution that is most clinically relevant. Most clinical assessment implicitly assumes a certain level of stability in the constructs being assessed. The most commonly assessed constructs are presumed to be moderately stable. This is due partly to the fact that stable variables only need to be assessed once, or once in a while, and thus they are less burdensome than variables that would need to be measured every session, day, or millisecond. For example, most of the variables in a typical intake procedure are generally presumed to be relatively stable (e.g., demography, personality traits) or to change substantially only with dedicated interventions (e.g., depression, therapeutic alliance).

Commonly assessed constructs are also usually nomothetic: They tell the clinician something about where a person ranks on some attribute in a population distribution. In contrast, many clinically relevant dynamic variables are idiographic, with the implication that they need to be selected based on their importance for the particular client being assessed. Dynamic idiographic assessment is important because an individual's standing on these constructs can vary across timescales ranging from milliseconds to months. For instance, mood can be affected by a moment's excitement, the course of a conversation, or the changing seasons. Considering carefully the sensitivity of different methods to these changes would permit more precise predictions and would help clinicians choose approaches that capture a level of stability that is most relevant to their assessment question.

Indeed, as Stanfill et al. remarked, "dynamic variables are relevant in management, supervision, and treatment. . . . However, many of these variables are quite changeable, and can fluctuate greatly over time. Moreover, the importance of each may vary from person to person" (Chapter 13, p. 384). Luckily, as emphasized in a number of chapters, "The use of moment-by-moment process assessments . . . represents a new frontier for research-informed treatment" (Pascual-Leone et al., Chapter 11, p. 324). Such assessments are among the most promising areas in assessment research today not only because of their clinical and heuristic value, but also because of the increasing availability of technology amenable to such methods. For instance, with the proliferation of smartphone technology, dynamic assessments of interpersonal and affective processes will be increasingly applicable to actual cases. Improvements in technology are also making on-line neurophysiological assessment more accessible, and in vivo behavioral assessments more sophisticated. Each of these innovations is demonstrated in several chapters.

Linking Assessment Domains to Assessment Methods

In light of the particular importance of thinking more carefully about time in clinical assessment, in this chapter we expand Bornstein's (2009, 2011) taxonomy of assessment methods to distinguish those methods that are capable of assessing more stable as opposed to more dynamic thoughts, feelings, and behaviors. Table 1 breaks down common assessment approaches into several broad classes including explicit self-attribution measures as well as more implicit measures such as constructive approaches, stimulus attribution instruments, behavioral observations, and informant reports. In some cases, broad classes of assessment methods are split up into different subclasses, such as interview and self-report methods within self-attribution tests.

Within each class, examples of measures designed to assess both relatively stable and more dynamic characteristics are given.[1] A cursory glance at Table 1 shows that, although some cells have a wider range of tests to choose from than others, there are no empty cells. This implies that valid assessment procedures are available to assess both stable traits and dynamic processes across each of the major classes of testing procedure.

Another fundamental distinction in Table 1 is between the explicit and the implicit. As one of the main goals of assessment is to help clients understand themselves better so that they can make more mindful, informed choices, it is critical to complement data derived from measures that rely on introspection and insight with those from measures that tap information that is likely to be outside the client's awareness. The organization of Table 1 assumes that explicit data tend to come most directly from self-attribution tests, whereas the other four classes of tests provide data that are to varying degrees implicit (see also Erdelyi, 2004, for a discussion of this issue). The variation in methods that can be used to assess content that might be outside of an individual's awareness is likely due to the fact, as Cogswell and Emmert write, that "personality researchers have long wanted to reliably assess unobservable phenomena that individuals cannot

---

[1]We acknowledge that a gray area exists between the stable and dynamic because stability is itself a dimensional construct—hence the difficulty in deciding the minimum interval that represents.

TABLE 1. Assessment Strategies for Stable and Dynamic Individual Differences

Class	Subclass	Stable trait or problem	Dynamic process
Explicit			
Self-attribution	Self-report	Trait questionnaires	Cross-level analysis
		Psychopathology questionnaires	Ecological momentary assessment
		Attitude, interest, and value measures	
	Interview	Diagnostic interviews	
		Q-sorts	
Implicit			
Constructive		Unstructured interviews	Temporally sensitive coding systems
		Drawings	
Stimulus attribution		Implicit Association Test	Temporally sensitive coding systems
		Rorschach Inkblot Method	
		Storytelling procedures	
Behavioral	Observation	Functional analysis	Interpersonal joystick
	Cognitive performance	Neurological and intelligence assessments	Continuous performance tests
	Neurophysiology	Positron emission tomography	Electroencephalogram
		Magnetic resonance imaging	Skin conductance
Informant		Trait questionnaires	Informant ecological momentary assessment
		Problem checklists	

Note. Assessment strategies in the Explicit class are shaped primarily by explicit (conscious, controlled) processes; those in the Implicit class are shaped primarily by implicit (unconscious, reflexive) processes (see Bornstein, 2009, and McGrath, 2008, for discussions of the interplay of implicit and explicit processes in psychological tests).

access through introspection" (Chapter 5, p. 154). Despite the availability of a wide variety of such techniques, self-attribution tests remain by far the most common assessment method, as discussed by several authors in this volume.

Self-attribution tests will be involved in most assessments that use standardized procedures because—as we noted in the Introduction—it is almost always critical to have some sense of the client's description of their difficulties and other factors relevant to the assessment question. Self-attribution tests also have a number of strengths, such as practicality, ease, cost, and minimization—in the case of questionnaires—of error associated with administration or interpretation of test behavior. Furthermore, many of the common criticisms of client self-report are often overstated, as this passage from Blonigen and Wytiaz exemplifies: "By and large, reviews support the reliability and validity of self-report methods to assess outcome data related to use of alcohol . . . and illicit drugs . . . by demonstrating high rates of concordance with, and low rates of underreporting relative to, biological indices (e.g., urinalysis)" (Chapter 7, p. 216). However, it is also the case that nearly any assessment that relies solely on self-attribution tests will be incomplete, as has been emphasized throughout this book.

Although interviews also involve self-attribution, they differ from questionnaires in a number of ways. First, because the clinician must interpret and score assessee responses, interviews introduce the potential for error associated with these processes (see Garb, 1998). As Blais and Bello note, "unstructured clinical interviews in particular tend to produce limited diagnostic agreement . . . and structured interviews are often used inconsistently across clinicians." Interviews also tend to be less sensitive to problems in living than are more direct self-reports. Although some in the field have interpreted this finding as suggesting that self-reports "overpathologize," evidence suggests that neither questionnaires nor interviews deserve privileged status as "gold standards" (e.g., Hopwood et al., 2008). Indeed, attributing such status to any instrument runs counter to the underlying thesis of multimethod assessment—that different assessment methods tap unique realms of information that are not fully accessible when other methods are used. Self-reports might be best used to provide initial assessments of difficulties in living from the client's perspective, which can be followed up with more conservative interviews. Regardless of how information from self-attribution tests is combined, researchers should not be "satisfied with considering an assessment 'multimethod' if questionnaires and diagnostic/clinical interviews are used" (Moser et al., Chapter 6, p. 179).

Constructive tests involving open-ended "online" behavior capture important aspects of client responding, but are also among the most difficult to validate because the client's test behavior is largely unconstrained. While one such procedure, the unstructured interview, is among the most commonly used assessment methods in applied settings, standardized scoring and interpretation are rarely applied, creating problems related to reliability and validity (see Rogers, 2003). Despite the importance of constructive assessment and the availability of standardized coding procedures, they were not emphasized heavily in this book.

The same cannot be said for stimulus attribution tests, which have long been a fundamental tool in the clinical armamentarium and are making an evidence-based resurgence in research and practice. Chief among these are the Rorschach inkblots, the use of which was emphasized in several chapters. Several authors commented on the important issue of how stimulus–attribution tests such as the Rorschach provide incremental information that is not available vwith other methods, which is critical given that they also usually involve more extensive effort in terms of training, administration, and scoring. For instance, Blonigen and Wytiaz noted that a recent meta-analysis by Mihura, Meyer, Dumitrascu, and Bombel (2013) "provided support for the validity of individual Rorschach variables and clarified that such validity is higher in relation to externally assessed characteristics (e.g., observer ratings) than introspectively assessed characteristics (e.g., self-report)" (Chapter 7, p. 215). Similarly, Smith and Finn reported that recent "neurobiological research suggests that different assessment methods tap into different areas of the brain," and they went on to note that "the verbal and nonemotionally arousing administration of common self-report instruments, such as the MMPI or PAI, appears to activate more left-hemisphere cortical functions, while tests such as the Rorschach and the Adult Attachment Projective Picture System (AAP) activate more right-hemisphere and subcortical functioning due to their visual, emotionally arousing stimulus properties and the interpersonal demands of their administration" (Chapter 14, p. 406). This type of research provides a novel and compelling rationale for incorporating stimulus–attribution tests in applied clinical assessment (see also Meyer, Viglione, Mihura, Erard, & Erdberg, 2011, for an extensive discussion of this issue).

Consistent with Smith and Finn's forward-looking approach (see also Finn, 2012), we sought to include the tried and true methods of traditional adult assessment with significant evidence bases (e.g., MMPI, PAI, Rorschach), along with novel or pioneering methods from basic science that hold considerable promise for applied clinical assessment. A relative newcomer on the stimulus–attribution block is the Implicit Association Test (IAT), which Cogswell and Emmert reviewed in detail in Chapter 5 in terms of its evidence base and clinical potential. As the major challenge associated with this class of tests involves developing reliable and valid procedures that can be easily mastered and efficiently administered, this form of assessment has considerable potential as a stimulus–attribution method in clinical and research settings.

Behavioral tests include a wide variety of procedures, including the direct coding of observable behaviors, performance-based measures of cognitive and neuropsychological functioning, and neurophysiological assessments. Unfortunately, outside of specifically identified neuropsychological assessments, such procedures are less frequently used in applied settings than they probably should be, but improvements in technology are making their use more feasible. An exciting development in contemporary assessment science is the development of increasingly sophisticated behavioral coding paradigms (Durbin, 2010; Sadler, Ethier, Gunn, Duong, & Woody, 2009; Pincus et al., Chapter 2, this volume) and increasingly accessible neurophysiological assessments (Moser et al., Chapter 6, this volume). This is certainly a growth area in psychological assessment.

The last section of Table 1 involves informant reports, which were described in a number of chapters and are increasingly a staple of basic personality research. This work has produced some important evidence-based principles for the use of information provided by knowledgeable others in clinical practice. The first is that, all things equal, informants will tend to be most effective at assessing externally observable behavior, whereas individuals will tend to outperform informants in the assessment of internal experience (Vazire, 2010). Thus, it may be more useful to solicit informants to describe substance use problems than to evaluate an acquaintance's alexithymia or boredom. In this context, all things equal, informants who do not like the target tend to provide information that is less redundant than those who do like the target, and often more accurate (Leising, Erbs, & Fritz, 2010). This creates a challenge in clinical assessment, since informants are typically nominated by the person being assessed (though of course they need not be).

As Smith and Finn emphasize in Chapter 14, multimethod assessment "is most applicable when similar constructs (e.g., depression, self-esteem) are formally measured with different methods that have distinct sources of error (e.g., self-report and observational rating, or self-report and performance-based test)" (p. 404). Moreover, as Burchett and Bagby emphasize with respect to distortion, it is critical "to understand differences between these strategies" and to "employ several strategies during any given assessment" (Chapter 12, p. 349). In order to do this, Mihura and Graceffo suggest that "researchers and practitioners map the assessment method's response process (e.g., reporting morbid images to inkblots) onto the psychological characteristic of interest (e.g., having morbid images on one's mind)" (Chapter 10, p. 287). Taken together, the recommendations in this book imply that any single source of information can, at best, provide an incomplete picture. Thus the central question for clinical assessors is about the cost of more thorough assessment relative to the cost of making an incorrect inference—decisions that require a coherent and evidence-based conceptual model.

Conceptual Models

As Galione and Oltmanns point out, "Ideally, researchers and clinicians will be able to interpret redundant and nonredundant information from multiple personality assessments in a standardized and practical fashion" (Chapter 1, p. 44). Some conceptual models cross domain and method completely, such as Lang's (1968) three-system approach for the assessment of anxiety, which integrates subjective experience, behavior, and psychophysiological response. This logic fits well with the process–dissociation procedures emphasized in the Introduction (Bornstein and Hopwood, this volume), in which discontinuities in the data yielded by contrasting methods can be exploited to better understand the processes by which individuals produce test scores.

Historically, different theoretical models have been associated with preferences for one kind of data over another: Generally speaking behaviorists prefer observational data, trait psychologists prefer questionnaire data, psychiatrists prefer interview and neurophysiological data, and psychoanalysts prefer inferential data about implicit processes. Aspects of each of these orientations are represented in this book. However, one of the important messages we hope to convey is that as clinical science evolves, the boundaries between these perspectives are blurring. Although distinctive theoretical perspectives played an important role in establishing hypotheses for clinical research and practice in the 20th century, we would argue that in the 21st century it is no longer productive to constrain oneself to a particular perspective at the expense of a broader, more integrative view. Furthermore, traditional theoretical models have splintered to the degree that the lines between them have blurred and many hybrid approaches have been developed.

In 20th-century assessment, it was also common to have a preferred assessment tool or battery that might be applied routinely to all patients (e.g., Rappaport, Gill, & Schafer, 1945). One of us remembers well that in his graduate training in the early 1980s, he was taught that clinical assessment always involved a standard test battery consisting of WAIS, Rorschach, MMPI, and a brief neurological screen—regardless of the patient (or problem) being evaluated. Those days are gone, and with the press of efficiency coupled with the availability of a range of novel and specific assessment tools, clinicians will need to become more facile and thoughtful in the targeted application of different methods for different purposes.

An instructive example of the dangers of linking a method to a theoretical model comes from the Rorschach. Although the Rorschach inkblots were originally developed to study the underlying perceptual anomalies associated with psychotic disorders (and this is still perhaps their most distinctive and powerful application), they were adopted as a primary clinical assessment method by psychoanalytic ego psychologists in the middle of the 20th century. The reaction in the "dust bowl" of empiricism associated with the MMPI was skeptical and antagonistic. Over time, and despite the fact that both instruments have been evidence based from the start and continue to yield roughly similar results in terms of validity (Hiller, Rosenthal, Bornstein, Berry, & Brunell-Neuleib, 1999), the MMPI and Rorschach crystallized underlying theoretical tensions in the field between more versus less inferential perspectives. As the popularity of psychoanalysis waned in the late 20th century, critiquing the Rorschach became popular (e.g., Wood, Nezworski, Lilienfeld, & Garb, 2003). Many aspects of these critiques were valid and in those cases often led to notable improvements in Rorschach assessment as well as clearer demonstrations of its validity (Meyer et al., 2011; Mihura et al., 2013). However, the more polemic aspects of some critiques also helped reify widespread misconceptions about the instrument.

Historical baggage aside, the Rorschach is simply ink on cardboard, whose value derives from the fact that it can generate evidence-based inferences about how responses to the images relate to behaviors outside the consulting room (Bornstein & Masling, 2005; Mihura et al., 2013). This approach to assessment fits comfortably within basic cognitive science, despite the Rorschach having been marginalized widely in contemporary clinical psychology. As Cogswell and Emmert note, it is interesting that "many scholars and clinicians who have largely rejected the use of instruments such as the Rorschach and TAT have in recent years given increasing notice to unconscious, unobservable phenomena, albeit with those phenomena conceptualized in a different manner" (Chapter 5, p. 155). In other words, coupling standardized ambiguous stimuli with evidence-based scoring and interpretation procedures is not controversial among basic experimental scientists, so why should it be taboo in some clinical quarters?

Self-report assessments have likewise been criticized by some despite their extensive validity support. In the case of questionnaires, the criticism has involved the sense that they are "superficial" because patients are unlikely to have good insight about their difficulties and attributes. Nevertheless, self-report methods are uniquely powerful tools for assessing how people perceive and describe themselves—crucial information in any clinical encounter. The broader point here is that tethering assessment methods with potential for broad application to theoretical models that will wax and wane in popularity is not adaptive for the methods, and important techniques can get lost from the clinical toolbox in such a process. Assessment is too complex and difficult to forego valuable methods like perceptual tasks or self-reports because they are not aligned primarily with one's assumptions or favored theoretical perspective.

However, integrative theoretical models that can accommodate data from contrasting methods and different domains are sorely needed. There are a number of examples of potentially useful models in the literature (e.g., Millon, 1996; Blais & Hopwood, 2010; Harkness et al., 2014). In the context of our focus on multimethod assessment, we would emphasize three critical factors with respect to selecting and developing comprehensive models for organizing assessment content. First, returning to the theme of stable features and dynamic processes, Pincus and colleagues point out that "it is important to understand that the structural and temporal realms are, in principle, closely interrelated. In other words, it is the organization of dimensions within the individual that, at least in part, underlies oscillations and other patterns of variation over time in the person's behavior. . . . [These] underlying mental structures help to make temporal variation intelligible" (Chapter 2, pp. 53–54). In other words, conceptual models need to have a system for linking the stable and nomothetic to the dynamic and idiographic. Second, as Denckla and Mancini point out, "Before we can identify factors associated with resilience . . . we have to translate our operational definition of resilience into measurement strategies" (Chapter 9, p. 259). That is, theories must imply specific assessment procedures to be useful, and procedures need to map onto theory (cf. Loevinger, 1957). Third—and perhaps most important to the practicing clinician—ultimately, "Psychological assessment instruments are a means of getting into our client's shoes" (Smith & Finn, Chapter 14, p. 403). Simply put, if conceptual models do not speak to how assessment procedures facilitate the clinician's empathy and understanding, they are unlikely to enable clinicians to provide "durable benefit" (Sullivan, 1954) to clients.

A major take-home message of this volume is that in addition to employing empirically validated intervention strategies, evidence-based practice must also involve the use of multiple methods for psychological assessment to determine which strategies are best suited to a particular patient and that patient's problems. Tomko and Trull captured this theme succinctly: "A complete understanding of affective processes cannot be gained through reliance on any single assessment tool or method. . . . First, the strengths of one method may address limitations of a second method, reducing measurement error and increasing the predictive power of the latent construct. Second, discrepant findings between methods may provide important information that is unattainable using either method alone" (Chapter 3, p. 93).

The Challenge of Multimethod Assessment

As with all advances in clinical science and practice, incorporating novel assessment methods comes with a number of important challenges. For instance, although new methods are exciting and provide unique information, in the near term (and despite advancements in technology), it will be difficult to improve upon the efficiency and low cost of commonly used procedures such as questionnaires and interviews. This is a major challenge. For instance, Denckla and Mancini describe complex issues related to "resource burden, potential lack of compensation, training requirements, and assessee . . . fatigue" (Chapter 9, p. 272) that constrain the routine use of multimethod assessment.

Interestingly, Moser et al. point out that "in the 1970s and 1980s, multimodal assessment of anxiety in psychopathology and intervention research was fairly common. An analysis of assessment trends in the literature, however, indicates that . . . researchers have been relying more heavily on subjective reports of behavior and symptoms and single-response system assessment" (Chapter 6, p. 178). Indeed, the empirical review by Tomko and Trull suggests that multimethod assessment rates are troublingly low in psychological research on basic affective processes, let alone in clinical practice. As Pascual-Leone et al. note, "while standardized progress and process assessments have become an essential component of psychotherapy research, the proportion of clinicians who report using such measures in their independent practice remains low" (Chapter 11, p. 320). This pattern can almost certainly be attributed to issues of cost and resource burden to which Denckla and Mancini alluded, as well as the increasing focus on diagnostic issues in lieu of comprehensive assessment (Mihura & Graceffo, Chapter 10).

It is unlikely that either the cost factors related to mental health or the burden on practitioners to operate efficiently will improve in the near future. So the question becomes one of trade-offs and incremental gain. When are more complicated and costly methods justifiable from a clinical perspective? How much unique predictive value do they add to existing methods? How can clinically useful procedures and algorithms be developed to guide the interpretation of results from such methods? The chapters in this book provide a rich and compelling foundation from which researchers can begin answering these questions, and clinicians can begin gathering more nuanced multimethod data from their clients and patients.

Beyond the challenges that arise from integrating new clinical techniques into a managed care-driven environment, one of the major barriers to multimethod assessment involves training and expertise: There are simply many more assessment procedures available to the contemporary assessment psychologist than there were in the days of standard test batteries involving the same set of tried and true instruments. There may be motives for time-strapped clinicians (or understandably anxious trainees) to seek converging results that point toward the "right answer," and evidence that assessment is often more complicated than that can be unwelcome. Furthermore, as Mihura and Graceffo point out in Chapter 10, "Basic psychological assessment textbooks often organize the material by test. These tests may not be different—or only minimally different—in their method of assessment" (p. 285). That is, rather than promoting thoughtful integration of assessment data, most training texts reinforce the stereotype that psychological tests fit neatly into discrete categories. They also reinforce the tendency for trainees, clinicians, and researchers to pick favorites rather than combine methods to meet the particular needs of individual cases.

One apparent consequence of this test-focused approach to assessment is that there is little in the way of evidence regarding how to choose different assessment tools and integrate divergent test results. Any comprehensive algorithmic frameworks, decision trees, or specific protocols that might be offered at this time for how to combine tests—while potentially helpful for organizing clinical thinking—are thus bound to fall short from an empirical perspective. However, there are considerable advantages to pursuing this issue. Mental health problems place a tremendous strain on individuals and society, and our current assessment procedures continue to provide only a limited picture of patient functioning. The vastness of this problem—which not only impacts the individual patient, but also the health care system, the broader economy, and the legal system as well—should compel the field to continue searching for sources of deeper understanding that can help us relieve many longstanding problems and alleviate their associated cost and suffering. We hope this book contributes in some small part to this effort, helping set the stage for a future in which evidence-based multimethod assessment is routine in clinical practice.

REFERENCES

American Psychiatric Association. (2013). *Diagnostic and statistical manual of mental disorders* (5th ed.). Arlington, VA: Author.

Blais, M. A., & Hopwood, C. J. (2010). Personality-focused assessment in the PAI. In M. A. Blais, M. R. Baity, & C. J. Hopwood (Eds.), *Clinical applications of the Personality Assessment Inventory* (pp. 195–210). New York: Routledge Mental Health.

Bornstein, R. F. (2009). Heisenberg, Kandinsky, and the heteromethod convergence problem: Lessons from within and beyond psychology. *Journal of Personality Assessment, 91,* 1–8.

Bornstein, R. F. (2011). Toward a process-focused model of test score validity: Improving psychological assessment in science and practice. *Psychological Assessment, 23,* 532–544.

Bornstein, R. F., & Masling, J. M. (Eds.). (2005). *Scoring the Rorschach: Seven validated systems.* Mahwah, NJ: Erlbaum.

Cain, N. M., Ansell, E. B., Wright, A. G. C., Hopwood, C. J., Thomas, K. M., Pinto, A., et al. (2012). Interpersonal pathoplasticity in the course of major depression. *Journal of Consulting and Clinical Psychology, 80,* 78–86.

Campbell, D. T., & Fiske, D. W. (1959). Convergent and discriminant validation by the multitrait-multimethod matrix. *Psychological Bulletin, 56,* 81–105.

Clark, L. A. (2007). Assessment and diagnosis of personality disorder: Perennial issues and an emerging reconceptualization. *Annual Review of Psychology, 58,* 227–257.

Cramer, A. O. J., Waldorp, L. J., van der Maas, H., & Borsboom, D. (2010). Comorbidity: A network perspective. *Behavioral and Brain Sciences, 33,* 137–193.

Cronbach, L. J., & Meehl, P. E. (1955). Construct validity in psychological tests. *Psychological Bulletin, 52,* 281–302.

Durbin, C. E. (2010). Validity of young children's self-reports of their emotion in response to structured laboratory tasks. *Emotion, 10,* 519–535.

Erdelyi, M. H. (2004). Subliminal perception and its cognates: Theory, indeterminacy, and time. *Consciousness and Cognition, 13,* 73–91.

Garb, H. N. (1998). *Studying the clinician: Judgment research and psychological assessment.* Washington, DC: American Psychological Association.

Harkness, A. R., Reynolds, S. M., & Lilienfeld, S. O. (2014). A review of systems for psychology and psychiatry: Adaptive systems, personality Psychopathology-Five (PSY-5), and the DSM-5. *Journal of Personality Assessment, 96,* 121–139.

Hiller, J. B., Rosenthal, R., Bornstein, R. F., Berry, D. T. R., & Brunell-Neuleib, S. (1999). A comparative meta-analysis of Rorschach and MMPI validity. *Psychological Assessment, 11,* 278–296.

Hopwood, C. J., Morey, L. C., Edelen, M. O., Shea, M. T., Grilo, C. M., Sanislow, C. A., et al. (2008). A comparison of interview and self-report methods for the assessment of borderline personality disorder criteria. *Psychological Assessment, 20*, 81–85.

Lang, P. J. (1968): Fear reduction and fear behavior: Problems in treating a construct. In J. Schlien (Ed.), *Research in psychotherapy* (Vol. III, pp. 90–103). Washington, DC: American Psychiatric Press.

Leising, D., Erbs, J., & Fritz, U. (2010). The letter of recommendation effect in informant ratings of personality. *Journal of Personality and Social Psychology, 98*, 668–682.

Lenzenweger, M. F., Clarkin, J. F., Yeomans, F. E., Kernberg, O. F., & Levy, K. N. (2008). Refining the borderline personality disorder phenotype through finite mixture modeling: Implications for classification. *Journal of Personality Disorders, 22*, 313–331.

Loevinger, J. (1957). Objective tests as instruments of psychological theory. *Psychological Reports, 3*, 635–694.

McGrath, R. E. (2008). The Rorschach in the context of performance-based personality assessment. *Journal of Personality Assessment, 90*, 465–475.

Messick, S. (1995). Validity of psychological assessment: Validation of inferences from persons' responses and performances as scientific inquiry into score meaning. *American Psychologist, 50*, 741–749.

Meyer, G. J., Viglione, D. J., Mihura, J. L., Erard, R. E., & Erdberg, P. (2011). *Rorschach Performance Assessment System: Administration, coding, interpretation, and technical manual.* Toledo, OH: Rorschach Performance Assessment System.

Mihura, J. L., Meyer, G. J., Dumitrascu, N., & Bombel, G. (2013). The validity of individual Rorschach variables: Systematic reviews and meta-analyses of the comprehensive system. *Psychological Bulletin, 139*, 548–605.

Millon, T. (1996). *Personality and psychopathology: Building a clinical science.* New York: Wiley.

Patrick, C. J., & Bernat, E. M. (2010). Neuroscientific foundations of psychopathology. In T. Millon, R. F. Krueger, & E. Simonsen (Eds.), *Contemporary directions in psychopathology* (pp. 419–452). New York: Guilford Press.

Rappaport, D., Gill, M., & Schafer, R. (1945). *Diagnostic psychological testing.* Chicago: Year Book.

Rogers, R. (2003). Standardizing DSM-IV diagnoses: The clinical applications of structured interviews. *Journal of Personality Assessment, 81*, 220–225.

Sadler, P., Ethier, N., Gunn, G. R., Duong, D., & Woody, E. (2009). Are we on the same wavelength?: Interpersonal complementarity as shared cyclical patterns during interactions. *Journal of Personality and Social Psychology, 97*, 1005–1020.

Samuel, D. B., & Widiger, T. A. (2008). A meta-analytic review of the relationships between the five-factor model and DSM personality disorders: A facet level analysis. *Clinical Psychology Review, 28*, 1326–1342.

Sullivan, H. S. (1954). *The psychiatric interview.* New York: Norton.

Vazire, S. (2010). Who knows about a person?: The self–other knowledge asymmetry (SOKA) model. *Journal of Personality and Social Psychology, 98*, 281–300.

Wood, J. M., Nezworski, M. T., Lilienfeld, S. O., & Garb, H. N. (2003). *What's wrong with the Rorschach?: Science confronts the controversial inkblot test.* San Francisco: Jossey-Bass.

Wright, A. G. C., Krueger, R. F., Hobbs, M. J., Markon, K. E., Eaton, N. R., & Slade, T. (2013). The structure of psychopathology: Toward an expanded quantitative empirical model. *Journal of Abnormal Psychology, 122*, 281–294.

Author Index

Subject Index

464